Modern Approaches to Augmentation of Brain Function

Modern Approaches to Augmentation of Brain Function

Edited by Ryan Lewis

STATES
ACADEMIC PRESS
www.statesacademicpress.com

States Academic Press,
109 South 5th Street,
Brooklyn, NY 11249, USA

Visit us on the World Wide Web at:
www.statesacademicpress.com

ISBN: 978-1-63989-360-7

Cataloging-in-Publication Data

Modern approaches to augmentation of brain function / edited by Ryan Lewis.
p. cm.
Includes bibliographical references and index.
ISBN 978-1-63989-360-7
1. Brain. 2. Brain--Physiology. 3. Neurosciences. 4. Neurology. 5. Brain--Localization of functions.
6. Neurophysiology. I. Lewis, Ryan.

QP376 .M63 2021
612.82--dc23

Table of Contents

Preface

The purpose of the book is to provide a glimpse into the dynamics and to present opinions and studies of some of the scientists engaged in the development of new ideas in the field from very different standpoints. This book will prove useful to students and researchers owing to its high content quality.

Brain augmentation encompasses the various approaches which seek to supplement the functioning of the brain. Enhancements in the brain can be done using pharmacological methods or through neurostimulation. Techniques to exercise the brain through modern technologies such as virtual reality can be used to improve the functionality of the brain. Some of the major concepts which lie behind the modern approaches to augmenting brain function are decrypting information from the brain activity and utilizing this information for other purposes, and stimulating the brain through electrical or pharmacological means. A futuristic extension of this approach is a vision that in the future, brain-to-brain communication and immortality of consciousness can be achieved. This book includes some of the vital pieces of work being conducted across the world, on various topics related to the augmentation of brain function. It strives to provide a fair idea about this discipline and to help develop a better understanding of the modern approaches within this area of study. This book will help the readers in keeping pace with the rapid changes in this field.

At the end, I would like to appreciate all the efforts made by the authors in completing their chapters professionally. I express my deepest gratitude to all of them for contributing to this book by sharing their valuable works. A special thanks to my family and friends for their constant support in this journey.

Editor

1

Two is more than one: how to combine brain stimulation rehabilitative training for functional recovery?

Satoko Koganemaru[1,2]*, *Hidenao Fukuyama*[2] *and Tatsuya Mima*[2]

[1] *Brain Integrative Science, Kyoto University School of Medicine, Sakyo-ku, Kyoto, Japan,* [2] *Human Brain Research Center, Kyoto University School of Medicine, Sakyo-ku, Kyoto, Japan*

Edited by:
Mikhail Lebedev, Duke University, USA

Reviewed by:
Po-Yi Tsai, Yang-Ming National University, Taiwan
Anna-Katharine Brem, University of Oxford, UK
Marco Sandrini, University of Roehampton, UK

***Correspondence:**
Satoko Koganemaru
kogane@kuhp.kyoto-u.ac.jp

A number of studies have shown that non-invasive brain stimulation has an additional effect in combination with rehabilitative therapy to enhance functional recovery than either therapy alone. The combination enhances use-dependent plasticity induced by repetitive training. The neurophysiological mechanism of the effects of this combination is based on associative plasticity. However, these effects were not reported in all cases. We propose a list of possible strategies to achieve an effective association between rehabilitative training with brain stimulation for plasticity: (1) control of temporal aspect between stimulation and task execution; (2) the use of a shaped task for the combination; (3) the appropriate stimulation of neuronal circuits where use-dependent plastic changes occur; and (4) phase synchronization between rhythmically patterned brain stimulation and task-related patterned activities of neurons. To better utilize brain stimulation in neuro-rehabilitation, it is important to develop more effective techniques to combine them.

Keywords: use-dependent plasticity, associative plasticity, neuro-rehabilitation, transcranial magnetic stimulation (TMS), transcranial direct current stimulation (tDCS)

USE-DEPENDENT PLASTICITY ENHANCED BY THE COMBINATION OF REHABILITATIVE TRAINING AND BRAIN STIMULATION

Repetitive training is one of the fundamental strategies in neuro-rehabilitation regardless of what type of damage has occurred in the central or peripheral nervous system. Task-specific training induces task-specific neuronal changes lasting for a long period i.e., use-dependent plasticity that can lead to functional recovery (Butefisch et al., 1995; Nudo and Milliken, 1996; Nudo et al., 1996a,b; Hummelsheim, 1999; Masiero and Carraro, 2008; Richards et al., 2008; Dimyan and Cohen, 2011). Use-dependent plasticity induced by motor training has been demonstrated within the human primary motor cortex (M1). The long-term potentiation (LTP)-like changes in specific cortcospinal motoneurons were induced for the trained task after repetitive simple finger movements (Classen et al., 1998; Butefisch et al., 2000; Rossini and Pauri, 2000).

In recent decades, a number of studies have shown that non-invasive brain stimulation such as repetitive transcranial magnetic stimulation (rTMS) or transcranial direct current stimulation (tDCS) has an add-on effect in combination with rehabilitative therapy

(Platz and Rothwell, 2010; Edwardson et al., 2013; Sandrini and Cohen, 2013; Floel, 2014). Furthermore, this combination may better enhance functional recovery in post-stroke patients, as compared with rehabilitation training alone, which may not sufficiently induce functional recovery (Khedr et al., 2005, 2010; Kim et al., 2006, 2010; Takeuchi et al., 2008; Chang et al., 2010, 2012; Emara et al., 2010; Koganemaru et al., 2010; Conforto et al., 2012; Meehan et al., 2011; Nair et al., 2011; Stagg and Nitsche, 2011; Wang et al., 2012; Hsu et al., 2013), especially in the chronic phase when it is difficult to produce plastic changes (Nakayama et al., 1994; Verheyden et al., 2008). A single intervention of brain stimulation alone without rehabilitative therapy seems to have limited effects on patients with mild motor symptoms (Hummel and Cohen, 2005; Koganemaru et al., 2010) and insufficient sustainability of effects (Takeuchi et al., 2005; Kim et al., 2009). Whereas the combination may enhance use-dependent plasticity induced by repetitive training.

ASSOCIATIVE PLASTICITY TO PRODUCE THE COMBINATION EFFECTS

Although the exact neurophysiological mechanism of this combination effect is not known yet, it may be based on Hebbian associative plasticity (Hebb, 1949). For example, a post-synaptic neuron (A) receives low-frequency weak inputs from one pre-synaptic neuron (B) (the inputs themselves cannot induce LTP in a synaptic connection). Simultaneously, neuron (A) receives high-frequency weak inputs (the inputs themselves can induce LTP) from another pre-synaptic neuron (C). According to the Hebbian rule, LTP is also induced in the weak synaptic connection between neurons (A) and (B) as well as between neurons (A) and (C). A similar mechanism would work in the case of the combination of training with brain stimulation. Training alone may only produce a weak activation of neuronal circuits, which do not lead to long term changes. On the other hand, brain stimulation can induce LTP-like changes for synaptic strength in stimulated areas (Pascual-Leone et al., 1994; Hallett, 2000; Fritsch et al., 2010; Dayan et al., 2013; Karabanov et al., 2015). Therefore, simultaneous training with brain stimulation would enable weak synaptic connections to induce associative LTP-like effects through the Hebbian rule.

However, a recent study reported no additional effects of theta-burst stimulation (TBS) in combination with standardized rehabilitative therapy in chronic stroke patients. That might be possibly due to a failure to induce associative plasticity. Neuronal activities enhanced by TBS may not have been associated with task-specific neuronal activities produced by the rehabilitative therapy (Talelli et al., 2012).

We can speculate and make a list of possible factors that may have weakened the therapeutic effects of combined rehabilitation and brain stimulation:

1. Diversities in diseases, particularly the locations of lesions
   – The effects of facilitatory rTMS over M1 depended on lesion location in post-stroke hemiparetic patients. The deterioration of finger function was seen in the patients with cortical lesions, whereas improvement in finger function was seen in patients with subcortical lesions (Ameli et al., 2009).
2. Small sample size
   – The responses to brain stimulation show a large variability even if patients are similar in lesion location, severity of paresis and time after stroke onset in patients. Genetic factors are responsible for individual susceptibility to rTMS-induced plasticity (Cheeran et al., 2008).
3. Insufficient intensity and/or too short duration of the intervention
   – Patients with severe paresis show reduced or no motor evoked potentials (MEP) with TMS (Pennisi et al., 1999; Hendricks et al., 2002). If the intensity of brain stimulation is determined by the excitability of the healthy hemisphere, it may be too weak to induce plasticity in the affected hemisphere. Unless brain stimulation is repeated daily for days to weeks, its effects might not be sustainable (Khedr et al., 2009; Emara et al., 2010; Bolognini et al., 2011; Conforto et al., 2012; Edwardson et al., 2013).
4. Inappropriate affinity between rehabilitation task and brain stimulation modality
   – This will be discussed in detail in the following section.

Future clinical studies should give careful consideration to these factors. We have considered how effectively we can induce associative plasticity through the combination of training and brain stimulation.

EFFECTIVE METHODS OF COMBINING REHABILITATIVE TRAINING AND BRAIN STIMULATION

Control of the Temporal Aspect Between Stimulation and Task Execution

First, we should control the temporal aspect between stimulation and task execution. Spike timing-dependent associative plasticity has been proven in both animals (Hess and Donoghue, 1996; Hess et al., 1996; Egger et al., 1999) and humans (Stefan et al., 2000, 2002; Ueki et al., 2006; Koganemaru et al., 2009). Associative LTP occurs when a post-synaptic neuron fires less than 10–20 ms after a pre-synaptic neuron. Recently, we have demonstrated that associative plasticity is induced within human M1. The repetitive pairing of TMS and paired bihemispheric stimulation (PBS) applied at a time interval of 15 ms, produced an associative LTP-like effect within the targeted M1 and facilitated fine finger movements (Koganemaru et al., 2009). Furthermore, associative use-dependent plasticity has been demonstrated within human M1. Thabit et al. (2010) showed that associative LTP-like changes were induced by the repetitive paring of a unidirectional finger movement and a single TMS pulse over the contralateral M1 with a specific interval in healthy subjects. It resulted in a faster reaction in the trained direction. By decrease or increase of the interval, LTP-like effects can disappear or be reversed. Buetefisch et al. (2011) showed that the extensor-specific M1 reorganization was induced by robot-assisted training of paretic wrist extension combined with TMS over the ipsilesional M1 in a strict temporal relationship in chronic post-stroke patients. Particularly, a decrease of motor threshold and a shift of motor mapping for the extensor carpi ulnaris muscles, not the biceps muscles, were demonstrated in the combination therapy with TMS over the ipsilesional M1. The training alone and the simulation protocol with TMS over the contralesional M1 did not show those changes. The results suggest that temporal associative plasticity is induced specifically for the extensor-related activity in the ipsilesional M1. If we can associate brain stimulation and task execution with proper timing, a task-specific associative plasticity may be induced. There is a large variability in movement onset of the paretic limbs after neurological insults. The central motor conduction time is prolonged in stroke and other neurodegenerative diseases due to lesions in the corticospinal tract (Kaviraja and Robert, 2013). It is influenced by time after disease onset or disease progression. On the other hand, electromyogram (EMG) onsets are often variable since it is difficult to increase firing rate in central nervous diseases (Barnes, 1980). Therefore, when we do simultaneous TMS with training, we may as well be careful for both the timing for TMS and task execution.

Use of a Shaped Task for the Combination

An effective rehabilitative approach should consist of various types of training pertaining to body movements in enriched environments that encourage patterns and combinations of movement for improving recovery. Different types of task-specific training help their effects transfer into actual activities of daily life in patients (Teasell et al., 2005). However, a specific task or tasks for specific movements are better combined with brain stimulation. If a task consists of various gross and precise movements, it may evoke conflicting neuronal activities such as inhibition and activation. Then, it may reduce the effect of brain stimulation. In recent animal studies, it was shown that training general gross movements inhibited recovery of skilled movements (Garcia-Alias et al., 2009). Neural competition for newly available neural resources may occur when multiple tasks are trained (Reinkensmeyer and Boninger, 2012). In clinical studies, task-specificity of training is more important than the intensity of training (Page, 2003; Bayona et al., 2005). The repetition of task-specific training produced long-lasting cortical reorganization and use-dependent plasticity specific to the areas that were activated during the trained movements in healthy subjects (Classen et al., 1998; Butefisch et al., 2000). In post-stroke patients, shaped task-specific training resulted in a better recovery of their paretic upper-limb function as compared with general training (Butefisch et al., 1995; Woldag et al., 2010).

Recently, we have investigated the effect of repetitive motor tasks in the paretic upper-limb combined with brain stimulation in post-stroke patients (Koganemaru et al., 2010). Patients with chronic stroke with moderate-to-severe hemiparesis often suffer from motor deficits associated with flexor hypertonia. A possible therapeutic strategy is to selectively induce use-dependent plasticity in the extensors to counteract the flexor hypertonia. However, the beneficial effects of training in chronic-phase patients are relatively limited due to resistance to induction of use-dependent plasticity in the chronic phase (Nakayama et al., 1994; Verheyden et al., 2008). When 5 Hz rTMS over the ipsilesional M1 was combined with extensor training assisted by electrical neuromuscular stimulation, the combined intervention resulted in an improvement of extensor movement with a reduction of flexor hypertonia, whereas neither of the single interventions alone demonstrated any improvements. The extensor-specific change in M1 was likely attributable to a functional recovery of the paretic upper limb (Koganemaru et al., 2010). Our study is an exemplary case showing the relevance of task selection combined with brain stimulation to enhance use-dependent plasticity for functional recovery.

The Stimulation of Neuronal Circuits Where Use-Dependent Plastic Changes Occur

Stimulation should be given to neuronal circuits and brain areas where use-dependent plastic changes occur. Because use-dependent plasticity is task-specific, changed circuits and areas depend on what type of task was trained. For repetitive simple motor tasks, use-dependent plastic changes have been reported within M1 (Classen et al., 1998; Butefisch et al., 2000; Rossini and Pauri, 2000). However, it is unknown whether it occurs within M1 alone or in combination with the multi-regional functional reorganization of the motor-related brain network. If it occurs in a multi-regional brain network, other non-M1 regions would be the possible targets of stimulation.

Recently, we used neuroimaging to investigate whether use-dependent changes occurred in a multiregional brain network in chronic post-stroke patients (Koganemaru et al., 2015). In process of post-stroke recovery with rehabilitative

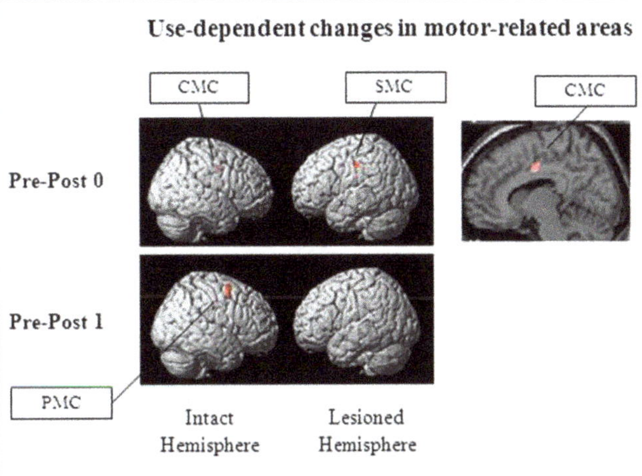

FIGURE 1 | Brain regions with use-dependent task-specific changes. Reduced activation was observed in the ipsilesional SMC, the contralesional cingulate motor cortex (CMC) and the contralesional premotor cortices (PMC), specifically for extensor movements of the paretic upper-limb after our combination therapy consisting of 5 Hz repetitive transcranial magnetic stimulation (rTMS) and the paretic extensor training in post-stroke patients with flexor hypertonia ("Post 0" and "Post 1", immediately after and 2 weeks after the combination therapy, respectively). Adapted from Koganemaru et al. (2015).

training, neuroimaging studies demonstrated that multi-regional brain reorganization occurred in several motor-related regions, including bilateral M1, premotor cortices (PMC), cingulate motor cortex (CMC), basal ganglia, and cerebellum (Nelles et al., 2001; Carey et al., 2002; Johansen-Berg et al., 2002a; Jang et al., 2003, 2005; Ward et al., 2003a, 2004; Luft et al., 2004; Ward and Cohen, 2004). The over-activity of non-M1 regions such as bilateral PMC in the acute stage was progressively decreased with an improvement in motor performance of the hemiparetic limbs (Calautti et al., 2001; Small et al., 2002; Ward et al., 2003a). In the chronic stage, the magnitude of brain activity in the non-M1 regions was negatively correlated with clinical outcome (Ward et al., 2003a,b) and positively correlated with the extent of damage in the corticospinal system (Ward et al., 2006). The findings suggest that the compensatory mechanism of these regions may be due to insufficient motor recovery (Feydy et al., 2002; Ward et al., 2003b). Those patients with larger brain damage and poorer clinical recovery may rely on activity in secondary motor areas to drive residual hand function (Johansen-Berg et al., 2002b). If a combination therapy of a task-specific training and brain stimulation could restore the ipsilesional M1 function by use-dependent plasticity, compensatory drive from secondary motor areas would be changed in post-stroke patients.

As previously described, we have developed a new combination therapy consisting of 5 Hz rTMS and an electrical neuromuscular stimulation assisted extensor training of the paretic upper-limb for stroke patients with flexor hypertonia. The extensor-specific plastic change in M1 was associated with beneficial functional effects (Koganemaru et al., 2010). We investigated whether extensor-specific multiregional brain reorganization occurred after our combination therapy by using functional magnetic resonance imaging (fMRI). The patients were scanned while performing upper-limb extensor movements. Untrained flexor movements were used as a control condition. Assessments were performed before, immediately after, and 2 weeks after the hybrid rehabilitation protocol. Analysis of the imaging data showed a significant reduction of brain activity in the ipsilesional SMC and the contralesional CMC immediately after (Post 0) and in the contralesional PMC 2 weeks after the intervention (Post 1; **Figure 1**). It suggests that the effects of the hybrid-rehabilitation appeared to differ temporally in each brain area. The process of motor learning consists of a fast learning stage and a slow learning stage. Specific neural representations are known in each stage (Karni et al., 1998; Kantak et al., 2012). The changes in activity in the ipsilesional SMC and the contralesional CMC may have shown combined effects of the fast learning stage, whereas the activity change in the contralesional PMC may have been involved in a consolidative process of the slow learning stage. Furthermore, the changes were associated with functional improvements of the paretic hands. They were not shown for the control condition (Koganemaru et al., 2015). Use-dependent plasticity induced by repetitive training may be related to the task-specific multi-regional brain reorganization. Thus, we expect that possible future targets for brain stimulation could include secondary motor areas. Artificial control of compensatory drive from secondary motor areas in accordance with the recovery process may be the next target for a combination therapy.

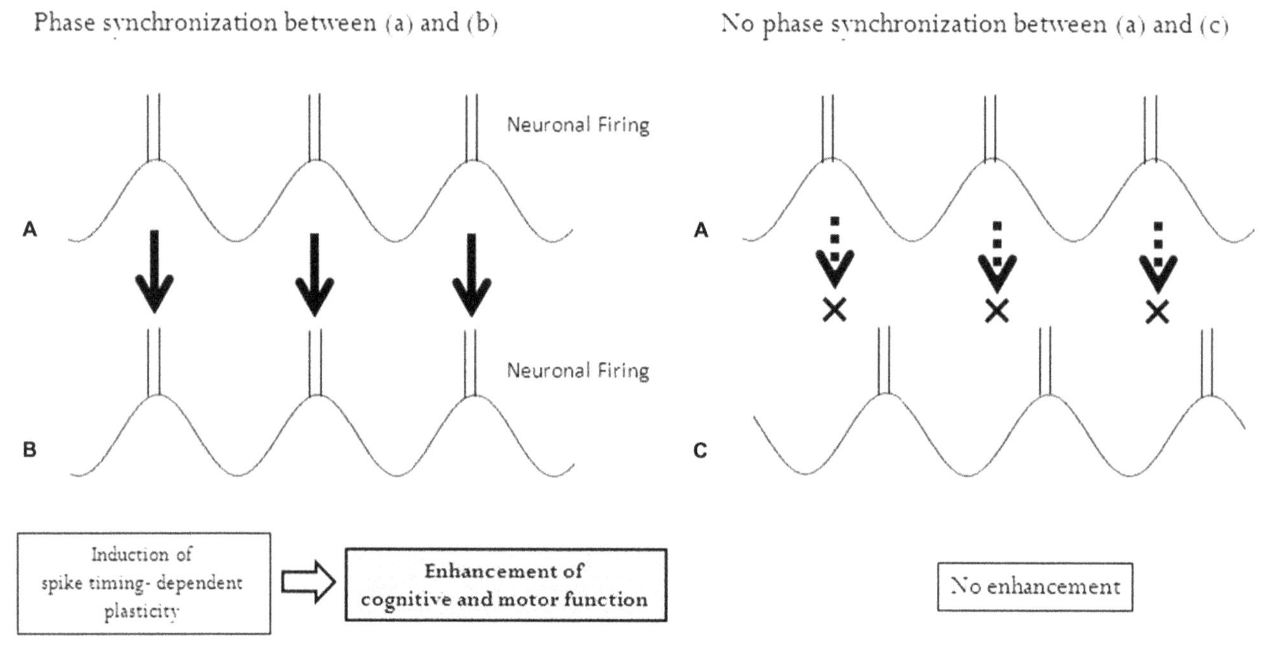

FIGURE 2 | Phase synchronization and temporal associative plasticity. Phase synchronization enables neurons in two different regions **(A)** and **(B)** to fire at the same timing, leading to an induction of spike-timing dependent plasticity between these regions. No synchronization of phases between the two regions **(A)** and **(C)** with different timing of neuronal firing does not induce any plasticity.

Phase Synchronization Between Rhythmically Patterned Brain Stimulation and Task-Related Patterned Activities of Neurons

In line with the theory of associative plasticity, we may be able to utilize the synchronization of phases between rhythmically patterned brain stimulation and task-related rhythmical activities of neurons. The phase synchronization of pre- and post-synaptic oscillations (wave-like neuronal signals) enabled researchers to correlate the timing of pre- and post-synaptic action potentials, resulting in the induction of temporal associative plasticity (Fell and Axmacher, 2011). Oscillatory non-invasive brain stimulation such as transcranial alternative current stimulation (tACS) and oscillatory tDCS (otDCS) has been reported to modulate oscillatory brain activity (Herrmann et al., 2013). Both tACS and otDCS use a sinusoidal form of electrical currents; however, tACS has no DC offset (net current = 0) and otDCS has a DC offset (net current = DC offset). In otDCS, the alternating current is superimposed onto a direct current. These protocols of stimulation may enhance neuronal circuits associated with intrinsic rhythmicity, leading to the enhancement of cognitive function (Marshall et al., 2006; Castro-Alamancos et al., 2007; Kanai et al., 2008, 2010; Kirov et al., 2009; Zaehle et al., 2010). In a recent study, phase-synchronized tACS suppressed Parkinson tremor by adjusting the phase to an abnormal cycle of the movements (Brittain et al., 2013). Rhythmical movements are produced with neuronal rhythmicity, a periodical repeat of excitation and inhibition. If oscillatory brain stimulation is synchronized with them at an appropriate phase, temporal associative plasticity may be induced (**Figure 2**).

One of the most familiar rhythmical movements in our daily life is locomotion, which requires the repeated patterned activation of specific neurons and muscles. Recently, in a preliminary experiment, we found that otDCS simulating gait rhythm induced gait-specific plasticity in healthy subjects (Koganemaru et al., 2014). Oscillatory patterned brain stimulation could be a new and powerful approach for the association of neuronal activities involved with training.

CONCLUSION

We have proposed the possible strategies for combination therapy of stimulation and rehabilitative trainings: (1) the control of temporal aspect between stimulation and task execution; (2) the use of a shaped task for the combination; (3) the appropriate stimulation of neuronal circuits where use-dependent plastic changes occur; and (4) phase synchronization between rhythmically patterned brain stimulation and task-related patterned activities of neurons. Associative brain plasticity induced by the combination therapy can bring functional improvements in patients.

There are still many diseases that are resistant to neuro-rehabilitative approaches. To better utilize brain stimulation in neuro-rehabilitation, we must explore more effective techniques for combining brain stimulation and rehabilitative training. An efficient association between brain stimulation and rehabilitative training could improve brain plasticity and promote functional recovery of patients.

ACKNOWLEDGMENTS

This study was partly supported by Grant-in-Aid for JSPS Fellows (25-5251), by Grant-in-Aid for Young Scientists (B) (26870321) from the Japan Society for the Promotion of Science, by the research grant (2015) from the Nakatomi Foundation (to SK), by Grant-in-Aid for Scientific Research (B) 15H03044, Grant-in-Aid for Scientific Research on Innovative Areas (15H05880, 15H05871) from the Japan Society for the Promotion of Science, STEP2 (15ek0109078h0001) from Japan Agency for Medical Research and development, AMED and the research grant (2015) from the Brain Science Foundation (to TM).

REFERENCES

Ameli, M., Grefkes, C., Kemper, F., Riegg, F. P., Rehme, A. K., Karbe, H., et al. (2009). Differential effects of high-frequency repetitive transcranial magnetic stimulation over ipsilesional primary motor cortex in cortical and subcortical middle cerebral artery stroke. *Ann. Neurol.* 66, 298–309. doi: 10.1002/ana.21725

Barnes, W. S. (1980). The relationship of motor-unit activation to isokinetic muscular contraction at different contractile velocities. *Phys. Ther.* 60, 1152–1158.

Bayona, N. A., Bitensky, J., Salter, K., and Teasell, R. (2005). The role of task-specific training in rehabilitation therapies. *Top Stroke Rehabil.* 12, 58–65. doi: 10.1310/bqm5-6ygb-mvj5-wvcr

Bolognini, N., Vallar, G., Casati, C., Latif, L. A., El-Nazer, R., Williams, J., et al. (2011). Neurophysiological and behavioral effects of tDCS combined with constraint-induced movement therapy in poststroke patients. *Neurorehabil. Neural Repair* 25, 819–829. doi: 10.1177/1545968311411056

Brittain, J. S., Probert-Smith, P., Aziz, T. Z., and Brown, P. (2013). Tremor suppression by rhythmic transcranial current stimulation. *Curr. Biol.* 23, 436–440. doi: 10.1016/j.cub.2013.01.068

Buetefisch, C., Heger, R., Schicks, W., Seitz, R., and Netz, J. (2011). Hebbian-type stimulation during robot-assisted training in patients with stroke. *Neurorehabil. Neural Repair* 25, 645–655. doi: 10.1177/1545968311402507

Butefisch, C., Hummelsheim, H., Denzler, P., and Mauritz, K. H. (1995). Repetitive training of isolated movements improves the outcome of motor rehabilitation of the centrally paretic hand. *J. Neurol. Sci.* 130, 59–68. doi: 10.1016/0022-510x(95)00003-k

Butefisch, C. M., Davis, B. C., Wise, S. P., Sawaki, L., Kopylev, L., Classen, J., et al. (2000). Mechanisms of use-dependent plasticity in the human motor cortex. *Proc. Natl. Acad. Sci. U S A* 97, 3661–3665. doi: 10.1073/pnas.97.7.3661

Calautti, C., Leroy, F., Guincestre, J. Y., and Baron, J. C. (2001). Dynamics of motor network overactivation after striatocapsular stroke: a longitudinal PET study using a fixed-performance paradigm. *Stroke* 32, 2534–2542. doi: 10.1161/hs1101.097401

Carey, J. R., Kimberley, T. J., Lewis, S. M., Auerbach, E. J., Dorsey, L., Rundquist, P., et al. (2002). Analysis of fMRI and finger tracking training in subjects with chronic stroke. *Brain* 125, 773–788. doi: 10.1093/brain/awf091

Castro-Alamancos, M. A., Rigas, P., and Tawara-Hirata, Y. (2007). Resonance (approximately 10 Hz) of excitatory networks in motor cortex: effects of voltage-dependent ion channel blockers. *J. Physiol.* 578, 173–191. doi: 10.1113/jphysiol.2006.119016

Chang, W. H., Kim, Y. H., Bang, O. Y., Kim, S. T., Park, Y. H., and Lee, P. K. (2010). Long-term effects of rTMS on motor recovery in patients after subacute stroke. *J. Rehabil. Med.* 42, 758–764. doi: 10.2340/16501977-0590

Chang, W. H., Kim, Y. H., Yoo, W. K., Goo, K. H., Park, C. H., Kim, S. T., et al. (2012). rTMS with motor training modulates cortico-basal ganglia-thalamocortical circuits in stroke patients. *Restor. Neurol. Neurosci.* 30, 179–189. doi: 10.3233/RNN-2012-110162

Cheeran, B., Talelli, P., Mori, F., Koch, G., Suppa, A., Edwards, M., et al. (2008). A common polymorphism in the brain-derived neurotrophic factor gene (BDNF) modulates human cortical plasticity and the response to rTMS. *J. Physiol. Lond.* 586, 5717–5725. doi: 10.1113/jphysiol.2008

Classen, J., Liepert, J., Wise, S. P., Hallett, M., and Cohen, L. G. (1998). Rapid plasticity of human cortical movement representation induced by practice. *J. Neurophysiol.* 79, 1117–1123.

Conforto, A. B., Anjos, S. M., Saposnik, G., Mello, E. A., Nagaya, E. M., Santos, W., et al. (2012). Transcranial magnetic stimulation in mild to severe hemiparesis early after stroke: a proof of principle and novel approach to improve motor function. *J. Neurol.* 259, 1399–1405. doi: 10.1007/s00415-011-6364-7

Dayan, E., Censor, N., Buch, E. R., Sandrini, M., and Cohen, L. G. (2013). Noninvasive brain stimulation: from physiology to network dynamics and back. *Nat. Neurosci.* 16, 838–844. doi: 10.1038/nn.3422

Dimyan, M. A., and Cohen, L. G. (2011). Neuroplasticity in the context of motor rehabilitation after stroke. *Nat. Rev. Neurol.* 7, 76–85. doi: 10.1038/nrneurol.2010.200

Edwardson, M. A., Lucas, T. H., Carey, J. R., and Fetz, E. E. (2013). New modalities of brain stimulation for stroke rehabilitation. *Exp. Brain Res.* 224, 335–358. doi: 10.1007/s00221-012-3315-1

Egger, V., Feldmeyer, D., and Sakmann, B. (1999). Coincidence detection and changes of synaptic efficacy in spiny stellate neurons in rat barrel cortex. *Nat. Neurosci.* 2, 1098–1105.

Emara, T. H., Moustafa, R. R., Elnahas, N. M., Elganzoury, A. M., Abdo, T. A., Mohamed, S. A., et al. (2010). Repetitive transcranial magnetic stimulation at 1Hz and 5Hz produces sustained improvement in motor function and disability after ischaemic stroke. *Eur. J. Neurol.* 17, 1203–1209. doi: 10.1111/j.1468-1331.2010.03000.x

Fell, J., and Axmacher, N. (2011). The role of phase synchronization in memory processes. *Nat. Rev. Neurosci.* 12, 105–118. doi: 10.1038/nrn2979

Feydy, A., Carlier, R., Roby-Brami, A., Bussel, B., Cazalis, F., Pierot, L., et al. (2002). Longitudinal study of motor recovery after stroke: recruitment and focusing of brain activation. *Stroke* 33, 1610–1617. doi: 10.1161/01.str.0000017100.68294.52

Floel, A. (2014). tDCS-enhanced motor and cognitive function in neurological diseases. *Neuroimage* 85, 934–947. doi: 10.1016/j.neuroimage.2013.05.098

Fritsch, B., Reis, J., Martinowich, K., Schambra, H. M., Ji, Y., Cohen, L. G., et al. (2010). Direct current stimulation promotes BDNF-dependent synaptic plasticity: potential implications for motor learning. *Neuron* 66, 198–204. doi: 10.1016/j.neuron.2010.03.035

Garcia-Alias, G., Barkhuysen, S., Buckle, M., and Fawcett, J. W. (2009). Chondroitinase ABC treatment opens a window of opportunity for task-specific rehabilitation. *Nat. Neurosci.* 12, 1145–1151. doi: 10.1038/nn.2377

Hallett, M. (2000). Transcranial magnetic stimulation and the human brain. *Nature* 406, 147–150. doi: 10.1038/35018000

Hebb, D. O. (1949). *The Organization of Behavior: A Neuropsychological Theory.* New York, NY: Wiley.

Hendricks, H. T., Van Limbeek, J., Geurts, A. C., and Zwarts, M. J. (2002). Motor recovery after stroke: a systematic review of the literature. *Arch. Phys. Med. Rehabil.* 83, 1629–1637. doi: 10.1053/apmr.2002.35473

Herrmann, C. S., Rach, S., Neuling, T., and Struber, D. (2013). Transcranial alternating current stimulation: a review of the underlying mechanisms and modulation of cognitive processes. *Front. Hum. Neurosci.* 7:279. doi: 10.3389/fnhum.2013.00279

Hess, G., Aizenman, C. D., and Donoghue, J. P. (1996). Conditions for the induction of long-term potentiation in layer II/III horizontal connections of the rat motor cortex. *J. Neurophysiol.* 75, 1765–1778.

Hess, G., and Donoghue, J. P. (1996). Long-term potentiation and long-term depression of horizontal connections in rat motor cortex. *Acta. Neurobiol. Exp. (Wars)* 56, 397–405.

Hsu, Y. F., Huang, Y. Z., Lin, Y. Y., Tang, C. W., Liao, K. K., Lee, P. L., et al. (2013). Intermittent theta burst stimulation over ipsilesional primary motor cortex of subacute ischemic stroke patients: a pilot study. *Brain Stimul.* 6, 166–174. doi: 10.1016/j.brs.2012.04.007

Hummel, F. C., and Cohen, L. G. (2005). Drivers of brain plasticity. *Curr. Opin. Neurol.* 18, 667–674. doi: 10.1097/01.wco.0000189876.37475.42

Hummelsheim, H. (1999). Rationales for improving motor function. *Curr. Opin. Neurol.* 12, 697–701. doi: 10.1097/00019052-199912000-00007

Jang, S. H., Kim, Y. H., Cho, S. H., Chang, Y., Lee, Z. I., and Ha, J. S. (2003). Cortical reorganization associated with motor recovery in hemiparetic stroke patients. *Neuroreport* 14, 1305–1310. doi: 10.1097/01.wnr.0000078700.79393.09

Jang, S. H., You, S. H., Hallett, M., Cho, Y. W., Park, C. M., Cho, S. H., et al. (2005). Cortical reorganization and associated functional motor recovery after virtual reality in patients with chronic stroke: an experimenter-blind preliminary study. *Arch. Phys. Med. Rehabil.* 86, 2218–2223. doi: 10.1016/j.apmr.2005.04.015

Johansen-Berg, H., Dawes, H., Guy, C., Smith, S. M., Wade, D. T., and Matthews, P. M. (2002a). Correlation between motor improvements and altered fMRI activity after rehabilitative therapy. *Brain* 125, 2731–2742. doi: 10.1093/brain/awf282

Johansen-Berg, H., Rushworth, M. F., Bogdanovic, M. D., Kischka, U., Wimalaratna, S., and Matthews, P. M. (2002b). The role of ipsilateral premotor cortex in hand movement after stroke. *Proc. Natl. Acad. Sci. U S A* 99, 14518–14523. doi: 10.1073/pnas.222536799

Kanai, R., Chaieb, L., Antal, A., Walsh, V., and Paulus, W. (2008). Frequency-dependent electrical stimulation of the visual cortex. *Curr. Biol.* 18, 1839–1843. doi: 10.1016/j.cub.2008.10.027

Kanai, R., Paulus, W., and Walsh, V. (2010). Transcranial alternating current stimulation (tACS) modulates cortical excitability as assessed by TMS-induced phosphene thresholds. *Clin. Neurophysiol.* 121, 1551–1554. doi: 10.1016/j.clinph.2010.03.022

Kantak, S. S., Stinear, J. W., Buch, E. R., and Cohen, L. G. (2012). Rewiring the brain: potential role of the premotor cortex in motor control, learning and recovery of function following brain injury. *Neurorehabil. Neural Repair* 26, 282–292. doi: 10.1177/1545968311420845

Karabanov, A., Ziemann, U., Hamada, M., George, M. S., Quartarone, A., Classen, J., et al. (2015). Consensus paper: probing homeostatic plasticity of human cortex with non-invasive transcranial brain stimulation. *Brain Stimul.* 8, 442–454. doi: 10.1016/j.brs.2015.01.404

Karni, A., Meyer, G., Rey-Hipolito, C., Jezzard, P., Adams, M. M., Turner, R., et al. (1998). The acquisition of skilled motor performance: fast and slow experience-driven changes in primary motor cortex. *Proc. Natl. Acad. Sci. U S A* 95, 861–868. doi: 10.1073/pnas.95.3.861

Kaviraja, U., and Robert, C. (2013). "Central motor conduction time," in *Handbook of Clinical Neurology, Brain Stimulation*, eds A. M. Lozano and M. Hallett (Amsterdam: Elsevier B.V.), 375–386. doi: 10.1007/978-3-540-29678-2_891

Khedr, E. M., Abdel-Fadeil, M. R., Farghali, A., and Qaid, M. (2009). Role of 1 and 3 Hz repetitive transcranial magnetic stimulation on motor function recovery after acute ischaemic stroke. *Eur. J. Neurol.* 16, 1323–1330. doi: 10.1111/j.1468-1331.2009.02746.x

Khedr, E. M., Ahmed, M. A., Fathy, N., and Rothwell, J. C. (2005). Therapeutic trial of repetitive transcranial magnetic stimulation after acute ischemic stroke. *Neurology* 65, 466–468. doi: 10.1212/01.wnl.0000173067.84247.36

Khedr, E. M., Etraby, A. E., Hemeda, M., Nasef, A. M., and Razek, A. A. (2010). Long-term effect of repetitive transcranial magnetic stimulation on motor function recovery after acute ischemic stroke. *Acta. Neurol. Scand.* 121, 30–37. doi: 10.1111/j.1600-0404.2009.01195.x

Kim, D. Y., Lim, J. Y., Kang, E. K., You, D. S., Oh, M. K., Oh, B. M., et al. (2010). Effect of transcranial direct current stimulation on motor recovery in patients with subacute stroke. *Am. J. Phys. Med. Rehabil.* 89, 879–886. doi: 10.1097/phm.0b013e3181f70aa7

Kim, D. Y., Ohn, S. H., Yang, E. J., Park, C. I., and Jung, K. J. (2009). Enhancing motor performance by anodal transcranial direct current stimulation in subacute stroke patients. *Am. J. Phys. Med. Rehabil.* 88, 829–836. doi: 10.1097/phm.0b013e3181b811e3

Kim, Y. H., You, S. H., Ko, M. H., Park, J. W., Lee, K. H., Jang, S. H., et al. (2006). Repetitive transcranial magnetic stimulation-induced corticomotor excitability and associated motor skill acquisition in chronic stroke. *Stroke* 37, 1471–1476. doi: 10.1161/01.str.000221233.55497.51

Kirov, R., Weiss, C., Siebner, H. R., Born, J., and Marshall, L. (2009). Slow oscillation electrical brain stimulation during waking promotes EEG theta activity and memory encoding. *Proc. Natl. Acad. Sci. U S A* 106, 15460–15465. doi: 10.1073/pnas.0904438106

Koganemaru, S., Mikami, Y., Fukuyama, H., and Mima, T. (2014). Slow oscillatory stimulation simulating gait rhythm induces LTP-like effects on corticospinal excitability in foot. *Clin. Neurophysiol.* 125, Suppl 1, Abstracts of the 30th International Congress of Clinical Neurophysiology (ICCN) of the IFCN, March 20–23 2014, Berlin, Germany, S223.

Koganemaru, S., Mima, T., Nakatsuka, M., Ueki, Y., Fukuyama, H., and Domen, K. (2009). Human motor associative plasticity induced by paired bihemispheric stimulation. *J. Physiol.* 587, 4629–4644. doi: 10.1113/jphysiol.2009.174342

Koganemaru, S., Mima, T., Thabit, M. N., Ikkaku, T., Shimada, K., Kanematsu, M., et al. (2010). Recovery of upper-limb function due to enhanced use-dependent plasticity in chronic stroke patients. *Brain* 133, 3373–3384. doi: 10.1093/brain/awq193

Koganemaru, S., Sawamoto, N., Aso, T., Sagara, A., Ikkaku, T., Shimada, K., et al. (2015). Task-specific brain reorganization in motor recovery induced by a hybrid-rehabilitation combining training with brain stimulation after stroke. *Neurosci. Res.* 92, 29–38. doi: 10.1016/j.neures.2014.10.004

Luft, A. R., Mccombe-Waller, S., Whitall, J., Macko, R., Sorkin, J. D., Schulz, J. B., et al. (2004). Repetitive bilateral arm training and motor cortex activation in chronic stroke: A randomized controlled trial. *JAMA* 292, 1853–1861. doi: 10.1001/jama.292.20.2470-b

Marshall, L., Helgadottir, H., Molle, M., and Born, J. (2006). Boosting slow oscillations during sleep potentiates memory. *Nature* 444, 610–613. doi: 10.1038/nature05278

Masiero, S., and Carraro, E. (2008). Upper limb movements and cerebral plasticity in post-stroke rehabilitation. *Aging Clin. Exp. Res.* 20, 103–108. doi: 10.1007/bf03324755

Meehan, S. K., Dao, E., Linsdell, M. A., and Boyd, L. A. (2011). Continuous theta burst stimulation over the contralesional sensory and motor cortex enhances motor learning post-stroke. *Neurosci. Lett.* 500, 26–30. doi: 10.1016/j.neulet.2011.05.237

Nair, D. G., Renga, V., Lindenberg, R., Zhu, L., and Schlaug, G. (2011). Optimizing recovery potential through simultaneous occupational therapy and non-invasive brain-stimulation using tDCS. *Restor. Neurol. Neurosci.* 29, 411–420. doi: 10.3233/RNN-2011-0612

Nakayama, H., Jorgensen, H. S., Raaschou, H. O., and Olsen, T. S. (1994). Recovery of upper extremity function in stroke patients: the Copenhagen Stroke Study. *Arch. Phys. Med. Rehabil.* 75, 394–398.

Nelles, G., Jentzen, W., Jueptner, M., Müller, S., and Diener, H. C. (2001). Arm training induced brain plasticity in stroke studied with serial positron emission tomography. *NeuroImage* 13, 1146–1154. doi: 10.1006/nimg.2001.0757

Nudo, R. J., and Milliken, G. W. (1996). Reorganization of movement representations in primary motor cortex following focal ischemic infarcts in adult squirrel monkeys. *J. Neurophysiol.* 75, 2144–2149.

Nudo, R. J., Milliken, G. W., Jenkins, W. M., and Merzenich, M. M. (1996a). Use-dependent alterations of movement representations in primary motor cortex of adult squirrel monkeys. *J. Neurosci.* 16, 785–807.

Nudo, R. J., Wise, B. M., Sifuentes, F., and Milliken, G. W. (1996b). Neural substrates for the effects of rehabilitative training on motor recovery after ischemic infarct. *Science* 272, 1791–1794. doi: 10.1126/science.272.5269.1791

Page, S. J. (2003). Intensity versus task-specificity after stroke: how important is intensity? *Am. J. Phys. Med. Rehabil.* 82, 730–732. doi: 10.1097/01.phm.0000078226.36000.a5

Pascual-Leone, A., Valls-Solé, J., Wassermann, E. M., and Hallett, M. (1994). Responses to rapid-rate transcranial magnetic stimulation of the human motor cortex. *Brain* 117, 847–858. doi: 10.1093/brain/117.4.847

Pennisi, G., Rapisarda, G., Bella, R., Calabrese, V., Maertens De Noordhout, A., and Delwaide, P. J. (1999). Absence of response to early transcranial magnetic stimulation in ischemic stroke patients: prognostic value for hand motor recovery. *Stroke* 30, 2666–2670. doi: 10.1161/01.str.30.12.2666

Platz, T., and Rothwell, J. C. (2010). Brain stimulation and brain repair–rTMS: from animal experiment to clinical trials–what do we know? *Restor. Neurol. Neurosci.* 28, 387–398. doi: 10.3233/RNN-2010-0570

Reinkensmeyer, D. J., and Boninger, M. L. (2012). Technologies and combination therapies for enhancing movement training for people with a disability. *J. Neuroeng. Rehabil.* 9, 17. doi: 10.1186/1743-0003-9-17

Richards, L. G., Stewart, K. C., Woodbury, M. L., Senesac, C., and Cauraugh, J. H. (2008). Movement-dependent stroke recovery: A systematic review and meta-analysis of TMS and fMRI evidence. *Neuropsychologia* 46, 3–11. doi: 10.1016/j.neuropsychologia.2007.08.013

Rossini, P. M., and Pauri, F. (2000). Neuromagnetic integrated methods tracking human brain mechanisms of sensorimotor areas 'plastic' reorganisation. *Brain Res. Rev.* 33, 131–154. doi: 10.1016/s0169-328x(00)00090-5

Sandrini, M., and Cohen, L. G. (2013). "Noninvasive brain stimulation in neurorehabilitation," in *Handbook of Clinical Neurology, Brain Stimulation*, eds A. M. Lozano and M. Hallett. (Amsterdam: Elsevier B.V.), 499–524. doi: 10.1016/b978-0-444-53497-2.00040-1

Small, S. L., Hlustik, P., Noll, D. C., Genovese, C., and Solodkin, A. (2002). Cerebellar hemispheric activation ipsilateral to the paretic hand correlates with functional recovery after stroke. *Brain* 125, 1544–1557. doi: 10.1093/brain/awf148

Stagg, C. J., and Nitsche, M. A. (2011). Physiological basis of transcranial direct current stimulation. *Neuroscientist* 17, 37–53. doi: 10.1177/1073858410386614

Stefan, K., Kunesch, E., Benecke, R., Cohen, L. G., and Classen, J. (2002). Mechanisms of enhancement of human motor cortex excitability induced by interventional paired associative stimulation. *J. Physiol. Lond.* 543, 699–708. doi: 10.1113/jphysiol.2002.023317

Stefan, K., Kunesch, E., Cohen, L. G., Benecke, R., and Classen, J. (2000). Induction of plasticity in the human motor cortex by paired associative stimulation. *Brain* 123, 572–584. doi: 10.1093/brain/123.3.572

Takeuchi, N., Chuma, T., Matsuo, Y., Watanabe, I., and Ikoma, K. (2005). Repetitive transcranial magnetic stimulation of contralesional primary motor cortex improves hand function after stroke. *Stroke* 36, 2681–2686. doi: 10.1161/01.str.0000189658.51972.34

Takeuchi, N., Tada, T., Toshima, M., Chuma, T., Matsuo, Y., and Ikoma, K. (2008). Inhibition of the unaffected motor cortex by 1 Hz repetitive transcranical magnetic stimulation enhances motor performance and training effect of the paretic hand in patients with chronic stroke. *J. Rehabil. Med.* 40, 298–303. doi: 10.2340/16501977-0181

Talelli, P., Wallace, A., Dileone, M., Hoad, D., Cheeran, B., Oliver, R., et al. (2012). Theta burst stimulation in the rehabilitation of the upper limb: a semirandomized, placebo-controlled trial in chronic stroke patients. *Neurorehabil. Neural Repair* 26, 976–987. doi: 10.1177/1545968312437940

Teasell, R., Bitensky, J., Foley, N., and Bayona, N. A. (2005). Training and stimulation in post stroke recovery brain reorganization. *Top Stroke Rehabil.* 12, 37–45. doi: 10.1310/e893-m0pr-njej-1gxm

Thabit, M. N., Ueki, Y., Koganemaru, S., Fawi, G., Fukuyama, H., and Mima, T. (2010). Movement-related cortical stimulation can induce human motor plasticity. *J. Neurosci.* 30, 11529–11536. doi: 10.1523/JNEUROSCI.1829-10.2010

Ueki, Y., Mima, T., Kotb, M. A., Sawada, H., Saiki, H., Ikeda, A., et al. (2006). Altered plasticity of the human motor cortex in Parkinson's disease. *Ann. Neurol.* 59, 60–71. doi: 10.3410/f.7018.349452

Verheyden, G., Nieuwboer, A., De Wit, L., Thijs, V., Dobbelaere, J., Devos, H., et al. (2008). Time course of trunk, arm, leg and functional recovery after ischemic stroke. *Neurorehabil. Neural Repair* 22, 173–179. doi: 10.1177/1545968307305456

Wang, R. Y., Tseng, H. Y., Liao, K. K., Wang, C. J., Lai, K. L., and Yang, Y. R. (2012). rTMS combined with task-oriented training to improve symmetry of interhemispheric corticomotor excitability and gait performance after stroke: a randomized trial. *Neurorehabil Neural Repair* 26, 222–230. doi: 10.1177/1545968311423265

Ward, N. S., Brown, M. M., Thompson, A. J., and Frackowiak, R. S. (2003a). Neural correlates of motor recovery after stroke: a longitudinal fMRI study. *Brain* 126, 2476–2496. doi: 10.1093/brain/awg245

Ward, N. S., Brown, M. M., Thompson, A. J., and Frackowiak, R. S. (2003b). Neural correlates of outcome after stroke: a cross-sectional fMRI study. *Brain* 126, 1430–1448. doi: 10.1093/brain/awg145

Ward, N. S., Brown, M. M., Thompson, A. J., and Frackowiak, R. S. (2004). The influence of time after stroke on brain activations during a motor task. *Ann. Neurol.* 55, 829–834. doi: 10.1002/ana.20099

Ward, N. S., and Cohen, L. G. (2004). Mechanisms underlying recovery of motor function after stroke. *Arch. Neurol.* 61, 1844–1848. doi: 10.1001/archneur.61.12.1844

Ward, N. S., Newton, J. M., Swayne, O. B., Lee, L., Thompson, A. J., Greenwood, R. J., et al. (2006). Motor system activation after subcortical stroke depends on corticospinal system integrity. *Brain* 129, 809–819. doi: 10.1093/brain/awl002

Woldag, H., Stupka, K., and Hummelsheim, H. (2010). Repetitive training of complex hand arm movements with shaping is beneficial for motor improvement in patients after stroke. *J. Rehabil. Med.* 42, 582–587. doi: 10.2340/16501977-0558

Zaehle, T., Rach, S., and Herrmann, C.S. (2010). Transcranial alternating current stimulation enhances individual alpha activity in human EEG. *PLoS One* 5:e13766. doi: 10.1371/journal.pone.0013766

2

Mechatronic wearable exoskeletons for bionic bipedal standing and walking: a new synthetic approach

Gelu Onose [1,2], Vladimir Cârdei [3], Ştefan T. Crăciunoiu [3], Valeriu Avramescu [3], Ioan Opriş [4], Mikhail A. Lebedev [5] and Marian Vladimir Constantinescu [6]*

[1] Department of Physical and Rehabilitation Medicine, University of Medicine and Pharmacy "Carol Davila", Bucharest, Romania, [2] Teaching Emergency Hospital "Bagdasar-Arseni", Bucharest, Romania, [3] Research and Technological Design Institute for Machines Construction, Bucharest, Romania, [4] Miller School of Medicine, University of Miami, Miami, FL, USA, [5] Department of Neurobiology, Duke University, Durham, NC, USA, [6] Holistic Dental Medicine Institute – ROPOSTURO, Bucharest, Romania

Edited by:
Mircea Dragoman, National Institute for Research and Development in Microtechnologies, Romania

Reviewed by:
Giuseppe D'Avenio, Istituto Superiore di Sanità, Italy
Giovanni Stellin, Telerobot Labs Srl, Italy

***Correspondence:**
Gelu Onose
geluonose@gmail.com

During the last few years, interest has been growing to mechatronic and robotic technologies utilized in wearable powered exoskeletons that assist standing and walking. The available literature includes single-case reports, clinical studies conducted in small groups of subjects, and several recent systematic reviews. These publications have fulfilled promotional and marketing objectives but have not yet resulted in a fully optimized, practical wearable exoskeleton. Here we evaluate the progress and future directions in this field from a joint perspective of health professionals, manufacturers, and consumers. We describe the taxonomy of existing technologies and highlight the main improvements needed for the development and functional optimization of the practical exoskeletons.

Keywords: mechatronic, portable/wearable exoskeletons, bipedal standing, bionic walk assistance, models

HUMAN POSTURE AND WALKING, AND THEIR RESTORATION TO THE DISABLED

Vertical posture and bipedal gait are two hallmarks of human biomechanics and motor physiology, which emerged over the millions of years of evolution. While our body size and overall physical performance are not particularly impressive compared to other animal species, having our hands relieved from body support against gravity gives us a number of advantages, dexterity being one of the most important ones. In addition to motor physiology, virtually any human physiological function is adapted to the bipedal posture and walking, for example breathing, digestion, and excretion (Uebelhart et al., 2000)[1]. Moreover, human bipedalism has had a great influence on our daily social interactions and the manmade habitat.

While the surrounding objects and structure of the buildings all fit the needs of healthy humans, the conditions are quite different for disabled, wheelchair bound people. No matter how many facilities would be made in order to overcome their numberless structural barriers, new hurdles are always to be expected. Wheelchair users will never be able to completely adapt to the habitat built for the people who walk bipedally and stand upright. By contrast, the cartoon of a person in the wheelchair is the worldwide used symbol for handicap.

[1]http://www.sci-info-pages.com/other_issues.html#Osteoporosis

Although there is no cure for many lesions of the spinal cord and the brain (Talley Watts et al., 2015)—the major causes of paralysis—essential improvements can be made to the quality of life of handicapped people using devices that assist vertical stance and bipedal walking (Louie et al., 2015). These assistive technologies are based on mechatronic, robotic, and bionic exoskeletons (Chen et al., 2013). Such devices clearly represent one of the most important developments in rehabilitation of paralysis, even though they are currently not expected to deliver a truly spectacular, translational progress. Rather, they are considered as viable intermediary solutions, which bring us closer to the long-awaited recovery of posture and gait to the paralyzed patients. While much work is still needed to improve these external aids, they already have shown effective daily use capabilities.

ASSISTIVE TECHNOLOGIES: MANUFACTURER AND CONSUMER PERSPECTIVES

In the last decade and mostly in its second half, a series of exoskeletons have been designed, built, clinically tested in small groups of subjects, and reviewed in the literature[2–9]. These previous publications have fulfilled the promotional and marketing objectives of the manufacturers, and several exoskeletons are currently commercially available. Yet, an optimal, fully functional assistive device has not yet emerged from this research and development[10,11] (Chen et al., 2013; Arazpour et al., 2015b; Lajeunesse et al., 2015; Louie et al., 2015).

An optimal, practical exoskeleton should fulfill the following requirements:

- The system should be safe.
- It should be effectively wearable[11] in the common sense of the term, mainly regarding don and doff issues. Additionally, it should be psychologically acceptable in terms of self-esteem, miniaturization, and esthetics. Ideally, the exo-suit should be thin and wearable like clothes or underwear.
- The exoskeleton should be appropriate for long time performance, including the performance in community (Louie et al., 2015).
- It should produce very low, practically imperceptible noise when functioning.
- The assistive device should be truly affordable and cost effective.

We believe that achieving these requirements should be the main goal of the field, so we focus on these practical, consumer-oriented objectives in this article. We start with proposing a taxonomy of exoskeletons. We then discuss the improvements of these assistive devices that need to be achieved in near-term and long-term. Our views reflect both the professional, multi-disciplinary expertise of the authors and consumer perspective. The first author (**Figure 1**) sees both sides of the coin: he is an academic physician in Physical and Rehabilitation Medicine (with special focus on Neurorehabilitation) and in Gerontology and Geriatrics, and also a chronic, complete paraplegic, dependent on the wheelchair.

Our multidisciplinary approach intends—without underestimating the legitimate competition between different technical solutions and producers—to foster the optimization of assistive and rehabilitation devices, so that they could eventually become suitable and available to as many people in need as possible. Being one of the consumers too, the first author is looking forward to welcome this long awaited accomplishment, no matter which exoskeleton model meets the expectations first.

MAIN INDICATIONS

The currently available wearable powered exoskeletons serve two main functions. The first function is medical: providing assistive and rehabilitation technology for disabled people[12]. The second function is non-medical: augmenting normal human physical capabilities.

As to the non-medical domain, we are covering it here only briefly. Noteworthy, non-medical exoskeletons have indirect linkages to medical issues, such as contributions to technology development and prevention of occupational injuries. The other uses encompass military devices for enhancement of soldier speed, power, and interactions with the equipment[13–15]; exoskeletons for people professionally involved in critical rescue situations, such transportation of wounded individuals to safety from the war or civil disaster areas[13–16]; civil applications for lifting and carrying heavy objects and patients[17]; and exoskeletons that augment human gait by assisting leg muscles and supporting a comfortable orthostatic posture. The target population for these applications includes the elderly with weak legs, personnel engaged in long-distance walking and/or performing flexion and extension movements with their lower limbs, and people utilizing exoskeleton appliances for entertainment[18].

[2]http://www.cyberdyne.jp/company/download/20160212_financialresultssummary.pdf
[3]http://www.digitaltrends.com/cool-tech/rewalk-6-0-exoskeleton/
[4]http://www.rexbionics.com/investors/
[5]http://www.engadget.com/2011/05/02/new-zealand-paralympian-buys-first-rex-bionics-exoskeleton-take/
[6]http://www.fastcompany.com/1822791/eksos-exoskeletons-let-paraplegics-walk-will-anyone-actually-wear-one
[7]http://world.honda.com/news/2015/p150721eng.html
[8]http://www.indego.com/indego/en/Product
[9]http://www.fastcodesign.com/3056049/a-budget-exoskeleton-allows-parapalegics-to-walk-for-the-price-of-a-car7
[10]http://www.b-temia.com/category/press_releases/
[11]https://www.cadth.ca/sites/default/files/pdf/htis/july-2015/RA0784%20Powered%20Wearable%20Walking%20Assistive%20Devices%20Final.pdf
[12]http://www.keeogo.com/biomechatronics/
[13]http://bleex.me.berkeley.edu/research/exoskeleton/bleex/
[14]http://bleex.me.berkeley.edu/research/exoskeleton/exohiker/
[15]http://bleex.me.berkeley.edu/research/exoskeleton/hulc/
[16]http://www.b-temia.com/defense-security-soldier-protection/
[17]http://www.cyberdyne.jp/english/products/Lumbar_LaborSupport.html
[18]http://asimo.honda.com/innovations/feature/body-weight-support-assist/

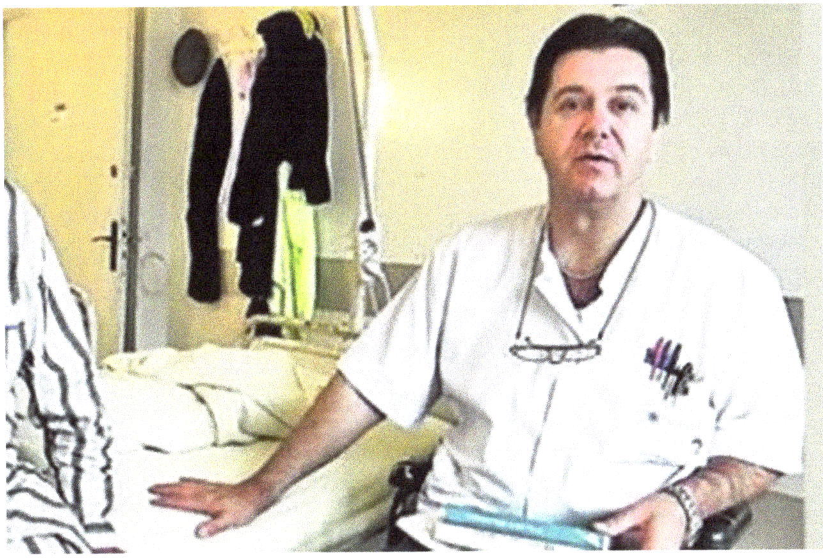

FIGURE 1 | The picture of the first author Prof. Dr. Gelu Onose in wheelchair visiting patients in the NeuroRehabilitation Clinic Division of the 'Bagdasar-Arseni' Teaching Emergency Hospital, Bucharest, Romania. Reproduced with permission of the TV producer, Romanian Television.

The medical domain includes wearable devices utilized for prophylactic, rehabilitation, and assistance to disabled people. Taxonomy of these devices reflects the needs of different types of patients. A complete paraplegic would need a device that performs a set of sophisticated tasks, and there is currently no device with these capabilities. Such a device would require no effort from the paralyzed patient, and would do almost everything for the patient.

The device for a complete paraplegic would have to ensure:

- Complete assistance to orthostatic posture and walking, including the very difficult task of maintaining balance in order to avoid falls with severe consequences (Kannape and Lenggenhager, 2016).
- Prevention of spasticity and contractures (Arazpour et al., 2013) and related articular stiffness and pain.
- Prevention of venous and lymphatic stasis in the lower limbs, which could result in lower extremity edema and related complications due to prolonged standing (Louie et al., 2015).
- Partial compensation of the body weight to avoid injuries, such as fracture of the talus (Louie et al., 2015).

The complete paraplegia is classified by the scales of American Spinal Injury Association (ASIA) and International Spinal Cord Society (ISCoS) ("Standard Neurological Classification of Spinal Cord Injury"[19], Frankel et al., 1969). Mechatronic wearable exoskeletons can be very useful as assistive devices in these cases because in complete chronic lesions of the spinal cord, as a rule, there are not enough remaining neural-muscular units to be trained. The possibility that exoskeletons could be used for rehabilitation in such cases, for example for rehabilitation of muscle activity, is still unclear (Arazpour et al., 2015b). The use of exoskeletons still can induce neuroplasticity (Muresanu et al., 2012; Bryce et al., 2015; Louie et al., 2015) that improved patient interaction with the device[20]. Additionally, a supplementary input from the patient's collected and decoded cortical activity might improve the man-machine interaction and the overall functional outcome.

The indications are different for incomplete paraplegics classified as AIS/ Frankel B-D, tetraplegics with low cervical spinal cord lesions classified as AIS/ Frankel C, and for hemiplegics and hemiparetics with fully preserved functionality of the non-affected hemi-body and limbs, and no sensorial, cognitive and balance serious impairments. The other potential beneficiaries of such exoskeletons are patients with neuromuscular and somatic impairments, including patients with polyneuropathia in lower limbs (Zeilig et al., 2012), multiple sclerosis, Parkinson's disease, hip or knee osteoarthritis[21], limb fractures, and amputated limbs (Chen et al., 2013).

In hemiplegia cases, an H2 (Technaid S.L., Spain) robotic exoskeleton is more appropriate for gait rehabilitation (Bortole et al., 2015)—an exoskeleton based on two control strategies: (i) adaptive trajectory control for guiding the patient's limb within a desired path, the strategy that facilitates patient interaction with the device, and (ii) admittance control strategy that captures the user's movements during assistive training phase and reproduces it during active training phase (Bortole et al., 2013). The main feature of the wearable exoskeletons indicated to approach these kinds of patients is usually not an assistive control of the trunk. An essential feature of using such devices is training induced rehabilitation, where the exercise outcomes are compared to the time spent exercising (Louie et al., 2015).

[19] http://www.scribd.com/doc/37064936/2006-Classif-Worksheet

[20] http://who.int/disabilities/policies/actionplan/disability_action_plan_en.docx

[21] http://www.keeogo.com/keeogo-in-action/

The choice of the exoskeleton system and training regime critically depend on the extent of neurological impairment, the affected neural site (central, peripheral, or both), and the state of muscles (which can change with training). Additionally, it is important to take into account and correct by training such conditions as pain, contracture, osteoporosis, bed sores, and edema (Arazpour et al., 2013).

In the disabled elderly, the degree and characteristics of multimorbidity should be considered (Salive, 2013), particularly balance disorders, cardio-respiratory impairments, and para-physiological sarcopenia (Morley, 2012). The assistive and rehabilitation devices should be adjusted to these conditions. For instance, if an older adult has preserved, although altered, ability to stand-up and walk, extended trunk stabilization may not be needed. However, if the senior beneficiary has marked sensory and/or balance impairment, a maximally assistive devices might be more appropriate, in order to avoid frequent falls in the older population[22]. The frequency of falls is variable (6–34%) in different countries and regions: (Kalache et al., 2007). Falls represent some of the most serious negative events with considerable pathological consequences, including disabilities and life threatening conditions. Such negative events result in economic burden for the patients, their families, and the society[22] (Kalache et al., 2007). These considerations will become progressively more important in the future, as the global process of demographic ageing intensifiers[22] (Kalache et al., 2007; Chen et al., 2013).

CURRENT TECHNOLOGIES

Currently popular wearable powered exoskeletons include Isocentric Reciprocating Gait Orthosis (IRGO), Hybrid Assistive Leg/Limb (HAL), ReWalk, Ekso, Mina, Wearable Power-Assist Locomotor (WPAL), Rex, Indego, Keeogo, Kickstart, Stride Management Assist, and ExoAtlet[23]. These devices have been recently reviewed[11] (Arazpour et al., 2013, 2015a,b; Chen et al., 2013; Lajeunesse et al., 2015; Louie et al., 2015). These review articles documented the following characteristics of the existing systems:

- Benefits, including compared to the robotic exoskeletons fixed to treadmills (Chen et al., 2013; Louie et al., 2015).
- Safety (Lajeunesse et al., 2015).
- Efficacy in restoring walking[11] (Louie et al., 2015), including the performense in community settings (Lajeunesse et al., 2015).
- Clinical effectiveness outcomes, imcluding such parameters as stair climbing performance, speed, mobility, quaility of life, and independence[11] (Chen et al., 2013; Lajeunesse et al., 2015; Louie et al., 2015; Arazpour et al., 2015a,b; Lajeunesse et al., 2015).
- Walking distance (Benson et al., 2016).
- Vertical ground reaction force (vGRF) that quantifies the pattern and magnitude of mechanical loading (Fineberg et al., 2013). This characteristic is particularly important for exoskeletons used by completely paralyzed persons.
- Training protocols (Lajeunesse et al., 2015; Louie et al., 2015).
- User satisfaction and secondary benefits and skills achieved with the exoskeleton (Lajeunesse et al., 2015).
- Level of scientific evidence (Lajeunesse et al., 2015).
- Cost-effectiveness outcomes[11].

Overall, the current literature reports both successes of exoskeleton technology and remaining problems. One important achievement is that wearable exoskeletons enable patients with complete paralysis of the lower part of the body to stand and walk. The speed of walking is modest; it varies with the level of injury and training duration (Louie et al., 2015). In addition to paraplegics, wearable exoskeletons can be used by patients with post-stroke hemiparesis (Bortole et al., 2015), as well as non-stroke neurological pathologies[24] (Esquenazi et al., 2012), such as cerebral palsy, myelome-ningocele, traumatic brain injury and Guillain Barré syndrome (Zeilig et al., 2012).

Wearable exoskeletons have advantages compared to Hip-Knee-Ankle-Foot-Orthoses (KHAFO). For example, powered gait orthosis (PGO) and the IRGO outperform HKAFO, as evident from the improvements in physiological cost index (PCI), distance walked, and walking speed (Arazpour et al., 2013). Additionally, wearable exoskeletons have certain advantages compared to the treadmill-based ones. With wearable exoskeletons, patients get much greater autonomy. The autonomy in turn facilitates rehabilitative training because the device can be used at home in addition to specialized facilities (Chen et al., 2013; Louie et al., 2015). Yet, autonomous use of wearable exoskeletons in community settings still has to be demonstrated (Lajeunesse et al., 2015). Overall, there is still a discrepancy between the consumer high expectations of autonomy and versatility and the actual effectiveness of using wearable exoskeletons (Benson et al., 2016).

A critical analysis of the assessments of exoskeletons as health technology[11] indicates the need for more research, particularly regarding long-term performance (Lajeunesse et al., 2015), assessment of training (Louie et al., 2015), randomized controlled trials, and economic analysis[11]. Overall, the level of scientific evidence remains low in clinical trials of exoskeletons (Lajeunesse et al., 2015). Prevention and detection of medical complications in the exoskeleton users is yet another area that needs more research (Benson et al., 2016). A unified framework is needed for assessment of exoskeleton performance (Bryce et al., 2015). Such a framework is needed to make different clinical trials comparable. The framework should include at least six modules: functional applications, personal factors, device factors, external factors, activities, and health outcomes (Bryce et al., 2015).

Current exoskeletons (**Figure 2**) provide several secondary skills and benefits (Lajeunesse et al., 2015). Exoskeleton with compact design and small backpacks are particularly useful

[22]http://www.cdc.gov/Features/OlderAmericans/

[23]http://www.exoatlet.com/

[24]http://www.parker.com/literature/Exoskeleton/Parker%20Indego%20Brochure.pdf

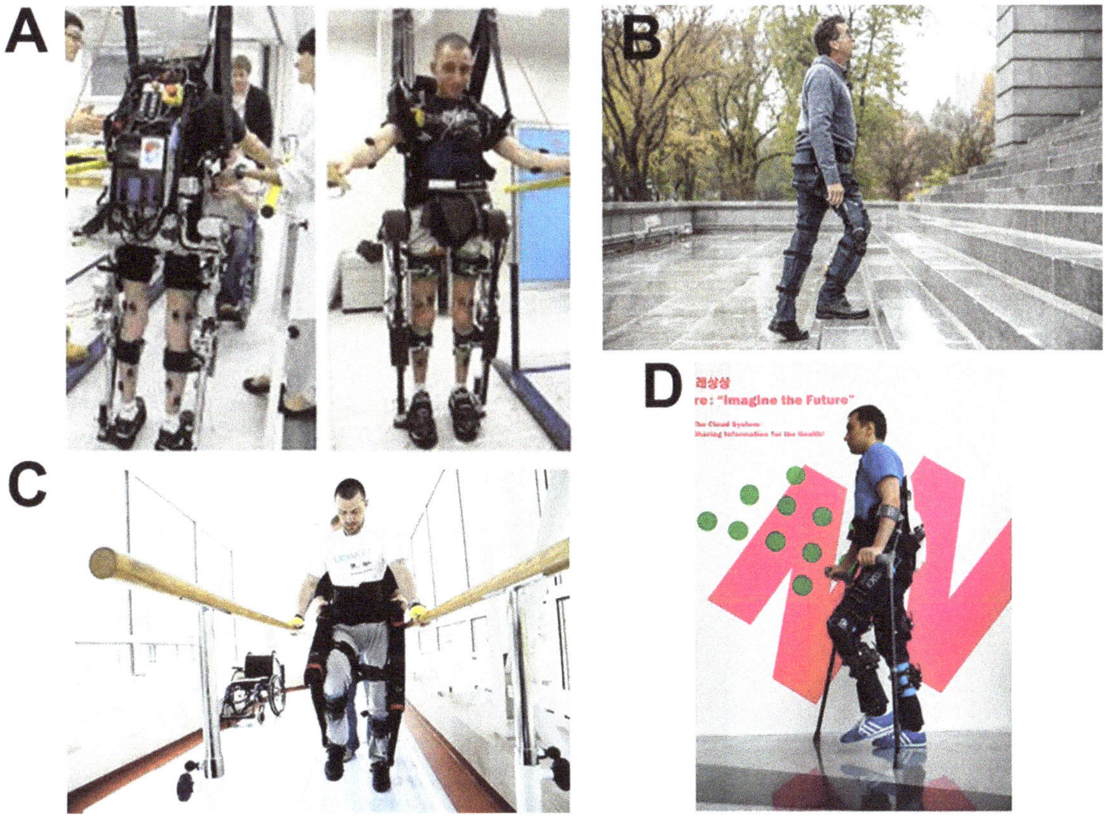

FIGURE 2 | Images of several types of exoskeletons. (A) Mindwalker mind-controlled exoskeleton could help the disabled walk again. With courtesy from Professor van der Kooij at University of Twente, NL. **(B)** The Keeogo^{TM} exoskeleton from B- TEMIA reveals the latest in an increase of the human systems (human augmentation systems) designed to help people walk more and better. Keeogo^{TM} eliminates several problems in patients with Parkinson's disease. With courtesy from Danielle Beaudoin at b-termia.com. **(C,D)** The ExoAtlet is a powered exoskeleton designed to assist patients during their rehabilitation after stroke, injury, or unsuccessful operation. ExoAtlet automatically repeats the natural patterns of walking, has electrical stimulation system, and physiological sensors. The control system of the ExoAtlet is unique: it collects data from body angles, allows to set the height and length of the step, which provides: (i) standing still; (ii) classic walking; (iii) walking on angled surface; (iv) stepping over obstacles; and (v) comfortable walking up & down stairs. ExoAtlet can be used in rehabilitation centers and at home[24]. ExoAtlet can be controlled with the app on tablet when used in clinics. Experienced user of ExoAtlet use "thinking" crutch for control. With courtesy from Ekaterina Bereziy at exoatlet.ru.

in this respect (Chen et al., 2013) because they allow don, doff and wearing an exoskeleton while sitting in a wheelchair. These operations are possible using electrically actuated ReWalk and ExoAtlet, hydraulically actuated Ekso, and Indego, which combines electriaclly actuated hip and knee joints for both legs (Chen et al., 2013) with functional electrical stimulation (FES) of paralyzed, yet responsive muscles[23] (Chen et al., 2013). This combination of the exoskeleton action with FES training improves rehabilitation results.

FUTURE DIRECTIONS

Notwithstanding significant technological advancements in the field, the current exoskeleton systems still need much improvement for them to become practically efficient. The areas that need improvement remain almost the same as about one decade ago. Accordingly, our assessment made 8 years ago (Onose et al., 2008) remains of current interest: exoskeletons need further miniaturization, optimization of actuators and sensors. Ideally, exoskeletons should become robotic orthotic suits wearable beneath the clothes.

In our perspectives from 2007 to 2008 (**Figures 3**, **5**, **6**), we conceived a soft cable-driven exo-suit device that can apply forces to the body to assist walking. Unlike traditional exoskeletons which contain rigid framing elements, the soft exosuit is worn like clothing and uses geared motors to pull on Bowden cables connected to the suit near the ankle (Asbeck et al., 2013).

Some of the authors of this article have been involved in extensive scientific research on this topic for almost 15 years (Onose et al., 2008, 2012a), and were awarded with the Gold Medal at the Inventions Saloon, in Genève, Switzerland, in 2008 (**Figure 4**).

We have not finished all the necessary tests and improvements of our prototype (**Figure 5**). Because of this delay, several mechatronic wearable powered exoskeletons are in overall more advanced stage of development, including the clinical trials.

We re-emphasize ichnographically two important requirements to exoskeletons: (i) prevention of venous-lymphatic stasis in the lower limbs, and (ii) skin protection at the interface with the rigid structure of the exoskeleton.

Both issues can cause serious hurdles, especially during the long-time wearing of the assistive devices. Regarding the former issue, because of an impaired venous-lymphatic outflow in paralyzed persons (as well as patients with cardiovascular problems) (Guyton and Hall, 2006), regaining vertical posture with the aid of a wearable exoskeleton provokes regional stasis. This may cause discomfort and edema, including the risk of venous thrombosis, associated trophic somatic lesions, and secondary reactive heart conditions. As for the latter, an improper interface between the exoskeleton and the limb can result in mechanically generated lesions of the heel, respectively of the skin and subjacent soft tissue, which thus need for protection at the interface with the rigid structure of such devices (compressive, friction and tensile forces), as determined through performance metrics (van der Kooij et al., 2006). Therefore, we have conceived—for counteracting these problems—two components of our MOD.

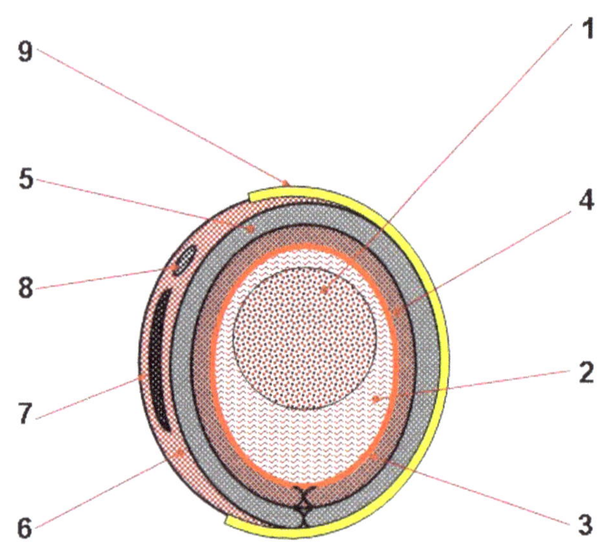

FIGURE 3 | Concept design of a cross section through lower limb(s)'module of the MOD. 1, Bony area; 2, Muscle area; 3, Skin and sucutaneous soft tissues; 4, Textile material for contact with the skin; 5, Pulsed air flow textile structure; 6, (Eeach) exoskeleton's external part, made of composite material; 7, Metallic insertion; 8, Tubular seating for pull and respectively, electric cables; 9, Fasten system. Reproduced with permission from the publisher (Onose et al., 2012a, pp. 1–99).

Furthermore, regarding the underwear exoskeleton, we consider it ambitious and difficult, but worth trying developmental direction. Such an underwear exoskeleton would require a soft supporting structure actuated by strengthening/relaxing device. Specifically, we have foreseen, since 2006–2007 (Onose, 2007) the usage of electro-active polymers (EAPs). EAP materials seem to be the most applicable because of their large actuation forces and highest robustness (Bar-Cohen, 2005). These materials could be improved to act as artificial muscles (Bar-Cohen, 2005; Mirfakhrai et al., 2007).

The development of such a device would be a revolutionary breakthrough, since the soft support structure in cadence with the artificial muscle contraction could not only move the lower limbs but also apply thrusts to the user's calf and thighs, thus mimicking a "muscle pump" and compensating for the returning, venous-lymphatic circulation (Onose, 2007; Onose et al., 2012a). However, during the last decade not enough progress has been made in the development and subsequent translational implementation of EAPs. We still need to improve the safety, controllability and energy supply for EAPs[25].

Another extremely challenging and still incompletely solved item, as mentioned above, is the problem of balance maintenance using advanced mechatronic wearable exoskeletons. Reliable balance is needed for prevention of falls during exoskeleton usage.

At least regarding the most difficult and demanding—in need for total assistance from the apparatus—but, at the same time, an essential category of potential beneficiaries, *the complete paraplegics*, all current devices require supplementary aids for securing the balance: walkers, crutches or—at

[25] http://sbdi.co.kr/cart/data/info/IDTechEx_Electroactive_Polymers_and_Devices_2013-2018_Sample.pdf?ckattempt=1

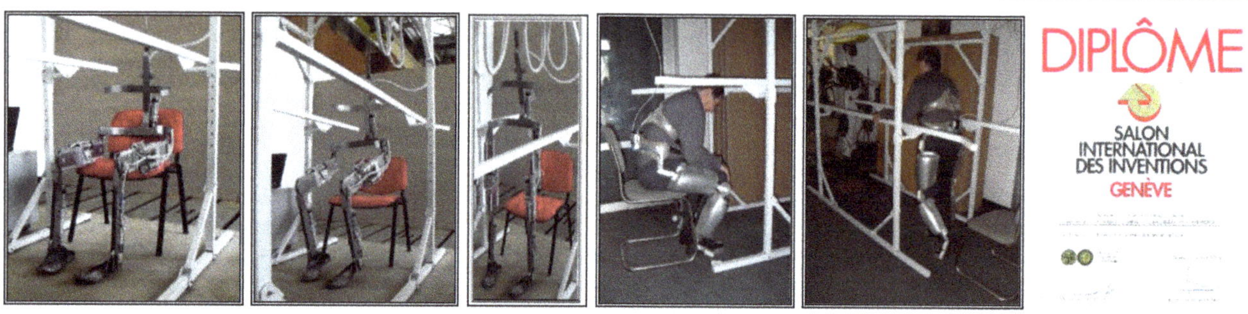

FIGURE 4 | Mechatronic Orthotic Device (MOD) Left: some relevant images of exoskeletons. Right: Award Diploma by the Geneva International Inventions Fair. Reproduced with permission from the publisher (Onose et al., 2012a, pp. 1–99).

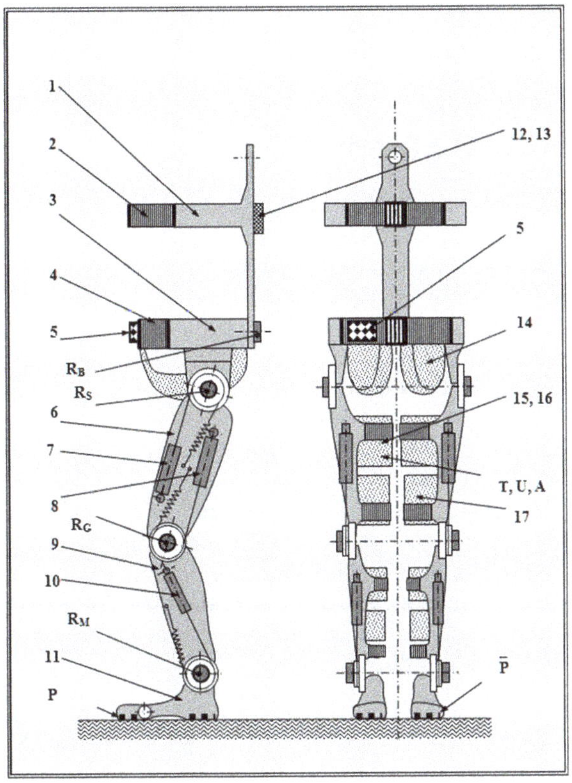

FIGURE 5 | General concept design of the MOD. 1, Back segment; 2, Chest belt; 3, Pelvis segment; 4, Pelvis belt; 5, Programs command box; 6, Thigh segment; 7, Hip actuator; 8, Knee actuator; 9, Ankle segment; 10, Foot actuator; 11, Foot segment; 12, Connections box; 13, Pneumatic connect fitting; 14, Bottom holder; 15, Drawer panty hose; 16, Pulsed air flow textile structure; 17, Attachment belt; R, Angular transducers (B, lumbar sacral; S, hip; G, knee; M, ankle); P, Pressure sensor; T, Temperature sensor; U, Humidity sensor; A, Compressed air pressure sensor. Reproduced with permission from the publisher (Onose et al., 2012a, pp. 1–99).

best—canes. In sum, the powered exoskeletons that assist over-ground walking require the user to maintain balance (Swinnen et al., 2014; Yoshimoto et al., 2015; Louie and Eng, 2016).

As an illustration of the current state of this problem, it is worth mentioning a study that reported loss of balance (LOB) and falls as the primary safety outcomes (Kolakowsky-Hayner et al., 2013). Additionally, the EU FP7 "BALANCE" project (Veneman, 2014) made an observation that "none of the devices available on the market use the exoskeleton itself to support postural balance." Therefore, the goal of the BALANCE project is to research the possibility of using the exoskeleton to maintain balance and prevent falls. The project is organized as a 4 year Specific Targeted Research Project (STREP)[26] and has the practical objectives to "create a human-cooperative robotic postural balance controller framework," in order to "implement the human-cooperative postural balance controller on a real exoskeleton" and to

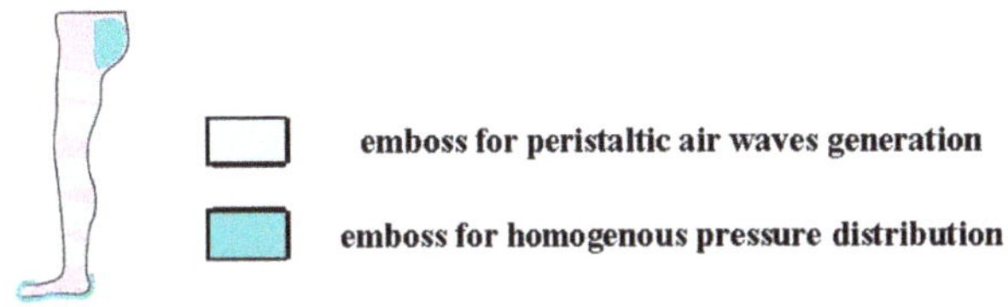

FIGURE 6 | MOD: plantar skin protection and pulsed air flow to mimic the "muscles' pump"—thus compensating the returning, venous-lymphatic circulation, in the lower limbs—concepts. Reproduced with permission from the publisher (Onose et al., 2012a, pp. 1–99).

"evaluate the developed concepts in subjects walking with the exoskeleton."[27]

Lastly, one more direction to improve the performances of a mechatronic wearable exoskeleton, is to empower it with brain's voluntary motor commands using a brain-machine-interface (BMI) (Onose et al., 2012b; Lebedev, 2014). The feasibility of such a BMI has been demonstrated in an experiment conducted in rhesus monkeys (Fitzsimmons et al., 2009). In this study, monkeys were implanted with invasive multielectrode arrays in the leg representation of the sensorimotor cortex. The animals were trained to walk bipedally on a treadmill. Activity of several hundred cortical neurons was recorded and converted into the kinematics of lower limb movements. This BMI was able to extract lower limb kinematics when monkeys walked both forward and backward on the treadmill.

These results justified the foundation of the Walk Again Project with the goal of the advancement of BMI-controlled exoskeletons (Nicolelis and Lebedev, 2009). An European project, called Mindwalker (**Figure 2A**), declared the goal of controlling an exoskeleton with electroencephalographic (EEG) and electromyographis (EMG) recordings (Cheron et al., 2012). Decoding of leg movements from EEGs have been demonstrated in humans walking on a treadmill (Presacco et al., 2012). Moreover, a BMI that decoded steady-state visual evoked potentials (SSVEP) from EEGs was employed to operate a lower-limb exoskeleton by healthy human subjects (Kwak et al., 2015).

The progress in BMIs for bipedal walking opens the perspective of neural control of exoskeleton-assisted walking by a completely paralyzed subject. While a slow control of walking could be provided by EEG-based BMIs, invasive BMIs hold promise to enable faster and more accurate control. However, invasive recordings are risky, so there have been no studies of invasive BMIs for walking control in humans. Additionally, it is unclear whether patients could become proficient enough to efficiently control an exoskeleton through an invasive or noinvasive BMI (Onose et al., 2012b). In this respect, we are satisfied of having deployed a clinical trial in the motor imagery BMI domain, by enrolling nine chronic tetraplegics volunteers (the largest lot for such type of trial, at that time), to control

[26] http://balance-fp7.eu/project_structure.php

[27] http://balance-fp7.eu/objectives.php

wirelessly a robotic arm by EEG commands (Onose et al., 2012b).

We have foreseen also the possibility of empowering MOD's actuating systems by voluntary commands extracted from EEGs (Onose et al., 2008). From this point of view, we have expressed our confidence in the success of the Walk Again[28] and Mindwalker projects[29] (**Figure 2**).

CONCLUSION

We suggest that the joint perspective of health professionals, manufacturers and consumers on the mechatronic wearable exoskeletons should contribute to a comprehensive agenda regarding the development of devices that assist and rehabilitate bipedal posture and walking to severely impaired people. The technological advances, together with collaborative endeavors of multidisciplinary teams of researchers, could foster the progress and pave the way to the long awaited optimized and practical exoskeleton.

[28]http://virtualreality.duke.edu/project/walk-again-project/

[29]https://www.utwente.nl/ctw/bw/research/projects/MINDWALKER/

AUTHOR CONTRIBUTIONS

All authors listed, have made substantial, direct and intellectual contribution to the work, and approved it for publication.

ACKNOWLEDGMENTS

The authors thank to: Florin Alexiuc, Ioana Andone, Aurelian Anghelescu, Cornel Baluţă, Ana Maria Bumbea, Eftalea Cărpuş, Crenguţa Coman, Cristina Daia, Alexandru Vlad Ciurea, Jean Ciurea, Radu Stefan Craciunoiu, Ionut Catalin Dimache, Constantin Dogariu, Angela Dorogan, Condurache Dumitru, Maria Gratiela Epureanu, Eva Gheorghiţă, Carmen Giuglea, Roxana Grejdanescu, Monica Haras, Gheorghe Huian, Noela Ionescu, Andrada Mirea, Marius Modreanu, Alexandru Moldovanu, Cristian Nicolau, Raluca Magdalena Niţă, Liliana Onose, Horia Catalin Orasanu, Loredana Theodora Păun, Vergil Racicovschi, Dorin Roşu, Aura Spînu, Olga Surdu, Emilia Visileanu, and Tudor Ursu—for their contribution to the inter-/multi-disciplinary scientific research project that has resulted in the achievement of the MOD and/or to the afferent monography (Onose et al., 2012a), which constitutes a valuable background resource, including for this article.

REFERENCES

Arazpour, M., Bani, M. A., Hutchins, S. W., and Jones, R. K. (2013). The physiological cost index of walking with mechanical and powered gait orthosis in patients with spinal cord injury. *Spinal Cord* 51, 356–359. doi: 10.1038/sc.2012.162

Arazpour, M., Hutchins, S. W., and Bani, M. A. (2015a). The efficacy of powered orthoses on walking in persons with paraplegia. *Prosthet. Orthot. Int.* 39, 90–99. doi: 10.1177/0309364613520031

Arazpour, M., Samadian, M., Bahramizadeh, M., Joghtaei, M., Maleki, M., Bani, M. A., et al. (2015b). The efficiency of orthotic interventions on energy consumption in paraplegic patients: a literature review. *Spinal Cord* 53, 168–175. doi: 10.1038/sc.2014.227

Asbeck, A. T., Dyer, R. J., Larusson, A. F., and Walsh, C. J. (2013). Biologically-inspired soft exosuit. *IEEE Int. Conf. Rehabil. Robot.* 2013:6650455. doi: 10.1109/icorr.2013.6650455

Bar-Cohen, Y. (2005). Current and future developments in artificial muscles using electroactive polymers. *Expert Rev. Med. Devices* 2, 731–740. doi: 10.1586/17434440.2.6.731

Benson, I., Hart, K., Tussler, D., and van Middendorp, J. J. (2016). Lower-limb exoskeletons for individuals with chronic spinal cord injury: findings from a feasibility study. *Clin. Rehabil.* 30, 73–84. doi: 10.1177/0269215515575166

Bortole, M., del Ama, A., Rocon, E., Moreno, J. C., Brunetti, F., and Pons, J. L. (2013). "A robotic exoskeleton for overground gait rehabilitation," in *Proceedings of 2013 IEEE International Conference on Robotics and Automation* (Karlsruhe), 3356–3361.

Bortole, M., Venkatakrishnan, A., Zhu, F., Moreno, J. C., Francisco, G. E., Pons, J. L., et al. (2015). The H2 robotic exoskeleton for gait rehabilitation after stroke: early findings from a clinical study. *J. Neuroeng. Rehabil.* 12:54. doi: 10.1186/s12984-015-0048-y

Bryce, T. N., Dijkers, M. P., and Kozlowski, A. J. (2015). Framework for assessment of the usability of lower-extremity robotic exoskeletal orthoses. *Am. J. Phys. Med. Rehabil.* 94, 1000–1014. doi: 10.1097/PHM.0000000000000321

Chen, G., Chan, C. K., Guo, Z., and Yu, H. (2013). A review of lower extremity assistive robotic exoskeletons in rehabilitation therapy. *Crit. Rev. Biomed. Eng.* 41, 343–363 doi: 10.1615/critrevbiomedeng.2014010453

Cheron, G., Duvinage, M., De Saedeleer, C., Castermans, T., Bengoetxea, A., Petieau, M., et al. (2012). From spinal central pattern generators to cortical network: integrated BCI for walking rehabilitation. *Neural Plast.* 2012:375148. doi: 10.1155/2012/375148

Esquenazi, A., Talaty, M., Packel, A., and Saulino, M. (2012). The ReWalk powered exoskeleton to restore ambulatory function to individuals with thoracic-level motor-complete spinal cord injury. *Am. J. Phys. Med. Rehabil.* 91, 911–921. doi: 10.1097/PHM.0b013e318269d9a3

Fineberg, D. B., Asselin, P., Harel, N. Y., Agranova-Breyter, I., Kornfeld, S. D., Bauman, W. A., et al. (2013). Vertical ground reaction force-based analysis of powered exoskeleton-assisted walking in persons with motor-complete paraplegia. *J. Spinal Cord Med.* 36, 313–321. doi: 10.1179/2045772313Y.0000000126

Fitzsimmons, N. A., Lebedev, M. A., Peikon, I. D., and Nicolelis, M. A. L. (2009). Extracting kinematic parameters for monkey bipedal walking from cortical neuronal ensemble activity. *Front. Integr. Neurosci.* 3:3. doi: 10.3389/neuro.07.003.2009

Frankel, H. L., Hancock, D. O., Hyslop, G., Melzak, J., Michaelis, L. S., Ungar, G. H., et al. (1969). The value of postural reduction in the initial management of closed injuries of the spine with paraplegia and tetraplegia. I. *Paraplegia* 7, 179–192. doi: 10.1038/sc.1969.30

Guyton, A. C., and Hall, J. E. (eds.). (2006). *Textbook of Medical Physiology 11th (International) Edition - Chap. 15 (Vascular Distensibility and Functions of the Arterial and Venous Systems) and 20 (Cardiac Output, Venous Return, and Their Regulation)*. Philadelphia, PA: Elsevier Inc.

Kalache, A., Fu, D., and Yoshida, S. (2007). *WHO Global Report on Falls Prevention in Older Age*. Geneva: WHO Press.

Kannape, O. A., and Lenggenhager, B. (2016). Engineered embodiment: Comment on "The embodiment of assistive devices—from wheelchair to exoskeleton" by M. Pazzaglia and M. Molinari Oliver. *Phys. Life Rev.* 16, 181–183. doi: 10.1016/j.plrev.2016.01.011

Kolakowsky-Hayner, S. A., Crew, J., Moran, S., and Shah, A. (2013). Safety and feasibility of using the EksoTM bionic exoskeleton to aid ambulation after spinal cord injury. *J. Spine* S4:003. doi: 10.4172/2165-7939.S4-003

Kwak, N. S., Müller, K. R., and Lee, S. W. (2015). A lower limb exoskeleton control system based on steady state visual evoked potentials. *J. Neural Eng.* 12:056009. doi: 10.1088/1741-2560/12/5/056009

Lajeunesse, V., Vincent, C., Routhier, F., Careau, E., and Michaud, F. (2015). Exoskeletons' design and usefulness evidence according to a systematic review of lower limb exoskeletons used for functional mobility by people with spinal cord injury. *Disabil. Rehabil. Assist. Technol.* 4, 1–13. doi: 10.3109/17483107.2015.1080766

Lebedev, M. (2014). Brain-machine interfaces: an overview. *Transl. Neurosci.* 5, 99–110. doi: 10.2478/s13380-014-0212-z

Louie, D. R., and Eng, J. J. (2016). Powered robotic exoskeletons in post-stroke rehabilitation of gait: a scoping review. *J. Neuroeng. Rehabil.* 13, 53. doi: 10.1186/s12984-016-0162-5

Louie, D. R., Eng, J. J., Lam, T., and Spinal Cord Injury Research Evidence (SCIRE) Research Team (2015). Gait speed using powered robotic exoskeletons after spinal cord injury: a systematic review and correlational study. *J. Neuroeng. Rehabil.* 12, 82. doi: 10.1186/s12984-015-0074-9

Mirfakhrai, T., Madden, J. D. W., and Baughman, R. H. (2007). Polymer artificial muscles. *Mater. Today* 10, 30–38. doi: 10.1016/S1369-7021(07)70048-2

Morley, J. E. (2012). Sarcopenia in the elderly. *Fam. Pract.* 29(Suppl. 1), i44–i48. doi: 10.1093/fampra/cmr063

Muresanu, D. F., Buzoianu, A., Florian, S. I., and von Wild, T. (2012). Towards a roadmap in brain protection and recovery. *J. Cell. Mol. Med.* 16, 2861–2871. doi: 10.1111/j.1582-4934.2012.01605.x

Nicolelis, M. A., and Lebedev, M. A. (2009). Principles of neural ensemble physiology underlying the operation of brain-machine interfaces. *Nat. Rev. Neurosci.* 10, 530–540. doi: 10.1038/nrn2653

Onose, G. (2007). *Manual de Recuperare, Medicină Fizică şi Balneoclimatologie - Noţiuni de Baza şi Actualităşi*, Vol. I. Bucureşti: Editura Medicală.

Onose, G., Cârdei, V., Ciurea, A. V., Ciurea, J., Onose, L., Anghelescu, A., et al. (2008). "Achievement of an experimental mechatronic orthotic device to assist/ rehabilitate orthostatism and walk in patients with complete paraplegia and other specific severe disabling conditions (short form)," in *Proceedings of the 7th Mediterranean Congress of Physical and Rehabilitation Medicine* (Portorose; Torino: Edizioni Minerva Medica), 40–42.

Onose, G., Cârdei, V., Crăciunoiu, Ş T., and Avramescu, V. (eds.). (2012a). *Mechatronic Orthotic Device. Concept, Sumptions and Functional-Construction Aspects.* Bucureşti: Editura ICTCM.

Onose, G., Grozea, C., Anghelescu, A., Daia, C., Sinescu, C. J., Ciurea, A. V., et al. (2012b). On the feasibility of using motor imagery EEG-based brain-computer interface in chronic tetraplegics for assistive robotic arm control: a clinical test and long-term post-trial follow-up. *Spinal Cord* 50, 599–608. doi: 10.1038/sc.2012.14

Presacco, A., Forrester, L. W., and Contreras-Vidal, J. L. (2012). Decoding intralimb and inter-limb kinematics during treadmill walking from scalp electroencephalographic (EEG) signals, IEEE Trans. *Neural Syst. Rehabil. Eng.* 20, 212–219. doi: 10.1109/TNSRE.2012.2188304

Salive, M. E. (2013). Multimorbidity in older adults. *Epidemiol. Rev.* 35, 75–83. doi: 10.1093/epirev/mxs009

Swinnen, E., Beckwée, D., Meeusen, R., Baeyens, J. P., and Kerckhofs, E. (2014). Does robot-assisted gait rehabilitation improve balance in stroke patients? A systematic review. *Top Stroke Rehabil.* 21, 87–100. doi: 10.1310/tsr2 102-87

Talley Watts, L., Long, J. A., Manga, V. H., Huang, S., Shen, Q., and Duong, T. Q. (2015). Normobaric oxygen worsens outcome after a moderate traumatic brain injury. *J. Cereb. Blood. Flow. Metab.* 35, 1137–1144. doi: 10.1038/jcbfm.2015.18

Uebelhart, D., Bernard, J., Hartmann, D. J., Moro, L., Roth, M., Uebelhart, B., et al. (2000). Modifications of bone and connective tissue after orthostatic bedrest. *Osteoporos. Int.* 11, 59–67 doi: 10.1007/s001980050007

van der Kooij, H., Veneman, J. F., Ekkelenkamp, R., (2006)."Compliant actuation of exoskeletons," in *Robots Towards New Applications*, ed A. Lazinica (Source: ISBN 978-3-86611-314-5, pp. 784, ARS/plV. I-Tech Education and Publishing; DOI: 10.5772/33). Available online at: https://core.ac.uk/download/files/363/ 11473533.pdf

Veneman, J. F. (2014). "Chapter: exoskeletons supporting postural balance - the balance project," in *Replace, Repair, Restore, Relieve - Bridging Clinical and Engineering Solutions in Neurorehabilitation. Vol. 7 of the Series Biosystems and Biorobotics*, eds W. Jensen, O. K. Andersen, and M. Akay (San Sebastian: Springer International Publishing Switzerland), 203–208.

Yoshimoto, T., Shimizu, I., Hiroi, Y., Kawaki, M., Sato, D., and Nagasawa, M. (2015). Feasibility and efficacy of high-speed gait training with a voluntary driven exoskeleton robot for gait and balance dysfunction in patients with chronic stroke: nonrandomized pilot study with concurrent control. *Int. J. Rehabil. Res.* 38, 338–343. doi: 10.1097/MRR.00000000000 00132

Zeilig, G., Weingarden, H., Zwecker, M., Dudkiewicz, I., Bloch, A., and Esquenazi, A. (2012). Safety and tolerance of the ReWalk^{TM} exoskeleton suit for ambulation by people with complete spinal cord injury: a pilot study. *J. Spinal Cord Med.* 35, 96–101. doi: 10.1179/2045772312Y.0000000003

Disclosures: GO, VC, ŞC, and VA have been the main researchers involved in achieving the aforementioned Romanian original experimental prototype of mechatronic orthotic device (MOD), but as it could be determined throughout this article, there hasn't been any intention at all to favor in description this model of device, including with the fact that it has been honestly acknowledged in the body text that currently, there are a series of other such models significantly closer to reach the optimal, desired form.

3

Wearable functional near infrared spectroscopy (fNIRS) and transcranial direct current stimulation (tDCS): expanding vistas for neurocognitive augmentation

*Ryan McKendrick[1], Raja Parasuraman[1] and Hasan Ayaz[2]**

[1] Center of Excellence in Neuroergonomics, Technology, and Cognition (CENTEC), George Mason University, Fairfax, VA, USA, [2] School of Biomedical Engineering, Science and Health Systems, Drexel University, Philadelphia, PA, USA

Edited by:
Mikhail Lebedev, Duke University, USA

Reviewed by:
Andrea Kübler, University of Würzburg, Germany
Makii Muthalib, Universite de Montpellier 1, France

***Correspondence:**
Hasan Ayaz, School of Biomedical Engineering, Science and Health Systems, Drexel University, 3508 Market Street, Monell Suite 101, Philadelphia, PA 19104, USA
hasan.ayaz@drexel.edu

Contemporary studies with transcranial direct current stimulation (tDCS) provide a growing base of evidence for enhancing cognition through the non-invasive delivery of weak electric currents to the brain. The main effect of tDCS is to modulate cortical excitability depending on the polarity of the applied current. However, the underlying mechanism of neuromodulation is not well understood. A new generation of functional near infrared spectroscopy (fNIRS) systems is described that are miniaturized, portable, and include wearable sensors. These developments provide an opportunity to couple fNIRS with tDCS, consistent with a neuroergonomics approach for joint neuroimaging and neurostimulation investigations of cognition in complex tasks and in naturalistic conditions. The effects of tDCS on complex task performance and the use of fNIRS for monitoring cognitive workload during task performance are described. Also explained is how fNIRS + tDCS can be used simultaneously for assessing spatial working memory. Mobile optical brain imaging is a promising neuroimaging tool that has the potential to complement tDCS for realistic applications in natural settings.

Keywords: HDtDCS, fNIRS, neuroergonomics, DLPFC, spatial working memory

Introduction

The rediscovery, over a decade ago (Nitsche and Paulus, 2000), of transcranial brain stimulation has led to a proliferation of research on brain and cognitive augmentation, both in healthy adults and in patients with neurological or psychiatric disease (Clark and Parasuraman, 2014). Augmentation refers to the improvement of cognitive functioning through task performance, or reversal of cognitive deficits that are normal consequences of performance in healthy adults (e.g., fatigue, stress) or those related to brain disorders. Ayaz et al., 2006; Hunter et al., 2013). Although the initial motivating rationale for the use of techniques such as transcranial Direct Current Stimulation (tDCS) was to develop alternative therapies for the treatment of neuropsychiatric diseases, augmentation effects were also seen in the healthy participants (Clark and Parasuraman, 2014; Flöel, 2014). These findings led to the current interest in developing methods of neurocognitive enhancement for healthy adults, for example to enhance human performance in complex tasks (such as air traffic control) or to accelerate skill acquisition in tasks (such as piloting unmanned vehicles) that typically require many hours or days of practice to master

(Coffman et al., 2014; Parasuraman and Mckinley, 2014). Contemporary tDCS studies have provided a growing base of evidence for enhancing cognition through the non-invasive delivery of weak electric currents to the brain (Coffman et al., 2014). The main effect of tDCS is to modulate cortical excitability, depending on the polarity of the applied current. However, the underlying mechanism for the neuromodulation, such as how it is induced, how longs it persists, and the ways in which such modulation translate into improvement in performance are still not well understood and are currently the object of much research interest. Combining tDCS with multimodal neuroimaging techniques can enhance knowledge of its neuromodulatory effects in the brain (Hunter et al., 2013).

Traditional neuroimaging modalities such as functional magnetic resonance imaging (fMRI) have also been successfully utilized for studying cognition and understanding the neural mechanisms that contribute to the acquisition, development, and use of cognitive skills in artificial, controlled and stand-alone settings. These can be referred as read-only settings where functional neuroimaging is used to record brain activation and hence the flow of information is from brain to a computer. Moreover, modulation of neural signals can also be achieved through a neurofeedback training where a computer presents some derivative of the acquired brain signal in real-time back to user in visual or auditory form to establish the feedback loop (Hanslmayr et al., 2005; Gruzelier, 2009; Miller et al., 2010; Slagter et al., 2011; Ninaus et al., 2013). Neurofeedback training aims to allow volitional control of specific brain activity and has been extensively used in clinical neurorehabilitation or brain disorders such as attention-deficit hyperactivity, autism, epilepsy and mood disorders (Lubar et al., 1995; Hoffman et al., 1996; Raymond et al., 2005; Angelakis et al., 2007; Kouijzer et al., 2009; Lim et al., 2012; Heinrich et al., 2014). Neurofeedback training has been shown to enhance performance in cognitive tasks (Angelakis et al., 2007; Gruzelier, 2009) however, in this manuscript, we focused on tDCS based neuromodulation as it does not require training and has been utilized for human computer interaction applications (Clark and Parasuraman, 2014). Neuroimaging methods based on the MRI technique, such as functional MRI, resting state functional connectivity, and diffusion tensor analysis, have provided important information on the gray matter, white matter, and brain connectivity changes that accompany skill acquisition (Lewis et al., 2009; Lövdén et al., 2010; Voss et al., 2012; Strenziok et al., 2014), thus setting the stage for the development of theories of neuroplasticity, specifically for functional reorganization of neural networks and adaptation. For a review, see Elbert and Rockstroh (2004). However, some limitations of MRI are its requirement for participant immobility and its high operational cost. These factors have stimulated a need for lower-cost neuroimaging techniques that are portable and can be used in freely moving participants performing everyday tasks (Gramann et al., 2011, 2014). Among these are electroencephalography (EEG) and functional near infrared spectroscopy (fNIRS), both of which can be used for mobile brain imaging (Makeig et al., 2009; Gramann et al., 2011; Mehta and Parasuraman, 2013). The use of mobile brain imaging and stimulation techniques also falls within the field of neuroergonomics, defined as the study of the human brain in relation to performance at work and everyday settings (Parasuraman, 2003, 2011; Parasuraman and Rizzo, 2007). The main goal of neuroergonomics is to advance knowledge of brain functions in complex tasks and naturalistic work settings.

Overview of Paper

The neuroergonomic approach has been considerably facilitated by the recent rise of development of portable and wearable neuroimaging devices, including EEG and fNIRS (Gramann et al., 2014). In this paper we review the potential uses of joint fNIRS and tDCS and describe wireless and battery operated fNIRS sensors (Ayaz et al., 2013) that provide new opportunities for brain and cognitive augmentation. We first briefly describe tDCS studies for enhancing skill acquisition in complex cognitive tasks. It is particularly important to assess and measure operator mental workload in situations where performance failures could result in catastrophic losses (e.g., military command and control, air traffic control, etc.). Improving operators' cognitive abilities (such as working memory or attention) would help improve overall safety and productivity in such systems. Next we review tDCS studies that have targeted and assessed human operator performance. We then describe how fNIRS can be used to monitor brain dynamics during cognitive tasks, with a focus on evaluating effects on cognitive load. As a wearable and continuous monitoring sensor, fNIRS provides a safe and practical approach for monitoring brain activity in natural environments. We review studies that demonstrate task load related activity in the fNIRS signal. Next, we examine the combined use of fNIRS and tDCS for monitoring and enhancement of spatial working memory. Moreover, fNIRS + tDCS can realize new applications that were not possible before, such as "read-write" Brain Computer Interfaces (BCI) which can acquire (read) brain signals and also provide feedback directly to the brain (write) through stimulation. In general, optical brain imaging techniques such as fNIRS are a promising neuroimaging method and as the instruments continue to evolve, have the potential to become a complementary tool to tDCS for neuroergonomic applications in complex work tasks and in natural settings.

Effects of tDCS on Complex Task Performance

Many noninvasive brain stimulation techniques for enhancing neurocognitive function exist, including transcranial magnetic stimulation (TMS) and tDCS (Clark and Parasuraman, 2014). In TMS an electric current is transiently passed through a magnetic coil positioned over the participant's scalp over a brain region of interest. This creates a changing magnetic field that passes through the skull and induces current flow in the underlying cortical tissue sufficient to alter neural firing (Walsh and Pascual-Leone, 2005). tDCS involves application of a weak direct current (DC) electric current (1–2 mA) with electrodes attached to the scalp. A positive polarity (anode) is typically used to facilitate neuronal firing whereas a negative polarity (cathode) is used to inhibit neuronal firing. Application of tDCS is safe for experimental use in healthy participants for up to 30 min of stimulation (Bikson et al., 2009).

Understanding the mechanisms by which the tDCS modulations are induced and persist is still an open question. Initially, it was thought that application of weak DC current increases the resting neuronal membrane potential and thus lowers the threshold for firing of neurons (Bindman et al., 1964), but subsequent work suggests that other mechanisms are probably involved, such as dynamic modulation of synaptic efficacy (Rahman et al., 2013) and changes in neurotransmitter concentrations (Clark et al., 2011). Pharmacological tDCS studies also suggest neuronal membrane depolarisation during anodal stimulation may be responsible for the after-effects on cortical excitability (Liebetanz et al., 2002).

tDCS can be applied to better understand brain mechanisms and their relation to cognitive processes, although tDCS is not as focal in activating or inhibiting brain regions in comparison to TMS given the diffusivity of current flow for anode over region of interest, extra-cephalic cathode montages ("ring" montages; anode over region of interest encircled by multiple cathodes provide more focal stimulation but not to the level implemented by TMS (Datta et al., 2009)). Recent tDCS studies have allowed researchers to make inferences regarding the neural basis of learning, memory, perception, and motor actions (Filmer et al., 2014). The study by Holland et al. (2011) investigated language function of healthy participants and aimed to help develop the approach for potential clinical deployment for rehabilitation of brain-damaged patients. Authors utilized fMRI to monitor and localize the effects of tDCS stimulation concurrently. Left frontal anodal tDCS was used during an overt picture-naming task and results provided important evidence of contribution of the left inferior frontal cortex in the naming task and identified Broca's area for tDCS based rehabilitation (Holland et al., 2011).

Another example is a study by Clarke et al. (2014) in which the role of dorsolateral prefrontal cortex in attention bias modification (ABM) was investigated. The exaggerated attention to mildly threatening conditions is defined as the attention bias to threat and has been reliably observed across a range of anxiety and mood disorders. Reducing attention to threat in high anxiety patients has been demonstrated to also reduce anxiety symptoms, and thus suggests the promise of treatment of anxiety pathology. The authors utilized tDCS to isolate and test fMRI findings reported earlier by Browning et al. (2010) which implicated lateral prefrontal cortex in inhibitory control of attention in relation to threatening information. This study by Clarke et al. (2014) demonstrated the complementary nature of neuroimaging and neurostimulation (as the finding verified the functional MRI results of Browning et al. (2010)); and, highlights the potential power of joint neuroimaging and neurostimulation for novel interventions while establishing a broad neurocognitive framework. Below we further examine such joint investigations by combining tDCS and fNIRS.

Many studies have found that stimulation of different brain regions with tDCS can enhance performance of basic cognitive tasks that recruit the corresponding brain regions. For example, stimulating the dorso-lateral prefrontal cortex (DLPFC), which has been shown in neuroimaging studies to be involved in working memory, accordingly enhances performance on working memory tasks (Fregni et al., 2005). Beyond working memory, tDCS has also been found to enhance learning and performance on a wide variety of perceptual, cognitive, and motor tasks (for reviews, see Jacobson et al. (2012) and Coffman et al. (2014)). Here we provide a few examples of the effects of tDCS on more complex tasks representative of work settings.

One example involves surveillance and security operations, as in threat detection (Parasuraman and Galster, 2013). Accurate and timely detection of obscured or concealed objects, or the actions and movements of other people, is a critical need in many such work environments, both in the military and in civilian organizations. Skill in such threat detection tasks typically develops only after extensive training lasting many days. Can the development of expertise be speeded up with tDCS? Recent studies provide a positive answer (Clark et al., 2012; Falcone et al., 2012). These studies involved use of a complex task requiring participants to watch videos of naturalistic scenes containing movements of soldiers and civilians. Still images were extracted from the videos and manipulated so that half were targets, defined as concealed objects (e.g., bombs), people engaging in threatening activity (e.g., snipers), and so on, whereas the same scene without the threat was a non-target. An fMRI study was first conducted to determine optimal sites for application of tDCS (Clark et al., 2012). A total of 104 participants volunteered for the study and were imaged as novices. A subset, 13 participants performed the task during fMRI data collection to identify the brain networks supporting the identification of concealed objects and changes with learning. The results indicated that the right inferior frontal gyrus was the major locus of a distributed brain network that mediated acquisition of the threat detection task and so was chosen as the optimal stimulation site.

Falcone et al. (2012) examined whether tDCS applied to this location enhanced perceptual sensitivity in threat detection. Participants were given four training blocks of and were required to indicate whether a threat was present or absent. Two test blocks were given before training and were similar to training blocks, except that no feedback was given after each response. Anodal tDCS was applied to the electrode site F10 in the EEG system, over the right sphenoid bone, corresponding to an area overlying the inferior frontal gyrus. Although this is not as precise as subject-fMRI guided location selection, anatomical landmarks using international 10–20 system provided a viable solution which was confirmed by the results of the study. The cathode was placed on the contralateral (left) upper arm. Participants were randomly assigned to either active (2 mA current) or sham stimulation (0.1 mA) for a total of 30 min during the first two training blocks.

Compared to the 0.1 mA sham stimulation control, 2 mA stimulation increased perceptual sensitivity in detecting targets and accelerated learning. Performance was near chance ($d' = 0$) in both groups at the beginning of training. However, skill acquisition with tDCS was both rapid and extensive: On completion of training, participants in the active stimulation group had more than double the d' of the control group. There were no group or training effects on the response bias measure β, indicating that tDCS improved the actual efficiency of threat detection. Furthermore, threat detection sensitivity remained at a high level immediately after training and, more importantly, 24 h later. This last finding bodes well for the use of tDCS as a training method with potentially lasting effects in naturalistic work tasks.

A second example involves intelligence analysis, McKinley et al. (2013) trained image analysts to find and correctly identify ground targets, such as tanks and surface-to-air missile launchers, in synthetic aperture radar imagery. Stimulation of the right frontal cortex, using the same anodal F10 scalp location (cathode on the contralateral bicep) as in the previously described study of Falcone et al. (2012), significantly improved object recognition learning rates. During the first phase of training, one group was given active tDCS for 30 min; another, sham tDCS (active tDCS for 30 s); and a third group, no tDCS. Participants were then given a second round of training with the stimulation conditions reversed (i.e., the active tDCS group switched to sham tDCS, whereas the sham tDCS group received active tDCS in the second round). Both groups experienced larger increases in target acquisition accuracy when given active tDCS when compared to sham or no stimulation in either session. The image analysis task also included a change detection task in both training sessions. After the target image was complete, one of the targets (randomly assigned) changed in orientation, position, target type, or disappeared completely. Change detection performance was improved only when tDCS was applied in the second session. Thus, tDCS aided in change detection only after the analyst gained some experience with the images and target types. A similar finding was reported by Coffman et al. (2012), who found that tDCS had a larger effect on threat detection for images that had been viewed previously. These findings may reflect tDCS-induced plasticity changes in the brain networks responsible for object encoding and retrieval.

These are just two examples of the effectiveness of tDCS as a neuroergonomic tool for accelerating skill acquisition in complex, work-relevant tasks. Other examples are reviewed by Parasuraman and Mckinley (2014). Prior neuroimaging evidence suggests that such performance gains probably resulted from activation of specific brain networks associated with the relevant cognitive functions. However, direct evidence of modulation of brain dynamics would provide stronger evidence for such an association. Below, we examine how the combined use of fNIRS and tDCS can help in this endeavor. We begin, however, with a brief overview of the use of fNIRS alone in studies of cognitive workload.

Using fNIRS to Monitor the Relationship of Cognitive Workload and Brain Dynamics

fNIRS provides an attractive method for continuous monitoring of brain dynamics in both seated or mobile participants. fNIRS is safe, highly portable, user-friendly and relatively inexpensive, with rapid application times and near-zero run-time costs (Villringer and Chance, 1997; Ferrari and Quaresima, 2012). The most commonly used form of fNIRS uses infrared light, introduced at the scalp, to measure changes in blood oxygenation as oxy-hemoglobin converts to deoxy-hemoglobin during neural activity, i.e., the cerebral hemodynamic response. fNIRS uses specific wavelengths of light to provide measures of cerebral oxygenated and deoxygenated hemoglobin that are correlated with the fMRI BOLD signal (Cui et al., 2011; Sato et al., 2013). Below we briefly review fNIRS studies of cognitive workload.

For objective measures of cognitive workload in naturalistic environments, fNIRS offers a number of advantages over other measurement techniques such as fMRI. In particular, the high operational costs of fMRI makes long-duration or longitudinal (e.g., training) studies impractical. Cost is less of an issue with fNIRS as the systems themselves are less expensive and once purchased require no extra costs to run. fNIRS also does not require the participant to be immobile and the use of wireless fNIRS allows for imaging brain dynamics during tasks that require a participant to move regularly, as in motor and other physical tasks (Mehta and Parasuraman, 2014) and in naturalistic settings (Ayaz et al., 2013). fNIRS also offers a compromise between the spatial resolution of fMRI and temporal resolution of EEG. The superior spatial resolution (localization of activation) of fNIRS relative to EEG allows for greater accuracy in identifying specific brain regions responding to changes in workload. The superior temporal resolution (higher sampling rate) of fNIRS relative to fMRI affords improved statistical power when analyzing changes in the shape of the hemodynamic response.

fNIRS has proven beneficial for measuring workload in a number of complex tasks. Examples include supervisory control, natural orifice surgery simulations, and driving. In a study of air traffic controllers, Ayaz et al. (2012) found that as the number of supervised aircraft increased there was an increase in cerebral oxygenation (oxygenated hemoglobin minus deoxygenated hemoglobin) in the left medial/orbito frontal cortex. The relationship was linear and corresponded with increased oxygenation observed in the same sample during a multi-load N-back working memory task (Ayaz et al., 2012). Similarly during natural orifice translumenal endoscopic surgery (NOTES) simulation experienced surgeons familiar with NOTES showed increases in oxygenated hemoglobin in bilateral ventral lateral prefrontal cortex (VLPFC) when the simulation required a more difficult navigation path through an orifice (James et al., 2011).

fNIRS measurement of mental workload has also been used within the context of driving. In two separate studies while individuals drove on a closed road it was observed that deceleration increased oxygenated hemoglobin in regions involved in eye movements and optic flow (Yoshino et al., 2013a,b). The results indicated that deceleration is more cognitively taxing on visual processing than acceleration or constant velocity driving. Increases in oxygenated hemoglobin in bilateral VLPFC during U-turns was also observed (Yoshino et al., 2013b), suggesting the need for increased executive control relative to acceleration, deceleration, and constant velocity driving. Other recent studies also demonstrated the potential of fNIRS for assessment of cognitive workload (Abibullaev and An, 2012; Naseer and Keum-Shik, 2013; Afergan et al., 2014; Bogler et al., 2014; Derosière et al., 2014; Herff et al., 2014; Schudlo and Chau, 2014; Solovey et al., 2015).

Although a linear relationship between task workload and hemodynamics has often been observed (Ayaz et al., 2012; Fishburn et al., 2014) where the difficulty of the task at hand does not exceed the cognitive capacity of participant, whereas when cognitive capacity is exceeded the observed effects on hemodynamics conform to the shape reported by the Yerkes--Dodson law (Yerkes and Dodson, 1908). On a supervisory control task a negative quadratic relationship (inverted U) between workload and DLPFC activation was found (Durantin et al., 2014). Individuals were asked to control remotely operated vehicles as they navigated through an airspace while avoiding no fly zones. Workload was manipulated by altering crosswinds, vehicle inertia and memory load regarding supervisory control. It was also noted that there was a strong correlation between increased DLPFC activation in the highest workload condition and performance. This actually suggests that workload alone does not have a quadratic relationship with functional hemodynamics, but instead once mental overload is reached functional activation decreases. Evidence from two other studies supports this claim. Yamauchi et al. (2013) had participants play a modified version of "rock, paper, scissors" against a computer, with the objective to actually lose each hand. The computer presented one of the three hands and the participant had to choose the losing hand. Workload was manipulated by decreasing the inter stimulus interval (ISI). Furthermore these decreases were adapted to each participants minimum effective ISI. When workload was manipulated as a function of an individual's maximum workload, only linear increases in oxygenated hemoglobin were observed in left lateral prefrontal cortex, premotor cortex and supplementary motor area (Yamauchi et al., 2013).

Similarly in a dual-working memory training study when task memory load increased as a function of participant's skill acquisition, a strong linear increase in total hemoglobin after an initial decrease in activation occurred while participants adapted to the task. However a different group of participants had their task memory load yoked to the performance of the other group, and they showed a negative quadratic relationship between memory load and total hemoglobin (McKendrick et al., 2014). Taken together these findings suggest that the presence of a negative quadratic slope during fNIRS monitoring of workload dynamics is indicative of task overload. This trend can be used to assess the points at which overload occurs for individuals, or as a means of ensuring that tests of workload only include load up to an individual's maximum effective capability. This can be used to optimize operator work periods, introducing adaptive automation (Byrne and Parasuraman, 1996), or delegation of tasks to other operators as methods of optimizing operator efficiency and system performance. It is also apparent that an individual's maximum effective workload can change with task training. Therefore this trend may occur concurrently with an individual's skill acquisition and non-linear components should be included within statistical models of workload dynamics to observe and utilize this quadratic trend.

The changes in oxygenated and deoxygenated hemoglobin representative of mental workload may not only arise from cognitive work. Both physical and emotional work can affect and potentially invalidate measures of cognitive workload. Submaximal physical effort can reduce mental performance, furthermore increasing submaximal physical effort has similar effects on oxygenated and deoxygenated hemoglobin as moving from a single cognitive task to a dual cognitive task (Mandrick et al., 2013). Mental and physical work to exhaustion may also cause cognitive interference resulting in decreased oxygenated and increased deoxygenated hemoglobin in prefrontal cortex (Mehta and Parasuraman, 2013).

Monitoring the Effects of tDCS on Brain Dynamics Using fNIRS

There is now considerable evidence that tDCS can boost brain plasticity processes and accelerate skill acquisition in complex cognitive tasks (Clark and Parasuraman, 2014). Less well known, however, is the neural changes that make such performance gains possible. There are only a few investigations of simultaneous neuroimaging and stimulation studies, such as using fMRI (Alon et al., 2011; Antal et al., 2011; Holland et al., 2011; Kwon and Jang, 2011). However, the electric current flow of tDCS can create confounds in simultaneous fMRI echo-planar imaging (Antal et al., 2014). For a review of neuroimaging artifacts and limitations during simultaneous tDCS and fMRI, see Saiote et al. (2013) and Antal et al. (2014). Hence, a neuroimaging tool is needed that is inherently independent of electrical stimulation. As an optical imaging technique fNIRS provides one such neuroimaging approach.

Combining fNIRS with tDCS can provide some insights for understanding brain plasticity associated with skill acquisition. An initial basic research direction for joint use of fNIRS and tDCS is for understating how tDCS effects the brain in both animal models (Han et al., 2014) and human studies (Merzagora et al., 2010; Khan et al., 2013; Muthalib et al., 2013; Ishikuro et al., 2014; Jones et al., 2015). Merzagora et al. (2010) reported on the anterior prefrontal cortex effects of tDCS before and after stimulation using a prefrontal sensor pad based fNIRS measurement. Results indicated that fNIRS successfully captured the activation changes induced by the tDCS stimulation. Khan et al. (2013) compared altered hemodynamic patterns in the sensorimotor cortex in response to bi-hemispheric tDCS polarities and their relationship to muscle activity and motor task performance. Muthalib et al. (2013) utilized anodal tDCS based motor cortex stimulation to study neuromuscular fatigue and task failure related prefrontal cortex activation measured by fNIRS. Ishikuro et al. (2014) studied the relationship between frontal and sensorimotor cortices and motor learning of tasks used in rehabilitation. Healthy participants performed the task using a whole head fNIRS system. The neuroimaging session was used to identify relevant brain area (anterior dorsomedial prefrontal cortex) for stimulation in a separate experiment. Participants performed the same task with and without tDCS. Authors reported significant effects of tDCS and improvement in performance with stimulation. Jones et al. (2015) investigated the role of motivation (incentives) and tDCS in improving performance for both high and low working memory capacity participants. Authors used fNIRS to assess the cortical effects and brain activity changes.due to tDCS stimulation. The underlying motivation of such joint stimulation and neuroimaging studies is to extend boundaries of knowledge on brain-behavior relationships and translate the acquired knowledge for potential clinical and neuroergonomic applications.

Combined tDCS-fNIRS: Neuroergonomics Pilot Study

We illustrate the utility of the combination of simultaneous tDCS and fNIRS techniques in a study examining the effects of tDCS on spatial working memory. The task involved recalling the location of 5–7 randomly spaced black disks on a computer display after a short retention period. Each trial began with 15 s of fixation followed by a 1 s presentation of 5–7 randomly spaced black disks. A 4 s random noise mask was displayed after the presentation of the stimulus, after which participants were instructed to respond and recall the number and positions of the stimulus. A more complete description of the task is presented in McKendrick et al. (2014).

Participants received a block of baseline trials, followed by two blocks of sham stimulation, one block of 1 mA stimulation using a high-density tDCS montage, and a final block of continued stimulation monitoring, with each block consisting of 33 trials. Participants were fitted with an elastomere cap with high density tDCS (HD-tDCS) electrode holders positioned at F2 and F10 in the 10–20 EEG system. A Ag/AgCl sintered ring electrode was placed in each holder along with electroconductive gel to conduct the current to the scalp (See Villamar et al., 2013 for a more detailed description of the Soterix HD-tDCS system). An fNIR Devices Model 1100 NIRS imaging device sensor that has 16 optodes (10 photodetectors and 4 light emitters each using 730 nm and 850 nm wavelengths of light) was attached to the forehead for monitoring changes in frontal oxygenated and deoxygenated hemoglobin (for a more complete description of the fNIR Devices Model 1100 NIRS see Ayaz et al., 2012).

A pilot study using this task had identified a region of right VLPFC that showed an increase in activity during the task period relative to fixation (McKendrick et al., 2014). This region also showed a correlation between increased performance and increased neural efficiency (increased performance negatively modulated increases in activity amplitude). As such this region was selected for stimulation via HDtDCS and is an example of fNIRS guided tDCS. Using the modeling software HD-explore (Soterix Medical), we constructed a montage that elicited maximum current flow to right VLPFC (**Figure 1**) by placing the anode at F10 and cathode at F2.

The current density of this montage is considerably higher than that traditionally observed with two electrode montages using saline soaked sponges. For this reason twice during the study participants were asked to report the current severity of sensations such as heat, tingling, and itching. No participants were removed from the study due to reports of severe sensations.

Linear mixed effects models were used to assess changes in task performance as a function of time and stimulus condition. Analysis was performed in R with package "LME4" and function "lmer". Model selection and control for over fitting were done with AIC and BIC log-likelihood weighting functions with BIC taking precedence if the two weighting functions selected a different model.

Raw NIRS time series data were low pass filtered and corrected for motion artifacts, after which relative concentrations of oxygenated and deoxygenated hemoglobin were calculated with the modified Beer Lambert law, with the first 10 s of fixation for a given block of trials used as the NIRS baseline. Oxygenated and deoxygenated hemoglobin time series for each optode were analyzed with linear mixed effects regression. Orthogonal regressors were constructed with boxcar time series representing hypotheses of interest and convolved with a canonical hemodynamic response function. The following regressors were constructed and entered into a design matrix: (1) increased activity during the task period relative to fixation; (2) correlation between task activity amplitude and performance; (3) increased task amplitude during stimulation relative to baseline; (4) increased task amplitude during stimulation relative to sham; (5) correlation between task performance and increased task activity during stimulation relative to baseline; and (6) correlation between task performance and increased task activity during stimulation relative to sham. Fixed effects were composed of the full design matrix of regressors and random effects were selected via the same methods used for behavioral model selection. Multiple comparisons were corrected for using the Hochberg false discovery rate correction. Final effects of increases or decreases in activation were determined by comparing the sign of beta coefficients for significant changes in oxygenated and deoxygenated hemoglobin. Opposite signs of oxygenated and deoxygenated hemoglobin, where the beta coefficient of oxygenated hemoglobin was positive were interpreted as increases in activity; where the coefficient of oxygenated hemoglobin was negative were interpreted as decreases in activity.

The most parsimonious behavioral model specified fixed effects of a linear and quadratic effect of experimental block, and random effects of participant intercept uncorrelated with experimental block. There was a significant linear effect of block (b = −0.38, SE = 0.16, $p < 0.05$). This suggests that increased time on the task lead to a decrement in performance. However there was also a significant quadratic effect of block (b = 0.06, SE = 0.02, $p < 0.05$). This positive quadratic effect counteracted the decline in performance following the first three blocks. The uptrend in performance also corresponds with the time at which participants began receiving stimulation, and continues even after stimulation was removed.

In the NIRS data there were a number of optodes that showed significant effects in oxygenated and deoxygenated hemoglobin for the design matrix regressors we constructed; however for the sake of brevity and clarity only effects where oxygenated hemoglobin and deoxygenated hemoglobin had opposite beta coefficients are reported. Visualization of brain activation patterns are described elsewhere (Ayaz et al., 2006) and more

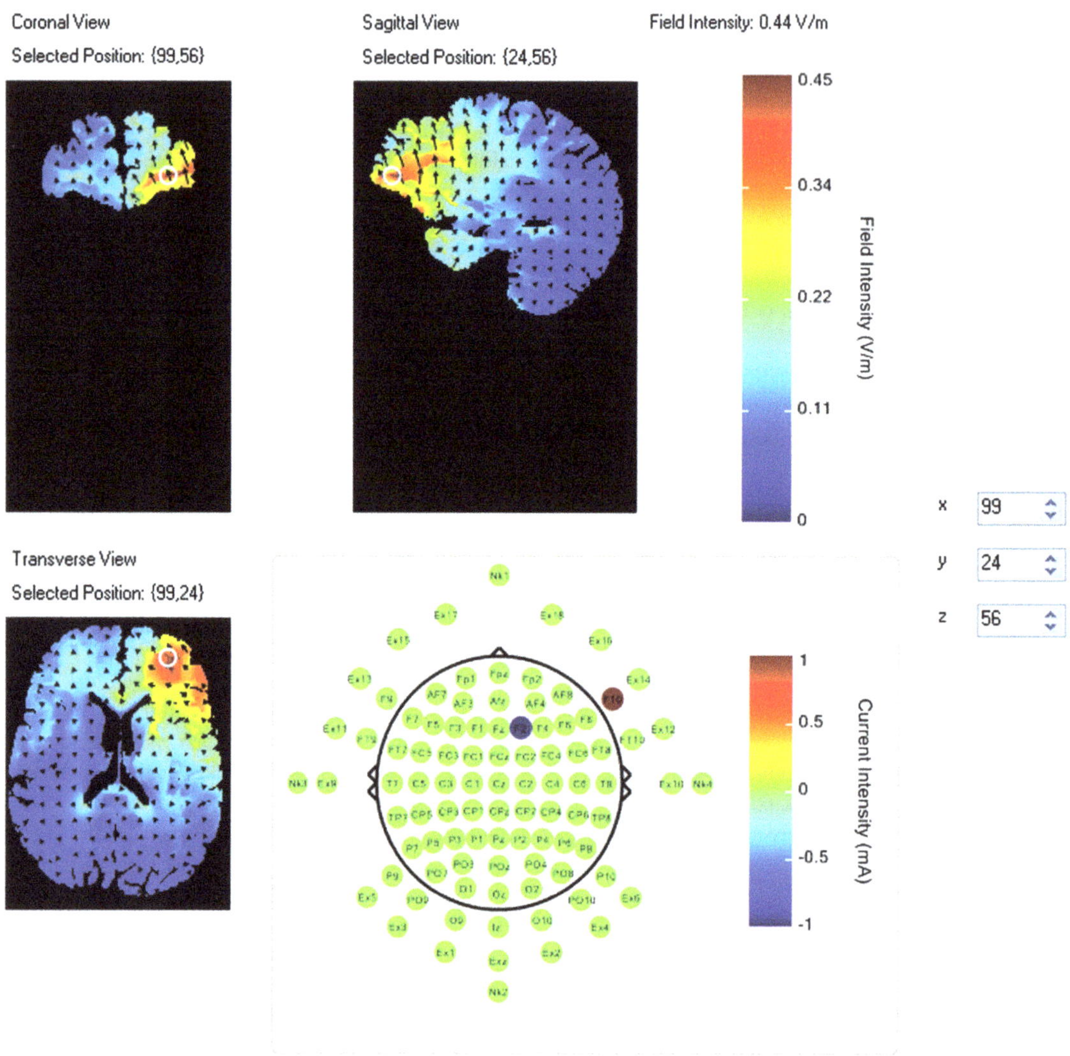

FIGURE 1 | Current flow model of tDCS montage (F10 anode, F2 cathode), field intensity of 0.44 V/m represented at white ring in coronal, sagittal and transverse views. Arrows represent direction of current flow.

information on placement of optodes, see Ayaz et al. (2012). Final models for each optode consisted of the full design matrix for fixed effects and random effects were participant intercept uncorrelated with time. There were no significant activation changes comparing task period to fixation, however optode 16 in coherence with our pilot findings showed a relationship between activity amplitude during the task period and subsequent performance (Oxy $b = 0.019$, SE = 0.008, $p < 0.05$, Deoxy $b = -0.008$, SE = 0.004, $p < 0.05$) (**Figure 2**).

Optodes 1, 3, 5, 6, 7, 11, 12, and 13 showed evidence of increased activation during the task period for stimulation blocks relative to the base line block. However these same regions and optode 14 showed a decrease in activation during the task period when comparing the stimulation blocks to the sham blocks (**Figure 3**).

We also observed that reduced positive activity in optodes 1 and 13 were associated with higher performance between the stimulation and baseline trials. Finally greater reduced activity in optodes 11 (Oxy $b = -0.058$, SE = 0.011, $p < 0.001$, Deoxy $b = 0.022$, SE = 0.005, $p < 0.001$) and 15 (Oxy $b = -0.118$, SE = 0.014, $p < 0.001$, Deoxy $b = 0.043$, SE = 0.009, $p < 0.001$) was associated with improved performance between the stimulation and sham trials, this was also accompanied by less negative activity in optode 6 (Oxy $b = 0.027$, SE = 0.012, $p < 0.05$, Deoxy $b = -0.017$, SE = 0.007, $p < 0.05$) correlating with improved performance (**Figure 4**).

1 mA of DC was applied with anode at F10 and cathode at F2 while participants performed a spatial memory task while being concurrently monitored with fNIRS. Task performance declined rapidly following baseline, possibly reflecting changes in vigilance or fatigue. However this decrement was overcome and almost eliminated following HDtDCS stimulation. The stimulation also had a number of effects on hemodynamic

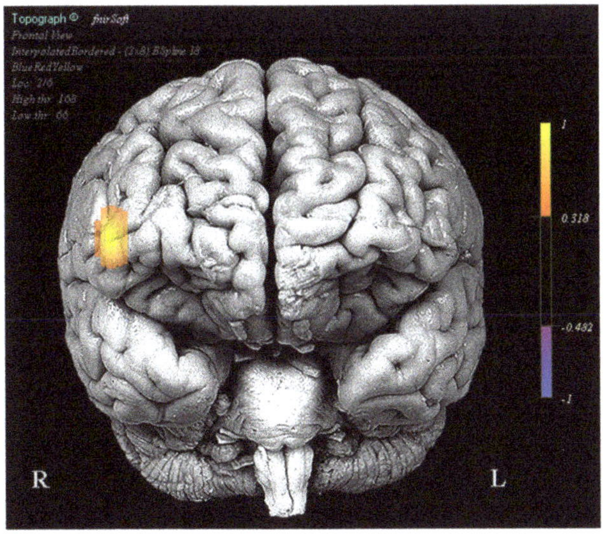

FIGURE 2 | Regions in which effects represent a correlation between increased activity and increased task performance. Legend represents the presence and direction of the effect, not *p* or *t* values.

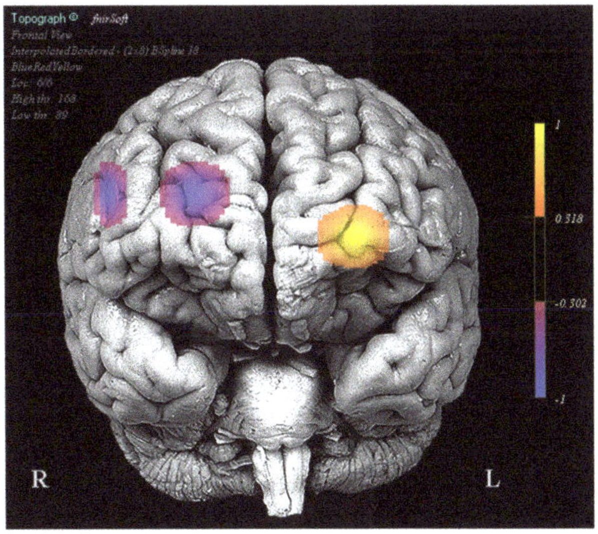

FIGURE 4 | Regions in which effects represent a correlation between activity and increases in performance in stimulation trials relative to the sham trials. Legend represents the presence and direction of the effect, not *p* or *t* values.

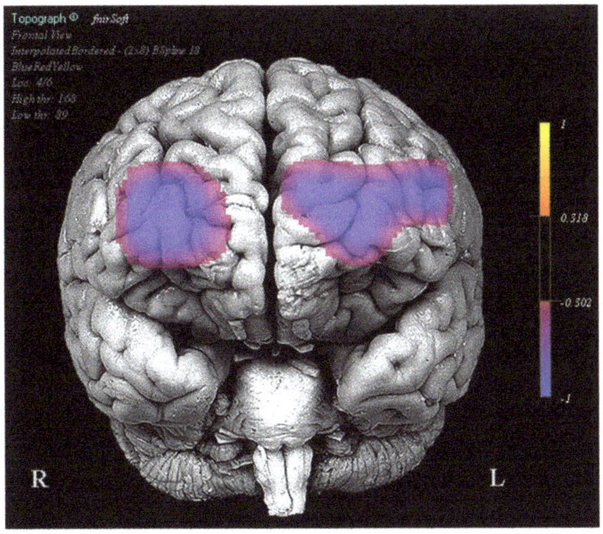

FIGURE 3 | Regions in which effects represent a decrease in activity during stimulation trials relative to the sham trials. Legend represents the presence and direction of the effect, not *p* or *t* values.

correlates of neural activity and their relationship to task performance. Specifically stimulation reduced the activity in bilateral prefrontal cortex, however most of these changes were unrelated to the effect of tDCS on task performance. Only continued decreased activity in right dorsal medial (optode 11), and right dorsolateral PFC (optode 15) were associated with the increase in performance experienced as participants shifted from the sham blocks to the stimulation blocks. This is particularly interesting as the cathode was placed directly above right dorsomedial PFC at the sight associated with performance recovery. Furthermore it is interesting to note that the region selected for modulation via our model of current flow was not actually modulated by stimulation, however its activity was still consistently associated with task performance. Taken together these results suggest that tDCS can modulate the neural activity of specific brain regions near the site of stimulation, however current models and protocol for determining tDCS montages are lacking, as it appears there are intimate interactions between stimulation montage, task and underlying hemodynamics that are complex. Additional joint tDCS and fNIRS studies are needed to further unravel these complexities and to better define the pattern of cortical excitation induced by tDCS during the performance of cognitive tasks.

Wireless Brain Imaging With tDCS

Significant progress has been made over the last decades in understanding the brain physiology and neural dynamics related to cognitive processes and behavior. However traditional neuroimaging tools such as fMRI severely restrict subject movements due to the inherent imaging operation (Makeig et al., 2009). Such technical limitations require brain imaging in more artificial settings separated from dynamic and multi-faceted natural environment (Gramann et al., 2014). To be able to capture brain dynamics related to natural cognition, mobile brain imaging systems are needed to operate in complex and partially unpredictable environments, consistent with mobile brain/body imaging (MoBI) and neuroergonomics approaches (Gramann et al., 2011; Parasuraman, 2011), A new generation of portable brain sensing technologies of EEG and fNIRS have begun to overcome the limitations of traditional neuroimaging through untethered measurements and wearable sensors (Liao et al., 2012; Ayaz et al., 2013; De Vos et al., 2014; Stopczynski et al., 2014; Mihajlovic et al., 2015). For a review of commercial available mobile EEG systems see (Mihajlovic et al., 2015) and recent studies demonstrated combined EEG and tDCS (Faria et al., 2012; Schestatsky et al., 2013; Mangia et al., 2014) as well as the combined fNIRS and tDCS studies (Khan et al., 2013; Ishikuro et al., 2014; Jones et al., 2015). However, joint use of EEG and tDCS is prone to artifacts, requires additional effort (such as extra reference electrodes and processing) to control and isolate the electrical fields to prevent contamination. Since fNIRS is optical (no electrical interference) and fNIRS sensor usually has an opening directly over the measurement area (light source and detectors are positioned around the measurement area, see **Figure 6**) there's a natural opportunity for integration. Potential applications of portable fNIRS were reviewed recently for neuroergonomics (Ayaz et al., 2013) and economics research (Kopton and Kenning, 2014). These developments have provided an opportunity for coupling mobile brain imaging sensors with wireless tDCS for monitoring and modulating brain activity in ecologically valid natural environments.

Recent comprehensive reviews on fNIRS technology (Ferrari and Quaresima, 2012) confirm that the vast majority of instrumentation development has been conducted on continuous wave (CW) type fNIRS. CW systems have a limitation in terms of their information content (i.e., it measures only changes of oxy and deoxy-Hb) compared to frequency and time-resolved fNIRS systems. However, CW fNIRS is also most appropriate for miniaturization and portable system development, because the signal type and acquisition timing requirements are less demanding.

The development of wearable and low cost fNIRS systems began in 1990s and by Chance et al. (1997) specifically for prefrontal cortex brain hemodynamics and muscle measurements. These systems, were later further developed into the portable systems at Drexel University for functional brain imaging using both desktop and miniaturized wireless versions (Ayaz et al., 2013) as well as breast tumor scanning (Sao et al., 2003), chronic wound monitoring (Weingarten et al., 2008) and brain hematoma scanning (Ayaz et al., 2011a).

fNIRS based wireless brain imaging systems have also been of interest and Hoshi (2003) reported use of one the earliest for assessing regional blood flow related to emotion in children. The system had one detector and two light sources, providing two optodes overall. Participants were carrying the equipment and transmitter in a backpack. Later, Yurtsever et al. (2006) reported a pocket PC integrated system that reduced the overall size considerably by using off-the-shelf embedded system as computational platform and featured up to 48 channels (16 optodes). Also, Muehlemann et al. (2008) described an *in vivo* measurement system that featured wireless data transfer with up to 32 channels and high sampling rate to reach fast optical signal. Holper et al. (2010) used that system for virtual reality based neurorehabilitation approach during observation and motor imagery tasks. Also, an EEG integrated prototype has been used in epilepsy research (Safaie et al., 2013). More recently, Muthalib et al. (2014) presented an HD-tDCS EEG/fNIRS capable experiment setup that was used for studying both electrophysiological and hemodynamic components of the modulation of cortical sensorimotor networks.

In previous work we have reported a custom miniaturized system (Rodriguez and Pourrezaei, 2011) that can be used for general purpose functional neuroimaging studies of prefrontal cortex (Ayaz et al., 2013). The device is a smart-phone size unit that can be carried in hand (See **Figure 5**), and drive up to 5 optodes (15 channels) at 4 Hz sampling rate. The system interfaces and transmits data wirelessly to a PC that runs the COBI Studio (Ayaz et al., 2011b). The implemented system is depicted in **Figure 5** below. The main advantage is further miniaturization of the hardware unit and hence no need for backpack, subjects can carry the system in their pocket or hand allowing more freedom in experimental design.

Integration of fNIRS sensors with tDCS also shows promise given that optical brain imaging is not influenced by electrical stimulation. Simultaneous use with fiber based fNIRS sensors is less of an issue as placement of fibers that run perpendicular to scalp leaves much space for other types of sensors. However, such sensors require laser light sources and larger hardware equipment, which are not as portable as LED based systems. Hence further miniaturization and customization of LED based sensor pads is needed. **Figure 6** below depicts a miniaturized prototype fNIRS sensor pad that is compatible with the fNIRS wireless unit described above (Ayaz et al., 2013) and a similar configuration was already tested with tDCS (Rodriguez and Pourrezaei, 2011). The combined tDCS fNIRS in that study was constructed by first molding the insulated fNIRS PCB in a skin safe silicon cast which was designed to hold tDCS electrodes in standard size (2″ × 3.5″) acting as a sleeve to the electrode. Systemic performance tests with varying power and gain parameters indicated that undesired interference is not introduced by the tDCS stimulation and that the fNIR sensor performs as expected. Similarly, there are also prototype fNIRS sensors that are already integrated with EEG electrodes for hybrid measurements (Lareau et al., 2011; Leamy et al., 2011; Safaie et al., 2013).

Since the fNIRS sensor positioning of the light source and detectors are around the measurement area (which is in between the light source and detector as illustrated in **Figure 6**) and not directly on top of the measurement area, combining with tDCS is feasible and practical from a hardware development perspective. Moreover recent developments in tDCS systems provide multi-channel tDCS systems that allow independent control of individual electrode currents, such as the HDtDCS systems developed by Soterix Medical and the wireless tDCS system Starstim (by NE Electrics) enabling potential ambulatory experimental protocols.

Future Directions

This paper reviews the potential joint use and future convergence of two technologies for neuroimaging and neurostimulation, fNIRS and tDCS, and how the two can be synergistically used together to enhance our current understanding of brain dynamics. Both technologies have complimentary capabilities, and both are built wearable and wireless that allow for application in natural environments and real world settings. Future neuroergonomics applications could range from

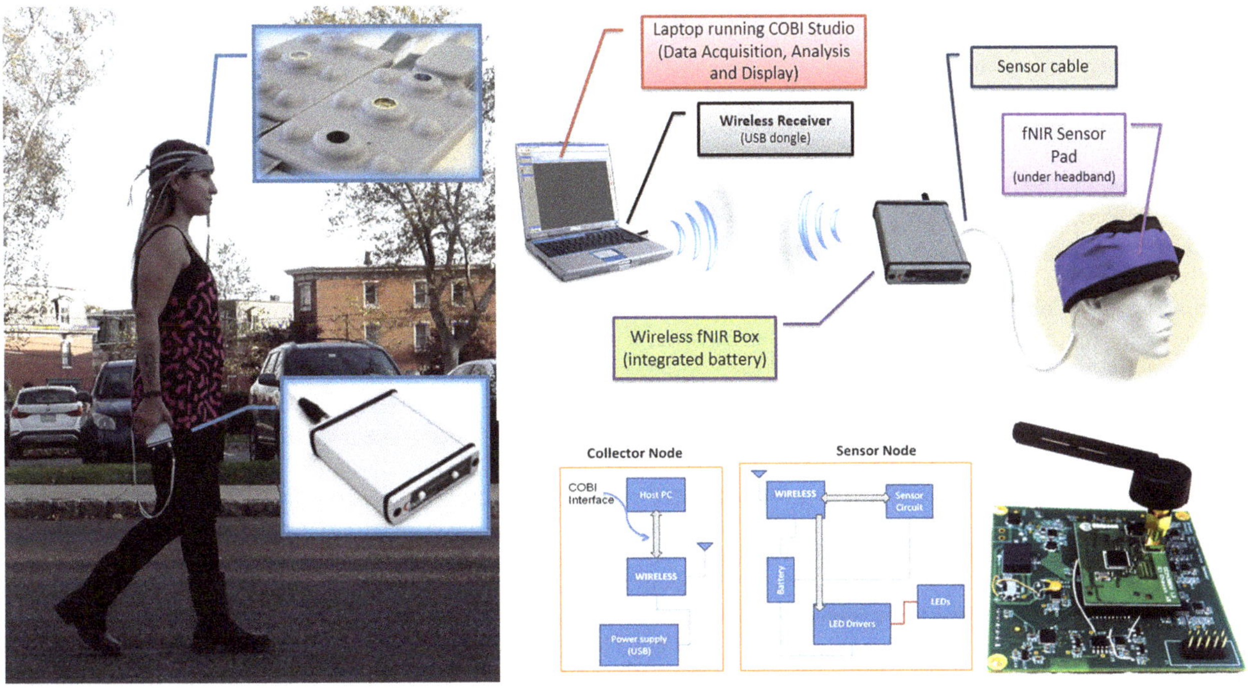

FIGURE 5 | Wireless fNIRS System. (left) Battery operated and wireless unit allows untethered outdoor measurement (right, up). Block diagram of the overall system (right, bottom), Building blocks and circuit representation (Ayaz et al., 2013).

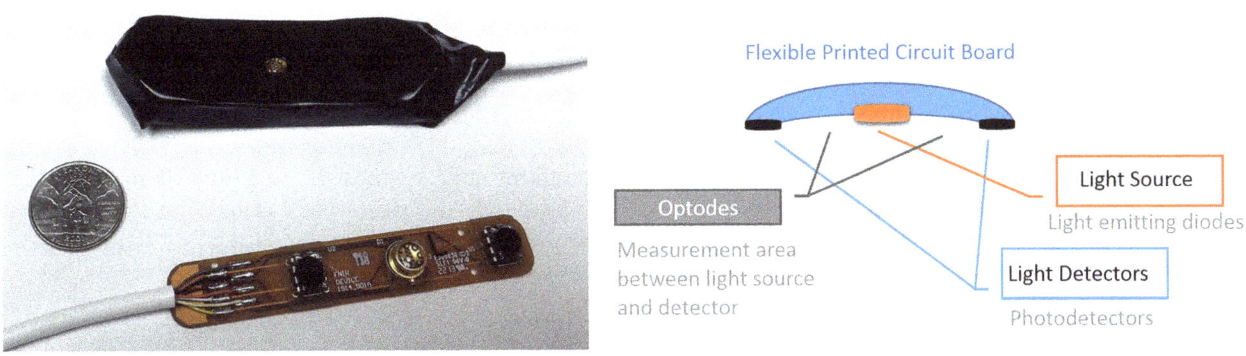

FIGURE 6 | Miniaturized and scalable fNIRS sensor pad with 2 optodes can be integrated with electrodes. (left) prototype sensor pad circuit board and covered with foam enclosure. A U.S. quarter is included for size. (right) The 2 optodes sensor pad parts.

enhanced/accelerated learning and training of complex human-machine systems to optimization of task load for improved safety and productivity.

Also, joint use of tDCS and fNIRS could enable new unique applications such as read-write BCI. A BCI is defined as a system that captures and transforms signals originating from the human brain into commands that can control external applications or instruments. In its most general form BCI provides a route for neural output that does not involve the neuromuscular system (Wolpaw et al., 2002; Lebedev, 2014). BCI systems have a wide range of potential applications, including rehabilitation and assistive use for severely paralyzed patients to help them communicate and interact with their environments, as well as monitoring brain activity for assessment of mental state or intervention in various psychiatric conditions and/or to augment the interactivity of healthy individuals.

Current noninvasive BCI systems are read-only as they capture brain activity and produce output/action for user. However, future portable and noninvasive BCI systems can also write to brain for direct communication and bypassing the peripheral nervous system and enhancing the brains' sensory input mechanism. Earlier studies in animal models achieved meaningful sensorimotor information in real time using invasive intracortical microstimulation to deliver sensory feedback signals in rats (Pais-Vieira et al., 2013) and monkeys (O'Doherty et al., 2011). This concept has been tested on humans recently after lab prototypes and demonstrations indicated feasibility and Grau et al. (2014) published their approach for Brain to Brain Communication which was made possible with dual use of noninvasive neuroimaging and neurostimulation. In the study, authors utilized EEG for capturing voluntary motor imagery related activations which were relayed as light perception to second brain by stimulating occipital lobe via TMS. Practical brain to brain communication would have profound impact on how we communicate and work, and as a portable system, tDCS is the natural candidate for closing the loop for future portable BCI systems.

As the potential use of future BCI systems has implications from individual to society at large, ethical aspects have also been a focus of discussion as part of the rising field of neuroethics (Illes and Bird, 2006; Haselager et al., 2009; Schermer, 2009; Clausen, 2011; Nijboer et al., 2011; Vlek et al., 2012). One of the immediate concerns is related to "treatment vs. research" which is related to the decision of using new systems on clinical and vulnerable populations such as locked-in patients. As in all new medical technologies, clinical utility and benefit vs. the risk (e.g., when using invasive neuroimaging or burden of engaging with the system) has to be evaluated with due process (informed consent) (Vlek et al., 2012). Also, privacy has been a core concern (Nijboer et al., 2011; Fairclough, 2014) and mostly attributed to keeping ones' physiological signals private. With the influence of contemporary science-fiction, write-only or read-write BCI have often been considered akin to mind control. Writing to the brain has been used here in terms of modification/modulation of brain signals and is a physiological effect with immediate clinical uses (e.g., Parkinson treatment with deep brain stimulation). Current concepts of write-only or read-write BCI can only operate with the user's consent and engagement. And, the design of future BCI systems should be informed by neuroethics considerations from personal to societal perspectives. For a discussion of the near and long-term issues please see recent reviews by Clausen (2011), Nijboer et al. (2011), Vlek et al. (2012) and Attiah and Farah (2014).

Another interesting future direction could be the unification of neuroimaging and neurostimulation technology by using near infrared light. A novel integration of optics and genetics is the emerging field of optogenetics which uses light to control neurons that have been genetically modified to be sensitive to light (Deisseroth, 2011). Optogenetics studies has been exponentially growing to observe and perturb neural mechanisms from single cell level to animal brain models. The requirement of genetically encoded, protein-based probes to achieve experimental manipulation is a major limitation for human studies. Optical stimulation with near infrared lasers that are low powered but have high energy density could be a solution (Wells et al., 2005a,b; Shapiro et al., 2012). A recent study suggest that such lasers could be utilized to excite cells by changing their electrical capacitance (Shapiro et al., 2012). Although light sources for such lasers would be different for reading and writing, having a unified/fused wearable pad that can both record and stimulate brain activity could enable new applications in natural environments. In summary, the simultaneous use of tDCS and fNIRS, the development of wireless, portable fNIRS systems, and the potential development of optical systems for both stimulation and neuroimaging are opening up new vistas for neurocognitive augmentation, with exciting new clinical and neuroergonomic applications.

Disclosure

fNIR Devices, LLC manufactures the optical brain imaging instrument and licensed IP and know-how from Drexel University. H. Ayaz was involved in the technology development and thus offered a minor share in the new startup firm fNIR Devices, LLC.

References

Abibullaev, B., and An, J. (2012). Classification of frontal cortex haemodynamic responses during cognitive tasks using wavelet transforms and machine learning algorithms. *Med. Eng. Phys.* 34, 1394–1410. doi: 10.1016/j.medengphy.2012.01.002

Afergan, D., Peck, E. M., Solovey, E. T., Jenkins, A., Hincks, S. W., Brown, E. T., et al. (2014). "Dynamic difficulty using brain metrics of workload," in *Proc. ACM CHI 2014 Human Factors in Computing Systems Conference* (Toronto, Canada: ACM Press).

Alon, G., Roys, S., Gullapalli, R., and Greenspan, J. (2011). Non-invasive electrical stimulation of the brain (ESB) modifies the resting-state network connectivity of the primary motor cortex: a proof of concept fMRI study. *Brain Res.* 1403, 37–44. doi: 10.1016/j.brainres.2011.06.013

Angelakis, E., Stathopoulou, S., Frymiare, J. L., Green, D. L., Lubar, J. F., and Kounios, J. (2007). EEG neurofeedback: a brief overview and an example of peak alpha frequency training for cognitive enhancement in the elderly. *Clin. Neuropsychol.* 21, 110–129. doi: 10.1080/13854040600744839

Antal, A., Bikson, M., Datta, A., Lafon, B., Dechent, P., Parra, L. C., et al. (2014). Imaging artifacts induced by electrical stimulation during conventional fMRI of the brain. *Neuroimage* 85(Pt. 3), 1040–1047. doi: 10.1016/j.neuroimage.2012.10.026

Antal, A., Polania, R., Schmidt-Samoa, C., Dechent, P., and Paulus, W. (2011). Transcranial direct current stimulation over the primary motor cortex during fMRI. *Neuroimage* 55, 590–596. doi: 10.1016/j.neuroimage.2010.11.085

Attiah, M. A., and Farah, M. J. (2014). Minds and motherboards and money: futurism and realism in the neuroethics of BCI technologies. *Front. Syst. Neurosci.* 8:86. doi: 10.3389/fnsys.2014.00086

Ayaz, H., Ben Dor, B., Solt, D., and Onaral, B. (2011a). Infrascanner: cost effective, mobile medical imaging system for detecting hemotomas. *J. Med. Device.* 5:027540. doi: 10.1115/1.3591407

Ayaz, H., Izzetoglu, M., Platek, S. M., Bunce, S., Izzetoglu, K., Pourrezaei, K., et al. (2006). Registering fNIR data to brain surface image using MRI templates. *Conf. Proc. IEEE Eng. Med. Biol. Soc.* 1, 2671–2674. doi: 10.1109/iembs.2006.260835

Ayaz, H., Onaral, B., Izzetoglu, K., Shewokis, P. A., McKendrick, R., and Parasuraman, R. (2013). Continuous monitoring of brain dynamics with functional near infrared spectroscopy as a tool for neuroergonomic research: empirical examples and a technological development. *Front. Hum. Neurosci.* 7:871. doi: 10.3389/fnhum.2013.00871

Ayaz, H., Shewokis, P. A., Bunce, S., Izzetoglu, K., Willems, B., and Onaral, B. (2012). Optical brain monitoring for operator training and mental workload assessment. *Neuroimage* 59, 36–47. doi: 10.1016/j.neuroimage.2011.06.023

Ayaz, H., Shewokis, P. A., Curtin, A., Izzetoglu, M., Izzetoglu, K., and Onaral, B. (2011b). Using MazeSuite and functional near infrared spectroscopy to study learning in spatial navigation. *J. Vis. Exp.* 56:3443. doi: 10.3791/3443

Bikson, M., Datta, A., and Elwassif, M. (2009). Establishing safety limits for transcranial direct current stimulation. *Clin. Neurophysiol.* 120, 1033–1034. doi: 10.1016/j.clinph.2009.03.018

Bindman, L. J., Lippold, O., and Redfearn, J. (1964). The action of brief polarizing currents on the cerebral cortex of the rat (1) during current flow and (2) in the production of long-lasting after-effects. *J. Physiol.* 172, 369–382. doi: 10.1113/jphysiol.1964.sp007425

Bogler, C., Mehnert, J., Steinbrink, J., and Haynes, J. D. (2014). Decoding vigilance with NIRS. *PLoS One* 9:e101729. doi: 10.1371/journal.pone.0101729

Browning, M., Holmes, E. A., Murphy, S. E., Goodwin, G. M., and Harmer, C. J. (2010). Lateral prefrontal cortex mediates the cognitive modification of attentional bias. *Biol. Psychiatry* 67, 919–925. doi: 10.1016/j.biopsych.2009.10.031

Byrne, E. A., and Parasuraman, R. (1996). Psychophysiology and adaptive automation. *Biol. Psychol.* 42, 249–268. doi: 10.1016/0301-0511(95)05161-9

Chance, B., Luo, Q., Nioka, S., Alsop, D. C., and Detre, J. A. (1997). Optical investigations of physiology: a study of intrinsic and extrinsic biomedical contrast. *Philos. Trans. R. Soc. Lond. B Biol. Sci.* 352, 707–716. doi: 10.1098/rstb.1997.0053

Clark, V. P., Coffman, B. A., Mayer, A. R., Weisend, M. P., Lane, T. D., Calhoun, V. D., et al. (2012). TDCS guided using fMRI significantly accelerates learning to identify concealed objects. *Neuroimage* 59, 117–128. doi: 10.1016/j.neuroimage.2010.11.036

Clark, V. P., Coffman, B. A., Trumbo, M. C., and Gasparovic, C. (2011). Transcranial direct current stimulation (tDCS) produces localized and specific alterations in neurochemistry: A^1 H magnetic resonance spectroscopy study. *Neurosci. Lett.* 500, 67–71. doi: 10.1016/j.neulet.2011.05.244

Clark, V. P., and Parasuraman, R. (2014). Neuroenhancement: enhancing brain and mind in health and in disease. *Neuroimage* 85, 889–894. doi: 10.1016/j.neuroimage.2013.08.071

Clarke, P. J., Browning, M., Hammond, G., Notebaert, L., and MacLeod, C. (2014). The causal role of the dorsolateral prefrontal cortex in the modification of attentional bias: evidence from transcranial direct current stimulation. *Biol. Psychiatry* 76, 946–952. doi: 10.1016/j.biopsych.2014.03.003

Clausen, J. (2011). Conceptual and ethical issues with brain-hardware interfaces. *Curr. Opin. Psychiatry* 24, 495–501. doi: 10.1097/YCO.0b013e32834bb8ca

Coffman, B. A., Clark, V. P., and Parasuraman, R. (2014). Battery powered thought: enhancement of attention, learning and memory in healthy adults using transcranial direct current stimulation. *Neuroimage* 85, 895–908. doi: 10.1016/j.neuroimage.2013.07.083

Coffman, B. A., Trumbo, M., Flores, R., Garcia, C. M., van der Merwe, A., Wassermann, E. M., et al. (2012). Impact of tDCS on performance and learning of target detection: interaction with stimulus characteristics and experimental design. *Neuropsychologia* 50, 1594–1602. doi: 10.1016/j.neuropsychologia.2012.03.012

Cui, X., Bray, S., Bryant, D. M., Glover, G. H., and Reiss, A. L. (2011). A quantitative comparison of NIRS and fMRI across multiple cognitive tasks. *Neuroimage* 54, 2808–2821. doi: 10.1016/j.neuroimage.2010.10.069

Datta, A., Bansal, V., Diaz, J., Patel, J., Reato, D., and Bikson, M. (2009). Gyri-precise head model of transcranial direct current stimulation: improved spatial focality using a ring electrode versus conventional rectangular pad. *Brain Stimul.* 2, 201–207.e1. doi: 10.1016/j.brs.2009.03.005

Deisseroth, K. (2011). Optogenetics. *Nat. Methods* 8, 26–29. doi: 10.1038/nmeth.f.324

Derosière, G., Dalhoumi, S., Perrey, S., Dray, G., and Ward, T. (2014). Towards a near infrared spectroscopy-based estimation of operator attentional state. *PLoS One* 9:e92045. doi: 10.1371/journal.pone.0092045

De Vos, M., Kroesen, M., Emkes, R., and Debener, S. (2014). P300 speller BCI with a mobile EEG system: comparison to a traditional amplifier. *J. Neural Eng.* 11:036008. doi: 10.1088/1741-2560/11/3/036008

Durantin, G., Gagnon, J.-F., Tremblay, S., and Dehais, F. (2014). Using near infrared spectroscopy and heart rate variability to detect mental overload. *Behav. Brain Res.* 259, 16–23. doi: 10.1016/j.bbr.2013.10.042

Elbert, T., and Rockstroh, B. (2004). Reorganization of human cerebral cortex: the range of changes following use and injury. *Neuroscientist* 10, 129–141. doi: 10.1177/1073858403262111

Fairclough, S. (2014). Physiological data must remain confidential. *Nature* 505:263. doi: 10.1038/505263a

Falcone, B., Coffman, B. A., Clark, V. P., and Parasuraman, R. (2012). Transcranial direct current stimulation augments perceptual sensitivity and 24-hour retention in a complex threat detection task. *PLoS One* 7:e34993. doi: 10.1371/journal.pone.0034993

Faria, P., Fregni, F., Sebastião, F., Dias, A. I., and Leal, A. (2012). Feasibility of focal transcranial DC polarization with simultaneous EEG recording: preliminary assessment in healthy subjects and human epilepsy. *Epilepsy Behav.* 25, 417–425. doi: 10.1016/j.yebeh.2012.06.027

Ferrari, M., and Quaresima, V. (2012). A brief review on the history of human functional near-infrared spectroscopy (fNIRS) development and fields of application. *Neuroimage* 63, 921–935. doi: 10.1016/j.neuroimage.2012.03.049

Filmer, H. L., Dux, P. E., and Mattingley, J. B. (2014). Applications of transcranial direct current stimulation for understanding brain function. *Trends Neurosci.* 37, 742–753. doi: 10.1016/j.tins.2014.08.003

Fishburn, F. A., Norr, M. E., Medvedev, A. V., and Vaidya, C. J. (2014). Sensitivity of fNIRS to cognitive state and load. *Front. Hum. Neurosci.* 8:76. doi: 10.3389/fnhum.2014.00076

Flöel, A. (2014). tDCS-enhanced motor and cognitive function in neurological diseases. *Neuroimage* 85(Pt. 3), 934–947. doi: 10.1016/j.neuroimage.2013.05.098

Fregni, F., Boggio, P. S., Nitsche, M., Bermpohl, F., Antal, A., Feredoes, E., et al. (2005). Anodal transcranial direct current stimulation of prefrontal cortex enhances working memory. *Exp. Brain Res.* 166, 23–30. doi: 10.1007/s00221-005-2334-6

Gramann, K., Gwin, J. T., Ferris, D. P., Oie, K., Jung, T.-P., Lin, C.-T., et al. (2011). Cognition in action: imaging brain/body dynamics in mobile humans. *Rev. Neurosci.* 22, 593–608. doi: 10.1515/RNS.2011.047

Gramann, K., Jung, T. P., Ferris, D. P., Lin, C. T., and Makeig, S. (2014). Toward a new cognitive neuroscience: modeling natural brain dynamics. *Front. Hum. Neurosci.* 8:444. doi: 10.3389/fnhum.2014.00444

Grau, C., Ginhoux, R., Riera, A., Nguyen, T. L., Chauvat, H., Berg, M., et al. (2014). Conscious brain-to-brain communication in humans using non-invasive technologies. *PLoS One* 9:e105225. doi: 10.1371/journal.pone.0105225

Gruzelier, J. (2009). A theory of alpha/theta neurofeedback, creative performance enhancement, long distance functional connectivity and psychological integration. *Cogn. Process.* 10, S101–S109. doi: 10.1007/s10339-008-0248-5

Han, C.-H., Song, H., Kang, Y.-G., Kim, B.-M., and Im, C.-H. (2014). Hemodynamic responses in rat brain during transcranial direct current stimulation: a functional near-infrared spectroscopy study. *Biomed. Opt. Express.* 5, 1812–1821. doi: 10.1364/BOE.5.001812

Hanslmayr, S., Sauseng, P., Doppelmayr, M., Schabus, M., and Klimesch, W. (2005). Increasing individual upper alpha power by neurofeedback improves cognitive performance in human subjects. *Appl. Psychophysiol. Biofeedback* 30, 1–10. doi: 10.1007/s10484-005-2169-8

Haselager, P., Vlek, R., Hill, J., and Nijboer, F. (2009). A note on ethical aspects of BCI. *Neural Netw.* 22, 1352–1357. doi: 10.1016/j.neunet.2009.06.046

Heinrich, H., Busch, K., Studer, P., Erbe, K., Moll, G. H., and Kratz, O. (2014). EEG spectral analysis of attention in ADHD: implications for neurofeedback training? *Front. Hum. Neurosci.* 8:611. doi: 10.3389/fnhum.2014.00611

Herff, C., Heger, D., Fortmann, O., Hennrich, J., Putze, F., and Schultz, T. (2014). Mental workload during n-back task—quantified in the prefrontal cortex using fNIRS. *Front. Hum. Neurosci.* 7:935. doi: 10.3389/fnhum.2013.00935

Hoffman, D., Stockdale, S., and Van Egren, L. (1996). EEG neurofeedback in the treatment of mild traumatic brain injury. *Clin. Electroencephalogr.* 27, 105.

Holland, R., Leff, A. P., Josephs, O., Galea, J. M., Desikan, M., Price, C. J., et al. (2011). Speech facilitation by left inferior frontal cortex stimulation. *Curr. Biol.* 21, 1403–1407. doi: 10.1016/j.cub.2011.07.021

Holper, L., Muehlemann, T., Scholkmann, F., Eng, K., Kiper, D., and Wolf, M. (2010). Testing the potential of a virtual reality neurorehabilitation system during performance of observation, imagery and imitation of motor actions recorded by wireless functional near-infrared spectroscopy (fNIRS). *J. Neuroeng. Rehabil.* 7:57. doi: 10.1186/1743-0003-7-57

Hoshi, Y. (2003). Functional near-infrared optical imaging: utility and limitations in human brain mapping. *Psychophysiology* 40, 511–520. doi: 10.1111/1469-8986.00053

Hunter, M. A., Coffman, B. A., Trumbo, M. C., and Clark, V. P. (2013). Tracking the neuroplastic changes associated with transcranial direct current stimulation: a push for multimodal imaging. *Front. Hum. Neurosci.* 7:495. doi: 10.3389/fnhum.2013.00495

Illes, J., and Bird, S. J. (2006). Neuroethics: a modern context for ethics in neuroscience. *Trends Neurosci.* 29, 511–517. doi: 10.1016/j.tins.2006.07.002

Ishikuro, K., Urakawa, S., Takamoto, K., Ishikawa, A., Ono, T., and Nishijo, H. (2014). Cerebral functional imaging using near-infrared spectroscopy during repeated performances of motor rehabilitation tasks tested on healthy subjects. *Front. Hum. Neurosci.* 8:292. doi: 10.3389/fnhum.2014.00292

Jacobson, L., Koslowsky, M., and Lavidor, M. (2012). tDCS polarity effects in motor and cognitive domains: a meta-analytical review. *Exp. Brain Res.* 216, 1–10. doi: 10.1007/s00221-011-2891-9

James, D. R. C., Orihuela-Espina, F., Leff, D. R., Sodergren, M. H., Athanasiou, T., Darzi, A. W., et al. (2011). The ergonomics of natural orifice translumenal endoscopic surgery (NOTES) navigation in terms of performance, stress and cognitive behavior. *Surgery* 149, 525–533. doi: 10.1016/j.surg.2010.11.019

Jones, K. T., Gözenman, F., and Berryhill, M. E. (2015). The strategy and motivational influences on the beneficial effect of neurostimulation: a tDCS and fNIRS study. *Neuroimage* 105, 238–247. doi: 10.1016/j.neuroimage.2014.11.012

Khan, B., Hodics, T., Hervey, N., Kondraske, G., Stowe, A. M., and Alexandrakis, G. (2013). Functional near-infrared spectroscopy maps cortical plasticity underlying altered motor performance induced by transcranial direct current stimulation. *J. Biomed. Opt.* 18:116003. doi: 10.1117/1.JBO.18.11.116003

Kopton, I. M., and Kenning, P. (2014). Near-infrared spectroscopy (NIRS) as a new tool for neuroeconomic research. *Front. Hum. Neurosci.* 8:549. doi: 10.3389/fnhum.2014.00549

Kouijzer, M. E. J., de Moor, J. M. H., Gerrits, B. J. L., Congedo, M., and van Schie, H. T. (2009). Neurofeedback improves executive functioning in children with autism spectrum disorders. *Res. Autism Spectr. Disord.* 3, 145–162. doi: 10.1016/j.rasd.2008.05.001

Kwon, Y. H., and Jang, S. H. (2011). The enhanced cortical activation induced by transcranial direct current stimulation during hand movements. *Neurosci. Lett.* 492, 105–108. doi: 10.1016/j.neulet.2011.01.066

Lareau, E., Lesage, F., Pouliot, P., Nguyen, D., Le Lan, J., and Sawan, M. (2011). Multichannel wearable system dedicated for simultaneous electroencephalography/near-infrared spectroscopy real-time data acquisitions. *J. Biomed. Opt.* 16:096014. doi: 10.1117/1.3625575

Leamy, D., Collins, R., and Ward, T. (2011). "Combining fNIRS and EEG to improve motor cortex activity classification during an imagined movement-based task," in *Foundations of Augmented Cognition. Directing the Future of Adaptive Systems*, eds D. D. Schmorrow and C. M. Fidopiastis (Berlin Heidelberg: Springer), 177–185.

Lebedev, M. (2014). Brain-machine interfaces: an overview. *Transl. Neurosci.* 5, 99–110. doi: 10.2478/s13380-014-0212-z

Lewis, C. M., Baldassarre, A., Committeri, G., Romani, G. L., and Corbetta, M. (2009). Learning sculpts the spontaneous activity of the resting human brain. *Proc. Natl. Acad. Sci. U S A* 106, 17558–17563. doi: 10.1073/pnas.0902455106

Liao, L.-D., Lin, C.-T., McDowell, K., Wickenden, A. E., Gramann, K., Jung, T.-P., et al. (2012). Biosensor technologies for augmented brain-computer interfaces in the next decades. *Proc. IEEE* 100, 1553–1566. doi: 10.1109/jproc.2012.2184829

Liebetanz, D., Nitsche, M. A., Tergau, F., and Paulus, W. (2002). Pharmacological approach to the mechanisms of transcranial DC-stimulation-induced after-effects of human motor cortex excitability. *Brain* 125, 2238–2247. doi: 10.1093/brain/awf238

Lim, C. G., Lee, T. S., Guan, C., Fung, D. S., Zhao, Y., Teng, S. S., et al. (2012). A brain-computer interface based attention training program for treating attention deficit hyperactivity disorder. *PLoS One* 7:e46692. doi: 10.1371/journal.pone.0046692

Lövdén, M., Bodammer, N. C., Kühn, S., Kaufmann, J., Schütze, H., Tempelmann, C., et al. (2010). Experience-dependent plasticity of white-matter microstructure extends into old age. *Neuropsychologia* 48, 3878–3883. doi: 10.1016/j.neuropsychologia.2010.08.026

Lubar, J. F., Swartwood, M. O., Swartwood, J. N., and O'Donnell, P. H. (1995). Evaluation of the effectiveness of EEG neurofeedback training for ADHD in a clinical setting as measured by changes in TOVA scores, behavioral ratings and WISC-R performance. *Biofeedback Self Regul.* 20, 83–99. doi: 10.1007/bf01712768

Makeig, S., Gramann, K., Jung, T.-P., Sejnowski, T. J., and Poizner, H. (2009). Linking brain, mind and behavior. *Int. J. Psychophysiol.* 73, 95–100. doi: 10.1016/j.ijpsycho.2008.11.008

Mandrick, K., Derosiere, G., Dray, G., Coulon, D., Micallef, J.-P., and Perrey, S. (2013). Prefrontal cortex activity during motor tasks with additional mental load requiring attentional demand: a near-infrared spectroscopy study. *Neurosci. Res.* 76, 156–162. doi: 10.1016/j.neures.2013.04.006

Mangia, A. L., Pirini, M., and Cappello, A. (2014). Transcranial direct current stimulation and power spectral parameters: a tDCS/EEG co-registration study. *Front. Hum. Neurosci.* 8:601. doi: 10.3389/fnhum.2014.00601

McKendrick, R., Ayaz, H., Olmstead, R., and Parasuraman, R. (2014). Enhancing dual-task performance with verbal and spatial working memory training: continuous monitoring of cerebral hemodynamics with NIRS. *Neuroimage* 85(Pt. 3), 1014–1026. doi: 10.1016/j.neuroimage.2013.05.103

McKinley, R. A., McIntire, L., Bridges, N., Goodyear, C., and Weisend, M. P. (2013). Acceleration of image analyst training with transcranial direct current stimulation. *Behav. Neurosci.* 127, 936–946. doi: 10.1037/a0034975

Mehta, R. K., and Parasuraman, R. (2013). Neuroergonomics: a review of applications to physical and cognitive work. *Front. Hum. Neurosci.* 7:889. doi: 10.3389/fnhum.2013.00889

Mehta, R. K., and Parasuraman, R. (2014). Effects of mental fatigue on the development of physical fatigue: a neuroergonomic approach. *Hum. Factors* 56, 645–656. doi: 10.1177/0018720813507279

Merzagora, A. C., Foffani, G., Panyavin, I., Mordillo-Mateos, L., Aguilar, J., Onaral, B., et al. (2010). Prefrontal hemodynamic changes produced by anodal direct current stimulation. *Neuroimage* 49, 2304–2310. doi: 10.1016/j.neuroimage.2009.10.044

Mihajlovic, V., Grundlehner, B., Vullers, R., and Penders, J. (2015). Wearable, wireless EEG Solutions in daily life applications: what are we missing? *IEEE J. Biomed. Health Inform.* 19, 6–21. doi: 10.1109/JBHI.2014.2328317

Miller, K., Schalk, G., Fetz, E., den Nijs, M., Ojemann, J., and Rao, R. (2010). Cortical activity during motor execution, motor imagery and imagery-based online feedback. *Proc. Natl. Acad. Sci. U S A* 107, 4430–4435. doi: 10.1073/pnas.0913697107

Muehlemann, T., Haensse, D., and Wolf, M. (2008). Wireless miniaturized in-vivo near infrared imaging. *Opt. Express* 16, 10323–10330. doi: 10.1364/oe.16.010323

Muthalib, M., Dutta, A., Besson, P., Rothwell, J., Ward, T., and Perrey, S. (2014). "Comparison of online vs offline effects of HD-tDCS induced modulation of cortical sensorimotor networks using a combined fNIRS-EEG setup," in *Poster presented at the International Society on Oxygen Transport to Tissues (ISOTT) Conference* (London).

Muthalib, M., Kan, B., Nosaka, K., and Perrey, S. (2013). "Effects of transcranial direct current stimulation of the motor cortex on prefrontal cortex activation during a neuromuscular fatigue task: an fNIRS study," in *Oxygen Transport to Tissue XXXV*, eds S. Van Huffel G. Naulaers A. Caicedo D. F. Bruley and D. K. Harrison (New York: Springer), 73–79.

Naseer, N., and Keum-Shik, H. (2013). "Functional near-infrared spectroscopy based discrimination of mental counting and no-control state for development of a brain-computer interface," in *Engineering in Medicine and Biology Society (EMBC), 35th Annual International Conference of the IEEE*, 1780–1783.

Nijboer, F., Clausen, J., Allison, B. Z., and Haselager, P. (2011). The asilomar survey: stakeholders' opinions on ethical issues related to brain-computer interfacing. *Neuroethics* 6, 541–578. doi: 10.1007/s12152-011-9132-6

Ninaus, M., Kober, S. E., Witte, M., Koschutnig, K., Stangl, M., Neuper, C., et al. (2013). Neural substrates of cognitive control under the belief of getting neurofeedback training. *Front. Hum. Neurosci.* 7:914. doi: 10.3389/fnhum.2013.00914

Nitsche, M., and Paulus, W. (2000). Excitability changes induced in the human motor cortex by weak transcranial direct current stimulation. *J. Physiol.* 527, 633–639. doi: 10.1111/j.1469-7793.2000.t01-1-00633.x

O'Doherty, J. E., Lebedev, M. A., Ifft, P. J., Zhuang, K. Z., Shokur, S., Bleuler, H., et al. (2011). Active tactile exploration using a brain-machine-brain interface. *Nature* 479, 228–231. doi: 10.1038/nature10489

Pais-Vieira, M., Lebedev, M., Kunicki, C., Wang, J., and Nicolelis, M. A. L. (2013). A brain-to-brain interface for real-time sharing of sensorimotor information. *Sci. Rep.* 3:1319. doi: 10.1038/srep01319

Parasuraman, R. (2003). Neuroergonomics: research and practice. *Theor. Issues Ergon. Sci.* 4, 5–20. doi: 10.1080/14639220210199753

Parasuraman, R. (2011). Neuroergonomics brain, cognition and performance at work. *Curr. Dir. Psychol. Sci.* 20, 181–186. doi: 10.1177/0963721411409176

Parasuraman, R., and Galster, S. (2013). Sensing, assessing and augmenting threat detection: behavioral, neuroimaging and brain stimulation evidence for the critical role of attention. *Front. Hum. Neurosci.* 7:273. doi: 10.3389/fnhum.2013.00273

Parasuraman, R., and Mckinley, R. A. (2014). Using noninvasive brain stimulation to accelerate learning and enhance human performance. *Hum. Factors* 56, 816–824. doi: 10.1177/0018720814538815

Parasuraman, R., and Rizzo, M. (2007). *Neuroergonomics: The Brain at Work.* New York, NY: Oxford University Press.

Rahman, A., Reato, D., Arlotti, M., Gasca, F., Datta, A., Parra, L. C., et al. (2013). Cellular effects of acute direct current stimulation: somatic and synaptic terminal effects. *J. Physiol.* 591, 2563–2578. doi: 10.1113/jphysiol.2012.247171

Raymond, J., Varney, C., Parkinson, L. A., and Gruzelier, J. H. (2005). The effects of alpha/theta neurofeedback on personality and mood. *Brain Res. Cogn. Brain Res.* 23, 287–292. doi: 10.1016/j.cogbrainres.2004.10.023

Rodriguez, M., and Pourrezaei, K. (2011). *Development of a Versatile Wireless fNIR System.* Philadelphia, PA: Masters Degree, Drexel University.

Safaie, J., Grebe, R., Abrishami Moghaddam, H., and Wallois, F. (2013). Toward a fully integrated wireless wearable EEG-NIRS bimodal acquisition system. *J. Neural Eng.* 10:056001. doi: 10.1088/1741-2560/10/5/056001

Saiote, C., Turi, Z., Paulus, W., and Antal, A. (2013). Combining functional magnetic resonance imaging with transcranial electrical stimulation. *Front. Hum. Neurosci.* 7:435. doi: 10.3389/fnhum.2013.00435

Sao, V., Pourrezaei, K., Akin, A., and Ayaz, H. (2003). "Breast tumor imaging using NIR LED based handheld continuous-wave imager," in *Bioengineering Conference, IEEE 29th Annual, Proceedings of* (IEEE).

Sato, H., Yahata, N., Funane, T., Takizawa, R., Katura, T., Atsumori, H., et al. (2013). A NIRS-fMRI investigation of prefrontal cortex activity during a working memory task. *Neuroimage* 83, 158–173. doi: 10.1016/j.neuroimage.2013.06.043

Schermer, M. (2009). The mind and the machine. On the conceptual and moral implications of brain-machine interaction. *Nanoethics* 3, 217–230. doi: 10.1007/s11569-009-0076-9

Schestatsky, P., Morales-Quezada, L., and Fregni, F. (2013). Simultaneous EEG monitoring during transcranial direct current stimulation. *J. Vis. Exp.* 76:e50426. doi: 10.3791/50426

Schudlo, L. C., and Chau, T. (2014). Dynamic topographical pattern classification of multichannel prefrontal NIRS signals: II. Online differentiation of mental arithmetic and rest. *J. Neural Eng.* 11:016003. doi: 10.1088/1741-2560/11/1/016003

Shapiro, M. G., Homma, K., Villarreal, S., Richter, C.-P., and Bezanilla, F. (2012). Infrared light excites cells by changing their electrical capacitance. *Nat. Commun.* 3:736. doi: 10.1038/ncomms1742

Slagter, H. A., Davidson, R. J., and Lutz, A. (2011). Mental training as a tool in the neuroscientific study of brain and cognitive plasticity. *Front. Hum. Neurosci.* 5:17. doi: 10.3389/fnhum.2011.00017

Solovey, E. T., Afergan, D., Peck, E. M., Hincks, S. W., and Jacob, R. J. K. (2015). Designing implicit interfaces for physiological computing: guidelines and lessons learned using fNIRS. *ACM Trans. Comput. Hum. Interact.* 21, 1–27. doi: 10.1145/2687926

Stopczynski, A., Stahlhut, C., Petersen, M. K., Larsen, J. E., Jensen, C. F., Ivanova, M. G., et al. (2014). Smartphones as pocketable labs: visions for mobile brain imaging and neurofeedback. *Int. J. Psychophysiol.* 91, 54–66. doi: 10.1016/j.ijpsycho.2013.08.007

Strenziok, M., Parasuraman, R., Clarke, E., Cisler, D. S., Thompson, J. C., and Greenwood, P. M. (2014). Neurocognitive enhancement in older adults: comparison of three cognitive training tasks to test a hypothesis of training transfer in brain connectivity. *Neuroimage* 85, 1027–1039. doi: 10.1016/j.neuroimage.2013.07.069

Villamar, M. F., Volz, M. S., Bikson, M., Datta, A., Dasilva, A. F., and Fregni, F. (2013). Technique and considerations in the use of 4x1 ring high-definition transcranial direct current stimulation (HD-tDCS). *J. Vis. Exp.* e50309. doi: 10.3791/50309

Villringer, A., and Chance, B. (1997). Non-invasive optical spectroscopy and imaging of human brain function. *Trends Neurosci.* 20, 435–442. doi: 10.1016/s0166-2236(97)01132-6

Vlek, R. J., Steines, D., Szibbo, D., Kubler, A., Schneider, M. J., Haselager, P., et al. (2012). Ethical issues in brain-computer interface research, development and dissemination. *J. Neurol. Phys. Ther.* 36, 94–99. doi: 10.1097/npt.0b013e31825064cc

Voss, M. W., Prakash, R. S., Erickson, K. I., Boot, W. R., Basak, C., Neider, M. B., et al. (2012). Effects of training strategies implemented in a complex videogame on functional connectivity of attentional networks. *Neuroimage* 59, 138–148. doi: 10.1016/j.neuroimage.2011.03.052

Walsh, V., and Pascual-Leone, A. (2005). *Transcranial Magnetic Stimulation: A Neurochronometrics of Mind.* Cambridge, MA: Bradford.

Weingarten, M. S., Papazoglou, E. S., Zubkov, L., Zhu, L., Neidrauer, M., Savir, G., et al. (2008). Correlation of near infrared absorption and diffuse reflectance spectroscopy scattering with tissue neovascularization and collagen concentration in a diabetic rat wound healing model. *Wound Repair Regen.* 16, 234–242. doi: 10.1111/j.1524-475x.2008.00364.x

Wells, J., Kao, C., Jansen, E. D., Konrad, P., and Mahadevan-Jansen, A. (2005a). Application of infrared light for in vivo neural stimulation. *J. Biomed. Opt.* 10:064003. doi: 10.1117/1.2121772

Wells, J., Kao, C., Mariappan, K., Albea, J., Jansen, E. D., Konrad, P., et al. (2005b). Optical stimulation of neural tissue in vivo. *Opt. Lett.* 30, 504–506. doi: 10.1364/ol.30.000504

Wolpaw, J. R., Birbaumer, N., Mcfarland, D. J., Pfurtscheller, G., and Vaughan, T. M. (2002). Brain-computer interfaces for communication and control. *Clin. Neurophysiol.* 113, 767–791. doi: 10.1016/S1388-2457(02)00057-3

Yamauchi, Y., Kikuchi, S., Miwakeichi, F., Matsumoto, K., Nishida, M., Ishiguro, M., et al. (2013). Relation between parametric change of the workload and prefrontal cortex activity during a modified version of the 'rock, paper, scissors' task. *Neuropsychobiology* 68, 24–33. doi: 10.1159/000350948

Yerkes, R. M., and Dodson, J. D. (1908). The relation of strength of stimulus to rapidity of habit-formation. *J. Comp. Neurol. Psychol.* 18, 459–482. doi: 10.1002/cne.920180503

Yoshino, K., Oka, N., Yamamoto, K., Takahashi, H., and Kato, T. (2013a). Correlation of prefrontal cortical activation with changing vehicle speeds in actual driving: a vector-based functional near-infrared spectroscopy study. *Front. Hum. Neurosci.* 7:895. doi: 10.3389/fnhum.2013.00895

Yoshino, K., Oka, N., Yamamoto, K., Takahashi, H., and Kato, T. (2013b). Functional brain imaging using near-infrared spectroscopy during actual driving on an expressway. *Front. Hum. Neurosci.* 7:882. doi: 10.3389/fnhum.2013.00882

Yurtsever, G., Ayaz, H., Kepics, F., Onaral, B., and Pourrezaei, K. (2006). *Wireless, Continuous Wave Near Infrared Spectroscopy System for Monitoring Brain Activity.* Philadelphia, PA: Drexel University.

4

Predictive technologies: can smart tools augment the brain's predictive abilities?

Giovanni Pezzulo[1]*, *Alessandro D'Ausilio*[2] *and Andrea Gaggioli*[3,4]

[1] Institute of Cognitive Sciences and Technologies, National Research Council, Rome, Italy, [2] IIT - Istituto Italiano di Tecnologia, CTNSC@UniFe - Center of Translational Neurophysiology for Speech and Communication, Ferrara, Italy, [3] Department of Psychology, Università Cattolica del Sacro Cuore, Milan, Italy, [4] Applied Technology for Neuro-Psychology Lab, I.R.C.C.S. Istituto Auxologico Italiano, Milan, Italy

Edited by:
Mikhail Lebedev,
Duke University, USA

Reviewed by:
Victor Manuel Pulgar,
Wake Forest School of Medicine, USA
Emiliano Macaluso,
Fondazione Santa Lucia, Italy

***Correspondence:**
Giovanni Pezzulo
giovanni.pezzulo@istc.cnr.it

The ability of "looking into the future"—namely, the capacity of anticipating future states of the environment or of the body—represents a fundamental function of human (and animal) brains. A goalkeeper who tries to guess the ball's direction; a chess player who attempts to anticipate the opponent's next move; or a man-in-love who tries to calculate what are the chances of her saying yes—in all these cases, people are simulating possible future states of the world, in order to maximize the success of their decisions or actions. Research in neuroscience is showing that our ability to predict the behavior of physical or social phenomena is largely dependent on the brain's ability to integrate current and past information to generate (probabilistic) simulations of the future. But could predictive processing be augmented using advanced technologies? In this contribution, we discuss how computational technologies may be used to support, facilitate or enhance the prediction of future events, by considering exemplificative scenarios across different domains, from simpler sensorimotor decisions to more complex cognitive tasks. We also examine the key scientific and technical challenges that must be faced to turn this vision into reality.

Keywords: predictive processing, planning, robotics, augmented reality, brain stimulation

INTRODUCTION

Modern cognitive neuroscience describes the brain as a predictive device, not a stimulus-response system. In this "predictive brain" perspective, the brain continuously predicts environmental dynamics and anticipates action effects, and this permits animals to be "ahead of time" when it takes decisions, rather than just react to what it currently senses (Pezzulo, 2008; Bar, 2009; Friston, 2010). Predictive abilities range from short-term predictions, which target (say) the few hundreds of milliseconds—the timescale of the sensorimotor loop, which is relevant to predict (say) whether or not to cross a busy road—to medium- or long-term predictions, which are useful for distal decisions such as the road to take to go home or the career to choose.

Recent research is shedding light on the neuronal underpinnings of these diverse abilities. For example, a growing literature studies predictive dynamics in sensorimotor control, highlighting the importance of so-called forward models: internal models that the brain uses to predict action consequences and plan accurate movements (Wolpert and Ghahramani, 2000). Even more interesting, research in "motor cognition" has shown that these forward models can be widely reused outside motor control, in more cognitive such as domains action recognition, action simulation and imagery (Jeannerod, 2006). Predictive domains, have been widely studied in many other domains of cognition, such as perceptual processing and navigation. For example, growing evidence indicates that internally generated brain dynamics in the (rodent) hippocampus might support navigational planning: in fact, if one registers from the hippocampus of rodents at rest before a decision, one can find neuronal sequences of place cells assembled to form trajectories in T-mazes, which can be predictive of the actual trajectories that they will select immediately afterwards (Johnson and Redish, 2007; Pfeiffer and Foster, 2013; Pezzulo et al., 2014). Based on parallels between neurophysiological evidence and human neuroimaging studies, it has been (speculatively) proposed that the ability to internally generate and "mesh" dynamical events—especially in the hippocampus—might support sophisticated prospective abilities such as the mental simulation of future events and "mental time travel" (Schacter et al., 2012; Buzsáki et al., 2014).

From the "predictive brain" perspective, the ubiquity of predictive components across cognitive domains reflects the fact that brain processing is intrinsically predictive. The most comprehensive attempt to describe formally the "predictive brain" perspective is the *free energy principle* developed by Friston and collaborators (Friston, 2010; Pezzulo et al., 2015). In this perspective, the brain is a statistical machine that learns a so-called *generative model* of external dynamics (especially how the environment changes as a function of the agent's actions) and uses it for continuous prediction. Importantly, prediction can be at multiple timescales, where these timescales map to brain hierarchies (especially cortical hierarchies) and increase from motor and premotor areas to prefrontal areas (Badre, 2008). Here, cognition depends on the interplay of top-down and bottom-up signals across (brain) hierarchical layers, the former propagating predictions and the latter prediction errors. Minimizing prediction errors (the difference from what is expected and what is sensed) across layers—or more formally minimizing free energy—supports both perception (because perceptual hypotheses encoded at higher levels can be revised based on prediction errors) and action (because goals encoded at higher hierarchical layers generate a cascade of exteroceptive and proprioceptive predictions, say on the next desired hand position, and the latter are ultimately suppressed by engaged reflexes that—essentially—guide the hand to the desired position). The same principles of prediction error minimization have been extended to model the planning of action sequences—when, essentially, predictions stemming from the generative model (encoding the agent's knowledge of action-outcome contingencies) are "chained" to covertly simulate and evaluate possible action plans in advance, before the agent performs any actual action or receives external feedback (Friston et al., 2012, 2015).

In sum, the idea of a "predictive brain" is becoming dominant in cognitive neuroscience. In this article, we explore an intriguing technological side of this phenomenon: the possible development of "predictive technologies" that augment human prediction. We address questions such as: is it possible to augment predictive abilities in humans using technologies? Which kind of predictions can be enhanced? Is it possible to use enhanced predictive abilities to improve real-time decisions and actions? What are the key scientific/technological issues for developing predictive technologies? And what are their potential applications?

Of course, prediction-based technologies are already routinely used, for example, in weather or stock market forecast, or in the development of smart (e.g., self-guiding) cars. Here, however, we specifically focus on *predictive technologies that can be seamlessly integrated into real-time human cognition, and augment it.* We discuss, for example, new interfaces that help humans predict the movements of a car in order to decide when to cross a busy road. Below we consider this and other specific examples of predictive technologies that—we will argue—might be soon within our reach.

DOMAINS OF ENHANCED PREDICTION

Human cognitive tasks involve short-, medium- or long-term predictions—and at least in principle, predictive technologies can support all them. Here we focus our analysis on predictive technologies that can support real-time, embodied decisions (Cisek and Pastor-Bernier, 2014; Lepora and Pezzulo, 2015), such as for example those that we continuously face when we drive a car (should I accelerate or press the brake?), which are based on short-term predictions of the order of hundreds of milliseconds (am I risking a collision with a pedestrian?) or sometimes medium-term predictions; but we do not target decisions that unfold over longer-term timescales such as "which University or career should I select?".

It is important to distinguish between two potential outputs of predictive technologies. The first, direct output of a predictive technology is enhancing a person's prediction abilities. For example, the technology might help a goalkeeper predicting the trajectory of a penalty kick, on the basis of (say) statistical information about past penalty kicks and the movements of the attacker. A second, more indirect output of predictive technologies is aiding decision-making and/or planning (based on prediction). For example, the predictive technology might suggest the goalkeeper the action course that maximizes the probability to parry the penalty kick, given the predicted trajectory. Below we provide examples of both kinds.

Consider the case of a person who wants to cross a busy road. Deciding when to cross is a complex embodied decision that has to take into consideration several factors, from cognitive rules and knowledge (e.g., knowledge of traffic rules; presence of traffic lights) to situational facts (e.g., where are the cars and at what velocity they run; what my own velocity is; how long the road to be crossed is). Various predictions can be useful to solve this task, such as the prediction of "where" a car is going, "whether" it will stop or "when" it will arrive at the crossing point. There are cases when an augmentation technology may help, such as when the person who is crossing has impaired perceptual or cognitive abilities, or comes from another culture (think of a Chinese tourist crossing a busy road in Rome).

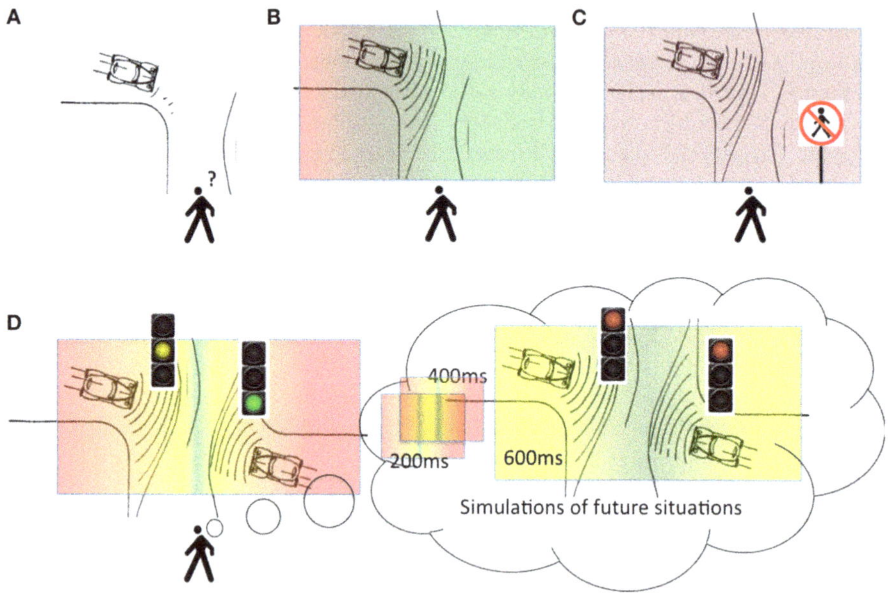

FIGURE 1 | How the affordance landscape changes as an effect of car movements and traffic signs. (A) An example situation: a pedestrian has to cross a road, with a car approaching. **(B)** The same situation, but now with the putative results of a predictive technology superimposed: here, the lines in front of the car represent its predicted future locations, and the colors represent a gradient of the "cross-ability" affordance (red = not crossable; green = crossable) ordered in a continuum. **(C)** The same situation with a traffic panel does not afford cross-ability anymore. **(D)** A more complex scenario, in which the predictive technology might simulate future simulated situations, e.g., display how the affordance landscape will change in the next 200, 400, and 600 ms.

How can we design a predictive technology that augments human cognition in this kind of situation? A useful starting point is the notion of an "affordance," which originates from ecological psychology (Gibson, 1979) but is also used in neuroscience (Cisek and Kalaska, 2010; Pezzulo and Cisek, 2016). In this perspective, an empty street *affords* "cross-ability," whereas a busy road does not. More generally, one can think of a "landscape" of affordances, which changes as an effect of environmental dynamics and our own actions. For example a car approaching fast in our direction (see **Figure 1**) modifies the landscape of "cross-ability" over time: when the car is far, the road is cross-able; but when it approaches, it becomes not cross-able. The concept of a landscape of affordances is dynamical and highly context-sensitive, in the sense that (for example) there is a gradient of "cross-ability" over time and it depends on both our and the car's velocity and direction, as well as the color of the traffic light (see **Figures 1B–D**).

While ecological psychology has often focused on the idea of exploiting available affordances (e.g., use the "sit-ability" of a chair to sit down), here we recast this concept in predictive terms, and discuss how the *prediction* of (for example) car movements permits to foresee how the affordance landscape will change in the immediate future - and to spot in advance the right time window to cross the road. **Figure 2B** exemplifies the potential benefits of a predictive technology: an augmented reality display that shows (predictively) the affordance landscape and signals that a good time frame for crossing the road is approaching (see later for a discussion of the feasibility of this technology and its required components). Coming back to our previous distinction between "prediction" and "prediction-based decision or planning," here the curved lines around the car represent its predicted future locations, while the colored parts represent the future predicted affordances (red = not crossable; green = crossable)—which can be considered as an aid to the decision (when and where to cross) based on the predicted car trajectory.

Another, more complex example concerns the decision of which path to take to cross a crossroad and reach a supermarket. This can be considered analogous to the "travel planning" functionality of Google maps (https://www.google.it/maps), which already takes several factors into account (e.g., length, size of streets, current traffic) to provide an estimate of "the best" or "the faster" road. Predictive technologies can extend these functionalities by considering various contextual factors, such as the current "cross-ability" affordances (as above) and the anticipated effort associated to the different paths (e.g., one path might require climbing stairs)—which in turn might require predicting energy expenditure based on physiological signals (e.g., heart rate) or other information (e.g., age). Here, different from the former example, the predictive technology would not (only) show a field of affordances, but—like Google maps—propose several paths and suggest the best one. Importantly, this exemplifies a medium-term decision, not a short-term decision as in road crossing case, and it can incorporate various elements and various predictions, at short and medium terms.

As a third example, let's consider a professional domain: an aircraft pilot who has to decide which buttons to press, which levers to pull, which indicators to look at, etc. A predictive technology might help pilots predict (for example) the outcome of different maneuver by directing attention to the controls

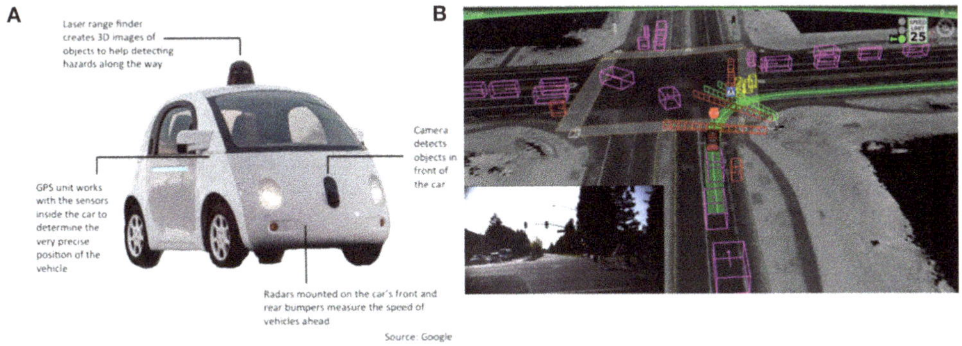

FIGURE 2 | Examples of enabling technologies. (A) Sensors of a self-driving car (source: Google). **(B)** Schematic of how objects are represented (from the self-guiding car's perspective) while approaching a turn; the inset shows what a human driver sees from inside the car. This representation can be used to generate predictions (e.g., of the trajectory of cars and pedestrians) based, for example, on probabilistic mechanisms (Thrun et al., 2006).

that are likely to show the most critical information. These functionalities might be useful for pilots but more critically to those who are learning to fly; the latter might learn faster if their attention is directed to the most relevant displays or controls.

As these examples illustrate, predictive technologies can augment human predictive abilities and be flexibly incorporated into human cognition, providing raw predictions (of car movements), suggestions (of a road to take) or guiding attention (to the most-likely-to-be-useful displays)—just to make a few examples.

ENABLING TECHNOLOGIES

In the previous section we have briefly discussed a few examples of predictive technologies and their use in everyday life. These examples are (on purpose) beyond the scope of the current state of the art. However, some components required by predictive technologies—software or hardware—are already available as components of existing technologies, or are currently studied as part of research programs. Here we provide some examples of enabling technologies that might support the future development of predictive technologies.

Self-driving cars are under development by many companies (e.g., Google, Tesla) and they might enter in the market in the near future. Self-driving cars already use many technologies—from sensors such as laser cameras and radars to dedicated processors—that can be integrated in future predictive technologies, see **Figure 2A**. Furthermore, at the software level, self-driving cars use prediction for control and planning—for example, to predict car trajectories that avoid collisions; and some of the solutions implemented in self-driving cars might be reused within human augmentation systems such as those that we described in the previous section.

Although self-driving cars use a range of diverse mechanisms, some solutions to key problems such as self-localization, path planning, data fusion and trajectory prediction are reused from robot navigation (Thrun et al., 2006) and most can be solved using probabilistic prediction methods (Thrun et al., 2006). Predictive mechanisms, and in particular methods for approximate-but-fast prediction figure prominently in both robot navigation (Montemerlo et al., 2002) and self-driving cars.

Another example of predictive algorithm that was initially developed for robotics but might be reused (or modified) within predictive technologies is the "internal world model" used by Ripley the robot (Roy et al., 2004). The system uses a physical engine to simulate or predict the robot movements, and to keep the "world model" of the robot updated—for example, to keep simulating the trajectory of a moving ball even if the robot is looking somewhere else. In this way, the robot's internal model is continuously "in register" with the external world. This software exemplifies the idea of using a physical engine—of the kind used, for example, in computer games—to run physically realistic simulations. Many widely-used physical engines are very accurate and can afford real-time simulation or prediction. Of course, they cannot simulate everything with the required level of accuracy (and in real time), thus their putative role within a predictive technology can only be evaluated case-by-case.

Physical engines have been also used for simulation in a series of studies on human physical scene understanding, such as how well humans predict how towers of wooden bricks will fall down (Battaglia et al., 2013). This study illustrates that a physical engine simulation can be used to predict in real time a challenging physical event that derives from the interaction of many components (here, many wooden bricks). This method might be extended to predict how other physical events (e.g., movements of objects such as cars) unfold in time.

Another example of a computational solution developed within robotics is the idea of "affordance gradients": a formalism that describes the transformations that can be applied on an object (e.g., how a triangular object rotates when it is pushed or pulled) and permits a robot to plan actions that exploit the affordances to achieve goals (e.g., plan a series of pushing actions that guide the triangular object to a desired or goal position, see Sanchez-Fibla et al., 2011). This method can be potentially reused outside robotics to represent e.g., the affordances of objects and infer their dynamics.

As these examples demonstrate, some component solutions of predictive technologies are available or under development. At the same time, these are still incomplete solutions to the problems of prediction, planning and decision, especially in real time (Geffner, 2013; Donnarumma et al., 2016). Thus, a key challenge for future research is integrating and extending these (and other) models to deliver predictive technologies that are effective and usable. Another key issue is making predictive technologies *usable*—a theme that we explore next.

REPRESENTING PREDICTIVE INFORMATION

A key challenge of predictive technologies is how to represent the information about an upcoming event (predictive cue). As suggested earlier, augmented reality may provide a viable solution. An augmented reality system allows superimposing digital information on the physical environment in real-time using a smartphone or head-mounted see-through displays coupled with a wearable computer. Thanks to recent progresses, current augmented reality systems afford real-time applications in which the user can interact with synthetic objects, manipulate them and receive additional information about the environment or the task at hand, in the form of images, text, video, audio components, etc.

Predictive information could be represented in augmented reality using various levels of abstraction, ranging from analog models to symbolic cues. For example, consider the question of how to represent the predicted trajectory of a ball. One could either visualize a virtual ball that precedes the actual ball (analog representation) or use a dynamic arrow (symbolic representation). In choosing the most appropriate representation of the predictive cue, a key requirement is the definition of temporal constraints. If the augmentation cue is too complex, its processing time may even exceed the timeframe available to complete the task, thus rendering the augmentation useless. For example, in rallying the pacenotes are a commonly used method of describing a route to be taken, in terms of turnings, junctions, the degree and severity of bends etc. The notes are designed to help the driver anticipating the conditions of the course ahead, but with a fast-moving vehicle, they are encoded to carry maximal information in minimum reading time. Relatedly, the design of AR interface should take into account user's cognitive requirements, i.e., by preventing split-attention between multiple predictive cues while preserving global situation awareness. This translates to the need for optimizing the trade-off between cue's maximal informativity about upcoming event(s) and least cognitive processing effort.

A further issue is whether, and in which ways, the presentation of the predictive cue could affect the course of the predicted event. For example, if a goalkeeper is shown the prediction that the penalty taker is going to place the ball at the lower right corner, he/she will jump as fast as possible to the lower right corner in order to reach the ball. However, if the goalkeeper initiates the movement too early, the penalty taker may notice the goalkeeper's intention and kick the ball in the opposite corner. Thus, in designing augmented predictions, it is necessary to model the complex interdependencies between the user's action and the context of his/her action, in order to prevent the predictive cue triggering behaviors that affect the course of events in (unpredictable) ways.

CONCLUSIONS

We have explored the idea of using technology to augment the human ability of predicting future events, by seamlessly integrating anticipatory information in the perception-action loop. The presentation of predictive cues is meant to facilitate perceptual, decision and action processes. Some key building blocks of predictive technology are available from developments in robotics and machine learning. In these fields, the need of accurately modeling the evolution of complex system has led to the deployment of computational solutions that could be eventually re-adapted to match the requirements of predictive cognition. However, the provision of external cues may not be the only possible approach to augment predictive processing. A rather more ambitious strategy could be to directly stimulating brain areas that are implicated in the computation of future events. Numerous studies have shown the possibility of modulating, and in some cases enhancing, cognitive processes by exciting brain regions involved in working memory and attention through transcranial electrical brain stimulation, including planning ability (Dockery et al., 2009). This approach could be justifiable within rehabilitation domains, where the goal would be to restore or support predictive functions in individuals suffering from neurocognitive impairments.

As the rehabilitation example suggests, predictive technologies hold the promise to enable a wide range of applications based on the extension of our prediction and planning abilities. Such application scenarios may include, but are not be limited to, anticipation of sources of dangers in natural or working environments for enhancing personal safety; support decision making and judgments in emergency situations; optimization of team coordination in complex collaboration tasks. Clearly, the exploitation of these possibilities require to address significant scientific and technological challenges, some of which have been outlined in this contribution. However, as understanding of cognitive mechanisms involved in predicting future progresses, so should the ability of enhancing these processes using advanced technologies.

AUTHOR CONTRIBUTIONS

GP and AG jointly conceived the main idea behind the article. GP drafted the manuscript. AD and AG gave conceptual advice and revised the manuscript critically for important intellectual content. GP and AG edited the manuscript. All authors read and approved the final manuscript.

ACKNOWLEDGMENTS

GP is funded by the EU's FP7 Initiative (grant FP7-270108) and the HFSP (grant RGY0088/2014).

REFERENCES

Badre, D. (2008). Cognitive control, hierarchy, and the rostro-caudal organization of the frontal lobes. *Trends Cogn. Sci.* 12, 193–200. doi: 10.1016/j.tics.2008.02.004

Bar, M. (2009). The proactive brain: memory for predictions. *Philos. Trans. R. Soc. Lond. B Biol. Sci.* 364, 1235–1243. doi: 10.1098/rstb.2008.0310

Battaglia, P. W., Hamrick, J. B., and Tenenbaum, J. B. (2013). Simulation as an engine of physical scene understanding. *Proc. Natl. Acad. Sci. U.S.A.* 110, 18327–18332. doi: 10.1073/pnas.1306572110

Buzsáki, G., Peyrache, A., and Kubie, J. (2014). Emergence of cognition from action. *Cold Spring Harb. Symp. Quant. Biol.* 79, 41–50. doi: 10.1101/sqb.2014.79.024679

Cisek, P., and Kalaska, J. F. (2010). Neural mechanisms for interacting with a world full of action choices. *Annu. Rev. Neurosci.* 33, 269–298. doi: 10.1146/annurev.neuro.051508.135409

Cisek, P., and Pastor-Bernier, A. (2014). On the challenges and mechanisms of embodied decisions. *Philos. Trans. R Soc. Lond. B Biol. Sci.* 369, 20130479. doi: 10.1098/rstb.2013.0479

Dockery, C. A., Hueckel-Weng, R., Birbaumer, N., and Plewnia, C. (2009). Enhancement of planning ability by transcranial direct current stimulation. *J. Neurosci.* 29, 7271–7277. doi: 10.1523/JNEUROSCI.0065-09.2009

Donnarumma, F., Maisto, D., and Pezzulo, G. (2016). Problem solving as probabilistic inference with subgoaling: explaining human successes and pitfalls in the Tower of Hanoi. *PLoS Comput. Biol.* 12:e1004864. doi: 10.1371/journal.pcbi.1004864

Friston, K. (2010). The free-energy principle: a unified brain theory? *Nat. Rev. Neurosci.* 11, 127–138. doi: 10.1038/nrn2787

Friston K., Rigoli, F., Ognibene, D., Mathys, C., Fitzgerald, T., and Pezzulo, G. (2015). Active inference and epistemic value. *Cogn. Neurosci.* 6, 187–214. doi: 10.1080/17588928.2015.1020053

Friston, K., Samothrakis, S., and Montague, R. (2012). Active inference and agency: optimal control without cost functions. *Biol. Cybern.* 106, 523–541. doi: 10.1007/s00422-012-0512-8

Geffner, H. (2013). Computational models of planning. *Wiley Interdiscip. Rev. Cogn. Sci.* 4, 341–356. doi: 10.1002/wcs.1233

Gibson, J. J. (1979). *The Ecological Approach to Visual Perception*. Mahwah, NJ: Lawrence Erlbaum Associates, Inc.

Jeannerod, M. (2006). *Motor Cognition*. Oxford: Oxford University Press.

Johnson, A., and Redish, A. D. (2007). Neural ensembles in CA3 transiently encode paths forward of the animal at a decision point. *J. Neurosci.* 27, 12176–12189. doi: 10.1523/JNEUROSCI.3761-07.2007

Lepora, N., and Pezzulo, G. (2015). Embodied Choice: how action influences perceptual decision making. *PLOS Comput. Biol.* 11:e1004110. doi: 10.1371/journal.pcbi.1004110

Montemerlo, M., Thrun, S., Koller, D., and Wegbreit, B. (2002). "FastSLAM: a factored solution to the simultaneous localization and mapping problem," in *Proceedings of the Eighteenth National Conference on Artificial Intelligence* (Edmonton, AB), 593–598.

Pezzulo, G. (2008). Coordinating with the future: the anticipatory nature of representation. *Minds Mach.* 18, 179–225. doi: 10.1007/s11023-008-9095-5

Pezzulo, G., Rigoli, F., and Friston, K. (2015). Active Inference, homeostatic regulation and adaptive behavioural control. *Prog. Neurobiol.* 134, 17–35. doi: 10.1016/j.pneurobio.2015.09.001

Pezzulo, G., van der Meer, M. A., Lansink, C. S., and Pennartz, C. M. (2014). Internally generated sequences in learning and executing goal-directed behavior. *Trends Cogn. Sci.* 18, 647–657. doi: 10.1016/j.tics.2014.06.011

Pezzulo, G. and Cisek, P. (2016). Navigating the affordance landscape: feedback control as a process model of behavior and cognition. *Trends Cogn. Sci.* doi: 10.1016/j.tics.2016.03.013

Pfeiffer, B. E., and Foster, D. J. (2013). Hippocampal place-cell sequences depict future paths to remembered goals. *Nature* 497, 74–79. doi: 10.1038/nature12112

Roy, D., Hsiao, K. Y., and Mavridis, N. (2004). Mental imagery for a conversational robot. *IEEE Trans. Syst. Man. Cybern. B. Cybern.* 34, 1374–1383. doi: 10.1109/TSMCB.2004.823327

Sanchez-Fibla, M., Duff, A., and Verschure, P. F. (2011). "The acquisition of intentionally indexed and object centered affordance gradients: a biomimetic controller and mobile robotics benchmark," in *Intelligent Robots and Systems (IROS), 2011 IEEE/RSJ International Conference on. IEEE*, (San Francisco, CA), 1115–1121.

Schacter, D. L., Addis, D. R., Hassabis, D., Martin, V. C., Spreng, R. N., and Szpunar, K. K. (2012). The future of memory: remembering, imagining, and the brain. *Neuron* 76, 677–694. doi: 10.1016/j.neuron.2012.11.001

Thrun, S., Montemerlo, M., Dahlkamp, H., Stavens, D., Aron, A., Diebel, J. et al. (2006). Stanley: The robot that won the DARPA Grand Challenge. *J. Field Robot.* 23, 661–692. doi: 10.1002/rob.20147

Wolpert, D. M., and Ghahramani, Z. (2000). Computational principles of movement neuroscience. *Nat. Neurosci.* 3, 1212–1217. doi: 10.1038/81497

5

Direct electric stimulation to increase cerebrovascular function

Victor M. Pulgar[1, 2, 3*]

[1] Biomedical Research and Infrastructure Center, Faculty of Natural and Physical Sciences, Winston-Salem State University, Winston-Salem, NC, USA, [2] Hypertension and Vascular Research Center, Wake Forest School of Medicine, Winston-Salem, NC, USA, [3] Department of Obstetrics and Gynecology, Wake Forest School of Medicine, Winston-Salem, NC, USA

Keywords: brain Stimulation, cerebral blood flow (CBF), neurovascular coupling, functional hyperemia, transcranial direct current stimulation (tDCS)

Edited by:
Mikhail Lebedev, Duke University, USA

Reviewed by:
Prasad V. Katakam, Tulane University School of Medicine, USA
Hannah Lucy Filmer, University of Queensland, Australia
Justin Schultz Cetas, Oregon Health and Science University, USA

***Correspondence:**
Victor M. Pulgar, vpulgar@wakehealth.edu

Various conditions affecting the cerebral vasculature may lead to cumulative damage and thus deterioration of brain function, in what has been called vascular cognitive impairment (Gorelick et al., 2011). Consequently, it makes sense that an increase in glucose and oxygen produced by an increase in blood flow may augment brain function. Since its rediscovery some years ago transcranial direct electric stimulation (tDCS) has attracted interest as potential therapy for patients with neurological impairments. This opinion article aims to succinctly review the mechanisms involved in neurogenic control of the cerebral blood flow (CBF) highlighting the potential of direct electrical stimulation targeting cerebral micro vessels to enhance brain function.

With the highest oxygen consumption than any other organ in the body, the brain utilizes around 20% of the total resting oxygen, making it an organ highly dependent on blood supply (Hossmann, 1994). Moreover, a direct relationship between the development of neurodegenerative diseases and impairment of CBF has been postulated (Farkas and Luiten, 2001).

The appropriate delivery of nutrients and oxygen to the brain tissue is regulated by mechanisms including cerebral autoregulation, vascular reactivity and neurovascular coupling. The autoregulatory properties of cerebral circulation make CBF independent of systemic blood pressure. Therefore, over a physiological range of pressure cerebral arteries relax when systemic pressure decreases and constrict when systemic pressure increases (Heistad and Kontos, 1983). Similarly, reactivity of the brain blood vessels to pH and CO_2 has been suggested to link neuronal metabolic changes to cerebral blood flow.

The Neurovascular Unit

One of the unique characteristics of the brain circulation is the intimate contact between blood vessels, neurons, and glia. Thus, neurons, glia, and vascular cells are structurally and functionally related in what is called the "neurovascular unit" (Iadecola, 2004). Since brain PO_2 is tightly regulated in relation to local brain activity, the neurovascular unit provides a framework for the functional interactions responsible for this concerted regulation. Thereby, functional hyperemia means that blood flow will increase in brain areas with increased activity.

From an anatomical point of view, pial arteries traveling on the surface of the brain are highly innervated with terminals coming from the peripheral nervous system (extrinsic innervation) (Hamel, 2006). These vessels are surrounded by the Virchow-Robin's space which gradually disappears as vessels enter the brain parenchyma. Cerebral arteries entering the brain parenchyma lose extrinsic innervation and come into intimate contact with neuronal and glial cells (intrinsic innervation) (Iadecola, 2004). Functions of these two vascular compartments, macro and micro vessels, involve regulation of global blood supply, as wells as control of local CBF and brain blood barrier permeability respectively.

It is currently accepted that postsynaptic increases in $[Ca^{++}]_i$ due to activation of glutamate receptors during synaptic transmission activate the production of vasoactive mediators.

Several mediators such as neurotransmitters, adenosine, arachidonic acid metabolites, nitric oxide (NO), hydrogen and potassium, have been suggested to mediate increases in CBF (Iadecola, 2004).

Due to their close contact with blood vessels, astrocytes are suggested to play an important role in functional hyperemia. Astrocyte's end-feet surround brain micro capillaries, and may mediate neuron-blood vessel communication and thus neuronal activity-induced blood flow changes (Zonta et al., 2003). Vasodilatory as well as vasoconstrictor activities have been ascribed to glial cells (Metea and Newman, 2006), with an important role for glial eNOS in mediating vasodilatation (Stobart et al., 2013). New evidences also point to astrocytes as relevant components of the recently described "glymphatic pathway," an important mechanism for clearance of solutes from the brain (Iliff et al., 2012). Thus, aquaporin water channels in astrocyte's end feet would couple paravascular pathways for the vectorial convective flow of waste products from arterial toward venous routes, with solutes ultimately clearing the brain through the lymphatic system (Nedergaard, 2013).

The brain endothelium is a highly specialized tissue mediating several physiological functions, such as thrombosis, adhesion, permeability and angiogenesis (Daneman and Prat, 2015). A protective function against cerebral dysfunction has been proposed for the brain vessel's endothelium consistent with the predominant role of endothelial dysfunction in several cerebrovascular diseases. Importantly, *in vivo* experiments have shown that endothelial cell-derived NO mediates cortical hyperemia induced by basal forebrain electrical stimulation (Zhang et al., 1995).

Pericytes, cells located outside of the microvessels in intimate contact with endothelium and astrocyte end-feet, are more frequent on microvessels of the retina and brain and thought to regulate blood flow (Kutcher and Herman, 2009). Pericytes are considered important components of the neurovascular unit as regulators of the brain blood barrier function and also potential mediators of brain vascular dysfunction (Hamilton et al., 2010). Among the properties identified include contraction, hemostasis and angiogenesis. Given their contractile properties, pericytes may act as surrogates of smooth muscle cells in brain microvessels.

Dysfunctional interactions within the neurovascular unit have the potential to lead to brain pathophysiological alterations. Impaired endothelial cell-astrocytes or endothelial cell-pericytes signaling may cause brain blood barrier disruption (Zlokovic, 2008), whereas altered coupling between neuronal activity and vascular responses may contribute to spreading depression (Dreier, 2011).

tDCS and Brain Perfusion

Effects of electrical stimulation on the brain have been known for centuries (Priori, 2003). Work in the rat primary motor region showed that electrical stimulation may increase, decrease, or silence neuron's firing (Bindman et al., 1964; Purpura and McMurtry, 1965). These animal studies showed that anodal stimulation caused depolarization, whereas cathodal stimulation caused hyperpolarization, thus increasing the probability for a neuron to produce an action potential. tDCS has been rediscovered as a non-invasive promising tool to modulate brain activity and as a potential treatment for psychiatric and neurological disorders (Priori, 2003; Filmer et al., 2014). An increasing number of studies have reported that tDCS modulates synaptic transmission by regulating levels of neurotransmitters such as GABA, glutamate, serotonin, and dopamine, among others (Nitsche et al., 2008).

Reports showing that stimulation of cerebellar neurons increased diameter of both adjacent arterioles and the upstream vessels, provided a demonstration of the propagation of vascular responses induced by increased neural activity (Iadecola et al., 1997). Importantly, cerebellar stimulation at the fastigial nucleus, reduced ischemia induced by medial cerebral artery occlusion in rats through NO-mediated hemodynamic mechanisms (Zhang and Iadecola, 1993).

tDCS in humans is performed by applying direct current over the scalp using electrodes and its effects depend on the size, polarity and position of the electrodes, current intensity, duration of stimulation, and tissue properties (DaSilva et al., 2011). Given the intimate relationship between neuronal activity and CBF, it is expected that tDCS will increase brain perfusion, as shown in animal (Han et al., 2014) and human (Zheng et al., 2011) studies. The opinion presented in this article is that in addition to the changes in neuronal-derived metabolites, evidences showing responses to electrical stimulation in non-neuronal cells suggest that tDCS acting on these cells has also the potential to modulate brain perfusion (**Figure 1**). Thus, understanding the vascular effects of tDCS may improve the treatment of diseases associated with vascular dysfunction.

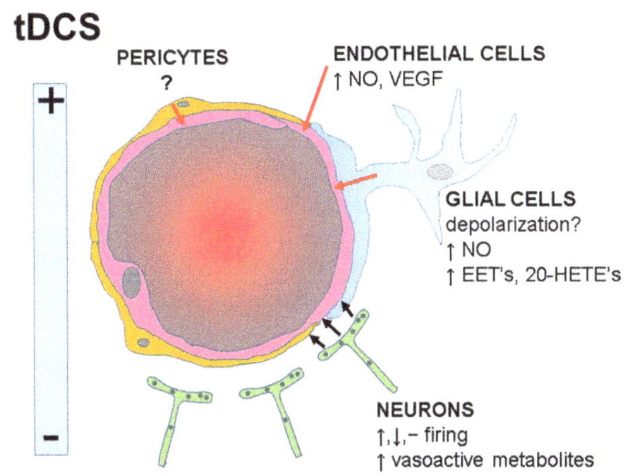

FIGURE 1 | Functional interactions within the neurovascular unit and potential influences of tDCS on specific cell types. tDCS-induced electrical fields may increase, decrease or have no effects on neuronal firing rates. Neuronal-derived metabolites directly or indirectly activate endothelial cells (black arrows), inducing vasodilatation. Potential direct effects of tDCS on glial, endothelial cells, and pericytes are indicated (red arrows). NO, nitric oxide; VEGF, vascular endothelial growth factor; EET's, epoxyeicosatrienoic acids; 20-HETE's, 20-hydroxyeicosatetraeonic acids.

Direct effects of electric stimulation on neurons *in vitro* include alignment of neurites perpendicular to the electric field, increased growth and migration (Pan and Borgens, 2012). In mouse coronal slices, a role for electrical stimulation-induced synaptic plasticity was demonstrated, an effect that may underlie implications of tDCS on motor learning (Fritsch et al., 2010). Results obtained in rat brain slices suggested that electrical stimulation modulates long term potentiation in a polarity-specific manner supporting a regulatory role of tDCS on synaptic plasticity (Ranieri et al., 2012).

Described effects of electrical stimulation on astrocytes *in vitro* include changes in metabolism depending on field polarization and applied voltage (Huang et al., 1997), as well as migration and perpendicular alignment (Pelletier et al., 2014). A theoretical analysis concluded that tDCS has the potential to directly stimulate glial cells since the tDCS-induced changes in membrane potential are similar to the changes induced in astrocytes during neuronal activation (Ruohonen and Karhu, 2012).

The effects of electric stimulation on endothelial cells *in vitro* include the alignment perpendicular to the direction of the electrical field, migration, and elongation (Zhao et al., 2012). These effects are associated with increases in VEGF production, suggesting that electrical stimulation may modulate angiogenesis (Zhao et al., 2012). Conversely, the data from brain slices, including effects on synaptic plasticity (Fritsch et al., 2010) are obtained in the absence of circulation, which may indicate that there is no endothelial contribution to the neuronal effects of electric stimulation. However, endothelial cells in culture exposed to a low physiological electrical field (3.3 mV/mm) showed increased NO production (Trivedi et al., 2013), suggesting a direct route by which electric stimulation may increase brain perfusion. Modeling of the electric properties of the brain suggests that the electric field generated during tDCS in humans is around 1 mV/mm (Neuling et al., 2012) indicating that endothelial cell-dependent responses may be triggered during tDCS.

The proposed role of pericytes in the neurovascular unit suggests that pericytes may transduce signals from neurons to endothelial cells (Hall et al., 2014). Thus, during neuronal activation glutamate release produces prostaglandin E_2 which in turn will induce capillaries vasodilatation by activating K^+ currents in pericytes. These are excitable cells and a direct effect of tDCS on pericyte's membrane potential may hyperpolarize it and induce vasodilatory signals. Whether pericyte-mediated responses to tDCS are playing a role in the tDCS effects remains to be elucidated.

Although general agreement has been observed between animal and human studies (Bennabi et al., 2014), it is necessary to note that stimulating parameters used in animal *in vivo* and in *in vitro* protocols are higher than those used in humans where a maximum current density of $\sim$0.28 A/m^2 is used (Im et al., 2012). In contrast a maximum safe stimulation in rats was reported at 142.9 A/m^2 (Liebetanz et al., 2009).

tDCS and Augmentation of Brain Function

In humans, evidences indicate the potential of tDCS to increase cognitive, motor and memory function. For example, tDCS may enhance gesture comprehension by improving gesture and language integration (Cohen-Maximov et al., 2014), a result especially relevant in cases of autism where patients have difficulties processing symbolic gestures (Baron-Cohen, 1988). Anodal tDCS administered repeatedly facilitates language (Meinzer et al., 2014) and motor skill learning (Zimerman et al., 2013). tDCS has also been shown to produce long-lasting effects on number processing (Cohen Kadosh et al., 2010) and there is increasing interest in the applicability of tDCS for memory enhancement (Bennabi et al., 2014).

However, not all tDCS studies have observed positive effects. Thus, the rate of motor sequence learning is increased by anodal tDCS and decreased by cathodal stimulation, whereas tDCS applied prior to the motor task slowed learning (Stagg et al., 2011). Also cerebellar tDCS has been shown to impair practice-dependent improvement in a working memory task (Ferrucci et al., 2008), whereas tDCS applied to pre-frontal cortex disrupts sensory-motor training (Filmer et al., 2013). Clearly, the research describing the efficacy of tDCS for motor and cognitive improvement is still inconclusive.

Brain blood flow responses to specific tasks may involve cortical and subcortical structures, as seen in the attention-derived effects on flow in both the visual cortex and the lateral geniculate nucleus (O'Connor et al., 2002). Thus, it is relevant to point out that tDCS may also modulate blood flow in subcortical structures (Lang et al., 2005; Nonnekes et al., 2014) demonstrating broader effects of tDCS on CBF.

Recent technical developments applying tDCS simultaneously with electroencephalography and brain blood flow measurements (Dutta et al., 2015) will help to integrate tDCS with modulation of vascular function and ultimately changes in human behavior.

Perspectives and Future Directions

In order to expand direct therapeutic applicability, tDCS needs to overcome the challenges related to inter- and intra-subject variability and parameters of stimulation impacting neuroplasticity (i.e., short *vs.* long term stimulation), among others. Simultaneous determination of vascular signals and cognitive performance during tDCS will help to integrate electrical stimulation with vascular functioning and changes in behavior. The relationships between neuronal and vascular effects are complex and it is proven difficult to differentiate between the effects of electrical stimulation on those two tissues, it is however conceivable that in addition to the vascular effects of neuronal-derived metabolites, direct effects of tDCS on non-neuronal cells especially glial and endothelial cells modulate brain perfusion. Thus, a deeper understanding of the effects tDCS have on non-neuronal members of the neurovascular unit is essential.

Acknowledgments

The author thanks Anne Jeffers for language revision of the article.

References

Baron-Cohen, S. (1988). Social and pragmatic deficits in autism: cognitive or affective? *J. Autism Dev. Disord.* 18, 379–402. doi: 10.1007/BF02212194

Bennabi, D., Pedron, S., Haffen, E., Monnin, J., Peterschmitt, Y., and Van Waes, V. (2014). Transcranial direct current stimulation for memory enhancement: from clinical research to animal models. *Front. Syst. Neurosci.* 8:159. doi: 10.3389/fnsys.2014.00159

Bindman, L. J., Lippold, O. C. J., and Redfearn, J. W. T. (1964). The action of brief polarizing currents on the cerebral cortex of the rat (1) during current flow and (2) in the production of long-lasting after-effects. *J. Physiol.* 172, 369–382. doi: 10.1113/jphysiol.1964.sp007425

Cohen Kadosh, R., Soskic, S., Iuculano, T., Kanai, R., and Walsh, V. (2010). Modulating neuronal activity produces specific and long-lasting changes in numerical competence. *Curr. Biol.* 20, 2016–2020. doi: 10.1016/j.cub.2010.10.007

Cohen-Maximov, T., Avirame, K., Flöel, A., and Lavidor, M. (2014). Modulation of gestural-verbal semantic integration by tDCS. *Brain Stimul.* doi: 10.1016/j.brs.2014.12.001. [Epub ahead of print]

Daneman, R., and Prat, A. (2015). The Blood-Brain Barrier. *Cold Spring Harb. Perspect. Biol.* 7:a020412. doi: 10.1101/cshperspect.a020412

DaSilva, A. F., Volz, M. S., Bikson, M., and Fregni, F. (2011). Electrode positioning and montage in transcranial direct current stimulation. *J. Vis. Exp.* 51:e2744. doi: 10.3791/2744

Dreier, J. P. (2011). The role of spreading depression, spreading depolarization and spreading ischemia in neurological disease. *Nat. Med.* 17, 439–447. doi: 10.1038/nm.2333

Dutta, A., Jacob, A., Chowdhury, S., Das, A., and Nitsche, M. (2015). EEG-NIRS based assessment of neurovascular coupling during anodal transcranial direct current stimulation - a stroke case series. *J. Med. Syst.* 39, 1–9. doi: 10.1007/s10916-015-0205-7

Farkas, E., and Luiten, P. G. M. (2001). Cerebral microvascular pathology in aging and Alzheimer's disease. *Prog. Neurobiol.* 64, 575–611. doi: 10.1016/S0301-0082(00)00068-X

Ferrucci, R., Marceglia, S., Vergari, M., Cogiamanian, F., Mrakic-Sposta, S., Mameli, F., et al. (2008). Cerebellar transcranial direct current stimulation impairs the practice-dependent proficiency increase in working memory. *J. Cogn. Neurosci.* 20, 1687–1697. doi: 10.1162/jocn.2008.20112

Filmer, H. L., Dux, P. E., and Mattingley, J. B. (2014). Applications of transcranial direct current stimulation for understanding brain function. *Trends Neurosci.* 37, 742–753. doi: 10.1016/j.tins.2014.08.003

Filmer, H. L., Mattingley, J. B., Marois, R., and Dux, P. E. (2013). Disrupting prefrontal cortex prevents performance gains from sensory-motor training. *J. Neurosci.* 33, 18654–18660. doi: 10.1523/JNEUROSCI.2019-13.2013

Fritsch, B., Reis, J., Martinowich, K., Schambra, H. M., Ji, Y., Cohen, L. G., et al. (2010). Direct current stimulation promotes BDNF-dependent synaptic plasticity: potential implications for motor learning. *Neuron* 66, 198–204. doi: 10.1016/j.neuron.2010.03.035

Gorelick, P. B., Scuteri, A., Black, S. E., DeCarli, C., Greenberg, S. M., Iadecola, C., et al. (2011). Vascular contributions to cognitive impairment and dementia: a statement for healthcare professionals from the American Heart Association/American Stroke Association. *Stroke* 42, 2672–2713. doi: 10.1161/STR.0b013e3182299496

Hall, C. N., Reynell, C., Gesslein, B., Hamilton, N. B., Mishra, A., Sutherland, B. A., et al. (2014). Capillary pericytes regulate cerebral blood flow in health and disease. *Nature* 508, 55–60. doi: 10.1038/nature13165

Hamel, E. (2006). Perivascular nerves and the regulation of cerebrovascular tone. *J. Appl. Physiol.* 100, 1059–1064. doi: 10.1152/japplphysiol.00954.2005

Hamilton, N. B., Attwell, D., and Hall, C. N. (2010). Pericyte-mediated regulation of capillary diameter: a component of neurovascular coupling in health and disease. *Front. Neuroenergetics* 2:5. doi: 10.3389/fnene.2010.00005

Han, C. H., Song, H., Kang, Y. G., Kim, B. M., and Im, C. H. (2014). Hemodynamic responses in rat brain during transcranial direct current stimulation: a functional near-infrared spectroscopy study. *Biomed. Opt. Express* 13, 1812–1821. doi: 10.1364/BOE.5.001812

Heistad, D., and Kontos, H. (1983). *Handbook of Physiology: The Cardiovascular System III.* Bethesda, MD: American Physiological Society.

Hossmann, K. A. (1994). Viability thresholds and the penumbra of focal ischemia. *Ann. Neurol.* 36, 557–565. doi: 10.1002/ana.410360404

Huang, R., Peng, L., and Hertz, L. (1997). Effects of a low-voltage static electric field on energy metabolism in astrocytes. *Bioelectromagnetics* 18, 77–80. doi: 10.1002/(SICI)1521-186X(1997)18:1<77::AID-BEM11>3.0.CO;2-N

Iadecola, C. (2004). Neurovascular regulation in the normal brain and in Alzheimer's disease. *Nat. Rev. Neurosci.* 5, 347–360. doi: 10.1038/nrn1387

Iadecola, C., Yang, G., Ebner, T., and Chen, G. (1997). Local and propagated vascular responses evoked by focal synaptic activity in cerebellar cortex. *Neurophysiol* 78, 651–659.

Iliff, J. J., Wang, M., Liao, Y., Plogg, B. A., Peng, W., Gundersen, G. A., et al. (2012). A paravascular pathway facilitates CSF flow through the brain parenchyma and the clearance of interstitial solutes, including amyloid β. *Sci. Transl. Med.* 4:147ra111. doi: 10.1126/scitranslmed.3003748

Im, C. H., Park, J. H., Shim, M., Chang, W. H., and Kim, Y. H. (2012). Evaluation of local electric fields generated by transcranial direct current stimulation with an extracephalic reference electrode based on realistic 3D body modeling. *Phys. Med. Biol.* 57:2137. doi: 10.1088/0031-9155/57/8/2137

Kutcher, M. E., and Herman, I. M. (2009). The pericyte: cellular regulator of microvascular blood flow. *Microvasc. Res.* 77, 235–246. doi: 10.1016/j.mvr.2009.01.007

Lang, N., Siebner, H. R., Ward, N. S., Lee, L., Nitsche, M. A., Paulus, W., et al. (2005). How does transcranial DC stimulation of the primary motor cortex alter regional neuronal activity in the human brain? *Eur. J. Neurosci.* 22, 495–504. doi: 10.1111/j.1460-9568.2005.04233.x

Liebetanz, D., Koch, R., Mayenfels, S., König, F., Paulus, W., and Nitsche, M. A. (2009). Safety limits of cathodal transcranial direct current stimulation in rats. *Clin. Neurophysiol.* 120, 1161–1167. doi: 10.1016/j.clinph.2009.01.022

Meinzer, M., Jähnigen, S., Copland, D. A., Darkow, R., Grittner, U., Avirame, K., et al. (2014). Transcranial direct current stimulation over multiple days improves learning and maintenance of a novel vocabulary. *Cortex* 50, 137–147. doi: 10.1016/j.cortex.2013.07.013

Metea, M. R., and Newman, E. A. (2006). Glial cells dilate and constrict blood vessels: a mechanism of neurovascular coupling. *J. Neurosci.* 26, 2862–2870. doi: 10.1523/JNEUROSCI.4048-05.2006

Nedergaard, M. (2013). Garbage truck of the brain. *Science* 340, 1529–1530. doi: 10.1126/science.1240514

Neuling, T., Wagner, S., Wolters, C. H., Zaehle, T., and Herrmann, C. S. (2012). Finite element model predicts current density distribution for clinical applications of tDCS and tACS. *Front. Psychiatry* 3:83. doi: 10.3389/fpsyt.2012.00083

Nitsche, M. A., Cohen, L. G., Wassermann, E. M., Priori, A., Lang, N., Antal, A., et al. (2008). Transcranial direct current stimulation: State of the art 2008. *Brain Stimul.* 1, 206–223. doi: 10.1016/j.brs.2008.06.004

Nonnekes, J., Arrogi, A., Munneke, M. A. M., van Asseldonk, E. H. F., Oude Nijhuis, L. B., Geurts, A. C., et al. (2014). Subcortical structures in humans can be facilitated by transcranial direct current stimulation. *PLoS ONE* 9:e107731. doi: 10.1371/journal.pone.0107731

O'Connor, D. H., Fukui, M. M., Pinsk, M. A., and Kastner, S. (2002). Attention modulates responses in the human lateral geniculate nucleus. *Nat. Neurosci.* 5, 1203–1209. doi: 10.1038/nn957

Pan, L., and Borgens, R. B. (2012). Strict perpendicular orientation of neural crest-derived neurons *in vitro* is dependent on an extracellular gradient of voltage. *J. Neurosci. Res.* 90, 1335–1346. doi: 10.1002/jnr.22809

Pelletier, S. J., Lagacé, M., St-Amour, I., Arsenault, D., Cisbani, G., Chabrat, A., et al. (2014). The morphological and molecular changes of brain cells exposed to direct current electric field stimulation. *Int. J. Neuropsychopharmacol.* 18. doi: 10.1093/ijnp/pyu090

Priori, A. (2003). Brain polarization in humans: a reappraisal of an old tool for prolonged non-invasive modulation of brain excitability. *Clin. Neurophysiol.* 114, 589–595. doi: 10.1016/S1388-2457(02)00437-6

Purpura, D. P., and McMurtry, J. G. (1965). Intracellular activities and evoked potential changes during polarization of motor cortex. *J. Neurophysiol.* 28, 166–185.

Ranieri, F., Podda, M. V., Riccardi, E., Frisullo, G., Dileone, M., Profice, P., et al. (2012). Modulation of LTP at rat hippocampal CA3-CA1 synapses by direct current stimulation. *J. Neurophysiol.* 107, 1868–1880. doi: 10.1152/jn.00319.2011

Ruohonen, J., and Karhu, J. (2012). tDCS possibly stimulates glial cells. *Clin. Neurophysiol.* 123, 2006–2009. doi: 10.1016/j.clinph.2012.02.082

Stagg, C. J., Jayaram, G., Pastor, D., Kincses, Z. T., Matthews, P. M., and Johansen-Berg, H. (2011). Polarity and timing-dependent effects of transcranial direct current stimulation in explicit motor learning. *Neuropsychologia* 49, 800–804. doi: 10.1016/j.neuropsychologia.2011.02.009

Stobart, J. L. L., Lu, L., Anderson, H. D. I., Mori, H., and Anderson, C. M. (2013). Astrocyte-induced cortical vasodilation is mediated by D-serine and endothelial nitric oxide synthase. *Proc. Natl. Acad. Sci. U.S.A.* 110, 3149–3154. doi: 10.1073/pnas.1215929110

Trivedi, D. P., Hallock, K. J., and Bergethon, P. R. (2013). Electric fields caused by blood flow modulate vascular endothelial electrophysiology and nitric oxide production. *Bioelectromagnetics* 34, 22–30. doi: 10.1002/bem.21741

Zhang, F., and Iadecola, C. (1993). Fastigial stimulation increases ischemic blood flow and reduces brain damage after focal ischemia. *J. Cereb. Blood Flow Metab.* 13, 1013–1019. doi: 10.1038/jcbfm.1993.127

Zhang, F., Xu, S., and Iadecola, C. (1995). Role of nitric oxide and acetylcholine in neocortical hyperemia elicited by basal forebrain stimulation: evidence for an involvement of endothelial nitric oxide. *Neuroscience* 69, 1195–1204. doi: 10.1016/0306-4522(95)00302-Y

Zhao, Z., Qin, L., Reid, B., Pu, J., Hara, T., and Zhao, M. (2012). Directing migration of endothelial progenitor cells with applied DC electric fields. *Stem Cell Res.* 8, 38–48. doi: 10.1016/j.scr.2011.08.001

Zheng, X., Alsop, D. C., and Schlaug, G. (2011). Effects of transcranial direct current stimulation (tDCS) on human regional cerebral blood flow. *Neuroimage* 58, 26–33. doi: 10.1016/j.neuroimage.2011.06.018

Zimerman, M., Nitsch, M., Giraux, P., Gerloff, C., Cohen, L. G., and Hummel, F. C. (2013). Neuroenhancement of the aging brain: restoring skill acquisition in old subjects. *Ann. Neurol.* 73, 10–15. doi: 10.1002/ana.23761

Zlokovic, B. V. (2008). The blood-brain barrier in health and chronic neurodegenerative disorders. *Neuron* 57, 178–201. doi: 10.1016/j.neuron.2008.01.003

Zonta, M., Angulo, M. C., Gobbo, S., Rosengarten, B., Hossmann, K. A., and Pozzan, T., et al. (2003). Neuron-to-astrocyte signaling is central to the dynamic control of brain microcirculation. *Nat. Neurosci.* 6, 43–50. doi: 10.1038/nn980

6

Design, fabrication, and packaging of an integrated, wirelessly-powered optrode array for optogenetics application

Ki Yong Kwon[1], *Hyung-Min Lee*[2], *Maysam Ghovanloo*[2], *Arthur Weber*[3] *and Wen Li*[1]*

[1] Department of Electrical and Computer Engineering, Michigan State University, East Lansing, MI, USA, [2] School of Electrical and Computer Engineering, Georgia Institute of Technology, Atlanta, GA, USA, [3] Department of Physiology, Michigan State University, East Lansing, MI, USA

Edited by:
Ioan Opris,
Wake Forest University School of Medicine, USA

Reviewed by:
Stelios M. Smirnakis,
Baylor College of Medicine, USA
Oana D. Jurchescu,
Wake Forest University School of Medicine, USA

***Correspondence:**
Wen Li,
Department of Electrical and Computer Engineering, Michigan State University, 428 S Shaw Ln, RM 2120 Engineering Building, East Lansing, MI 48824, USA
wenli@egr.msu.edu

The recent development of optogenetics has created an increased demand for advancing engineering tools for optical modulation of neural circuitry. This paper details the design, fabrication, integration, and packaging procedures of a wirelessly-powered, light emitting diode (LED) coupled optrode neural interface for optogenetic studies. The LED-coupled optrode array employs microscale LED (μLED) chips and polymer-based microwaveguides to deliver light into multi-level cortical networks, coupled with microelectrodes to record spontaneous changes in neural activity. An integrated, implantable, switched-capacitor based stimulator (SCS) system provides high instantaneous power to the μLEDs through an inductive link to emit sufficient light and evoke neural activities. The presented system is mechanically flexible, biocompatible, miniaturized, and lightweight, suitable for chronic implantation in small freely behaving animals. The design of this system is scalable and its manufacturing is cost effective through batch fabrication using microelectromechanical systems (MEMS) technology. It can be adopted by other groups and customized for specific needs of individual experiments.

Keywords: optrode array, implantable neural interface, optogenetics, microelectromechanical systems, switched-capacitor based stimulators, wireless power transfer

Introduction

Optogenetics is an emerging technique that combines optical and genetic tools for light modulation of neural activity. A key advantage of optogenetics in neuroscience is the ability to excite or inhibit specific cell types with millisecond precision and rapid reversibility (Boyden et al., 2005; Zhang et al., 2007; Deisseroth, 2011; Gerits and Vanduffel, 2013; Zalocusky and Deisseroth, 2013). Recently, neural transfection with substantially red-shifted channelrhodopsin or halorhodopsin genes has demonstrated the potential for deep transcranial optogenetic excitation and inhibition non-invasively (Zhang et al., 2008; Lin et al., 2013; Chuong et al., 2014). Recent emphasis on use of optogenetics has created an increased demand for optical devices targeting delivery of light not only to the surface, but also into deeper subregions of the brain. Examples of surface light delivery systems are acousto-optic deflectors (Losavio et al., 2011), digital micro-mirror devices (DMDs; Arrenberg et al., 2010; Zhu et al., 2012), and computer-generated holograms

(CGHs; Reutsky-Gefen et al., 2013). To deliver light to deeper regions of neural tissue, laser- or light-emitting-diode (LED) coupled optical fibers were initially implanted within the brain (Aravanis et al., 2007; Han et al., 2009; Zhang et al., 2010). Recently, more advanced methods, based on micro-/nanofabrication technologies, have been developed to increase the spatial resolution of optogenetic light stimulation of the three-dimensional neural networks of the brain. Such devices include, multichannel silicon oxynitride waveguide arrays (Zorzos et al., 2012), arrayed optical fibers (Royer et al., 2010; Stark et al., 2012), multi-waveguides fabricated on a single substrate (Zorzos et al., 2010), multipoint-emitting optical fibers (Pisanello et al., 2014), optrodes (Wang et al., 2012; Wu et al., 2013), and polymer-based flexible micro-LEDs arrays (Kim et al., 2013).

Despite the aforementioned development of light delivery devices, only limited methods currently are available for use in experiments with freely behaving subjects. These include, laser- or LED-coupled optical fibers, a polymer-based micro-LED array (Kim et al., 2013), and a head-mountable LED system (Iwai et al., 2011). The poor spatial resolution of such systems limits their functionality, and the tethered optical fiber greatly restricts the natural behaviors of the subjects. In addition, since most optogenetic neural probes integrate rigid silica fibers, their mechanical reliability is compromised by optoelectronic integration. As a solution to the current demand for multichannel, bi-directional optogenetic tools, our group has developed a series of flexible, hybrid neural interfacing devices for simultaneous optical modulation and electrical recording of neural activity at multiple levels of cortex. Depending on the interface location, three different devices are available: an Opto-μECoG array for epidural stimulation (Kwon et al., 2012, 2013c), a three dimension (3-D) waveguide array for deep cortical stimulation (Kwon and Li, 2013), and a slanted 3-D waveguide array for multi cortical layers stimulation (Kwon et al., 2013b). Such devices are microfabricated using Parylene-C as the flexible substrate and as the packaging material, thus ensuring biocompatibility while maintaining mechanical compliance (Takeuchi et al., 2005; Rodger et al., 2008; Li et al., 2010, 2011). Using microscale LEDs (μLEDs) as light sources provides several unique advantages compared to the use of external lasers and/or array-based diode lasers, including low power consumption, illumination stability, and fast light switching ability (Mohanty and Thakor, 2013). Integration of individually addressable μLEDs with microwaveguides allows for precise light delivery to the target neurons in individual cortical layers. Furthermore, electronically driven LEDs are particularly suitable for integration with wireless telemetry systems.

Building on the device development, most recently we have implemented a wireless neural interface system. Unlike standard optogenetic approaches that rely on rigid fiber optics tethered to external light sources, our system integrates a microfabricated LED-coupled optrode array with a switched-capacitor stimulator (SCS) and wireless telemetry on a single polymer platform toward a truly untethered bi-directional neural interface for optogenetic application (Kwon et al., 2014a; Lee et al., 2014). This system is flexible, miniaturized and lightweight, and thus suitable for use in small freely behaving animals. The design of our system is scalable and its manufacturing is cost effective, owing to the advantages of batch microfabrication technologies. In this paper, we present the detailed design principle and microfabrication protocols of the slanted LED-coupled optrode array, integration and packaging processes with the wireless system, and demonstration of *in vivo* neural recording and stimulation in rats. The methods described here provide a completely customizable approach for other groups and researchers to design and implement devices for specific needs of individual experiments.

Materials and Methods

Design of the Proposed System

As depicted in **Figure 1**, our wireless neural interfacing system contains three key components: a LED-coupled slanted optrode array, a wireless switched-capacitor based stimulator (SCS), and an inductive link for power transfer. The array has 32 embedded μLED light sources, with 4 × 4 channels per hemisphere on a 2.5 × 2.5 mm^2 flexible substrate to cover the rat visual cortices bilaterally. The μLED chips are coupled to slanted SU-8 microwaveguide cores, fabricated separately on a polydimethylsiloxane (PDMS) substrate. The design of the needle-shaped waveguide is simulated using a numerical ray-tracing method in TracePro (TracePro®, Lambda Research Co., MA, USA), as reported previously in Kwon et al. (2014b). The simulation results suggest that, given the same base size, the illumination range of the optrode is determined by the tip size of the waveguide core. In particular, a small tip results in divergent irradiance and low output light intensity due to the secondary reflection of light beams along the sidewalls of the tapered waveguide. Optrode with a large tip will enable high irradiance with a confined beam shape. For example, the radius of the illumination area increases from ~0.2 mm to ~0.6 mm when the tip diameter decreases from 100 μm to 10 μm. On the other hand, a large tip may cause more damage to brain tissue during implantation. Based on the simulation results, we designed the needle-shaped waveguides with various lengths ranging from 300–1500 μm in order to target neurons located in different cortical layers, a tip diameter of 30 μm to facilitate device implantation, and a base diameter of ~300 μm to match the dimensions of the μLED chip (220 μm (W) × 270 μm (L) × 50 μm (H)). The cladding layer provided with each individual microwaveguide makes it possible to record electrophysiological signals in response to optical stimulation while preventing light leakage through the sidewalls of the tapered microneedles. To minimize the light-induced artifacts during recording, the cladding layer of the waveguide is specifically designed with four layers of an oxide-polymer-metal-polymer sandwich structure, as depicted in **Figure 1B**. Starting from the inner layer, transparent indium tin oxide (ITO) is used as the electrical shielding layer to eliminate photoelectrical artifact without compromising

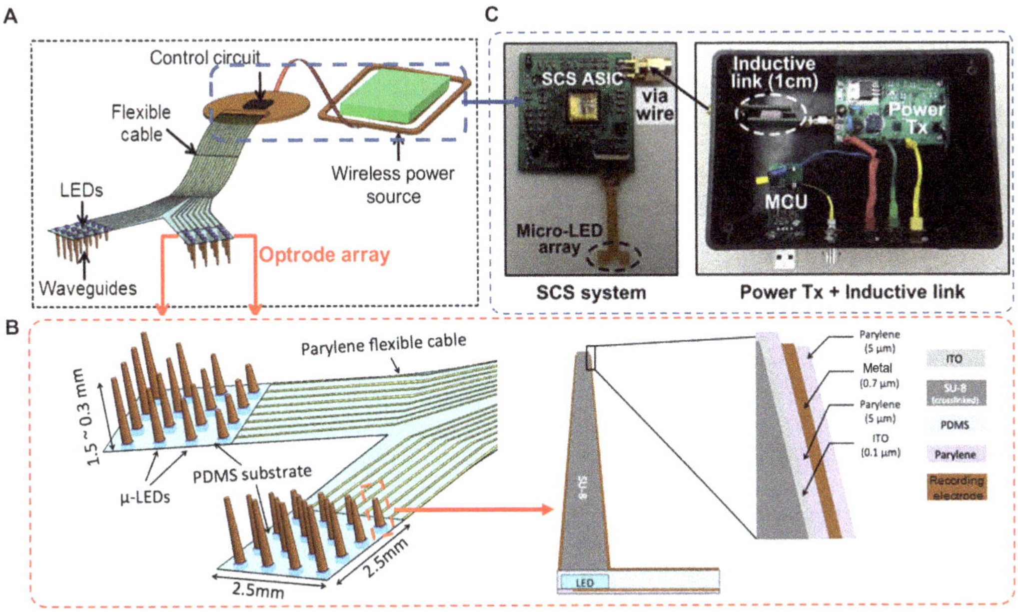

FIGURE 1 | (A) Conceptual illustration of the wireless optrode neural interface. **(B)** Overall design of the LED-coupled optrode array with 32 μLEDs, microwaveguides, and microelectrodes integrated on a Parylene-C substrate. **(C)** The inductively-powered telemetry and switched-capacitor based stimulating (SCS) system used to wirelessly drive the μLED array.

light throughput. After an insulating layer of Parylene-C, an opaque metallic layer is constructed to block out light side-leakage, with the tip being etched to allow light delivery to adjacent neurons expressing optogenetic opsins. This layer also is used for constructing the recording electrodes and leads to interconnect with the peripheral elements. The outermost layer is made of Parylene-C for encapsulation. The tip is selectively etched to expose the electrode side for neural recording.

The optrode array is inductively powered and controlled by a wireless switched-capacitor based stimulation (SCS) system, designed at Georgia Institute of Technology to improve power efficiency over traditional current-controlled stimulators, while being capable of delivering instantaneous high power to the μLEDs (Lee et al., 2013). During optical stimulation, the SCS system charges a small array of storage capacitors directly from the inductive link and periodically discharges them into the μLED array at the stimulation onsets, providing high instantaneous current without burdening the inductive link and system supply. To control stimulation parameters, a custom-designed PC interface wirelessly sends data to the SCS system through the inductive link, while a commercial neural recording system simultaneously detects the evoked neural signals from the same optrode array. For a chronically implantable system, all electronic components can be assembled on a mechanically flexible printed circuit board (PCB) substrate and encapsulated with Parylene-C to improve biocompatibility of the system by protecting the electronics from the corrosive biological environment. We graphically designed the masks of the optrode array and the PCB substrate in the AutoCAD environment (Autodesk Inc.), constructed the optrode array using polymer-based microelectromechanical systems (MEMS) techniques, and assembled the components on the PCB substrate using a customized assembly method. Details of the microfabrication and integration are described in the following sections.

Microfabrication Methods

To reduce fabrication complexity and improve the production yield, the multi-LED array and the slanted optrode array are fabricated and calibrated separately, then bonded together using SU-8 adhesive.

Fabrication of the LED Array

A process flow for making the multi-LED array has been developed previously in Kwon et al. (2013c), based on microfabrication and self-assembly techniques. (a-1) A 3-inch glass carrying wafer was cleaned by sonication in acetone, isopropyl alcohol (IPA), and de-ionized (DI) water (3 mins each), followed by Parylene-C deposition (5 μm thick) in a chemical vapor deposition (CVD) system (PDS2010 Parylene Coater, Specialty Coating System, IN, USA). (a-2) A 0.3 μm copper layer was deposited in a thermal evaporator (Edward Auto306, Edwards, UK) and patterned by wet etching to form contact pads and interconnection leads. A photoresist (PR) mask was selectively patterned to expose only the metal contacts for μLED connections. Copper was used to prove the concept, but can be replaced with gold or other conductive materials to improve chemical resistance and biocompatibility. (a-3) Low melting point (LMP) solder (melting point ~62°C, 144 ALLOY Field's Metal, Rotometals, Inc., CA, USA) was applied on the contacts. The substrate then was rinsed with acetone, IPA, and DI water to remove the PR layer. (a-4) A PDMS (Sylgard 184, Dow Corning, MI, USA) stamp with the embedded blue μLEDs (Cree® TR2227TM die-form LED, peak wavelength at 460 nm, Cree, NC, USA)[1] was aligned to match the pre-soldered receiver sites on the carrying substrate. Different color LED chips (e.g., green, yellow, or red) can be used for optogenetic inhibition or excitation. (a-5) The substrate with the aligned PDMS stamp was heated on a hot plate at 90°C for 30 s. The PDMS stamp was removed carefully after the substrate had cooled to 40°C, leaving the LEDs attached to the contact pads of the substrate. The substrate then was submerged into an acidic water bath (90°C, pH of 2.0) for 1 min. This step permits fine adjustment of LED alignment and the formation of an electrical connection in a self-assembly manner, utilizing the surface tension of the LMP solder.

The PDMS stamp facilitates the assembly of multiple LEDs on the carrying substrate in a precise and time-efficient way. To fabricate the PDMS stamp, (b-1) a 3-inch glass wafer was first cleaned and went through a dehydration bake. A ~30 μm SU-8 layer was spun onto the wafer and patterned as the mold for fabricating a PDMS stamp. (b-2) PDMS was poured over the SU-8 mold to form the stamp, which contained cavities matching the shape of the μLED chip. (b-3) After curing the PDMS for 40 min on a 95°C hotplate, the stamp was peeled off the mold. (b-4) Thirty-two LED chips were aligned in the cavities of the stamp, with metal pads facing outward. The assembly method using the PDMS stamp was adapted from Onoe et al. (2009), and the yield of the chip assembly was above 96%.

Fabrication of the Optrode Array and Assembly

As described in **Figure 2**, (1) a 3-inch glass wafer was cleaned and put through a dehydration bake, and a ~50 μm SU-8 (SU-8 3025, MicroChem Corp, MA, USA) layer was spun onto the wafer and patterned as the mock LEDs; (2) A thin layer of PDMS was spun onto the SU-8 master to create cavities matching the shape of the LED; (3) After the PDMS was cured for 40 min at 95°C, PR was patterned on the PDMS substrate to expose 7 mm-diameter circles, followed by oxygen plasma treatment to convert the exposed hydrophobic areas to hydrophilic ones; (4) After removal of the PR mask, ~45 μL SU-8 (SU-8 3005) was dispensed on top of the plasma treated PDMS surface using a micropipette; and (5) patterned with a backside droplet backside exposure (DBE) method that utilizes the height variance in a dome-shaped SU-8 structure to create out-of-plane microneedles of varying lengths (Kwon et al., 2013a, 2014b); (6) After SU-8 development, the array was polished by O_2 plasma etching; (7) DC sputtering of a 0.1-μm-thick ITO layer was performed in a Kurt Lesker Axiss PVD System, followed by deposition of 5 μm Parylene-C. Then a 0.2-μm-thick Au layer was deposited in the thermal evaporator, and the tip of the waveguide was chemically etched for light delivery, followed by deposition of 5 μm Parylene-C as a protective layer. The Parylene-C film at the tip of the optrode was removed using reactive-ion etching (RIE); and (8) The optrode array then was released from the glass wafer, and the microneedles with the matched LED cavities were aligned onto the corresponding LEDs. Finally, (9) the LED array and optrode array were bonded together, with a ~50 μm SU-8 (SU-8 3025) layer spun on the LED array as an adhesive.

System Integration and Packaging

SCS System and Inductive Telemetry

Integrated LED light sources powered by the wireless SCS system enable a truly untethered optogenetic stimulation system. Inductive power transmission across the skin has been a viable solution to provide sufficient power to the implantable medical devices (IMDs), while overcoming size, cost, and longevity constraints of embedded primary batteries. Light sources in optogenetics, however, typically require high instantaneous power to emit sufficient light for optical neural stimulation, which can be a significant limiting factor in conventional IMDs (Wentz et al., 2011). **Figure 3A** shows the conceptual block diagram of a conventional inductively-powered array of LEDs for wireless optogenetics, where a rectifier and a regulator convert AC voltage across a secondary coil, L_2, to DC output voltage to supply a LED driver. Power losses in these stages result in poor overall power efficiency from L_2 to the LED. Moreover, high instantaneous power that flows to the LEDs when they are on, leads to large load variation, which affects the impedance matching with the inductive link. This will significantly increase the required inductive power level, creating safety issues, and degrading the inductive link power efficiency as well as supply voltage for the rest of the IMD. To address these limitations in implantable optogenetics stimulators, the SCS system has been designed and implemented for power-efficient wireless optical stimulation, as shown in **Figure 3B**. The proposed SCS system efficiently charges a bank of storage capacitors, C_S, directly from V_{COIL} through the inductive link without using any rectifiers or regulators, improving the capacitor charging efficiency. Moreover, the charge stored in capacitors is delivered to the load through large switches, efficiently creating high current stimulation pulses.

Integration and Hermetic Package for Chronic Implants

Figure 4 illustrates the process flow for integration and hermetic packaging of a chronic implant on a flexible polyimide PCB substrate for experiments using freely behaving animals. The flexible polyimide PCB substrate was constructed using Pyralux®AP (AP7163E, DuPont) with the following steps: (1) A 3-inch Pyralux® wafer was cut and cleaned, and a 3-μm thick PR layer was spin coated; (2) The circuit design was transferred on to the PR using a lithography technique; (3) The circuit was patterned by wet etching of copper; (4) Through holes were made by a laser cutter; (5) Vias were made by filling the through holes with solder; (6) Solder paste was applied on the contact pads and the SCS chip, and other

[1]Cree LED Datasheet. http://www.cree.com/~/media/Files/Cree/LED%20 Components%20and%20Modules/XLamp/Data%20and%20 Binning/XLamp MCE_BL.pdf

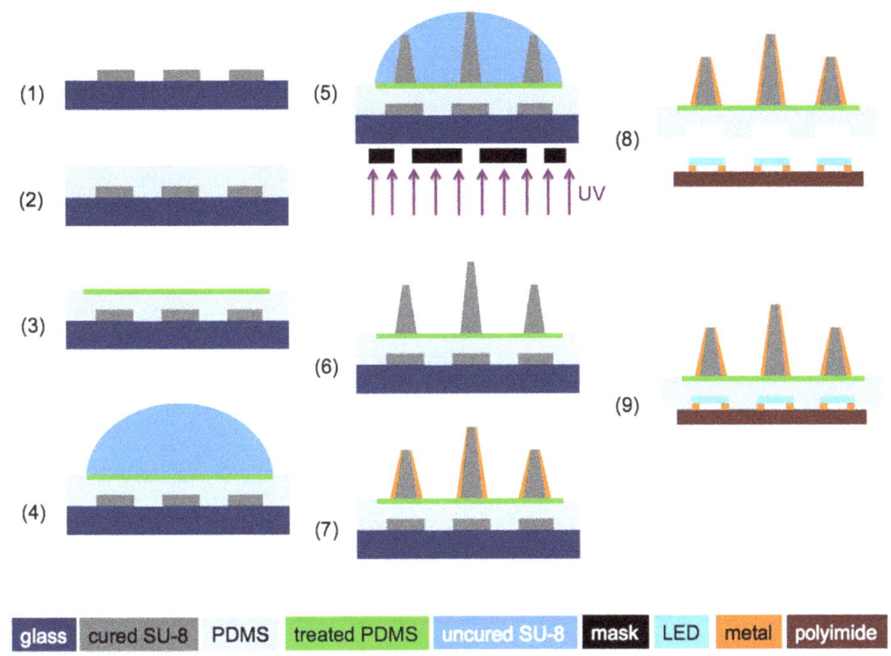

FIGURE 2 | Fabrication process flow for making the slanted optrode array (steps 1–7) and microassembly of the optrode array with the LED array (steps 8 and 9). ©[2014] IEEE. Reprinted, with permission, from Kwon et al. (2014a).

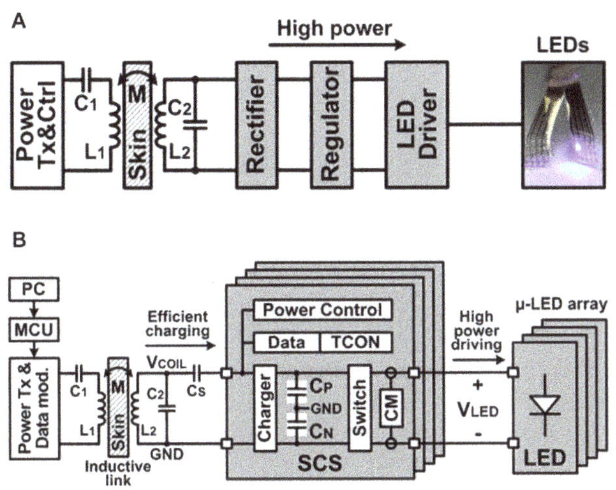

FIGURE 3 | (A) Simplified block diagram of a conventional inductively-powered device combined with an array of LEDs for wireless optogenetics and **(B)** simplified block diagram of the wireless switched-capacitor based stimulating (SCS) system to efficiently drive the μLED-coupled optrode array. ©[2014] IEEE. Reprinted, with permission, from Lee et al. (2014).

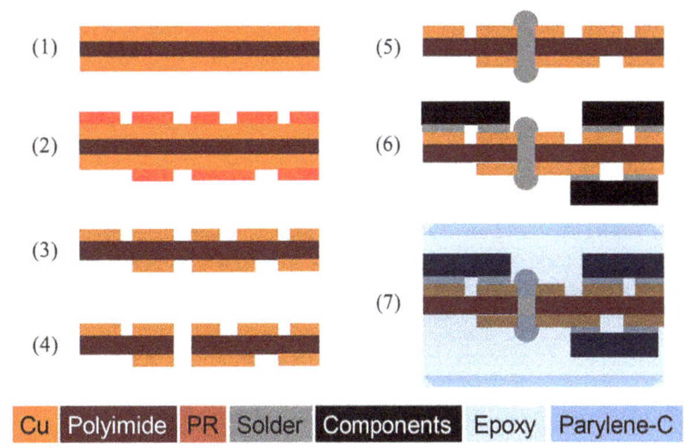

FIGURE 4 | Fabrication process of a hermetically-sealed chronic implant on a flexible polyimide circuit. ©[2014] IEEE. Reprinted, with permission, from Lee et al. (2014).

surface mount devices (SMDs) were populated on the pads. The circuit was baked at 200°C for 5 min, and extra flux was applied for reflow soldering, if necessary; and (7) Once all components were populated, a thick layer of medical-grade epoxy (200∼500 μm, EP21LVMed, Master Bond) was applied, followed by a 10 μm Parylene-C coating as a biocompatible package.

In Vivo Experiment in Rats

In vivo acute animal experiments have been conducted to demonstrate the ability of the LED-coupled optrode array to simultaneously modulate and record neural activities in the primary visual cortex (V1) of a rat. All procedures were approved by the Institutional Animal Care and Use Committee (IACUC) at Michigan State University. Two weeks prior to the experiments, rodent subjects (Sprague-Dawley rats: 250–400 g) had neurons in their V1 transfected with the AAV-hSyn-hChR2(H134R)-mCherry viral vector ($10 \times 10^{11} \sim 10 \times 10^{12}$ vector genome (vg)/mL; UNC Vector Core, NC, USA). During the viral injection, each animal was anesthetized with ketamine/xylazine

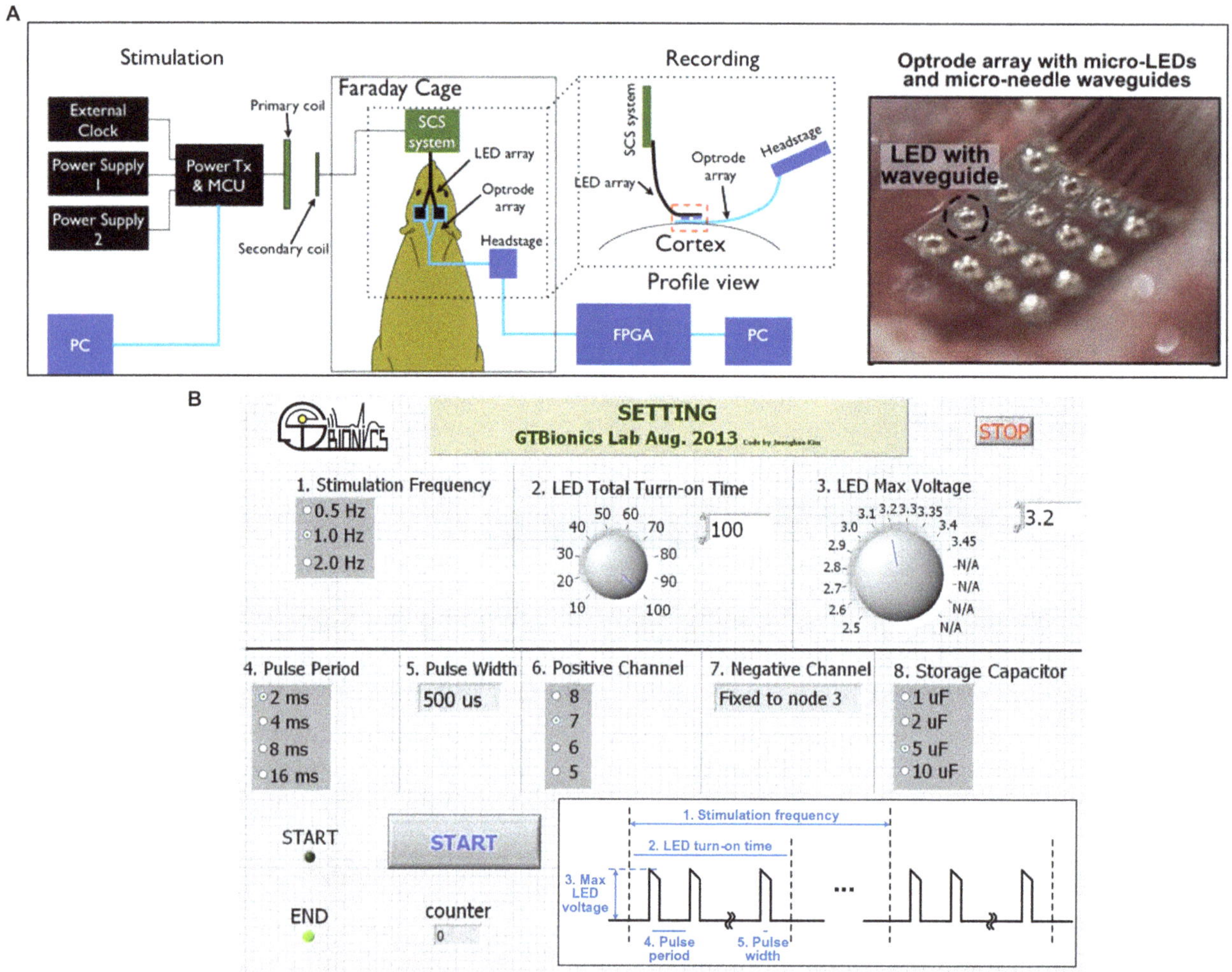

FIGURE 5 | (A) *In vivo* animal experiment setup with the wireless SCS system. **(B)** A SCS system GUI in LabVIEW to wirelessly control the SCS parameters. Inset shows the LED driving voltage waveform and its controllable parameters.

(80 mg/kg: 5 mg/kg i.m.) and anesthesia maintained with ketamine (20 mg/kg i.m.) as needed. The eyes were treated with 1% methylcellulose to prevent corneal drying. Using sterile surgical procedures, a 3–4 cm incision was made in the skin overlying the skull and small holes were drilled through the bone over V1. Using a glass pipette and a pressure injection system, 1.0 μL of the virus solution was injected at 3–4 equidistant locations. Injections occurred over a 2–3 min period, and the glass pipette was left in place for an additional 10 min to allow the vector to diffuse away from the injection site. The cortex then was covered with Gelfoam and the skin overlying the skull was sutured closed. Post-surgery, the animal received pain medication (buprenorphine; 0.05 mg/kg s.c.) and fluids (10–12 cc sterile saline, s.c.) subcutaneously and was placed in a cage on a heating pad until fully recovered, after which the animal was returned to the animal care facility. For device implantation, the animal expressing ChR2 (2–4 weeks after virus injection) was anesthetized using the procedure described above. The anesthetized animal was placed in a stereotaxic apparatus and a small region (4 × 4 mm^2) of the skull over V1 was removed. The optrode array was surgically implanted over V1, with the LEDs staying on the surface of the cortex and the waveguides inserted in the cortical tissues.

After device implantation, acute experiments were conducted in one transfected animal to validate the functionality of the implanted device. The experimental setup is shown in **Figure 5A**, where the SCS system was used to power and control the 32-channel LED array and a 32-channel headstage (Intan RHD2132) was used to receive and process the neural signals recorded through the optrode. A Faraday cage was used to isolate the animal, the optrode array, the integrated SCS system, and the recording headstage from the environmental interference in order to improve the signal-to-noise ratio of the neural recordings. The SCS system receives wireless power and data through the inductive link and drives μLEDs in the optrode array. The proof-of-concept prototype of the SCS system occupies 3.9 × 3.9 cm^2 on the PCB, and includes off-chip components for testing and optrode connectors. Key components of this prototype are the SCS chip (5 × 2.4 mm^2)

and four pairs of 1∼5 μF off-chip storage capacitors (SMD-0402, 1 × 0.5 mm^2 each). The SCS system can be miniaturized further using a single flex-PCB method described previously in **Figure 4**, which can connect directly to the LED array and include the receiver coil, L_2, without connectors or testing components. Storage capacitors can be placed on the opposite side of the SCS chip, minimizing the PCB size for chronically implantable optogenetics. Neural signals were recorded simultaneously from the penetrating electrodes on the same optrode array through an Intan RHD2132 evaluation board and its commercial hardwired recording setup (Intan Technologies, CA, USA).

To selectively turn on the LEDs and facilitate the adjustment of stimulation parameters, a graphical user interface (GUI) has been implemented in the LabVIEW environment (National Instruments, Austin, TX) to send data packets from the PC to the microcontroller unit (MCU) in the power transmitter (Tx) module, as shown in **Figure 5B**. Several parameters of the LED driving signal can be adjusted in this setup: (1) stimulation frequency, 0.5∼2 Hz; (2) LED total turn-on time, 10∼100 ms; (3) LED peak voltage, 2.5∼3.45 V; (4) pulse period, 2∼16 ms; (5) pulse width, 512 μs; (6) positive output connections, 4 channels; (7) negative output connections, fixed; and (8) storage capacitance, 1∼10 μF. While the pulse train periodically turns the LEDs on and off, the effective turn-on time can be simply calculated as (total turn-on time) × (pulse width/pulse period).

Results and Discussions

Fabrication Results

Figure 6 shows the photo images of a LED-coupled optrode array. The electrode-electrolyte interface impedances of the optrode array were measured at 1 kHz using a built-in electrode-impedance-testing circuitry in an Intan evaluation board (RHD2132 and RHD2000-EVAL, Intan Tech. LLC, CA, USA). The impedances of the recording electrodes ranged from 10–500 kΩ, suitable for local field potential (LFP) recordings. The impedance of the optrode can be adjusted by controlling the size of the Parylene-C opening, using the process in **Figures 2–7**.

Power consumption of the μLED at various operating conditions was investigated (**Figure 7A**) to provide useful guidelines for optical stimulation in *in vivo* experiments and future integration of the LED array with wireless power telemetry. The nonlinear current-voltage characteristic of a single μLED was measured with an impedance analyzer (HP 4191A RF, Hewlett Packard, CA, USA). Since a minimum light-energy density of 1 mW/mm^2 must be delivered onto the target area to effectively excite channelrhodopsin-2 (ChR2; Grossman et al., 2010), a minimum input voltage of ∼3.2 V is required to drive a single μLED, resulting in electrical power consumption of 27 mW and average light intensity of 1.4 mW/mm^2 from the waveguide tip. The temperature variation of the LED array was measured using a high definition infrared camera (Delta Therm. HS1570 and its software (DT v.2.19)) with different input voltages (2.7–3.2 V) and activation duration of 100 ms, as shown in **Figure 7B**. Thermal images were taken in air under an environment (at room temperature of 22.7°C) where ventilation was strictly controlled to minimize ambient thermal noise, and the array was suspended in the air during the LED activation. As expected, the localized temperature of the LED increases dramatically as the increase of the input voltage. The relatively high input voltage of the LED (3.2 V) can be attributed to inefficient light coupling between the LED chip and the tapered microwaveguide, which typically has a coupling efficiency of ∼10% for the butt coupling (Keiser, 2008). It is of note that, in **Figure 7B**, the pulse train of 3.2 V and 100 ms resulted in the temperature rise by more than ∼10°C, which may affect neural function and even cause tissue damage. However, this experiment was carried out in air without the thermoregulation effect of the cerebral circulation. To evaluate the safety of our simulation paradigm, we measured the temperature variation of the cortical region close to the implantation site using a thermocouple, when the LED was driven by a continuous train of 3.2 V, 100 ms pulse width, and 2 Hz frequency. Preliminary results show that the maximal temperature rise was approximately 0.1–0.4°C, which satisfies the safety requirement for implantable neuroprosthetics. Comprehensive investigation will be performed in the future to fully characterize the thermal properties of the integrated system.

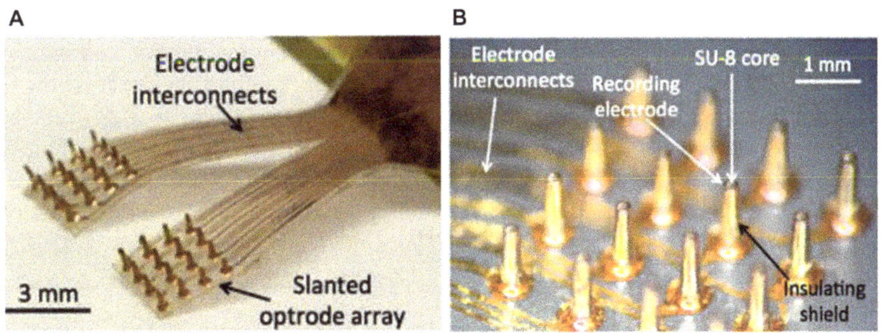

FIGURE 6 | Fabricated prototypes of (A) a 32-channel LED-coupled optrode array; and (B) microscopic image of individual optrodes.

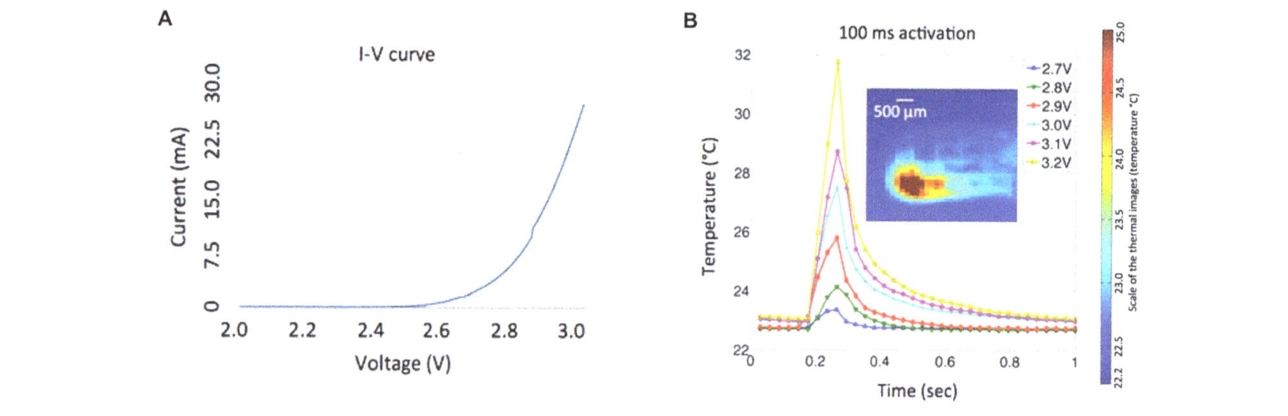

FIGURE 7 | (A) Measured I-V characteristic of a µLED chip. **(B)** Temperature variances of the LED array at various input voltages (2.7–3.2 V) for 100 ms activations. The inset shows the corresponding thermal image of a single LED activation taken at the maximum temperature with 3.2 V input voltage and activation duration of 100 ms.

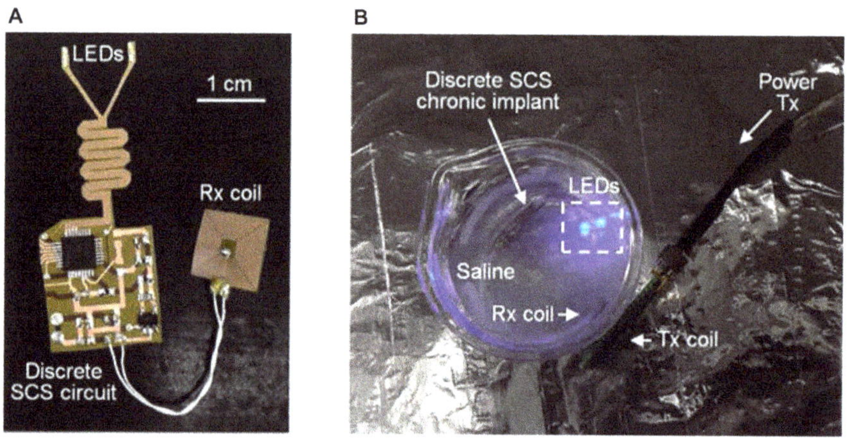

FIGURE 8 | (A) Discrete SCS chronic implant and **(B)** accelerated soak testing in saline with wireless power and data transfer. ©[2014] IEEE. Reprinted, with permission, from Lee et al. (2014).

To evaluate the performance of epoxy-Parylene-C packages and the possible electrical failure of the chronic implant, active accelerated-lifetime soak testing was performed in saline (a solution of 0.90% w/v of NaCl) at a higher than body temperature. For soak testing, a discrete version of the SCS circuit was designed using a MCU (MSP430, Texas Instruments, TX, USA), and constructed using the process described in **Figure 4**. This circuit was programmed to mimic SCS stimulation patterns, once it received wireless power and data through the inductive link. Dimensions and fabrication process of the discrete circuit were identical to the SCS system. Four LEDs (LB QH9G, blue 466 nm, OSRAM, Germany) were integrated on the flexible PCB, and each LED was individually controlled by the MCU. A MEMS-based receiver (Rx) coil was fabricated separately to be placed on the back of the animal and connected to the SCS with flexible wires (392 F high-flex miniature wire, 36 AWG, McMaster-Carr. OH, USA).

Five discrete SCS devices were prepared and immersed in saline at 75°C, as shown in **Figure 8B**. Each individual device was activated by coupling the Rx and Tx coils, and daily the samples were visually monitored for possible device failure. No delamination, major physical corrosion, or performance degradation occurred after 14 days in accelerated lifetime testing conditions. Using the Arrhenius relationship, preliminary results show that the implant lifetime can be the equivalent of 3.5 years at body temperature of 37°C, sufficient for one-year duration requirement in the animal study. Further improvements can be achieved by optimizing temperature and duration of heat treatment for the Parylene/metal thin-film skin or by using additional chemical treatments.

In Vivo Experimental Results

Figure 9 shows the LED driving voltage waveforms, V_{LED}, for optical stimulation with SCS as well as light-induced *in*

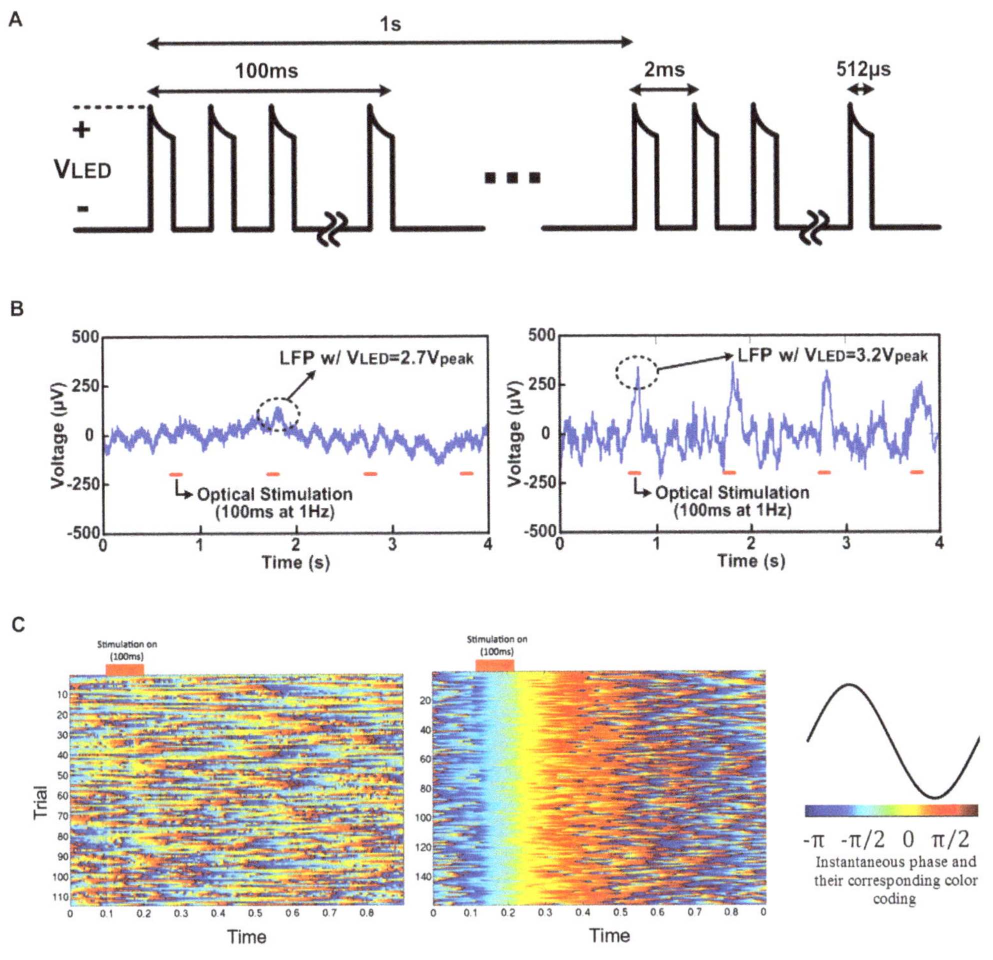

FIGURE 9 | Light-induced LFP recording driven by 2.7 V_{peak} and 3.2 V_{peak} for 100 ms: (A) LED driving voltage, V_{LED}, for *in vivo* optogenetics with SCS, (B) light-induced local field potentials (LFP) with V_{LED} = 2.7 V_{peak} and 3.2 V_{peak}, and (C) instantaneous phase with V_{LED} = 2.7 V_{peak} (top) and 3.2 V_{peak} (bottom) in low frequency band (1–25 Hz), and their corresponding color-coding.

TABLE 1 | Comparison between our LED-coupled optrode array and other laser-coupled optical/electrical devices.

	Optical neurostimulation		Electrical recording		Wireless-enabled	Ref
Light source	#of waveguides	Fiber size	#of electrodes	Electrode size		
Laser	4 or 8	Tip size: 5~20 μm	8 per probe	~160 μm^2	No	Royer et al. (2010)
Laser	1	50~100 μm	36	50~100 μm	No	Wang et al. (2012)
Laser	1	Tip size: 14~28 μm	8	20 μm × 20 μm	No	Wu et al. (2013)
Laser	7	~400 μm	16	N.A.	No	Pisanello et al. (2014)
LED	32	Base size: 300 μm Tip size: ~30 μm	32	~30 μm	Yes	Our Optrode Array

vivo LFP results. The LFPs below 500 Hz were recorded using the optrode array with microwaveguides in the rat's V1 when the SCS system drove μLEDs with a 512 μs pulse train for 100 ms at 1 Hz and V_{LED} = 2.7 V_{peak} and 3.2 V_{peak}, as shown in **Figure 9A**. For each V_{LED}, in total 150 trials of optical stimulation and simultaneous recording were performed. A clear and stable light-induced neural activity was observed in LFPs (1–500 Hz) in time domain driven by 3.2 V_{peak} input voltage (**Figure 9B**). The high input voltage of 3.2 V_{peak} results in an average irradiance of 1.4 mW/mm^2 at the tip of the waveguide, which is above the minimal irradiance (1 mW/mm^2) required for light-evoked neural responses. Lower input voltage (for example, 2.7 V_{peak} resulting in the average irradiance of 0.35 mW/mm^2) was also tried, but no significant neural modulation was observed.

To clearly visualize neural oscillations induced by the optrode array, instantaneous phases of the two datasets (with 2.7 V_{peak} and 3.2 V_{peak} input voltages) of light-evoked LFPs (1–25 Hz) were measured based on Hilbert transform. Each trial was truncated to a ~100 ms pre-stimulation period and an ~800 ms post-stimulation period. The instantaneous phases of each individual trial (1 s with 100 ms light stimulation), labeled with different colors according to **Figure 9C**, were aligned based on the stimulus ON time and stacked. With 3.2 V_{peak} input voltage, light-evoked neural activity shows strong phase synchronization, while no phase synchrony was observed in neural recording data with 2.7 V_{peak} input voltage. The neural modulation and recording was extremely reliable across over 100 trials during the *in vivo* experiments. The cortically optical stimulation generated almost deterministic phase-locked neuronal oscillations without any latency for ~0.3 s as validated with a nonparametric test ($p < 0.05$, Wilcoxon signed rank test for each pair of channels). This experiment, while still preliminary, has verified the feasibility of wirelessly powered optical stimulation and simultaneous recording of neural activity via the LED-coupled optrode array.

Discussion and Outlook

Table 1 compares the presented LED-coupled optrode array with some microfabricated, laser-coupled optical/electrical implants reported by other group. As can be seen, our LED-coupled optrode array provides several unique advantages over laser-coupled devices. First, the devices are manufactured using advanced microfabrication techniques, therefore enabling high channel count and fine spatial resolution for optical stimulation and electrical recording. The design of our system is scalable and the developed manufacturing method is cost effective and reliable. In addition, In addition, our approach uses commercially available LED chips coupled to microfabricated SU-8 waveguides, which eliminates the need for tethered optical fibers and thus is suitable for integration with wireless power and data telemetries. While this work is primarily focused on the neural excitation, the wide selection of the LED chips makes it possible to switch the colors of the LED chips to yellow or red for applications in optogenetic neural inhibition.

For chronic implantation the most critical aspects are certainly the aging behavior of the device and the stability of neural recordings. We anticipate that the performance degradation may be caused by two factors: failure of Parylene-C package and aging of SU-8 waveguide cores. The biocompatible package of the current prototype used 10 μm Parylene-C, which has lower moisture permeability over PDMS and polyimide, and is suitable for packaging of chronic neural implants (Loeb et al., 1977; Schmidt et al., 1988; Takeuchi et al., 2005; Rodger et al., 2008). SU-8 for constructing waveguides on implantable neural probes brings along advantages such as flexibility, optical clarity, and compatibility with conventional photolithography techniques. However, since SU-8 is a photosensitive resist, continuous exposure to blue light may cause the degradation of the material flexibility and optical transparency due to cross-linking of the resin (Fiedler et al., 2014), which will lead to increased coupling loss of light along the waveguides. In this paper, the accelerated short-term soak testing of the optrode prototype has shown good reliability and stability of the Parylene-C package. Although we have not observed any performance degradation of the device in short-term experiments, further long-term studies have to be performed to fully characterize the reliability and stability of the optrode array. More detailed investigation is necessary to optimize the fabrication processes, where, for example, the influence of PR exposure and hard baking should be examined carefully.

Conclusions

In conclusion, design, fabrication, and testing procedures of the wireless LED-coupled slanted optrode array for a really untethered bi-directional neural interface were presented. The array was inductively powered and controlled by the wireless SCS system, designed to improve power efficiency. The SCS system for implantable wireless optogenetics provides high instantaneous power through the inductive link to emit sufficient light and evoke neural activities. The LabVIEW PC interface and custom-designed power Tx module provide wireless power and data to the SCS system, while electrodes embedded in the optrode array enable simultaneous neural recording. The self-assembled LED array on a single substrate can reduce manufacturing cost. Acute *in vivo* experiments with optical stimulation and LFP recording have verified the efficacy of our system for wireless optogenetics application.

Acknowledgments

This work was supported by the National Science Foundation under the Award Numbers CBET-1264772 and ECCS-1407880. The authors would like to Dr. Baokang Bi for the help on microfabrication.

References

Aravanis, A. M., Wang, L.-P., Zhang, F., Meltzer, L. A., Mogri, M. Z., Schneider, M. B., et al. (2007). An optical neural interface: *in vivo* control of rodent motor cortex with integrated fiberoptic and optogenetic technology. *J. Neural. Eng.* 4, S143–S156. doi: 10.1088/1741-2560/4/3/s02

Arrenberg, A. B., Stainier, D. Y. R., Baier, H., and Huisken, J. (2010). Optogenetic control of cardiac function. *Science* 330, 971–974. doi: 10.1126/science.1195929

Boyden, E. S., Zhang, F., Bamberg, E., Nagel, G., and Deisseroth, K. (2005). Millisecond-timescale, genetically targeted optical control of neural activity. *Nat. Neurosci.* 8, 1263–1268. doi: 10.3410/f.1026686.335763

Chuong, A. S., Miri, M. L., Busskamp, V., Matthews, G. A. C., Acker, L. C., Sørensen, A. T., et al. (2014). Noninvasive optical inhibition with a red-shifted microbial rhodopsin. *Nat. Neurosci.* 17, 1123–1129. doi: 10.3410/f.718482076.793498459

Deisseroth, K. (2011). Optogenetics. *Nat. Methods* 8, 26–29. doi: 10.1038/nmeth.f.324

Fiedler, E., Haas, N., and Stieglitz, T. (2014). Suitability of SU-8, EpoClad and EpoCore for flexible waveguides on implantable neural probes. *Conf. Proc. IEEE Eng. Med. Biol. Soc.* 2014, 438–441. doi: 10.1109/EMBC.2014.6943622

Gerits, A., and Vanduffel, W. (2013). Optogenetics in primates: a shining future?. *Trends Genet.* 29, 403–411. doi: 10.1016/j.tig.2013.03.004

Grossman, N., Poher, V., Grubb, M. S., Kennedy, G. T., Nikolic, K., McGovern, B., et al. (2010). Multi-site optical excitation using ChR2 and micro-LED array. *J. Neural. Eng.* 7:016004. doi: 10.1088/1741-2560/7/1/016004

Han, X., Qian, X., Bernstein, J. G., Zhou, H.-H., Franzesi, G. T., Stern, P., et al. (2009). Millisecond-timescale optical control of neural dynamics in the nonhuman primate brain. *Neuron* 62, 191–198. doi: 10.1016/j.neuron.2009.03.011

Iwai, Y., Honda, S., Ozeki, H., Hashimoto, M., and Hirase, H. (2011). A simple head-mountable LED device for chronic stimulation of optogenetic molecules in freely moving mice. *Neurosci. Res.* 70, 124–127. doi: 10.1016/j.neures.2011.01.007

Keiser, G. (2008). *Optical Fiber Commn.* 4th Edn. New York: McGraw-Hill Education.

Kim, T. I., Mccall, J. G., Jung, Y. H., Huang, X., Siuda, E. R., Li, Y. H., et al. (2013). Injectable, cellular-scale optoelectronics with applications for wireless optogenetics. *Science* 340, 211–216. doi: 10.1126/science.1232437

Kwon, K. Y., Bi, X., and Li, W. (2013a). Droplet backside exposure for making slanted SU-8 microneedles. *Conf. Proc. IEEE Eng. Med. Biol. Soc.* 2013, 767–770. doi: 10.1109/EMBC.2013.6609613

Kwon, K. Y., Khomenko, A., Haq, M., and Li, W. (2013b). Integrated slanted microneedle-LED array for optogenetics. *Conf. Proc. IEEE Eng. Med. Biol. Soc.* 2013, 249–252. doi: 10.1109/EMBC.2013.6609484

Kwon, K. Y., Lee, H.-M., Ghovanloo, M., Weber, A., and Li, W. (2014a). "A wireless slanted optrode array with integrated micro leds for optogenetics," in *Micro Electro Mechanical Systems (MEMS), 2014 IEEE 27th International Conference on* (San Francisco, CA), 813–816.

Kwon, K. Y., and Li, W. (2013). "Integrated multi-LED array with three-dimensional polymer waveguide for optogenetics," in *the IEEE 26th International Conference on Micro Electro Mechanical Systems (IEEE MEMS 2013)* (Taipei), 1017–1020.

Kwon, K. Y., Sirowatka, B., Weber, A., and Li, W. (2012). "Opto-μECoG array: transparent μECoG electrode array and integrated LEDs for optogenetics," in *BioCAS 2012* (Hsinchu), 164–167.

Kwon, K. Y., Sirowatka, B., Weber, A., and Li, W. (2013c). Opto-μECoG array: a hybrid neural interface with transparent μECoG electrode array and integrated LEDs for optogenetics. *IEEE Trans. Biomed. Circuits Syst.* 7, 593–600. doi: 10.1109/TBCAS.2013.2282318

Kwon, K. Y., Weber, A., and Li, W. (2014b). Varying-length polymer microneedle arrays fabricated by droplet backside exposure. *J. Microelectromech. Syst.* 23, 1272–1280. doi: 10.1109/jmems.2014.2352412

Lee, H.-M., Kwon, K. Y., Li, W., and Ghovanloo, M. (2014). A wireless implantable switched-capacitor based optogenetic stimulating system. *Conf. Proc. IEEE Eng. Med. Biol. Soc.* 2014, 878–881. doi: 10.1109/EMBC.2014.6943731

Lee, H.-M., Park, H., and Ghovanloo, M. (2013). A power-efficient wireless system with adaptive supply control for deep brain stimulation. *IEEE J. Solid-State Circuits* 48, 2203–2216. doi: 10.1109/jssc.2013.2266862

Li, W., Rodger, D. C., Meng, E., Weiland, J. D., Humayun, M. S., and Tai, Y.-C. (2010). Wafer-level parylene packaging with integrated RF electronics for wireless retinal prostheses. *IEEE/ASME J. Microelectromech. Syst.* 19, 735–742. doi: 10.1109/jmems.2010.2049985

Li, W., Rodger, D. C., Pinto, A., Meng, E., Weiland, J. D., Humayun, M. S., et al. (2011). Parylene-based integrated wireless single-channel neurostimulator. *Sens. Actuators. A Phys.* 166, 193–200. doi: 10.1016/j.sna.2010.03.003

Lin, J. Y., Knutsen, P. M., Muller, A., Kleinfeld, D., and Tsien, R. Y. (2013). ReaChR: a red-shifted variant of channelrhodopsin enables deep transcranial optogenetic excitation. *Nat. Neurosci.* 16, 1499–1508. doi: 10.1038/nn.3502

Loeb, G. E., Bak, M. J., Salcman, M., and Schmidt, E. M. (1977). Parylene as a chronically stable, reproducible microelectrode insulator. *IEEE Trans. Biomed. Eng.* 24, 121–128. doi: 10.1109/tbme.1977.326115

Losavio, B. E., Iyer, V., Patel, S., and Saggau, P. (2011). Acousto-optic laser scanning for multi-site photo-stimulation of single neurons *in vitro*. *J. Neural. Eng.* 7:045002. doi: 10.1088/1741-2560/7/4/045002

Mohanty, S. K., and Thakor, N. V. (2013). Optogenetics: optical methods for cellular control. *Proc. of SPIE* 8586. doi: 10.1117/12.2021444

Onoe, H., Nakai, A., Iwase, E., Matsumoto, K., and Shimoyama, I. (2009). Temperature-controlled transfer and self-wiring for multi-color light-emitting diode arrays. *J. Micromech. Microeng.* 19:075015. doi: 10.1088/0960-1317/19/7/075015

Pisanello, F., Sileo, L., Oldenburg, I. A., Pisanello, M., Martiradonna, L., Assad, J. A., et al. (2014). Multipoint-emitting optical fibers for spatially addressable *in vivo* optogenetics. *Neuron* 82, 1245–1254. doi: 10.1016/j.neuron.2014.04.041

Reutsky-Gefen, I., Golan, L., Farah, N., Schejter, A., Tsur, L., Brosh, I., et al. (2013). Holographic optogenetic stimulation of patterned neuronal activity for vision restoration. *Nat. Commun.* 4:1509. doi: 10.1038/ncomms2500

Rodger, D. C., Fong, A. J., Li, W., Ameri, H., Ahuja, A. K., Gutierrez, C., et al. (2008). Flexible parylene-based multielectrode array technology for high-density neural stimulation and recording. *Sens. Actuators B Chem.* 132, 449–460. doi: 10.1016/j.snb.2007.10.069

Royer, S., Zemelman, B. V., Barbic, M., Losonczy, A., Buzsáki, G., and Magee, J. C. (2010). Multi-array silicon probes with integrated optical fibers: light-assisted perturbation and recording of local neural circuits in the behaving animal. *Eur. J. Neurosci.* 31, 2279–2291. doi: 10.1111/j.1460-9568.2010.07250.x

Schmidt, E. M., Mcintosh, J. S., and Bak, M. J. (1988). Long-term implants of Parylene-C coated microelectrodes. *Med. Biol. Eng. Comput.* 26, 96–101. doi: 10.1007/bf02441836

Stark, E., Koos, T., and Buzsáki, G. (2012). Diode probes for spatiotemporal optical control of multiple neurons in freely moving animals. *J. Neurophysiol.* 108, 349–363. doi: 10.1152/jn.00153.2012

Takeuchi, S., Ziegler, D., Yoshida, Y., Mabuchi, K., and Suzuki, T. (2005). Parylene flexible neural probes integrated with microfluidic channels. *Lab Chip* 5, 519–523. doi: 10.1039/b417497f

Wang, J., Wagner, F., Borton, D. A., Zhang, J. Y., Ozden, I., Burwell, R. D., et al. (2012). Integrated device for combined optical neuromodulation and electrical recording for chronic *in vivo* applications. *J. Neural Eng.* 9:016001. doi: 10.1088/1741-2560/9/1/016001

Wentz, C. T., Bernstein, J. G., Monahan, P., Guerra, A., Rodriguez, A., and Boyden, E. S. (2011). A wirelessly powered and controlled device for optical neural control of freely-behaving animals. *J. Neural. Eng.* 8:046021. doi: 10.1088/1741-2560/8/4/046021

Wu, F., Stark, E., Im, M., Cho, I. J., Yoon, Y. S., Buzsáki, G., et al. (2013). An implantable neural probe with monolithically integrated dielectric waveguide and recording electrodes for optogenetics applications. *J. Neural. Eng.* 10:056012. doi: 10.1088/1741-2560/10/5/056012

Zalocusky, K., and Deisseroth, K. (2013). Optogenetics in the behaving rat: integration of diverse new technologies in a vital animal model. *Optogenetics* 1, 1–17. doi: 10.2478/optog-2013-0001

Zhang, F., Gradinaru, V., Adamantidis, A. R., Durand, R., Airan, R. D., De Lecea, L., et al. (2010). Optogenetic interrogation of neural circuits: technology for probing mammalian brain structures. *Nat. Protoc.* 5, 439–456. doi: 10.1038/nprot.2009.226

Zhang, F., Prigge, M., Beyrière, F., Tsunoda, S. P., Mattis, J., Yizhar, O., et al. (2008). Red-shifted optogenetic excitation: a tool for fast neural control derived from Volvox carteri. *Nat. Neurosci.* 11, 631–633. doi: 10.1038/nn.2120

Zhang, F., Wang, L.-P., Brauner, M., Liewald, J. F., Kay, K., Watzke, N., et al. (2007). Multimodal fast optical interrogation of neural circuitry. *Nature* 446, 633–639. doi: 10.1038/nature05744

Zhu, P., Fajardo, O., Shum, J., Zhang Schärer, Y.-P., and Friedrich, R. W. (2012). High-resolution optical control of spatiotemporal neuronal activity patterns in zebrafish using a digital micromirror device. *Nat. Protoc.* 7, 1410–1425. doi: 10.1038/nprot.2012.072

Zorzos, A. N., Boyden, E. S., and Fonstad, C. G. (2010). Multiwaveguide implantable probe for light delivery to sets of distributed brain targets. *Opt. Lett.* 35, 4133–4135. doi: 10.1364/ol.35.004133

Zorzos, A. N., Scholvin, J., Boyden, E. S., and Fonstad, C. G. (2012). Three-dimensional multiwaveguide probe array for light delivery to distributed brain circuits. *Opt. Lett.* 37, 4841–4843. doi: 10.1364/ol.37.004841

7

Constraints and adaptation of closed-loop neuroprosthetics for functional restoration

Robert Bauer and Alireza Gharabaghi**

Division of Functional and Restorative Neurosurgery, Centre for Integrative Neuroscience, Eberhard Karls University Tuebingen, Tuebingen, Germany

Edited by:
Mikhail Lebedev, Duke University, USA

Reviewed by:
ShiNung Ching, Washington University in St. Louis, USA
Aysegul Gunduz, University of Florida, USA

***Correspondence:**
Robert Bauer
robert.bauer@cin.uni-tuebingen.de
Alireza Gharabaghi
alireza.gharabaghi@uni-tuebingen.de

Closed-loop neuroprosthetics aim to *compensate* for lost function, e.g., by controlling external devices such as prostheses or wheelchairs. Such assistive approaches seek to maximize speed and classification accuracy for high-dimensional control. More recent approaches use similar technology, but aim to restore lost motor function in the long term. To achieve this goal, *restorative* neuroprosthetics attempt to facilitate motor re-learning and to strengthen damaged and/or alternative neural connections on the basis of neurofeedback training within rehabilitative environments. Such a restorative approach requires reinforcement learning of self-modulated brain activity which is considered to be beneficial for functional rehabilitation, e.g., improvement of β-power modulation over sensorimotor areas for post-stroke movement restoration. Patients with motor impairments, however, may also have a compromised ability for motor task-related regulation of the targeted brain activity. This would affect the estimation of feature weights and hence the classification accuracy of the feedback device. This, in turn, can frustrate the patients and compromise their motor learning. Furthermore, the feedback training may even become erroneous when unconstrained classifier adaptation—which is often used in assistive approaches—is also applied in this rehabilitation context. In conclusion, the conceptual switch from assistance toward restoration necessitates a methodological paradigm shift from classification accuracy toward instructional efficiency. Furthermore, a constrained feature space, a priori regularized feature weights, and difficulty adaptation present key elements of restorative brain interfaces. These factors need, therefore, to be addressed within a therapeutic framework to facilitate reinforcement learning of brain self-regulation for restorative purposes.

Keywords: assistive technology, neurorehabilitation, stroke, rehabilitation robotics, brain-computer interface, brain-machine interface, brain-robot interface

RESTORATION INSTEAD OF ASSISTANCE

Brain self-regulation has recently been applied in the context of motor rehabilitation after stroke by providing contingent feedback of motor imagery (Buch et al., 2012; Ang et al., 2014; Morone et al., 2015; Pichiorri et al., 2015). In these approaches, specific brain states (i.e., rest vs. motor imagery) are often separated using an online analysis of sensorimotor power in a cue-paced trial-structure. When used in conjunction with robotic rehabilitation technology, these devices are also referred to as brain-robot interfaces (BRI; Bauer et al., 2015; Naros and Gharabaghi, 2015; Kraus et al., 2016).

While *assistive* BRIs aim to replace lost function by controlling external devices (Hochberg et al., 2012; Collinger et al., 2013), *restorative* BRIs aim to rehabilitate an impaired function (Gharabaghi, 2016; Krucoff et al., 2016). In such a restorative framework, BRIs adhere to an operant conditioning rationale (Sherlin et al., 2011; Bauer and Gharabaghi, 2015b). They provide contingent feedback to facilitate the self-regulation of specific brain activity. This reinforcement learning-based approach is considered to be beneficial for recovery and might ultimately lead to functional gains on the basis of motor re-learning and strengthening of damaged and/or alternative neural connections (Daly and Wolpaw, 2008). Restorative BRIs might be additionally supported by brain state dependent stimulation to strengthen cortico-spinal connectivity (Gharabaghi et al., 2014a; Royter and Gharabaghi, 2016; Kraus et al., 2016).

METHODOLOGICAL ADJUSTMENTS

We propose that, on account of their different goals, these restorative techniques require a different methodological approach than assistive BRIs, i.e., modifying brain physiology vs. controlling extremal devices. We acknowledge that different strategies may be adopted to achieve modified neurophysiology and, ultimately, behavioral gains. However, on the basis of empirical evidence acquired in our lab, we propose the following adjustments: constrained feature space, regularized feature weights, and difficulty adaptation.

Instead of analyzing all acquired signals for optimal classification, we propose that the feature space be intentionally constrained to reinforce a specific oscillatory pattern in accordance with the respective treatment rationale (*constrained feature space*). In a next step, to differentiate between the classes, assistive BRIs use classifier calibration to weight features according to their relevance. However, learning brain self-regulation may lead to non-stationarity of these classes in the course of the training (Vidaurre et al., 2011a; Sugiyama et al., 2013; Naros and Gharabaghi, 2015). Unsupervised adaptation of the feature weights may therefore lead to a switch in the mental strategy (Vidaurre et al., 2011b; Bryan et al., 2013). This approach may even result in artefactual control (Gharabaghi et al., 2014b). We, therefore, propose that *feature weight regularization* be applied to address this issue. Furthermore, cognitive, sensory, and motor impairments may limit the ability to modulate brain activity, perceive, and/or process feedback. This may cause frustration, which, in turn, may be exacerbated due to the low classification accuracy caused by the constrained and regularized feature space (Nijboer et al., 2008; Fels et al., 2015). In this context, we propose that *difficulty adaptation* be applied to overcome cognitive load issues (Bauer and Gharabaghi, 2015a; Bauer et al., 2016a,b). Such an approach may also improve the instructional efficiency of feedback (Bauer and Gharabaghi, 2015b) and maintain motivation (Bauer et al., 2016a,b).

In the following paragraphs, we discuss these methodological adjustments in greater detail.

CONSTRAINED FEATURE SPACE

In high-dimensional feature spaces, some regions may be sparsely populated with data, thereby, impairing the classifier setup (Theodoridis and Koutroumbas, 2009). Under these circumstances, constraining the feature space provides a way of dealing with this *curse of dimensionality*. However, if the feature space is constrained a priori, some useful features for classification may also be discarded. A classifier based on a constrained feature set therefore usually performs less well than a classifier based on a full feature set.

Restorative BRIs, which apply this approach, therefore appear inferior in comparison to their assistive counterparts. The latter use more flexible algorithms to select and weight all available features and to maximize classification accuracy (Ang et al., 2009; Theodoridis and Koutroumbas, 2009). An a priori constraint should therefore be well considered. It is tempting to assume that the brain will find the best combination of features by itself. Such an approach is therefore implicitly followed during standard or robotic neurorehabilitation, when the feedback that is provided by the therapist or the training device is independent of specific brain features. This strategy, however, has not been successful until now, at least when considering severely motor-impaired stroke patients with persistent deficits. Moreover, the features (α-desynchronization) identified as most useful for classification between different states in the post-stroke brain, e.g., rest vs. motor imagery, are not necessarily those that are most therapeutically relevant (β-desynchronization): Synchronization/Desynchronization describe the (often task-induced) increase/reduction in power in specific frequency bands. The α-band usually ranges from 8–14 Hz, while the β-band ranges from 15–30 Hz. Specifically, movement-related β-desynchronization (β-ERD) is compromised in the contralateral primary cortex in comparison to healthy controls; the more severe the patient's motor impairment, the less β-ERD (Rossiter et al., 2014). And so β-ERD remains inferior to other features for classification purposes in stroke patients, e.g., in differentiating movement-related brain states for the control of external devices (Gomez-Rodriguez et al., 2011). In this context, we argue that the fact that β-oscillations are less optimal for classification purposes does not compromise—but rather qualifies—this physiological marker as a therapeutic target (Naros and Gharabaghi, 2015). Here, we see an analogy to the concept of constraint-induced movement therapy in stroke patients, where the affected rather than the healthy side of the body is trained to facilitate restoration instead of compensation of motor function. Notably, such an approach does not exclude the possibility that alternative cortico-spinal pathways which do not originate from the contralateral primary motor cortex take over lost function. These pathways would be facilitated on the basis of cortical disinhibition and coherent interaction with the muscles in the β-band as well (Mima et al., 2001; Kilavik et al., 2012; Aumann and Prut, 2015; Brittain et al., 2014; Rossiter et al., 2014; Kraus et al., 2016).

Furthermore, an approach based on a constrained feature space allows making a direct, hypothesis-driven comparison of different interventions based on specific oscillatory patterns. By way of example, an increase in the β-modulation range will improve cortico-spinal connectivity (Kraus et al., 2015, 2016) and motor function (Naros et al., 2016). This will enable us to empirically detect functionally relevant markers and mechanisms of restoration and to determine physiology-based strategies for further improvement. Such knowledge will also enable us to develop approaches for treatment matching, e.g., defining feature sets on the basis of specific functional impairments and/or lesion locations (Shelton and Reding, 2001; Stinear et al., 2012). By contrast, an approach based on an unconstrained feature space would be based on the assumption that the most accurate detection of motor intention/imagery and provision of feedback is in itself sufficient to restore function.

REGULARIZED FEATURE WEIGHTS

Regularization can be considered a penalty term to prevent feature weights from reaching implausibly high values (Theodoridis and Koutroumbas, 2009; Bishop, 2013) caused by the empirical estimation of class parameters (e.g., mean and covariance). Such estimates can be biased, especially when the sample size is low. Due to the large variety of classification approaches (Theodoridis and Koutroumbas, 2009), several regularization approaches have been suggested, e.g., pooled covariance estimation (Friedman, 1989), rejection of eigenvectors (Blankertz et al., 2008), shrinkage estimators (Beltrachini et al., 2010), or feature subset selection (Friedman, 1989).

Even when recognizing that a constrained feature space can already be considered a form of regularization, the empirical determination of feature weights during the calibration period may pose a particular challenge for restorative brain-interface approaches, e.g., when estimating mean and covariance of two classes (rest vs. motor imagery). When patients are able to desynchronize sensorimotor oscillations (Pfurtscheller et al., 2005; Neuper et al., 2006; Kaiser et al., 2011), the estimation of feature weights is usually straightforward. In such a case, several approaches for regularization have been discussed (Yuan and Bentler, 1998; Beltrachini et al., 2010). If, however, the volitional modulation of sensorimotor oscillations has not been learned (Brauchle et al., 2015; Bauer and Gharabaghi, 2015b; Naros and Gharabaghi, 2015), or when it is impaired due to the underlying pathology (Buch et al., 2012; Bundy et al., 2012; Rossiter et al., 2014), the estimation might become noisy or even false. More formally, if one class (i.e. motor imagery) is not sufficiently expressed, its parameters (e.g., mean and covariance) cannot be measured. If, however, the mean during motor imagery is not sufficiently different from the mean during rest, a noisy estimate can result in the classifier being calibrated toward the wrong direction of modulation. Subsequently, the patient might receive feedback for synchronizing instead of desynchronizing.

Novelty detection has been suggested as a solution, if no information about a second class is available (Pimentel et al., 2014). Such a one-class approach might base mean and covariance estimation on the rest class only. However, without a priori information about the targeted direction of modulation, data-driven regularization approaches cannot be sufficient.

Furthermore, when a patient alters the mental strategy in the course of the intervention, a classifier trained on the initial strategy can become misaligned. In classical brain-interface approaches, the adaptation of feature weights has been proposed for such cases (Vidaurre et al., 2011b; Bryan et al., 2013; Sugiyama et al., 2013). But such data-driven approaches can be problematic for restorative approaches; classifier adaptation might condition the patients to explore alternative, i.e., therapeutically non-desired strategies (Bauer and Gharabaghi, 2015a,b). When the patient becomes frustrated with motor imagery, he/she may use artifacts for control, e.g., muscle contractions (Gharabaghi et al., 2014b).

Bearing these points in mind, we suggest employing informed regularization determined by a priori selected feature weights, thereby, ensuring the targeted direction of modulation. In our lab, we currently employ a variant of novelty classification by using a linear discriminant analysis with a fixed direction. In that regard, we base the mean and covariance estimation on the rest class only, with the parameter estimation pooled across several electrodes. Thereby, we provide feedback for the reduction of the mean, i.e., desynchronization, only.

DIFFICULTY OF ADAPTATION

Lotte and colleagues have pointed out that most neurofeedback protocols are limited with regard to their instructional design. They suggested adaptive training approaches, i.e., the use of difficulty levels which are challenging, but still achievable (Lotte et al., 2013). A similar idea was postulated by the cognitive load theory (Schnotz and Kürschner, 2007). On the basis of these concepts, both under- and over-challenge must be avoided to facilitate learning (Schnotz and Kürschner, 2007; Bauer and Gharabaghi, 2015a). In classifiers, which are constrained, regularized and linear, item response theory enables us to directly relate the threshold used for classification to the difficulty level (Bauer and Gharabaghi, 2015a). By using a linear discriminant analysis with a fixed direction, thresholding allows us to provide reward for desynchronization only when it is sufficiently strong. Within this framework, the shape of classification accuracy CA across different threshold can be interpreted as the zone of proximal development (ZPD). This argument, with detailed examples, has been clarified elsewhere (Bauer and Gharabaghi, 2015a). The ZPD is an indirect measure of a subject's cognitive resources (Schnotz and Kürschner, 2007). It also constitutes the range of threshold, where learning may occur because subjects are able to compensate for the extraneous load caused by the mismatch of ability and difficulty (Bauer and Gharabaghi, 2015a). Along these lines, two recent studies with healthy subjects provided empirical evidence that dynamic threshold adaptation is instrumental in facilitating learning (Bauer et al., 2016b; Naros et al., 2016).

Unconstrained and unregularized classifiers do not offer an accessible, one-dimensional parameter to fine-tune the difficulty of the task. It might therefore be problematic to adapt the difficulty within these approaches. In particular, a multi-dimensional or even non-linear theory of difficulty adaptation appears to be challenging. We instead explored the difficulty threshold of a linear, a priori constrained and regularized classifier and found evidence of a direct correlation between the subjects' perceived mental effort and the task difficulty (Bauer et al., 2016b). Further empirical evidence suggests that there is a link between classification accuracy and cognitive load; classification performance has been linked to mood and mastery confidence (Nijboer et al., 2008), as well as to the degree of concentration on the task and the ability to ignore distracting stimuli (Hammer et al., 2012). The sensation of challenge might therefore be linked to the ratio of true to false positives returned by the classifier. This hypothesis is supported by a Bayesian simulation study of reinforcement learning under adaptive changes of true and false positive rates (Bauer and Gharabaghi, 2015b). A generalized concept of difficulty adaptation might, therefore, be based on controlling the relationship between true and false positive rates by asking the patients to self-rate the perceived effort and/or applying non-cued training.

Nonetheless, further factors may affect the difficulty of the training: the challenge of achieving a sense of cognitive and internal control (Burde and Blankertz, 2006; Wood et al., 2014), the appropriate processing of cues to reduce impairments in mental chronometry (Liepert et al., 2012), and to increase the quality of motor imagery (Heremans et al., 2009, 2012), the specific sensory impairments of patients and their interaction with the feedback modality (e.g., visual, haptic, auditory) (Nijboer et al., 2008; Gomez-Rodriguez et al., 2011; Parker et al., 2011; Sollfrank et al., 2015), or the repetitive and fatiguing nature of training (Lee et al., 1991; Page et al., 2011). Dealing with these aspects by proper instructional design is more important for restorative than for assistive approaches (Lotte et al., 2013).

CONCLUSION

We propose that restorative approaches should apply prior information about beneficial features (e.g., β-power desynchronization over sensorimotor areas) to constrain the feature space and regularize their direction. Such an approach may reduce the classification accuracy in comparison to unconstrained or unregularized approaches, particularly in patients who are only partially able to self-regulate the targeted brain state. At the same time, this method would increase the likelihood that feedback is provided for the therapeutically targeted modulation of brain activity only. The threshold selection in restorative approaches should therefore not be misled by the goal of maximum classification accuracy. Instead, it should follow instructional demands to maximize learning.

Accordingly, several methods have been proposed for locating the threshold for maximum learning (Ivanova et al., 2005; Cegarra and Chevalier, 2008; Naros et al., 2016; Bauer et al., 2016a,b). Moreover, physiological parameters, e.g., distributed cortical patterns in the α-range (Vukelić et al., 2014; Vukelić and Gharabaghi, 2015a,b) and the θ-range (Fels et al., 2015) which were linked to β-band self-regulation may also be used in the long term for this purpose.

The conceptual switch from assistive to restorative neuroprosthetics necessitates methodological adjustments (constrained feature space, a priori regularized feature weights, difficulty adaptation) which ultimately represent a paradigm switch from classification accuracy toward instructional efficiency to facilitate reinforcement learning of brain self-regulation.

AUTHOR CONTRIBUTIONS

All authors listed, have made substantial, direct and intellectual contribution to the work, and approved it for publication.

ACKNOWLEDGMENTS

RB was supported by the Graduate Training Centre of Neuroscience, International Max Planck Research School for Cognitive and Systems Neuroscience, Tuebingen, Germany. AG was supported by grants from the German Federal Ministry of Education and Research [BMBF IMONAS 13GW0119B] and the Baden-Württemberg Stiftung [NemoPlast NEU005]. There are no conflicts of interests.

REFERENCES

Ang, K. K., Chin, Z. Y., Zhang, H., and Guan, C. (2009). "Robust filter bank common spatial pattern (RFBCSP) in motor-imagery-based brain-computer interface," in *Conference Proceedings Annual International Conference of the IEEE Engineering in Medicine and Biology Society* (Minneapolis, MN), 578–581. doi: 10.1109/IEMBS.2009.5332817

Ang, K. K., Guan, C., Phua, K. S., Wang, C., Zhou, L., Tang, K. Y., et al. (2014). Brain-computer interface-based robotic end effector system for wrist and hand rehabilitation: results of a three-armed randomized controlled trial for chronic stroke. *Front. Neuroeng.* 7:30. doi: 10.3389/fneng.2014.00030

Aumann, T. D., and Prut, Y. (2015). Do sensorimotor β-oscillations maintain muscle synergy representations in primary motor cortex? *Trends Neurosci.* 38, 77–85. doi: 10.1016/j.tins.2014.12.002

Bauer, R., Fels, M., Royter, V., Raco, V., and Gharabaghi, A. (2016a). Closed-loop adaptation of neurofeedback based on mental effort facilitates reinforcement learning of brain self-regulation. *Clin. Neurophysiol.* 127, 3156–3164. doi: 10.1016/j.clinph.2016.06.020

Bauer, R., Fels, M., Vukelić, M., Ziemann, U., and Gharabaghi, A. (2015). Bridging the gap between motor imagery and motor execution with a brain-robot interface. *Neuroimage* 108, 319–327. doi: 10.1016/j.neuroimage.2014.12.026

Bauer, R., and Gharabaghi, A. (2015a). Estimating cognitive load during self-regulation of brain activity and neurofeedback with therapeutic brain-computer interfaces. *Front. Behav. Neurosci.* 9:21. doi: 10.3389/fnbeh.2015.00021

Bauer, R., and Gharabaghi, A. (2015b). Reinforcement learning for adaptive threshold control of restorative brain-computer interfaces: a Bayesian simulation. *Front. Neurosci.* 9:36. doi: 10.3389/fnins.2015.00036

Bauer, R., Vukelić, M., and Gharabaghi, A. (2016b). What is the optimal task difficulty for reinforcement learning of brain self-regulation? *Clin. Neurophysiol.* 127, 3033–3041. doi: 10.1016/j.clinph.2016.06.016

Beltrachini, L., von Ellenrieder, N., and Muravchik, C. H. (2010). Shrinkage approach for EEG covariance matrix estimation. *Conf. Proc. IEEE Eng. Med. Biol. Soc.* 2010, 1654–1657. doi: 10.1109/iembs.2010.5626668

Bishop, C. M. (2013). *Pattern Recognition and Machine Learning*. New Delhi: Springer.

Blankertz, B., Tomioka, R., Lemm, S., Kawanabe, M., and Muller, K. (2008). Optimizing spatial filters for robust EEG single-trial analysis. *IEEE Signal Process. Mag.* 25, 41–56. doi: 10.1109/MSP.2008.4408441

Brauchle, D., Vukelić, M., Bauer, R., and Gharabaghi, A. (2015). Brain state-dependent robotic reaching movement with a multi-joint arm exoskeleton: combining brain-machine interfacing and robotic rehabilitation. *Front. Hum. Neurosci.* 9:564. doi: 10.3389/fnhum.2015.00564

Brittain, J.-S., Sharott, A., and Brown, P. (2014). The highs and lows of beta activity in cortico-basal ganglia loops. *Eur. J. Neurosci.* 39, 1951–1959. doi: 10.1111/ejn.12574

Bryan, M. J., Martin, S. A., Cheung, W., and Rao, R. P. (2013). Probabilistic co-adaptive brain–computer interfacing. *J. Neural Eng.* 10:66008. doi: 10.1088/1741-2560/10/6/066008

Buch, E. R., Modir Shanechi, A., Fourkas, A. D., Weber, C., Birbaumer, N., and Cohen, L. G. (2012). Parietofrontal integrity determines neural modulation associated with grasping imagery after stroke. *Brain J. Neurol.* 135, 596–614. doi: 10.1093/brain/awr331

Bundy, D. T., Wronkiewicz, M., Sharma, M., Moran, D. W., Corbetta, M., and Leuthardt, E. C. (2012). Using ipsilateral motor signals in the unaffected cerebral hemisphere as a signal platform for brain-computer interfaces in hemiplegic stroke survivors. *J. Neural Eng.* 9:36011. doi: 10.1088/1741-2560/9/3/036011

Burde, W., and Blankertz, B. (2006). "Is the locus of control of reinforcement a predictor of brain-computer interface performance?," in *Proceedings of the 3rd International Brain-Computer Interface Workshop and Training Course* (Graz), 76–77.

Cegarra, J., and Chevalier, A. (2008). The use of Tholos software for combining measures of mental workload: toward theoretical and methodological improvements. *Behav. Res. Methods* 40, 988–1000. doi: 10.3758/BRM.40.4.988

Collinger, J. L., Wodlinger, B., Downey, J. E., Wang, W., Tyler-Kabara, E. C., Weber, D. J., et al. (2013). High-performance neuroprosthetic control by an individual with tetraplegia. *Lancet* 381, 557–564. doi: 10.1016/S0140-6736(12)61816-9

Daly, J. J., and Wolpaw, J. R. (2008). Brain-computer interfaces in neurological rehabilitation. *Lancet Neurol.* 7, 1032–1043. doi: 10.1016/S1474-4422(08)70223-0

Fels, M., Bauer, R., and Gharabaghi, A. (2015). Predicting workload profiles of brain-robot interface and electromygraphic neurofeedback with cortical resting-state networks: personal trait or task-specific challenge? *J. Neural Eng.* 12:046029. doi: 10.1088/1741-2560/12/4/046029

Friedman, J. H. (1989). Regularized Discriminant Analysis. *J. Am. Stat. Assoc.* 84, 165–175. doi: 10.1080/01621459.1989.10478752

Gharabaghi, A. (2016). What turns assistive into restorative brain-machine interfaces? *Front. Neurosci.* 10:456. doi: 10.3389/fnins.2016.00456

Gharabaghi, A., Kraus, D., Leão, M. T., Spüler, M., Walter, A., Bogdan, M., et al. (2014a). Coupling brain-machine interfaces with cortical stimulation for brain-state dependent stimulation: enhancing motor cortex excitability for neurorehabilitation. *Front. Hum. Neurosci.* 8:122. doi: 10.3389/fnhum.2014.00122

Gharabaghi, A., Naros, G., Khademi, F., Jesser, J., Spüler, M., Walter, A., et al. (2014b). Learned self-regulation of the lesioned brain with epidural electrocorticography. *Front. Behav. Neurosci.* 8:429. doi: 10.3389/fnbeh.2014.00429

Gomez-Rodriguez, M., Peters, J., Hill, J., Schölkopf, B., Gharabaghi, A., and Grosse-Wentrup, M. (2011). Closing the sensorimotor loop: haptic feedback facilitates decoding of motor imagery. *J. Neural Eng.* 8:36005. doi: 10.1088/1741-2560/8/3/036005

Hammer, E. M., Halder, S., Blankertz, B., Sannelli, C., Dickhaus, T., Kleih, S., et al. (2012). Psychological predictors of SMR-BCI performance. *Biol. Psychol.* 89, 80–86. doi: 10.1016/j.biopsycho.2011.09.006

Heremans, E., Helsen, W. F., De Poel, H. J., Alaerts, K., Meyns, P., and Feys, P. (2009). Facilitation of motor imagery through movement-related cueing. *Brain Res.* 1278, 50–58. doi: 10.1016/j.brainres.2009.04.041

Heremans, E., Nieuwboer, A., Feys, P., Vercruysse, S., Vandenberghe, W., Sharma, N., et al. (2012). External cueing improves motor imagery quality in patients with Parkinson disease. *Neurorehabil. Neural Repair* 26, 27–35. doi: 10.1177/1545968311411055

Hochberg, L. R., Bacher, D., Jarosiewicz, B., Masse, N. Y., Simeral, J. D., Vogel, J., et al. (2012). Reach and grasp by people with tetraplegia using a neurally controlled robotic arm. *Nature* 485, 372–375. doi: 10.1038/nature11076

Ivanova, G., Perez, D., and Both, R. (2005). Threshold adaptation for mean value based operant conditioning. *Conf. Proc. Annu. Int. Conf. IEEE Eng. Med. Biol. Soc.* 4, 3612–3615. doi: 10.1109/iembs.2005.1617263

Kaiser, V., Kreilinger, A., Müller-Putz, G. R., and Neuper, C. (2011). First steps toward a motor imagery based stroke BCI: new strategy to set up a classifier. *Front. Neurosci.* 5:86. doi: 10.3389/fnins.2011.00086

Kilavik, B. E., Zaepffel, M., Brovelli, A., MacKay, W. A., and Riehle, A. (2012). The ups and downs of beta oscillations in sensorimotor cortex. *Exp. Neurol.* 15–26. doi: 10.1016/j.expneurol.2012.09.014

Kraus, D., Naros, G., Bauer, R., Khademi, F., Leão, M. T., Ziemann, U., et al. (2016). Brain state-dependent transcranial magnetic closed-loop stimulation controlled by sensorimotor desynchronization induces robust increase of corticospinal excitability. *Brain Stimul.* 9, 415–424. doi: 10.1016/j.brs.2016.02.007

Kraus, D., Naros, G., Bauer, R., Leão, M. T., Ziemann, U., and Gharabaghi, A. (2015). Brain-robot interface driven plasticity: distributed modulation of corticospinal excitability. *Neuroimage* 125, 522–532. doi: 10.1016/j.neuroimage.2015.09.074

Krucoff, M. O., Rahimpour, S., Slutzky, M. W., Edgerton, V. R., and Turner, D. A. (2016). Enhancing nervous system recovery through neurobiologics, neural interface training, and neurorehabilitation. *Front. Neurosci.* 10:584. doi: 10.3389/fnins.2016.00584

Lee, T. D., Swanson, L. R., and Hall, A. L. (1991). What is repeated in a repetition? Effects of practice conditions on motor skill acquisition. *Phys. Ther.* 71, 150–156.

Liepert, J., Greiner, J., Nedelko, V., and Dettmers, C. (2012). Reduced upper limb sensation impairs mental chronometry for motor imagery after stroke: clinical and electrophysiological findings. *Neurorehabil. Neural Repair* 26, 470–478. doi: 10.1177/1545968311425924

Lotte, F., Larrue, F., and Mühl, C. (2013). Flaws in current human training protocols for spontaneous Brain-Computer Interfaces: lessons learned from instructional design. *Front. Hum. Neurosci.* 7:568. doi: 10.3389/fnhum.2013.00568

Mima, T., Matsuoka, T., and Hallett, M. (2001). Information flow from the sensorimotor cortex to muscle in humans. *Clin. Neurophysiol. Off. J. Int. Fed. Clin. Neurophysiol.* 112, 122–126. doi: 10.1016/S1388-2457(00)00515-0

Morone, G., Pisotta, I., Pichiorri, F., Kleih, S., Paolucci, S., Molinari, M., et al. (2015). Proof of principle of a brain-computer interface approach to support poststroke arm rehabilitation in hospitalized patients: design, acceptability, and usability. *Arch. Phys. Med. Rehabil.* 96, S71–S78. doi: 10.1016/j.apmr.2014.05.026

Naros, G., and Gharabaghi, A. (2015). Reinforcement learning of self-regulated β-oscillations for motor restoration in chronic stroke. *Front. Hum. Neurosci.* 9:391. doi: 10.3389/fnhum.2015.00391

Naros, G., Naros, I., Grimm, F., Ziemann, U., and Gharabaghi, A. (2016). Reinforcement learning of self-regulated sensorimotor β-oscillations improves motor performance. *NeuroImage* 134, 142–152. doi: 10.1016/j.neuroimage.2016.03.016

Neuper, C., Wörtz, M., and Pfurtscheller, G. (2006). ERD/ERS patterns reflecting sensorimotor activation and deactivation. *Prog. Brain Res.* 159, 211–222. doi: 10.1016/S0079-6123(06)59014-4

Nijboer, F., Furdea, A., Gunst, I., Mellinger, J., McFarland, D. J., Birbaumer, N., et al. (2008). An auditory brain–computer interface (BCI). *J. Neurosci. Methods* 167, 43–50. doi: 10.1016/j.jneumeth.2007.02.009

Page, S. J., Dunning, K., Hermann, V., Leonard, A., and Levine, P. (2011). Longer versus shorter mental practice sessions for affected upper extremity movement after stroke: a randomized controlled trial. *Clin. Rehabil.* 25, 627–637. doi: 10.1177/0269215510395793

Parker, J., Mountain, G., and Hammerton, J. (2011). A review of the evidence underpinning the use of visual and auditory feedback for computer technology in post-stroke upper-limb rehabilitation. *Disabil. Rehabil. Assist. Technol.* 6, 1–8. doi: 10.3109/17483107.2011.556209

Pfurtscheller, G., Neuper, C., Brunner, C., and da Silva, F. L. (2005). Beta rebound after different types of motor imagery in man. *Neurosci. Lett.* 378, 156–159. doi: 10.1016/j.neulet.2004.12.034

Pichiorri, F., Morone, G., Petti, M., Toppi, J., Pisotta, I., Molinari, M., et al. (2015). Brain-computer interface boosts motor imagery practice during stroke recovery. *Ann. Neurol.* 77, 851–865. doi: 10.1002/ana.24390

Pimentel, M. A. F., Clifton, D. A., Clifton, L., and Tarassenko, L. (2014). A review of novelty detection. *Signal Process.* 99, 215–249. doi: 10.1016/j.sigpro.2013.12.026

Royter, V., and Gharabaghi, A. (2016). Brain state-dependent closed-loop modulation of paired associative stimulation controlled by sensorimotor desynchronization. *Front Cell Neurosci.* 10:115. doi: 10.3389/fncel.2016.00115

Rossiter, H. E., Boudrias, M.-H., and Ward, N. S. (2014). Do movement-related beta oscillations change following stroke? *J. Neurophysiol.* 112, 2053–2058. doi: 10.1152/jn.00345.2014

Schnotz, W., and Kürschner, C. (2007). A reconsideration of cognitive load theory. *Educ. Psychol. Rev.* 19, 469–508. doi: 10.1007/s10648-007-9053-4

Shelton, F. N., and Reding, M. J. (2001). Effect of lesion location on upper limb motor recovery after stroke. *Stroke* 32, 107–112. doi: 10.1161/01.STR.32.1.107

Sherlin, L. H., Arns, M., Lubar, J., Heinrich, H., Kerson, C., Strehl, U., et al. (2011). Neurofeedback and basic learning theory: implications for research and practice. *J. Neurother.* 15, 292–304. doi: 10.1080/10874208.2011.623089

Sollfrank, T., Ramsay, A., Perdikis, S., Williamson, J., Murray-Smith, R., Leeb, R., et al. (2015). The effect of multimodal and enriched feedback on SMR-BCI performance. *Clin. Neurophysiol.* 127, 490–498. doi: 10.1016/j.clinph.2015.06.004

Stinear, C. M., Barber, P. A., Petoe, M., Anwar, S., and Byblow, W. D. (2012). The PREP algorithm predicts potential for upper limb recovery after stroke. *Brain* 135, 2527–2535. doi: 10.1093/brain/aws146

Sugiyama, M., Yamada, M., and du Plessis, M. C. (2013). Learning under nonstationarity: covariate shift and class-balance change: learning under nonstationarity. *Wiley Interdiscip. Rev. Comput. Stat.* 5, 465–477. doi: 10.1002/wics.1275

Theodoridis, S., and Koutroumbas, K. (2009). *Pattern Recognition.* Burlington, MA; London: Academic Press.

Vidaurre, C., Kawanabe, M., von Bünau, P., Blankertz, B., and Müller, K. R. (2011a). Toward unsupervised adaptation of LDA for brain-computer interfaces. *IEEE Trans. Biomed. Eng.* 58, 587–597. doi: 10.1109/TBME.2010.2093133

Vidaurre, C., Sannelli, C., Müller, K.-R., and Blankertz, B. (2011b). Co-adaptive calibration to improve BCI efficiency. *J. Neural Eng.* 8:25009. doi: 10.1088/1741-2560/8/2/025009

Vukelić, M., Bauer, R., Naros, G., Naros, I., Braun, C., and Gharabaghi, A. (2014). Lateralized alpha-band cortical networks regulate volitional modulation of beta-band sensorimotor oscillations. *NeuroImage* 87, 147–153. doi: 10.1016/j.neuroimage.2013.10.003

Vukelić M., and Gharabaghi, A. (2015a). Oscillatory entrainment of the motor cortical network during motor imagery is modulated by the feedback modality. *Neuroimage* 1, 1–11. doi: 10.1016/j.neuroimage.2015.01.058

Vukelić, M., and Gharabaghi, A. (2015b). Self-regulation of circumscribed brain activity modulates spatially selective and frequency specific connectivity of distributed resting state networks. *Front. Behav. Neurosci.* 9:181. doi: 10.3389/fnbeh.2015.00181

Wood, G., Kober, S. E., Witte, M., and Neuper, C. (2014). On the need to better specify the concept of "control" in brain-computer-interfaces/neurofeedback research. *Front. Syst. Neurosci.* 8:171. doi: 10.3389/fnsys.2014.00171

Yuan, K. H., and Bentler, P. M. (1998). Robust mean and covariance structure analysis. *Br. J. Math. Stat. Psychol.* 51 (Pt 1), 63–88. doi: 10.1111/j.2044-8317.1998.tb00667.x

8

Sensitivity to microstimulation of somatosensory cortex distributed over multiple electrodes

*Sungshin Kim[1], Thierri Callier[1], Gregg A. Tabot[2], Francesco V. Tenore[3] and Sliman J. Bensmaia[1,2]**

[1] Department of Organismal Biology and Anatomy, University of Chicago, Chicago, IL, USA, [2] Committee on Computational Neuroscience, University of Chicago, Chicago, IL, USA, [3] Research and Exploratory Development Department, Johns Hopkins University Applied Physics Laboratory, Laurel, MD, USA

Edited by:
Mikhail Lebedev,
Duke University, USA

Reviewed by:
Emilio Salinas,
Wake Forest University, USA
Joseph E. O'Doherty,
University of California,
San Francisco, USA
Christian Klaes,
Caltech, USA

***Correspondence:**
Sliman J. Bensmaia,
Department of Organismal Biology and Anatomy, University of Chicago,
1027 East 57th Street, Chicago,
IL, USA
sliman@uchicago.edu

Meaningful and repeatable tactile sensations can be evoked by electrically stimulating primary somatosensory cortex. Intracortical microstimulation (ICMS) may thus be a viable approach to restore the sense of touch in individuals who have lost it, for example tetraplegic patients. One of the potential limitations of this approach, however, is that high levels of current can damage the neuronal tissue if the resulting current densities are too high. The limited range of safe ICMS amplitudes thus limits the dynamic range of ICMS-evoked sensations. One way to get around this limitation would be to distribute the ICMS over multiple electrodes in the hopes of intensifying the resulting percept without increasing the current density experienced by the neuronal tissue. Here, we test whether stimulating through multiple electrodes is a viable solution to increase the dynamic range of ICMS-elicited sensations without increasing the peak current density. To this end, we compare the ability of non-human primates to detect ICMS delivered through one vs. multiple electrodes. We also compare their ability to discriminate pulse trains differing in amplitude when these are delivered through one or more electrodes. We find that increasing the number of electrodes through which ICMS is delivered only has a marginal effect on detectability or discriminability despite the fact that 2–4 times more current is delivered overall. Furthermore, the impact of multielectrode stimulation (or lack thereof) is found whether pulses are delivered synchronously or asynchronously, whether the leading phase of the pulses is cathodic or anodic, and regardless of the spatial configuration of the electrode groups.

Keywords: neuroprosthetics, intracortical microstimulation, discrimination task, detection performance, non-human primates

Introduction

One approach to restoring sensorimotor function to patients with upper spinal cord injury consists of measuring signals from motor areas of their brains to control anthropomorphic robotic arms (Hochberg et al., 2012; Collinger et al., 2013). However, our ability to use our limbs relies heavily on somatosensory signals, which convey information about the consequences of our movements and about the objects with which we interact. With this in mind, it is necessary not only to re-establish the ability to send commands to the limb but also to restore the ability to receive sensory signals back from the limb. One strategy to restore somatosensation consists of electrically stimulating neurons in somatosensory cortex through chronically implanted electrode arrays in the hopes of eliciting meaningful tactile and proprioceptive sensations (London et al., 2008; O'Doherty et al., 2011; Berg et al., 2013; Tabot et al., 2013b, 2014; Thomson et al., 2013; Bensmaia and Miller, 2014; Dadarlat et al., 2014). One limitation of intracortical microstimulation (ICMS) is that high levels of current can damage neuronal tissue if the resulting current densities are too high. However, ICMS has been found to have a negligible effect on tissue over a range of current densities (up to about 1.0 mC/cm^2; Rajan et al., unpublished observations), unless it is applied continuously for long periods of time (McCreery et al., 2010). One strategy to expand the dynamic range of elicited sensations without increasing the current density experienced by any one population of neurons, and thus to avoid damaging the brain, is to distribute the injected current over multiple electrodes (Zaaimi et al., 2013). That way, we might be able to achieve a wider dynamic range of sensations without subjecting neurons to higher peak current densities.

To investigate this possibility, we had two non-human primates perform detection or discrimination tasks in a two-alternative forced choice paradigm (**Figure 1A**) to probe their sensitivity to ICMS delivered through one or more electrodes. Electrodes in each group were chosen such that their receptive fields were largely overlapping to ensure that the sensations evoked resulted in tactile sensations that were localized to a single location on the skin (cf. Tabot et al., 2013b). We wished to determine the degree to which stimulation through multiple electrodes (1) reduces the minimum amplitude required to achieve a percept (the absolute threshold) and (2) increases the number of discriminable amplitude increments [just noticeable differences (JNDs)] that can be achieved between absolute threshold and the maximum current per electrode (100 μA).

To these ends, we first investigated whether animals could better detect pulse trains delivered simultaneously through multiple electrodes (2 or 4) than they could the same pulse trains delivered through a single electrode. We also compared the animals' sensitivity to multi-electrode stimulation when pulses were delivered synchronously or asynchronously within each stimulus cycle (**Figure 1B**). Moreover, we probed the effect on sensitivity of polarity (that is, whether the leading phase is cathodic or anodic) and of the spatial configuration of the electrodes on the array (**Figure 1C**). Finally, we investigated how multi-electrode stimulation affects the discriminability of ICMS pulse trains that differ in amplitude. We conclude that multi-electrode stimulation only provides a modest improvement in the dynamic range and does not justify its energetic cost.

Results and Discussion

Effect of Multi-Electrode Stimulation on Detectability

We compared detection performance for ICMS pulse trains delivered through 1, 2, or 4 electrodes with cathodic phase-first current pulses delivered synchronously across electrodes (**Figure 1B**, left). In these experiments, two and four times as much current was delivered in the double and quad conditions as was delivered in the single electrode condition, respectively. We found that the absolute threshold – defined as the ICMS amplitude that yielded 75% detection performance – decreased as the number of stimulated electrodes increased (**Figures 2A,B**;

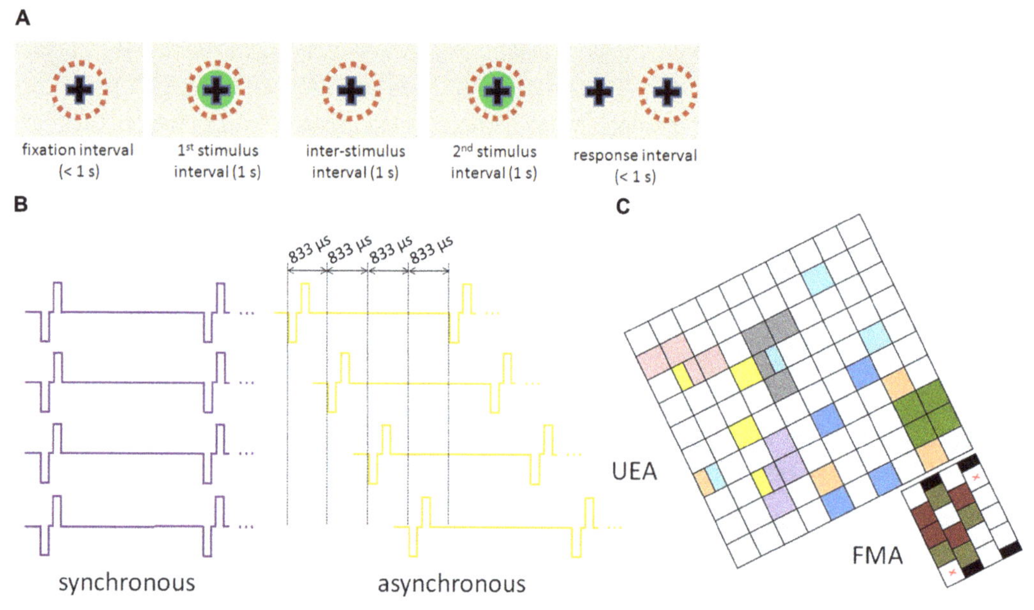

FIGURE 1 | Experimental design. (A) Structure of a trial. The red dashed circle denotes the animal's direction of gaze; on this example trial, the animal responded right. **(B)** Timing of synchronous and asynchronous ICMS for a quad of electrodes. **(C)** Spatial configuration of electrode quads from one monkey. Each square represents an electrode; electrodes that share a color were part of a quad (some electrodes were used in two quads).

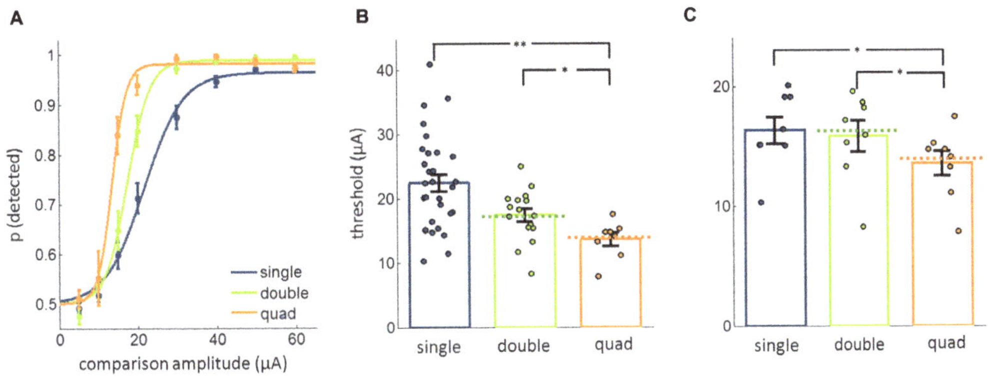

FIGURE 2 | Detectability of ICMS delivered through varying number of electrodes (20,577 trials from 54 electrodes). In these experiments, pulses occurred synchronously (**Figure 1B**, left). **(A)** Psychometric functions, averaged across single electrodes, electrode pairs, and electrode quads. **(B)** Measured and theoretically calculated thresholds. The bars and error bars denote the mean and SEs, respectively, and each point corresponds to a different single electrode, electrode pair, or quad. The dashed lines denote the expected threshold assuming that each electrode independently contributes to detectability. **(C)** Comparison of the most sensitive single electrode, best pair of electrodes, and the quad with pulses delivered synchronously in the multi-electrode conditions (9,520 trials from 24 electrodes). Error bars denote the SE of the mean. *$p < 0.05$, **$p < 0.01$.

Kruskal–Wallis test, $\chi^2_{(2,51)} = 14.8$, $p < 0.001$), as might be expected given that more current was delivered to the brain (see Ghose and Maunsell, 2012; Zaaimi et al., 2013). A *post hoc* analysis revealed that, while single-electrode thresholds were not significantly different from electrode-pair thresholds (rank-sum test, Bonferroni corrected, $p = 0.07$), single thresholds were significantly higher than quad thresholds ($p = 0.003$), and double thresholds were significantly higher than quad thresholds ($p = 0.04$). Furthermore, thresholds measured in the multi-electrode conditions closely matched theoretical predictions based on the assumption that each electrode exerts an independent effect on detectability (signed rank test, $p > 0.5$, dashed lines in **Figure 2B**).

Next, we wished to assess the extent to which stimulation through multiple electrodes improves detectability beyond that achieved through stimulation of the most sensitive electrode. To this end, we compared performance with four electrodes to that with the best (most sensitive) electrode and with the best pair of electrodes in the quad. We found that, while not completely eliminated, the apparent advantage of multi-electrode stimulation was substantially reduced. Indeed, while detection performance remained significantly different between single electrodes and multiple electrodes (Friedman test, $\chi^2_{(2,14)} = 9.25$, $p < 0.01$, **Figure 2C**), the mean difference in threshold between groups was less than 3 μA (mean ± SEM: single vs. double: 0.50 ± 0.50 μA, single vs. quad: 2.76 ± 1.02 μA, double vs. quad: 2.26 ± 0.82 μA, mean ± SEM), representing a decrease of less than 10%. Importantly, the detectability of subthreshold stimuli (5 and 10 μA) did not improve significantly with multiple electrodes (Friedman test, $\chi^2_{(2,30)} = 1.94$, $p = 0.4$), which stands in contrast with previous findings (Zaaimi et al., 2013).

Synchronous vs. Asynchronous Stimulation

In the multi-electrode conditions described above, electrical pulses were delivered synchronously through different electrodes. We wished to determine whether the effect of multi-electrode stimulation on sensitivity might be different when pulses are staggered rather than synchronous. To this end, we repeated the experiments described above, but interleaved trials in which pulses were delivered synchronously across electrodes with trials in which pulses were staggered (**Figure 1B**). First, we found that synchrony did not have a significant overall effect on thresholds [paired *t*-test, $t_{(23)} = 1.03$, $p = 0.31$] (**Figure 3A**), consistent with previous findings in optogenetic experiments with mice (Histed and Maunsell, 2014). Second, asynchronous multi-electrode ICMS had a similar effect on detectability as did its synchronous counterpart, with thresholds decreasing with more electrodes (Friedman test, $\chi^2_{(2,18)} = 14.6$, $p < 0.001$); a *post hoc* analysis revealed significant differences across all three groups (signed rank test, Bonferroni corrected, $p < 0.05$; **Figure 3B**). Additionally, as was the case with synchronous stimulation, measured thresholds were indistinguishable from theoretically estimated thresholds assuming independent contributions of each electrode to detection performance (signed rank test, double: $p = 0.063$, quad: $p > 0.5$). Again, the mean difference in threshold was small (single vs. double: 1.35 ± 0.32 μA, single vs. quad: 2.96 ± 0.43 μA, double vs. quad: 1.61 ± 0.38 μA) and the detectability of subthreshold stimuli did not improve significantly (Friedman test, $\chi^2_{(2,38)} = 1.85$, $p = 0.40$).

Effect of Pulse Polarity on Detectability

Next, we investigated whether changing the polarity of the pulses might modulate how stimulation through multiple electrodes affects detectability. That is, we compared the effect of multi-electrode stimulation when the leading phase was anodic to that when leading phase was cathodic. First, as has been previously shown (Ranck, 1975; Schmidt et al., 1996; Koivuniemi and Otto, 2011), detection thresholds were significantly higher for anodic-first pulses than for cathodic-first pulses [**Figure 4A**; *t*-test: $t_{(70)} = 12.2$, $p < 10^{-18}$]. As was the case for cathodic-first pulses,

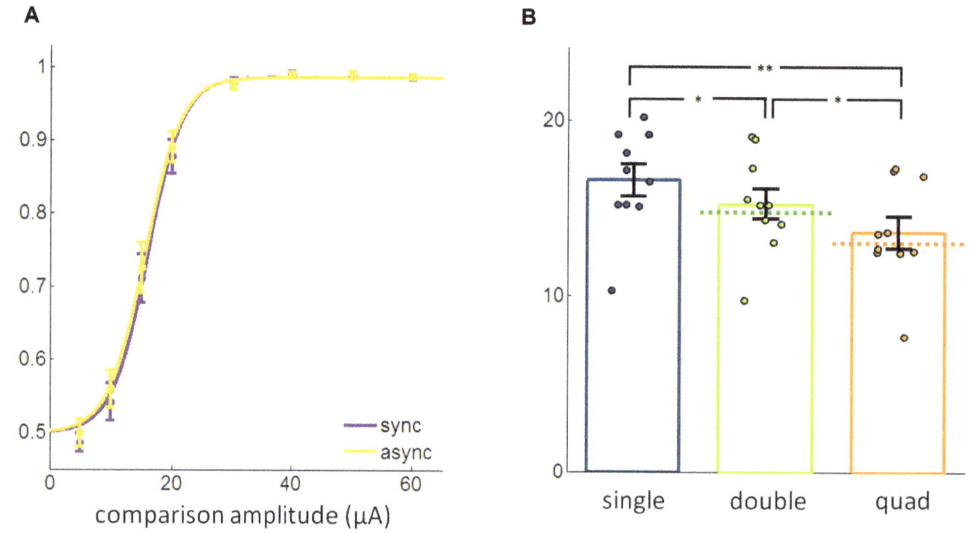

FIGURE 3 | (A) Detection performance with synchronous and asynchronous stimulation (13,202 trials from 48 electrodes). **(B)** Comparison of the most sensitive single electrode, best pair of electrodes, and the quad with pulses delivered asynchronously in the multi-electrode conditions (19,400 trials from 30 electrodes). Error bars denote the SE of the mean. *$p < 0.05$, **$p < 0.01$.

thresholds for anodic-first stimulation decreased as the number of electrodes increased (Kruskal–Wallis test, $\chi^2_{(2,45)} = 6.68$, $p = 0.036$). However, the increase in sensitivity with increasing number of electrodes was eliminated when the best single electrode and the best pair were compared to the quad [Friedman test, $\chi^2_{(2,10)} = 2.33$, $p = 0.31$, single/double/quad: 23.6 ± 1.70 μA/28.9 ± 1.08 μA/27.2 ± 1.64 μA; **Figure 4B**]. Thus, results using multi-electrode ICMS with anodic phase leading did not conform with theoretical predictions based on the assumption of independence.

Effect of Electrode Spacing on Detectability

Electrodes that formed each quad were selected to have largely overlapping receptive fields. In some cases the electrodes were physically adjacent, but in others they were not (**Figure 1C**). We wished to assess whether the spatial configuration of the electrode groups might impact how stimulation through these is combined to culminate in a behavioral outcome. Using ICMS with cathodic phase leading, we found that spatial configuration had no impact on sensitivity to multi-electrode stimulation: threshold decreased as the number of electrodes increased, whether these

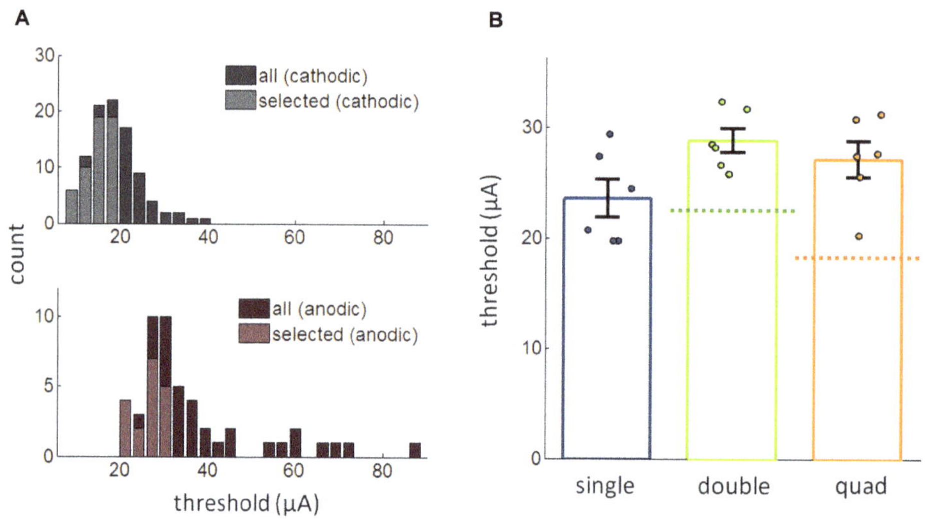

FIGURE 4 | (A) Distribution of thresholds for anodic phase leading and cathodic phase leading ICMS (56,021 trials from 97 electrodes). The distribution of thresholds for the best electrodes is shown in the lighter hue. **(B)** Comparison of the most sensitive single electrode, best pair of electrodes, and the quad with pulses in the multi-electrode conditions with anodic phase leading (12,661 trials from 18 electrodes). Error bars denote the SE of the mean.

were adjacent (Friedman test, $\chi^2_{(2,18)} = 18.2, p < 0.001$) or not ($\chi^2_{(2,14)} = 6.75, p = 0.03$). In both conditions (adjacent vs. non-adjacent), observed thresholds were consistent with the assumption of independence; that is, these were not significantly different from predicted ones regardless of spatial separation (signed rank test, $p > 0.1$). The effect of separation was similar whether stimulation was presented synchronously or asynchronously, as might be expected from **Figure 3**.

Multi-Electrode Stimulation for Discrimination

Based on results from the detection experiments, we concluded that the detectability of ICMS improves only slightly when stimulation is delivered through multiple electrodes despite the fact that more current is injected. Next, we wished to examine whether the discriminability of ICMS pulse trains differing in amplitude increased when these were delivered through multiple electrodes simultaneously. To this end, we had animals discriminate ICMS that differed in amplitude, with stimuli delivered through single electrodes, pairs, or quads of electrodes. That is, we compared discrimination performance when both stimuli were presented through one, two, or four electrodes. In these experiments, pulses were anodic phase leading. We found that there was no significant difference in discrimination performance across the three conditions with either the 30-μA standard [Friedman test, $\chi^2_{(2,59)} = 0.03, p = 0.99$] or the 100-μA standard ($\chi^2_{(2,59)} = 1.12, p = 0.57$; **Figure 5**).

Implications for Neuroprosthetics

The results of our detection experiments are consistent with the hypothesis that each electrode exerts an independent effect on sensitivity, except perhaps when the anodic phase leads, where no effect was observed (though the sample was relatively small for that condition). As such, the advantage of multi-electrode stimulation is relatively modest when compared to the "best" electrode, with four electrodes yielding a mean decrease in threshold of less than 10%. There was no effect of multi-electrode stimulation on discrimination, likely reflecting the fact that discrimination is generally less sensitive to stimulus parameters than is detection. The lack of effect on discrimination performance was probably exacerbated by the fact that these experiments were carried out with anodic phase leading.

At first glance, our results seem generally inconsistent with those reported in a previous study (Zaaimi et al., 2013), in which a supra-additive effect of multi-electrode stimulation on sensitivity was reported. Furthermore, in this previous study, the synergistic effects of multi-electrode stimulation were observed even for subthreshold stimuli, which was not the case here. However, in that study, the supra-additive effect was strongest when five or more electrodes were simultaneously stimulated, so perhaps we did not stimulate a sufficient number of electrodes in the present study to observe it. The discrepancy regarding the effect of multi-electrode stimulation on subthreshold stimuli may be attributable to differences in somatosensory areas that were stimulated (areas 3b/1 vs. area 2), in the relevant sensory modalities (tactile vs. proprioceptive), or in the behavioral protocols (one stimulus interval vs. two, 360-ms vs. 1000-ms stimulus duration, etc.).

Whether pulses were delivered synchronously or asynchronously did not affect their detectability, a result that is consistent with previous findings in mice using optogenetic stimulation (Histed and Maunsell, 2014). At peri-threshold, amplitudes, the current may spread to a volume with a radius of 200–300 μm or less (Stoney et al., 1968; Tehovnik et al., 2006; Zaaimi et al., 2013), so the different electrodes may have activated mostly non-overlapping populations of neurons. Even if the fields do interact, it may be that both synchronous and asynchronous stimulation have their respective advantages: with synchronous stimulation, the fields interact, allowing intervening neurons to experience stronger stimulation, thereby increasing their probability of firing; with asynchronous stimulation, neurons experience more continuous stimulation, thereby increasing their probability of firing; the two effects may then be approximately equivalent.

Given its limited effect on sensitivity, stimulation through multiple electrodes is not a very promising way to extend the dynamic range of sensations achievable through ICMS, at

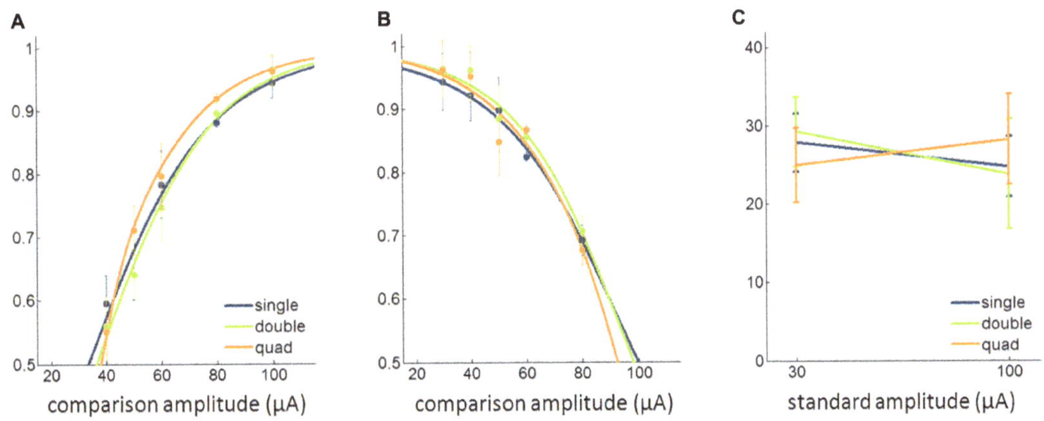

FIGURE 5 | Effect of multi-electrode stimulation on the discriminability of ICMS. (A,B) Psychometric functions with a 30-μA and 100-μA standard, respectively (9,280 trials from 12 sets of electrodes). **(C)** JNDs with different standard amplitudes. Error bars denote the SEM.

least for artificial touch and given current electrode technologies. Indeed, stimulating through the "best" electrode yields nearly equivalent results and requires a fraction of the current as does stimulating through four electrodes. One might argue that, given an independent contribution of each electrode, performance should improve as the number of stimulated electrodes increases. However, more electrodes will likely evoke more diffuse percepts (cf. Tabot et al., 2013b), so gains in dynamic range will be at the expense of spatial localization. On the other hand, for more distributed representations, such as proprioceptive ones, multi-electrode stimulation may be more practical (cf. Zaaimi et al., 2013). As technology develops, and implanted electrodes get closer together, the multi-electrode approach may be viable for touch as well. In the meantime, manipulations of phase width, pulse frequency, and pulse train duration may be more promising avenues to extend the dynamic range (Tabot et al., 2013a; Kim et al., 2014).

Materials and Methods

Animals

Procedures were approved by the University of Chicago Animal Care and Use Committee. Each of two male Rhesus macaques (6 years of age, around 10 kg in weight) was implanted with three electrode arrays: one Utah electrode array (UEA; Blackrock Microsystems, Inc., Salt Lake City, UT, USA) in the hand representation of areas 1 and 2 in the right hemisphere, flanked by two FMAs (Microprobes for Life Science, Gaithersburg, MD, USA) in area 3b (For more detail, see Berg et al., 2013; Tabot et al., 2013b). We mapped the receptive field of each electrode by identifying which areas of skin evoked multiunit activity (monitored through speakers).

Experimental Design

Each trial consisted of two sequentially presented stimulus intervals, one (detection) or both (discrimination) of which contained a stimulus (**Figure 1A**). In the detection task, the animal indicated which of the two stimulus intervals contained the stimulus; in the discrimination task, the animal indicated which of the two intervals contained the more intense stimulus. In both tasks, the animals responded by making a saccade to one of two visual targets. Animals were first trained on these tasks with mechanical indentations delivered to their skin until their performance leveled off. Mechanical stimuli were then replaced with ICMS; importantly, the animals performed at a high level on the very first block of ICMS, suggesting that the ICMS detection and discrimination were very similar to their mechanical counterparts.

Intracortical microstimulation consisted of 1-s long trains of symmetric biphasic pulses with a phase duration of 200 μs, an interphase interval of 53 μs, and a frequency of 300 Hz (**Figure 1B**). In the multi-electrode conditions, ICMS was either delivered synchronously (with all pulses in a given cycle occurring simultaneously) or asynchronously, such that pulses were evenly distributed throughout the cycle (that is, with an interpulse interval of 1667 μs for pairs and 833 μs for quads of electrodes; **Figure 1B**). In each experimental block, trials with a single electrode were interleaved with trials with pairs or quads of electrodes. In all cases, all of the electrodes in a quad had largely overlapping receptive fields on the palmar surface of the hand. Each quad was broken down into pairs, so that we could compare performance with quad stimulation to that with stimulation through electrode pairs or through single electrodes using repeated measures statistics.

In the detection experiments, ICMS amplitude was 5, 10, 15, 20, 30, 40, 50, or 80 μA and varied from trial to trial in pseudorandom order. In the discrimination experiments, the same number of electrodes was used in both intervals of each trial; the animal was comparing ICMS delivered through one, two, or four electrodes. On each trial, the amplitude of the standard stimulus was 30 or 100 μA. The 30-μA standard was paired with comparison stimuli at 40, 50, 60, 80, or 100 μA. The 100-μA standard was paired with comparison stimuli at 30, 40, 50, 60, or 80 μA. The standard stimulus was presented in either the first or the second interval and trials with both standards were interleaved so the animal would have to pay attention to both intervals to perform the task correctly.

Analysis

In the detection task, we estimated the detection threshold as the stimulus amplitude that yielded a performance of 75% correct. Similarly, in the discrimination task, we estimated the JND as the difference between comparison and standard amplitude that yielded a performance of 75% correct. Thresholds and JNDs were estimated using a standard sigmoid function. To compare sensitivity across conditions, we used parametric tests (e.g., *t*-tests) or non-parametric ones (e.g., Kruskal–Wallis test, Friedman test and signed rank test) depending on the sample size and variance of the data.

We also wished to quantify the expected performance if we assume that each electrode independently contributes to perception (cf. Zaaimi et al., 2013):

$$\begin{aligned} P_D &= 1 - (1 - P_{S1})(1 - P_{S2}) \\ P_Q &= 1 - (1 - P_{S1})(1 - P_{S2})(1 - P_{S3})(1 - P_{S4}) \end{aligned} \tag{1}$$

Where P_D and P_Q indicate the probability of detection with pairs and quads of electrodes, respectively, and P_{S1}, P_{S2}, P_{S3}, and P_{S4} denote the detection probability with each of the individual electrodes in the pair or quad. The proportion correct observed in the detection task, P_{obs}, is related to the probability of detection, P_{det}, as follows:

$$P_{\text{obs}} = P_{\text{det}} + 0.5(1 - P_{\text{det}}) \tag{2}$$

So the probability of detection is given by $P_{\text{det}} = 2P_{\text{obs}} - 1$. We computed P_{det} for each electrode and plugged the resulting value into Equation 1 to obtain the theoretical detection probability for double and quad electrodes. Finally, we used Equation 2 to convert the probabilities back to task performance metrics.

Acknowledgments

We would like to thank Lee Miller and Ricardo Ruiz Torres for helpful comments on a previous version of this manuscript. This material is based on work supported by the Defense Advanced Research Projects Agency under Contract N66001-10-C-4056. GT. was supported by National Science Foundation Grant DGE-0903637.

References

Bensmaia, S. J., and Miller, L. E. (2014). Restoring sensorimotor function through intracortical interfaces: progress and looming challenges. *Nat. Rev. Neurosci.* 15, 313–325. doi: 10.1038/nrn3724

Berg, J. A., Dammann, J. F. III, Tenore, F. V., Tabot, G. A., Boback, J. L., Manfredi, L. R., et al. (2013). Behavioral demonstration of a somatosensory neuroprosthesis. *IEEE Trans. Neural Syst. Rehabil. Eng.* 21, 500–507. doi: 10.1109/TNSRE.2013.2244616

Collinger, J. L., Wodlinger, B., Downey, J. E., Wang, W., Tyler-Kabara, E. C., Weber, D. J., et al. (2013). High-performance neuroprosthetic control by an individual with tetraplegia. *Lancet* 381, 557–564. doi: 10.1016/S0140-6736(12)61816-9

Dadarlat, M. C., O'Doherty, J. E., and Sabes, P. N. (2014). A learning-based approach to artificial sensory feedback leads to optimal integration. *Nat. Neurosci.* 18, 138–144. doi: 10.1038/nn.3883

Ghose, K., and Maunsell, J. H. (2012). A strong constraint to the joint processing of pairs of cortical signals. *J. Neurosci.* 32, 15922–15933. doi: 10.1523/JNEUROSCI.2186-12.2012

Histed, M. H., and Maunsell, J. H. (2014). Cortical neural populations can guide behavior by integrating inputs linearly, independent of synchrony. *Proc. Natl. Acad. Sci. U.S.A.* 111, E178–E187. doi: 10.1073/pnas.1318750111

Hochberg, L. R., Bacher, D., Jarosiewicz, B., Masse, N. Y., Simeral, J. D., Vogel, J., et al. (2012). Reach and grasp by people with tetraplegia using a neurally controlled robotic arm. *Nature* 485, 372–375. doi: 10.1038/nature11076

Kim, S. S., Callier, T., Tabot, G. A., Tenore, F. V., and Bensmaia, S. J. (2014). "Discrimination of electrical stimulation to primary somatosensory cortex," in *Proceedings of the Annual Meeting of the Society for Neuroscience*, Washington, DC.

Koivuniemi, A. S., and Otto, K. J. (2011). Asymmetric versus symmetric pulses for cortical microstimulation. *IEEE Trans. Neural Syst. Rehabil. Eng.* 19, 468–476. doi: 10.1109/TNSRE.2011.2166563

London, B. M., Jordan, L. R., Jackson, C. R., and Miller, L. E. (2008). Electrical stimulation of the proprioceptive cortex (area 3a) used to instruct a behaving monkey. *IEEE Trans. Neural Syst. Rehabil. Eng.* 16, 32–36. doi: 10.1109/TNSRE.2007.907544

McCreery, D., Pikov, V., and Troyk, P. R. (2010). Neuronal loss due to prolonged controlled-current stimulation with chronically implanted microelectrodes in the cat cerebral cortex. *J. Neural Eng.* 7:036005. doi: 10.1088/1741-2560/7/3/036005

O'Doherty, J. E., Lebedev, M. A., Ifft, P. J., Zhuang, K. Z., Shokur, S., Bleuler, H., et al. (2011). Active tactile exploration using a brain-machine-brain interface. *Nature* 479, 228–231. doi: 10.1038/nature10489

Ranck, J. B. Jr. (1975). Which elements are excited in electrical stimulation of mammalian central nervous system: a review. *Brain Res.* 98, 417–440. doi: 10.1016/0006-8993(75)90364-9

Schmidt, E., Bak, M., Hambrecht, F., Kufta, C., O'rourke, D., and Vallabhanath, P. (1996). Feasibility of a visual prosthesis for the blind based on intracortical micro stimulation of the visual cortex. *Brain* 119, 507–522. doi: 10.1093/brain/119.2.507

Stoney, S. D. Jr., Thompson, W. D., and Asanuma, H. (1968). Excitation of pyramidal tract cells by intracortical microstimulation: effective extent of stimulating current. *J. Neurophysiol.* 31, 659–669.

Tabot, G. A., Boback, J. L., and Dammann J. F. III, Tenore, F. V., and Bensmaia, S. J. (2013a). "Restoring touch using a brain interface: dependence of artificial percepts on stimulation parameters," in *Proceedings of the Annual Meeting of the Society for Neuroscience,* San Diego, CA.

Tabot, G. A., Dammann, J. F., Berg, J. A., Tenore, F. V., Boback, J. L., Vogelstein, R. J., et al. (2013b). Restoring the sense of touch with a prosthetic hand through a brain interface. *Proc. Natl. Acad. Sci. U.S.A.* 110, 18279–18284. doi: 10.1073/pnas.1221113110

Tabot, G. A., Kim, S. S., Winberry, J. E., and Bensmaia, S. J. (2014). Restoring tactile and proprioceptive sensation through a brain interface. *Neurobiol. Dis.* doi: 10.1016/j.nbd.2014.08.029 [Epub ahead of print].

Tehovnik, E., Tolias, A., Sultan, F., Slocum, W., and Logothetis, N. (2006). Direct and indirect activation of cortical neurons by electrical microstimulation. *J. Neurophysiol.* 96, 512–521. doi: 10.1152/jn.00126.2006

Thomson, E. E., Carra, R., and Nicolelis, M. A. (2013). Perceiving invisible light through a somatosensory cortical prosthesis. *Nat. commun.* 4: 1482.

Zaaimi, B., Ruiz-Torres, R., Solla, S. A., and Miller, L. E. (2013). Multi-electrode stimulation in somatosensory cortex increases probability of detection. *J Neural Eng.* 10:056013. doi: 10.1088/1741-2560/10/5/056013

9

Advancing brain-machine interfaces: moving beyond linear state space models

Adam G. Rouse[1, 2, 3] *and Marc H. Schieber*[1, 2, 3*]

[1] *Department of Neurology, University of Rochester, Rochester, NY, USA,* [2] *Department of Neurobiology and Anatomy, University of Rochester, Rochester, NY, USA,* [3] *Department of Biomedical Engineering, University of Rochester, Rochester, NY, USA*

Edited by:
Mikhail Lebedev, Duke University, USA

Reviewed by:
Ioan Opris, Wake Forest University School of Medicine, USA
Aaron Batista, University of Pittsburgh, USA

***Correspondence:**
Marc H. Schieber, Department of Neurology, University of Rochester Medical Center, 601 Elmwood Avenue, Box 673, Rochester, NY 14642, USA
mhs@cvs.rochester.edu

Advances in recent years have dramatically improved output control by Brain-Machine Interfaces (BMIs). Such devices nevertheless remain robotic and limited in their movements compared to normal human motor performance. Most current BMIs rely on transforming recorded neural activity to a linear state space composed of a set number of fixed degrees of freedom. Here we consider a variety of ways in which BMI design might be advanced further by applying non-linear dynamics observed in normal motor behavior. We consider (i) the dynamic range and precision of natural movements, (ii) differences between cortical activity and actual body movement, (iii) kinematic and muscular synergies, and (iv) the implications of large neuronal populations. We advance the hypothesis that a given population of recorded neurons may transmit more useful information than can be captured by a single, linear model across all movement phases and contexts. We argue that incorporating these various non-linear characteristics will be an important next step in advancing BMIs to more closely match natural motor performance.

Keywords: brain-computer interface, hand, kinematic synergy, motor cortex, movement phase, muscle synergy, neuroprosthetics, null space

Introduction

Research and development of brain-machine interfaces (BMIs) to restore lost motor function has expanded dramatically in recent years. Whereas, not long ago the state of the art in both non-human primates (Serruya et al., 2002; Taylor et al., 2002) and humans (Hochberg et al., 2006) consisted of controlling a cursor on a computer screen, recent advances in restoring upper limb function have incorporated robotic arms with the ability to grip and manipulate objects using either virtual (Carmena et al., 2003; Chadwick et al., 2011) or robotic (Velliste et al., 2008; Hochberg et al., 2012; Collinger et al., 2013; Wodlinger et al., 2015) hands and digits. In addition to restoring upper limb function, innovative exoskeletons are being used to restore trunk and leg function (Fitzsimmons et al., 2009; Lebedev and Nicolelis, 2011). Functional electrical stimulation also has made possible restoration of movement of the subject's own limbs (Moritz et al., 2008; Pancrazio and Peckham, 2009; Ethier et al., 2012). Many of these advances have transitioned from the research laboratory with non-human primates to the clinical world with human subjects.

Different but inter-related improvements have contributed to these advances. Better recording systems that allow chronically implanted electrodes to record an increasing number of channels of neural activity simultaneously have had a major impact (Stieglitz et al., 2009; Homer et al., 2013).

Better understanding of how to extract various neural signals, paradoxically including less focus on precise spike sorting and more use of simple detection methods like threshold crossings (Fraser et al., 2009; Chestek et al., 2011; Hochberg et al., 2012; Wodlinger et al., 2015), the application of statistical models to better estimate firing rates (Cunningham et al., 2010), and the implementation of Kalman filtering (Wu et al., 2003; Li et al., 2009), all have improved BMI performance as well. Better appreciation of the neural adaptation that occurs under BMI conditions has led to dynamic updating of decoding algorithms that enable BMI learning to be both faster and more robust to external changes (Gilja et al., 2012; Orsborn et al., 2012; Zhang and Chase, 2013; Shanechi et al., 2014). A focus on overcoming the technical challenges of chronically monitoring larger and larger amounts of neural activity and on controlling increasingly complex devices has advanced the field substantially and quickly.

Over the same period during which these advances have been made, relatively little has changed in how our understanding of natural motor physiology is applied to BMI control. Current BMI designs almost always assume that neural encoding is a linear, time-invariant system with independent degrees of freedom (DOFs), and therefore implement control algorithms that map neural inputs to a constant set of output variables with a fixed gain. Yet neural control of mammalian motor systems and the behaviors they produce cannot be explained fully with such an idealized model.

Here we examine selected aspects of motor behavior and physiology to explore ways in which current scientific understanding might be exploited to advance the design of BMIs toward achieving performance closer to that of natural human movement. We discuss four different topics. First, we consider differences in motor performance for very fast or very slow movements and examine how BMI decoding might better emulate similar principles. Second, we address evidence that cortical activity—even in areas with significant spinal projections—differs considerably from a veridical representation of actual movement of the body and we consider the implications of these differences for continuous BMI operation. Third, we explore the evidence that natural movement is not statistically independent across different joints or muscles but rather is coordinated and we ask how this might be incorporated more extensively in BMI design. And fourth, we explore the implications of having a large neuronal population to generate movement, examining whether such a system can be modeled effectively with a single, linear state space, and asking whether adhering to such a model has become a limiting oversimplification in current BMI designs. Although the four topics we explore may appear diverse and unrelated, they share the common theme that incorporating a deeper understanding of the non-linear dynamics of normal motor behavior and physiology—during different phases of movement and in different contexts—can advance BMI design. Whereas, scientists generally seek to identify the simplest explanation for the largest set of observations and engineers seek to provide the simplest design to achieve a specific function (Müller et al., 2003), here we argue that the next wave of advances in BMI technology will require incorporating additional levels of complexity.

Dealing with a Wide Dynamic Range of Movement

Humans are capable of performing skilled movements on a wide range of spatial and temporal scales, from the athletic prowess of throwing or kicking a ball at speeds approaching 100 miles per hour (44.7 m/s) to the fine motor skills required for watchmaking and surgery. But throwing a ball is not necessarily controlled in the same fashion as knotting a suture. We therefore consider how control might vary depending on the extent to which a subject intends to make a gross movement quickly vs. a fine movement accurately.

Dynamic Range of Movements

In natural movements, Fitts's law (Fitts, 1954) describes a tradeoff between speed and accuracy: The faster the movement, the less accurate it will be; greater accuracy is achieved with slower movement. This principle has been documented in numerous natural movement tasks and under many different conditions (Card et al., 1978; Jagacinski and Monk, 1985; Epps, 1986; MacKenzie, 1992), in neural correlates (Ifft et al., 2011), and in BMI tasks with direct neural control (Felton et al., 2009).

Current BMIs, however, do little to emulate the robust range of behavior observed to follow Fitts's law for either very fast or very accurate movements, relying instead on the designer to pick a fixed gain between input neural signals and output magnitude. This practice effectively limits good BMI performance to a narrow range of the speed/accuracy trade-off. Enabling the user's neural activity to select the movement speed and the associated accuracy dynamically depending on the current phase or context of the task could improve BMI control, providing a range of performance closer to that of natural movements.

Improving the Precision of BMIs

Fine, skilled movements presumably require more precise neural control signals than gross movements, whether the control signal is encoding muscle activation, force, joint position, or velocity. A study by Slifkin and Newell (1999) found, for example, that whereas the average maximum voluntary contraction (MVC) of the index finger against a load cell was 31.07 N with a standard deviation of ~2.1 N, when producing forces of 5% MVC (~1.55 N) the standard deviation was only ~0.09 N. Variability in normal human force production thus scales with the magnitude of force being produced. Such signal-dependent noise appears in many natural motor behaviors (Harris and Wolpert, 1998). Smaller movements are made with smaller errors.

A system that linearly transforms an input to output with constant noise cannot be optimized for fine, accurate movement and for gross, fast movement simultaneously. Indeed, cortical microcircuits in the motor system recently have been proposed to adjust neuron tuning according to the level of precision required. By functionally varying the overall strength of excitatory/inhibitory drive and changing the tuning widths of individual M1 neurons, the accuracy and precision of movement encoding by a population of neurons might be adjusted dynamically (Mahan and Georgopoulos, 2013; Georgopoulos, 2014). Although natural adjustment of neuronal tuning may be present in the input neurons, current BMIs that rely on the linear sum of neural activity nevertheless show poor adjustment of precision compared to that found in natural movements. Such suboptimal adjustment of precision might result from the small number of input neurons compared to the natural motor system and/or the lack of adjustment for precision in the tuning and decoding models used currently.

BMIs therefore might be improved by creating decoding schemes that more explicitly allow for encoding of the speed-accuracy tradeoff from a recorded subpopulation. If we construct a BMI model that uses instantaneous neuronal firing rates to encode velocity in a single dimension with a simple linear encoder, the magnitude of the error is uniform for all encoded velocities (**Figure 1A**). If instead the neurons in the model are assigned to encode a rescaling of velocity, the square root of velocity for example, the errors near zero velocity are smaller than those for high velocity (**Figure 1B**), more closely emulating the signal-dependent noise of natural behavior (**Figure 1C**). Applying such approaches to create noise profiles that more closely match natural behavior is likely to create BMI controlled movements that appear more natural by allowing greater precision for fine movements.

The Relationship of Cortical Activity to Physical Movement

The majority of current BMIs that control motor output use neural activity recorded from motor and premotor areas of the cerebral cortex as input for two reasons. First, many aspects of natural movements are represented in the activity of neurons in these cortical areas. Second, the cerebral cortex can be accessed for neural recording relatively easily compared to deeper parts of the brain and spinal cord. But using only cortical activity has other advantages and disadvantages for BMI control: (i) certain features of cortical activity are not output to physical movement of the body, (ii) the tuning of cortical neurons changes when controlling a BMI, and (iii) certain aspects of physical movement may not be controlled directly from the cortex.

Motor Imagery, Mirror Neurons, and BMI Control

During motor imagery, when humans imagine themselves performing movements without actually making any movement, activation appears in many of the same cortical motor areas that are activated during physical movement performance, including the primary motor cortex (Ersland et al., 1996; Grafton et al., 1996; Porro et al., 1996; Pfurtscheller and Neuper, 1997; Anderson et al., 2011; Ajiboye et al., 2012). Likewise during action observation, when a monkey observes another individual performing a particular movement, a large subpopulation of neurons discharges in a fashion similar to their discharge when the monkey executes the same action itself. These "mirror neurons," as well as other neurons that are activated when the monkey observes a cursor moved by the investigator, have been observed not only in premotor cortex but in primary motor cortex as well (Cisek and Kalaska, 2004; Tkach et al., 2007; Dushanova and Donoghue, 2010; Casile, 2013; Vigneswaran et al., 2013). Many neurons in motor cortex thus discharge during motor imagery and/or action observation, when subjects are not making any physical movement.

BMI experiments with normal subjects are perhaps the most clear-cut demonstration that neurons active during natural movements can also be activated voluntarily in the absence of

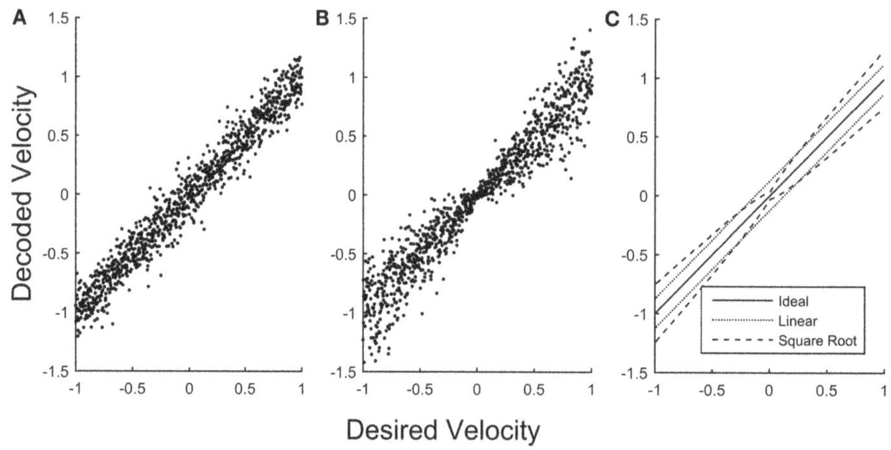

FIGURE 1 | Error in simulated velocity decoding. A simulated population of neurons was scaled to encode velocities (with a maximum system velocity equal to 1) using two different methods. **(A)** The simulated population encodes linear velocity, producing uniform error in the decoded velocity that is independent of the desired velocity. **(B)** The simulated population (with the same dynamic range and noise properties of the neurons) is now scaled to encode the square root of velocity, producing error in the decoded velocity that becomes smaller for velocities closer to zero. **(C)** The standard deviation of decoded velocity is plotted as a function of desired velocity for the linear model (**A**, dotted) and for the square root model (**B**, dashed), emphasizing that when decoding linear velocity the error is constant across desired velocities, whereas for the square root model the error is smaller close to zero velocity and larger for higher velocities.

physical movement. In such BMI experiments, normal monkeys typically first perform a task involving physical movement of their native limb while neural activity is recorded from the cortex. This activity then is used to calibrate a decoding algorithm that relates the recorded neuronal activity to the observed limb movements. But after switching to "brain-control"—now controlling a cursor or prosthesis directly through the decoding algorithm—the monkey often stops making any physical movement or producing any EMG activity, even though allowed to move freely (Taylor et al., 2002; Carmena et al., 2003). Meanwhile, the recorded neurons continue to modulate, voluntarily controlling the external BMI device. Like mirror neurons, these neurons are activated during physical movement of the native limb, but are not obligatorily coupled to physical movement. Though in most BMI experiments neurons have not been tested for such, many of them might have activity during action observation.

Indeed, we know that neurons activated during action observation can be used for voluntary BMI control, because in both normal monkeys and paralyzed humans neuronal activity recorded during action observation can be used effectively to develop the initial decoding algorithm (Velliste et al., 2008; Chadwick et al., 2011; Collinger et al., 2013). Although using neurons activated by action observation currently provides an advantage for calibrating BMIs in paralyzed or amputated subjects, using mirror neurons might have disadvantages as well. In one recent study, for example, having a particular object present during the initial calibration was needed to enable the subject subsequently to close the prosthetic hand optimally around that object (Wodlinger et al., 2015), possibly indicating that the recorded population included a substantial number of mirror neurons encoding that particular grasp shape. More detailed scientific understanding of the differences in neuronal activity during motor imagery vs. action observation vs. action execution may enable BMI decoding based on these differences to improve performance.

Changes in Cortical Activity during BMI Control

The change from "hand-control" to "brain-control" changes cortical activity. Many neurons, for example, show changes in their directional tuning (Taylor et al., 2002; Ganguly and Carmena, 2009). Such changes may result from alterations in proprioceptive feedback because a normal subject's native limb that moved during hand-control either moves differently or does not move at all during brain-control. Differences may exist as well in the descending regulation of sensory input to the spinal cord, which changes during voluntary movement as compared to rest (Seki et al., 2003). Visual inputs change too. If the subject is controlling a prosthetic arm, its visual representation obviously will differ from that of a native arm, as will incorporation of the prosthesis into the internal body schema (i.e., embodiment). Even if the subject is controlling a cursor on a computer screen, the visual motion of the cursor viewed by the subject will differ, being smoother and more accurate during hand-control but showing more jitter during brain-control. In addition, many changes in cortical activity may represent adaptation on the part of the subject to fit the linear model of the BMI decoder (Wolpaw, 2010; Chase and Schwartz, 2011). More detailed scientific understanding of such changes in cortical activity that occur upon switching to brain-control may improve BMI performance.

Transformations in the Spinal Cord and Phases of Motor Control

Though classically viewed as a simple communication channel between the brain and the motor periphery, the spinal cord now is known to contain complex circuits that make important contributions to natural movements. Beyond the basic reflex pathways that can elicit movement from sensory input through only one or two synapses without cortical interaction, central pattern generators in the spinal cord can produce complex rhythmic behaviors without patterned input from the brain or feedback from the periphery (Shik and Orlovsky, 1976; Stein, 1978; Grillner, 1985). Descending signals from the brain are likely to engage parts of this spinal circuitry for production of other, non-rhythmic movements as well (Georgopoulos and Grillner, 1989). Indeed, in most mammalian species, the descending fibers of the corticospinal tract end on spinal interneurons, not motoneurons. And in macaques, which do have direct cortico-motoneuronal (CM) projections, spinal interneurons output different information (Maier et al., 1998; Fetz et al., 2002). For example, whereas most CM-cells were active selectively when subjects exerted either flexion or extension wrist forces, a high percentage of spinal interneurons were active for both flexion and extension force production, as well as at rest. With such complexity in the spinal cord, it becomes apparent that spinal cord circuitry may be doing much more than simply relaying the current input of descending cortical signals to generate muscle activity.

An emerging distinction between motor signals in the cortex vs. those in the spinal cord has to do with relative degrees of dynamic vs. static function in controlling non-cyclical limb movements. Neurons in the motor cortex typically are relatively quiescent during maintenance of a steady posture, become intensely active leading limb movement, and then show declining activity as a new steady posture is established. In large part such observations are attributable to a stronger relationship to movement velocity than to position (Moran and Schwartz, 1999). Moreover, strong rotational dynamics of joint M1 neuron firing rate trajectories may reflect a complex, dynamical system responsible for the encoding of movement (Churchland et al., 2012; Hall et al., 2014). In comparison to cortical neurons, spinal interneurons show more static activity. In monkeys generating wrist forces isometrically and auxotonically, for example, cortical neurons produced relatively transient signals for ensuing motor actions while spinal neurons generated more sustained activity, suggesting that to some degree cortical signals to change state are integrated by spinal circuitry (Shalit et al., 2012). Indeed, recent models of spinal-like regulators have demonstrated that oversimplified step inputs from the brain could be transformed by spinal circuitry to replicate much of observed center-out reaching behavior (Tsianos et al., 2014). Implementing such spinal-like circuitry in BMIs may substantially improve the quality of the transitions between movement and posture.

The transition from movement to posture is but one example of what more generally might be considered different sequential phases of motor control. A single decoder cannot be expected to deal with all phases efficiently. Cortical neurons can be identified, for example, that are active specifically in relation to rest/posture in contrast to movement (Humphrey and Reed, 1983; Williams et al., 2013; Velliste et al., 2014). Including such neural activity in the same linear decoding algorithm that drives movement velocity would be counterproductive. But if one decoder used movement-related activity to drive motion during movement phases, and another decoder used posture-related activity to maintain position during postural phases, smoother and more efficient performance might be obtained. Such control would require yet another decoding algorithm to identify transitions between phases, sometimes referred to as changes of state (Kemere et al., 2008; Aggarwal et al., 2013; Kang et al., 2015). Sequential phases or states may include not just alternation between movement and posture, but also inattention, watchful waiting for an instructional cue, preparation of a specific motor plan, reaction time following a go cue, then reaching, grasping, manipulation, and others as well. Detecting these various phases and decoding them differently may be an important step toward achieving natural human performance with BMIs (see also section More Neurons than Controlled DOFs creates a Null Space, below).

Controlling Multiple Degrees of Freedom

Independent Degrees of Freedom

Analysis of voluntary movement consistently has shown that natural movement almost never occurs in isolation at a single joint or by activation of a single muscle, even the movement of a single finger (Hager-Ross and Schieber, 2000). For example, typists and pianists produce simultaneous movements of multiple digits even when striking a single key (Flanders and Soechting, 1992; Engel et al., 1997). Nevertheless, most of the variance of complex multi-joint movements can be reduced mathematically to a relatively small number of principal components, each of which captures a pattern of simultaneous motion at multiple joints (Santello et al., 1998; Mason et al., 2004). Such findings suggest that the number of DOFs being controlled actively during many natural movements might be less than the number of DOFs actually moving.

Bernstein (1967) first defined this problem of redundant DOFs in the musculoskeletal system: Many movements made in three-dimensional space engage more than three joint angles and more than three muscles. Mathematically, therefore, a given movement can be made in many different ways, i.e., infinite possible solutions can successfully accomplish a given movement task. Observing blacksmiths, for example, Bernstein noticed that while the joints of the arm might take quite different trajectories during a series of hammer strikes, the endpoint of contact was very consistent. This and other observations of considerable variation in certain DOFs while others are controlled precisely was formulated subsequently by Scholz and Schöner (1999) as the uncontrolled manifold hypothesis: Within the high dimensional configuration space that completely defines movements for a given task, there exists two orthogonal subspaces. Motion in a controlled subspace contains a set of actively controlled variables that are being monitored and controlled by the subject and are most important to completing the task. The other, uncontrolled subspace contains all motion orthogonal to the controlled variables and thus has no effect on successful task completion. Increased variability has been observed in the uncontrolled subspace compared to the controlled subspace in a wide variety of natural movement tasks (Scholz et al., 2001; Latash et al., 2002; Tseng et al., 2002; Kang et al., 2004), and recently in neuronal activity as well (Kaufman et al., 2014; Law et al., 2014).

Current BMI design, however, remains limited in strategies that take into account the relative importance of the various DOFs in different tasks, instead controlling the same fixed set of DOFs of the prosthetic device independently at all points in time. Likewise, regression and updating algorithms assume each DOF is encoded equally at all times. As the number of DOFs increase, BMI control becomes more difficult because more DOFs must be monitored and controlled by the subject. Models that more closely align BMI control at a given time with a subset of DOFs selected judiciously for the current task may enable more intuitive and precise control.

Kinematic and Muscular Synergies

One means of selecting subsets of multiple DOFs for BMI control is to look for naturally occurring patterns of simultaneous motion at multiple joints or patterns of simultaneous activation of multiple muscles. A small number of fixed patterns of multi-joint motion (Santello et al., 1998; Mason et al., 2004) or multi-muscle activity (d'Avella and Bizzi, 2005), each varying in amplitude and timing, in theory could produce a very large repertoire of smoothly coordinated motor output. Synergies that distribute forces across the fingers can also provide a balance between flexibility and stability (Latash et al., 2007).

Indeed, synergies identified with dimensionality reduction techniques—such as principal component analysis or non-negative matrix factorization—can provide a simplified view of complex movements. Two important scientific questions are (i) whether such synergies are, in fact, used by the nervous system in controlling natural movement, and if so, (ii) in what part(s) of the nervous system the synergies are instantiated. Recent studies indicate that many fundamental synergies may be organized in the brainstem and spinal cord, rather than the cortex (Buford and Davidson, 2004; Cheung et al., 2009; Baker, 2011; Roh et al., 2011; Giszter and Hart, 2013). Once these two questions have been answered, BMI performance might be enhanced by recording from these regions and using the decoded output to drive the relevant synergies rather than the individual degrees of freedom.

Whether or not synergies are used naturally by the nervous system, performance might be improved by incorporating synergies in BMI design. One synergy already in use involves control of arm endpoint in 3 dimensions (i.e., the location of the hand) with a robotic arm that has 4 rotational DOFs: 3 at the shoulder and 1 at the elbow (Lebedev et al., 2005; Velliste et al., 2008; Hochberg et al., 2012). Rather than providing the subject with independent control of all 4 DOFs, BMI output typically drives motion of the arm's endpoint in the

3 Cartesian coordinates (e.g., horizontal, vertical, depth), and this 3-dimensional output is partitioned across the 4 rotational DOFs by a fixed subroutine. Eliminating one DOF in this manner simplifies the control task for the subject at the cost of restricting the ways in which the robotic arm can move. Further incorporation of such simplifying synergies may enable the apparent complexity of movements achieved with BMIs to grow more rapidly than the complexity of control actually required of the subject.

Some synergies might be incorporated even in device hardware. For example, in the majority of hand motion for grasping, the four fingers extend roughly in parallel to open the hand. Rather than providing separate actuators (motors and cables) to extend each finger independently, a robotic hand could have one motor with a cable that divides to attach to each finger, reducing 4 DOFs to 1. Furthermore, extension of the fingers is rarely if ever used to apply substantial forces to objects, this being accomplished with finger flexion. If the extensor cable to each finger could be elastic, then independent flexion of each finger still could be achieved by independent flexion actuators for each finger.

Synergies may be especially useful in controlling a prosthetic hand. Whereas, motion of the shoulder, elbow, and wrist to transport and orient the hand involves 7 rotational DOFs, motion of the thumb and fingers involves 22. Yet even in sophisticated uses of the hand such as typing or piano playing, rarely if ever are individual DOFs moved independently (Soechting and Flanders, 1992, 1997; Engel et al., 1997). Current BMI decoding methods nevertheless assume separate channels for each individual digit, with no relationship between them. And state-of-the-art robotic hands now provide almost as many DOFs as are found in the natural hand (Dalley et al., 2010; Johannes et al., 2011; Resnik et al., 2013; Hutchinson, 2014). For most uses of the hand in activities of daily living, current BMI systems that attempt to control all the DOFs in the hand independently may, in fact, be overly complex.

Nevertheless, identifying an optimal set of synergies for controlling a prosthetic hand is far from simple. An orthogonal basis set of the multiple joints of the hand created with dimensionality reduction has obvious advantages both in its simplicity as well as straight-forward implementation in BMI applications (Ciocarlie et al., 2007; Vinjamuri et al., 2011; Velliste et al., 2012). Alternatively, observation can be used to select a limited set of basis functions. In one recent study, a human subject grasped a variety of objects by controlling a robotic hand through four independent basis functions identified by clinical observation of hand use: (i) pinch between the thumb and index, (ii) flexion and extension of the ring and little fingers in parallel, (iii) ab/adduction of all the fingers, and (iv) opposition of the thumb (Wodlinger et al., 2015). Yet such a simple, orthogonal basis set may fail to capture certain desirable features of hand motion. For example, while the flexion/extension of all five digits is a synergy commonly identified by analysis of hand movements, the thumb and index finger also move more independently than the other three digits. Thus, difficulty arises in trying to design a simple basis set that allows for a single degree of freedom that controls the opening and closing of all digits of the hand while also allowing independent control of the thumb and index finger.

While simplifying control, fixed synergies thus necessarily limit the ability to create all of the diverse movements of which humans are capable. An alternative model by Arbib and colleagues described "virtual fingers" and a schema that added or subtracted the number of digits to a central gripping controller depending on the size and shape of the object to be grasped (Arbib et al., 1985). This virtual fingers model essentially creates different synergies depending on the context of object size and shape. Extending the use of different sets of synergies depending on the particular task or context (e.g., throwing a ball vs. typing) may advance BMI control substantially toward normal human performance. Fully independent control of all the hand's DOFs may be valuable only for the most sophisticated uses of the hand.

More Inputs than Outputs

Redundancy in Neuron Populations

Of the roughly 100 billion neurons in the human cerebral cortex, approximately 1.4 million send axons through the corticospinal tract to synapse on motoneurons and interneurons in the spinal cord (Lassek, 1954). In achieving the remarkable performance of normal humans, these fibers convey much of natural cortical control to the "physical plant," which consists of approximately 600 muscles and 200 mechanical DOFs at the joints. At present, BMIs can sample only a small subset of any neuron population. As long as the sampling is reasonable, linear decoders can extract a representation of native limb motion and drive BMI end-effectors in multiple DOFs. A current trend, however, is to record increasing numbers of neural signals (Fitzsimmons et al., 2009; Lebedev and Nicolelis, 2011) with the goals not only of controlling more DOFs, but also of making the BMI more robust both to natural variability in neuron firing and to dropout of previously recorded neurons. How does the number of neurons used to control a BMI affect performance?

In the simplest BMI, a single neuron might be used to control each DOF (Fetz and Baker, 1973; Law et al., 2014). **Figure 2A** schematically illustrates 2 neurons (gray arrows) controlling 2 dimensions, using the familiar population vector approach. Each gray arrow represents a different neuron, the direction of the arrow represents that neuron's preferred direction, and the length of the arrow represents its firing rate. The black arrow represents the resulting population vector, and the cardioid curve indicates the idealized linear model of cosine tuning relative to the current output, i.e., the population vector. This arrangement has a major limitation: the noisiness of the individual neurons will produce equivalent noise in the resultant output.

Increasingly precise output can be obtained by linear summation of the observed firing rates of more neurons. **Figure 2B** illustrates such a situation, now using 20 neurons. In an idealized linear encoding model—where all neurons have the same noise properties and are independent—adding more neurons reduces error. Regardless of the specific partitioning of linear encoding across a population of n neurons, the predicted error decreases as $1/\sqrt{n}$, as follows from the central limit theorem. Adding more neurons thus progressively reduces

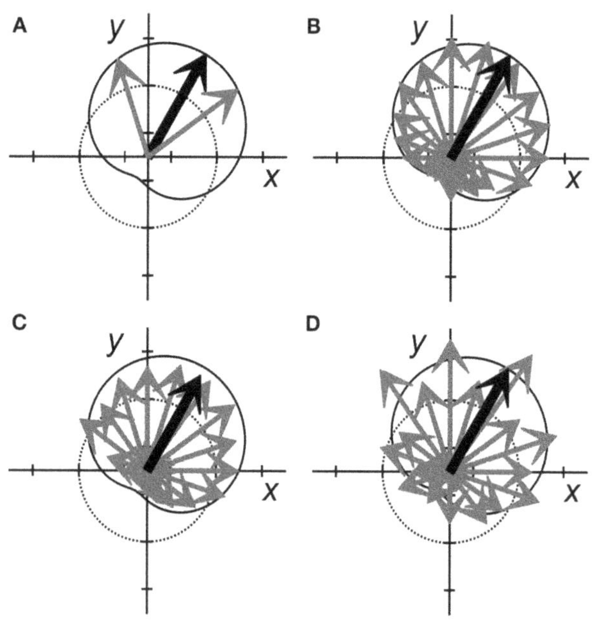

FIGURE 2 | Population vectors for neural encoding of two variables, *x* and *y*. Each neuron is represented by a gray arrow pointing in each cell's preferred direction. The length of each arrow represents the neuron's firing rate. The dotted circle represents a normalized baseline rate for each neuron, with arrow lengths greater than the dotted line representing increased firing rates and shorter lengths representing decreased firing rates. The black arrow represents the population vector sum that predicts the variables, *x* and *y*. The solid cardioid curve represents the expected firing rates of perfectly tuned neurons with various preferred directions when $x = 0.5$ and $y = 0.87$. **(A)** Two perfectly tuned neurons can encode *x* and *y* exactly, but the noise of the output will be equivalent to the noise of the two inputs. **(B)** More independently noisy neurons (here 20 neurons) can be combined to generate an accurate estimate of *x* and *y* with less noise. **(C)** When noise is correlated across neurons, adding more neurons to the population may not improve prediction. In this example, noise produced a correlated reduction in the firing rates of most neurons, resulting in a low amplitude prediction (small population vector). **(D)** In this example, although the neural activity does not match the tuning model (solid cardioid) as accurately as in **(B)**, the predicted *x* and *y* values nevertheless are similar. This departure from the tuning model for *x* and *y* might represent either increased noise, or the encoding of additional features.

error albeit requiring progressively increasing numbers of additional neurons for a given magnitude of reduction in error. In practice, as the number of neurons used for BMI control has increased, achieving BMI accuracy that matches idealized encoding behavior has become increasingly difficult. BMI performance tends to plateau once ~50 recorded neurons have been incorporated, after which much less improvement occurs as more neurons are added (Homer et al., 2013; Tehovnik et al., 2013).

This departure from ideal encoding results in part from the fact that neurons typically are not entirely independent of one another. Sampled neurons often have correlations related not only to the encoded signal, but also to other signals. The correlations produced by these other signals—signals that typically are unknown, unmonitored, and not experimentally controlled—constitute noise with respect to the signal being encoded (Lee et al., 1998). When the noise is correlated, even weakly as is typically observed in cortical recordings (Zohary et al., 1994), perfectly accurate linear encoding becomes impossible. Noise correlations, for example, could cause the estimate for a given trial to converge to an incorrect value. **Figure 2C** illustrates such an example in which a correlated decrease in firing amongst many members of a neuron population causes the magnitude of the resulting population vector to be too small. Even as more and more neurons are added to the decoded population, such noise correlations prevent converging toward perfect decoding.

As more and more neurons are added, incorporating some individual neurons to decode a given variable may actually be detrimental to BMI performance. The relative strength of various signals among different neurons may make adding some neurons corrupted by correlated noise worse than using only those with strong, independent signals. In a BMI application, the ability to generalize control from an initial regression is critical and runs the risk of overfitting if the amount of sampled data is too small for the number of neurons. Also, the ability of the user and/or the decoder to adapt and learn quickly may be diminished as the neural space that must be explored becomes larger. Recognizing such issues, algorithms have been developed to identify those neurons that provide the most independent information, permitting more parsimonious selection of neurons for input to the decoding algorithm (Singhal et al., 2010; Kahn et al., 2011; Xu et al., 2013).

Additionally, the noise levels across a population related to a given variable may not be stationary with time. **Figure 2D** illustrates a situation in which the individual neurons appear to be relatively noisy. Though the population vector is similar to that of **Figure 2B**, in **Figure 2D** the individual neurons appear to deviate randomly from the idealized cosine tuning model indicated by the cardioid curve. Yet this apparent noisiness might represent another signal encoded by the same neuron population (see section Selective Encoding of Variables at Different Times below). How can we make judicious choices regarding the number of neurons used for BMIs?

More Neurons than Controlled DOFs Creates a Null Space

Although the optimal trade-off between the number of neurons recorded and the number of DOFs being controlled by linear BMIs has yet to be well understood, some insight can be gained by considering the simultaneous firing rates of a population of n recorded neurons as an n-dimensional space. When used as a linear signal to control d DOFs, the n-dimensional neural signal is projected into a smaller d-dimensional active control sub-space, leaving a null space of dimensionality $m = n\text{-}d$. Neural activity that projects along the m null-space dimensions has no effect on the d output DOFs. If the neurons are independent predictors, then most noise tends to result in changes in this null space of the joint neural state, allowing an ensemble of "noisy" neural signals to encode the output more precisely.

Yet the null space may be more than a repository for noise. Much of what appears to be noise related to a given signal may represent neural activity related to other signals encoded by the same population of neurons. Below we explore two other potentially valuable aspects of the null space that permit: (i) motor learning with rapid flexibility, and (ii) non-linear encoding that repartitions the active control space vs. the null space depending on the phase of movement.

The Null Space and Motor Learning with Rapid Flexibility

While the null-space can be considered an "uncontrolled manifold" in a particular movement scenario (Scholz and Schöner, 1999; Latash et al., 2007), in the case of a neuronal state space, the uncontrolled manifold is not entirely uncontrolled. During both natural arm movements and BMI output, the joint neural state tends to follow a subset of preferred trajectories that use a subset of the null space, rather than using all possible trajectories distributed throughout the n-dimensional neural space that could provide an equivalent output (Kaufman et al., 2014; Law et al., 2014). Preferred trajectories through the neural state space may reflect the network architecture of pre-existing synaptic connections in which the neurons are embedded (Sadtler et al., 2014). Yet to control novel BMIs, monkeys can learn to use relatively novel neural trajectories (Jarosiewicz et al., 2008; Ganguly and Carmena, 2009; Ganguly et al., 2011; Law et al., 2014). A similar process of learning to use novel neural trajectories may underlie the natural process of learning new motor skills and then switching rapidly at will between one skill and another, according to the context. The relatively large number of neurons, $n > d$, is no longer entirely redundant when additional trajectories through the neural state space must be utilized in additional contexts. Finding and utilizing such additional trajectories might entail learning to associate a previously learned trajectory with a new context, modifying a previously learned trajectory for use in a new context, or learning an entirely new trajectory through the neural state space.

Some evidence that motor learning and rapid flexibility in various contexts involve changes in neural trajectories can be gleaned from studies that use spike-triggered averaging of EMG activity to assess functional connectivity among those neurons that provide last-order inputs to particular motoneuron pools. Broad synchrony facilitations in spike-triggered averages of EMG activity provide evidence that synchronous spikes are discharged by multiple neurons with inputs to the same motoneuron pool, indicating that groups of such neurons receive common or serial inputs (Baker and Lemon, 1998; Schieber and Rivlis, 2005). Among M1 cortico-motoneuronal (CM) cells, such spike synchronization is most common between CM-cells that have output effects in similar sets of muscles (muscle fields), suggesting that these groups of neurons may be recruited together to facilitate a particular set of muscles (Jackson et al., 2003). The prevalence of synchrony effects in M1 neurons increases with long-term training at an individuated finger movement task (Schieber, 2002), suggesting that such long-term training increases the common inputs to neurons that all input in turn to the same motoneuron pool. This change in common inputs will alter the neural trajectory during the practiced movements. Yet the size of synchrony effects also can change rapidly when novel motor behaviors are being performed (Davidson et al., 2007), suggesting that different common inputs to the population of neurons with last-order inputs to a given motoneuron pool become active in different contexts, again indicating different neural trajectories for different contexts. These rapid changes depending on context may involve processing in cortical minicolumns and corticostriatal circuits, where the level of functional connectivity (as measured by cross-correlations between simultaneously recorded spikes in layer 2/3 and layer 5 of a minicolumn, for example) has been found to vary with the type and difficulty of the task being performed (Opris et al., 2012, 2013; Santos et al., 2014). For optimal performance, BMIs will need to take into account such context-dependent changes in neuron activity and the changes in neural trajectories they represent.

Selective Encoding of Variables at Different Times

This idea that the firing of an individual neuron simultaneously carries representations of multiple motor parameters has been widely accepted in neurophysiological studies for some time (Humphrey et al., 1970; Thach, 1978). In general, however, neurophysiological studies make the implicit assumption that the relative weighting of the encoded motor variables remains stationary over the time course of single movements and entire sessions. The same assumption typically is made in current BMI controllers.

Yet some neurophysiological studies have indicated that the motor variables being encoded are not constant, even within a single movement. Time-resolved linear regression, for example, demonstrated that in single M1 and premotor cortex neurons, direction is represented most strongly early in the course of reaching movements, target position is represented most strongly later, and distance is represented most strongly still later in the same movements (Fu et al., 1995). Similarly, using time-resolved analysis of variance, we found recently that the firing rates of M1 neurons vary depending on location early in the course of reach-to-grasp movements, and then on the hand shape used to grasp the object later (Rouse and Schieber, 2014). Such changes in the strength of representation of different features can be viewed as rotations of the d controlled dimensions in the n-dimensional neural state space, which will repartition the m null-space dimensions across the time of a single movement. Hence different variables are represented more or less selectively at different phases of a single movement, and the apparent "null" space provides room for such rotations to occur.

Figure 3 and the Supplemental Video both illustrate this hypothetical repartitioning of the active control space vs. the null space, again using the familiar population vector approach. As in the 2-dimensional examples of **Figure 2**, each arrow represents a different neuron, the direction of the arrow represents that neuron's preferred direction, and the length of the arrow represents its firing rate. In **Figure 2**, the $d = 2$ active dimensions were represented as the ordinate and abscissa of the plot, and the output of the single, linear model depended only on the resulting population vector sum in those two dimensions. Similarly in **Figure 3A**, we plot a population of 20 neurons (colored arrows)

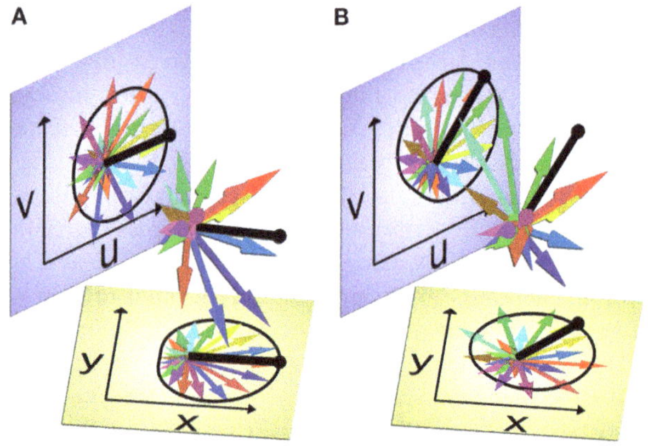

FIGURE 3 | Multi-dimensional population vector selectively encoding two pairs of variables at different times. Each of 20 neurons is represented by a colored arrow pointing in its preferred direction. The length of each arrow represents that neuron's firing rate. The two planes, $x \perp y$ (tan) and $u \perp v$ (blue), each show the individual neuron's firing rates and preferred directions projected into the two pairs of dimensions. The population vector sum (heavy black line) projected into each plane represents the population's estimate of the two pairs of variables: x and y, u and v. The black cardioid curve represents the predicted firing rates given the population vector if each neuron was ideally cosine-tuned to a given pair of variables (x and y, or u and v). The two panels **(A,B)** represent two different points in time. At the first time point **(A)**, the individual neuron firing rates are related most closely to x and y, matching the idealized cosine tuning to those two variables, as represented by the cardioid in that plane. But at the second time point **(B)**, the firing rates of the same 20 neurons are related most closely to u and v. The firing rates of these neurons may not be representing both pairs of variables equally at all points in time, but rather selectively encoding one pair of variables at each time. At either time point, if a single linear decoder were used to estimate all four dimensions—x, y, u, and v—simultaneously from the population, one pair would be estimated accurately and the other pair inaccurately. But using two different decoders—one to estimate x and y, the other to estimate u and v—and then selecting the currently decoded output by assessing which idealized model is better fit at the time, would enable more accurate decoding overall. The Supplemental Video provides an animated version of this Figure. (N.B. To illustrate a 4-dimensional space in 3-dimensions, we have made u linearly dependent on x and y in these images; but in the actual high-dimensional neural space, all four variables can be linearly independent).

projected into the plane of two output dimensions, x and y, and the resulting population vector (black). As in **Figure 2B**, at the point in time illustrated in **Figure 3A** each individual neuron's firing rate closely matches the idealized linear model represented by the cardioid curve drawn to indicate the cosine tuning of individual neurons to the variables x and y relative to the population vector.

The remaining $m = 20–2 = 18$-dimensional null space has no direct effect on the output (population vector) of this model in this $x \perp y$ plane. But consider the neural activity in two of these null dimensions, u and v. The neuron firing rates and resulting population vector projected in the $u \perp v$ plane also are illustrated in **Figure 3A**. A different cardioid curve is shown here to represent the cosine tuning that pertains when the population vector is calculated using a second idealized model based on the projections of the neuron firing rates in the $u \perp v$ plane. In the $u \perp v$ plane, the firing rates of the individual neurons match this second model poorly, not unlike the example of **Figure 2D**.

Now consider a different point in time when the individual neurons are firing at different rates, illustrated in **Figure 3B**. Now the firing rates match the cardioid in the $x \perp y$ plane poorly, but match the cardioid in the $u \perp v$ plane well. The same neuron population that encoded x and y previously, now is encoding u and v. We hypothesize that in this manner a given neuron population may encode different variables selectively during different phases of a single movement. In such a construct, treating the 20 neuron population as a 4-dimensional output space that continuously encodes x, y, u, and v plus a 16-dimensional null space would be suboptimal. For BMI purposes, decoding different variables at different points in time would provide more accurate output for the two variables as each becomes most relevant to the current phase (or context) of movement. At each point in time, the model most heavily weighted in the BMI output could be selected by having the computer assess which idealized model is better fit by the neuron firing rates currently being generated by the brain.

Such selective neural encoding of different sets of variables at different times might be dismissed as simply reflecting an inability to create a single linear model fitting all the observed firing rates well. An inaccurate single model might result from having insufficient data (numbers of trials), insufficient numbers of neurons (e.g., $n >> 20$ is needed), or insufficient sampling of the high-dimensional parameter space ($\ldots u, v, \ldots x, y \ldots$). Yet if a given population of neurons does indeed represent different output features at different times, applying a single linear model cannot achieve high accuracy at all points in time regardless of how many neurons or how much data are incorporated. Non-linear models will be needed to repartition the active control space vs. the null space.

As reviewed above (section The Null Space and Motor Learning with Rapid Flexibility), we envision that during natural behavior the nervous system achieves the non-linear repartitioning that selects different controlled variables by coactivating, or even synchronizing, various subpopulations of neurons at different times. In view of the wide range of inputs that impinge on a single α-motoneuron (including Ia afferents, Ia-inhibitory interneurons, excitatory spinal interneurons, and CM-cells) or that affect a single M1 neuron (including inputs from the primary somatosensory cortex, ventral premotor cortex, dorsal premotor cortex, supplementary motor area, and thalamus), we hypothesize that non-linear repartitioning may involve various inputs predominating at different times, with synaptic summation that is not necessarily linear. The extent to which the nervous system naturally uses non-linear repartitioning to output different features from the same neuron population at different times remains an open scientific question.

In any case, BMI performance might be improved by implementing methods that allow for selective encoding of the variables most relevant to the current phase of movement. This could be achieved by applying different decoding algorithms to sequentially capture different features of complex movements (Ethier et al., 2011; Jiang et al., 2011; Srinivasan and da Silva, 2011; Shanechi et al., 2012; Aggarwal et al., 2013; Kang et al., 2015). Rather than continuously decoding all DOF simultaneously, the BMI controller might use population neural activity to encode only a subset of variables while other variables are either passively dampened or even held constant by the BMI. Controlling a robotic arm and hand to reach and grasp, for example, might be improved by using neural activity sequentially, first to encode the reach location to which the arm transports the hand, and then as the hand arrives near the object, switching to encode the grasp while damping further movement of the arm. This could allow the user to focus on grasping the object precisely, without the distraction of simultaneously continuing to control the entire arm.

Conclusions

A general theme that emerges from our considerations is that natural motor control is not a single process that applies universally in all situations. The control of small, fine movements differs from that of large, gross movements. The control of posture is not achieved by producing movement with zero velocity. Many movements may be controlled through small numbers of synergies, and only the most sophisticated performances may require individuated control of large numbers of DOFs. In generating complex movements, the same neuronal population may transmit information on different sets of output variables sequentially rather than simultaneously. To advance the performance of BMIs further toward that of normal humans will require similar strategies that go beyond one-size-fits-all, linear state space models.

Achieving such advances necessarily will require increasing the complexity of BMI controllers. Decoding will need to be more flexible and applied differently at different times, possibly driven by inputs recorded from different parts of the nervous system. Moreover, supervisory algorithms will be needed to identify the contexts and movement phases that define this dynamic relationship between neural signals and output DOFs. Implementing such designs will go further to translate our knowledge of natural motor control physiology, advancing BMIs toward normal human performance.

Acknowledgments

This work was funded by National Institutes of Health R01s NS065902 and NS079664. The authors thank the anonymous reviewers for helpful suggestions and Marsha Hayles for editorial comments.

References

Aggarwal, V., Mollazadeh, M., Davidson, A. G., Schieber, M. H., and Thakor, N. V, (2013). State-based decoding of hand and finger kinematics using neuronal ensemble and LFP activity during dexterous reach-to-grasp movements. *J. Neurophysiol.* 109, 3067–3081. doi: 10.1152/jn.01038.2011

Ajiboye, A. B., Simeral, J. D., Donoghue, J. P., Hochberg, L. R., and Kirsch, R. F. (2012). Prediction of imagined single-joint movements in a person with high-level tetraplegia. *IEEE Trans. Biomed. Eng.* 59, 2755–2765. doi: 10.1109/TBME.2012.2209882

Anderson, W. S., Weiss, N., Lawson, H. C., Ohara, S., Rowland, L., and Lenz, F. A. (2011). Demonstration of motor imagery- and phantom-movement related neuronal activity in human thalamus. *Neuroreport* 22, 88–92. doi: 10.1097/WNR.0b013e328342c98a

Arbib, M. A., Iberall, T., and Lyons, D. (1985). "Coordinated control programs for movements of the hand," in *Hand Function and the Neocotex (Experimental Brain Research Series)*, eds A. W. Goodwin and I. Darian-Smith (Heidelberg: Springer–Verlag), 111–129.

Baker, S. N. (2011). The primate reticulospinal tract, hand function and functional recovery. *J. Physiol.* 589, 5603–5612. doi: 10.1113/jphysiol.2011.215160

Baker, S. N., and Lemon, R. N. (1998). Computer simulation of post-spike facilitation in spike-triggered averages of rectified EMG. *J. Neurophysiol.* 80, 1391–1406.

Bernstein, N. A. (1967). *The Co-ordination and Regulation of Movements*, 1st Edn. Oxford: Pergamon Press.

Buford, J. A., and Davidson, A. G. (2004). Movement-related and preparatory activity in the reticulospinal system of the monkey. *Exp. Brain Res.* 159, 284–300. doi: 10.1007/s00221-004-1956-4

Card, S. K., English, W. K., and Burr, B. J. (1978). Evaluation of mouse, rate-controlled isometric joystick, step keys, and text keys for text selection on a CRT. *Ergonomics* 21, 601–613. doi: 10.1080/00140137808931762

Carmena, J. M., Lebedev, M. A., Crist, R. E., O'Doherty, J. E., Santucci, D. M., Dimitrov, D. F., et al. (2003). Learning to control a brain-machine interface for reaching and grasping by primates. *PLoS Biol* 1:E42. doi: 10.1371/journal.pbio.0000042

Casile, A. (2013). Mirror neurons (and beyond) in the macaque brain: an overview of 20 years of research. *Neurosci. Lett.* 540, 3–14. doi: 10.1016/j.neulet.2012.11.003

Chadwick, E. K., Blana, D., Simeral, J. D., Lambrecht, J., Kim, S. P., Cornwell, A. S., et al. (2011). Continuous neuronal ensemble control of simulated arm reaching by a human with tetraplegia. *J. Neural Eng.* 8:034003. doi: 10.1088/1741-2560/8/3/034003

Chase, S. M., and Schwartz, A. B. (2011). "Inference from populations: going beyond models," in *Progress in Brain Research*, eds A. M. Green, C. E. Chapman, J. F. Kalaska, and F. Lepore (Amsterdam: Elsevier), 103–112. doi: 10.1016/B978-0-444-53355-5.00007-5

Chestek, C. A., Gilja, V., Nuyujukian, P., Foster, J. D., Fan, J. M., Kaufman, M. T., et al. (2011). Long-term stability of neural prosthetic control signals from silicon cortical arrays in rhesus macaque motor cortex. *J. Neural Eng.* 8:045005. doi: 10.1088/1741-2560/8/4/045005

Cheung, V. C. K., Piron, L., Agostini, M., Silvoni, S., Turolla, A., and Bizzi, E. (2009). Stability of muscle synergies for voluntary actions after cortical stroke in humans. *Proc. Natl. Acad. Sci. U. S. A.* 106, 19563–19568. doi: 10.1073/pnas.0910114106

Churchland, M. M., Cunningham, J. P., Kaufman, M. T., Foster, J. D., Nuyujukian, P., Ryu, S. I., et al. V (2012). Neural population dynamics during reaching. *Nature* 487, 51–56. doi: 10.1038/nature11129

Ciocarlie, M., Goldfeder, C., and Allen, P. (2007). Dimensionality reduction for hand-independent dexterous robotic grasping. *2007 IEEE/RSJ Int. Conf. Intell. Robot. Syst.* 20, 3270–3275. doi: 10.1109/IROS.2007.4399227

Cisek, P., and Kalaska, J. F. (2004). Neural correlates of mental rehearsal in dorsal premotor cortex. *Nature* 431, 993–996. doi: 10.1038/nature03005

Collinger, J. L., Wodlinger, B., Downey, J. E., Wang, W., Tyler-Kabara, E. C., Weber, D. J., et al. (2013). High-performance neuroprosthetic control by an individual with tetraplegia. *Lancet* 381, 557–564. doi: 10.1016/S0140-6736(12)61816-9

Cunningham, J. P., Gilja, V., Ryu, S. I., and Shenoy, K. V (2010). Methods for estimating neural firing rates, and their application to brain-machine interfaces. *Neural Netw.* 22, 249–266. doi: 10.1016/j.neunet.2009.02.004

Dalley, S. A., Wiste, T. E., Varol, H. A., and Goldfarb, M. (2010). A multigrasp hand prosthesis for transradial amputees. *Conf. Proc. IEEE Eng. Med. Biol. Soc.* 2010, 5062–5065. doi: 10.1109/iembs.2010.5626225

Davidson, A. G., Chan, V., O'Dell, R., and Schieber, M. H. (2007). Rapid changes in throughput from single motor cortex neurons to muscle activity. *Science* 318, 1934–1937. doi: 10.1126/science.1149774

d'Avella, A., and Bizzi, E. (2005). Shared and specific muscle synergies in natural motor behaviors. *Proc. Natl. Acad. Sci. U. S. A.* 102, 3076–3081. doi: 10.1073/pnas.0500199102

Dushanova, J., and Donoghue, J. P. (2010). Neurons in primary motor cortex engaged during action observation. *Eur. J. Neurosci.* 31, 386–398. doi: 10.1111/j.1460-9568.2009.07067.x

Engel, K. C., Flanders, M., and Soechting, J. F. (1997). Anticipatory and sequential motor control in piano playing. *Exp. brain Res.* 113, 189–199. doi: 10.1007/BF02450317

Epps, B. W. (1986). Comparison of six cursor control devices based on Fitts' law models. *Proc. Hum. Factors Ergon. Soc. Annu. Meet.* 30, 327–331. doi: 10.1177/154193128603000403

Ersland, L., Rosén, G., Lundervold, A., Smievoll, A. I., Tillung, T., Sundberg, H., et al. (1996). Phantom limb imaginary fingertapping causes primary motor cortex activation: an fMRI study. *Neuroreport* 8, 207–210. doi: 10.1097/00001756-199612200-00042

Ethier, C., Oby, E. R., Bauman, M. J., and Miller, L. E. (2012). Restoration of grasp following paralysis through brain-controlled stimulation of muscles. *Nature* 485, 368–371. doi: 10.1038/nature10987

Ethier, C., Sachs, N. A., Miller, L. E., and Collection, A. D. (2011). Continuous state-dependent decoders for brain machine interfaces. *Neural Eng. (NER), 2011 5th International IEEE/EMBS Conference on IEEE* (Cancun), 473–477. doi: 10.1109/NER.2011.5910589

Felton, E. A., Radwin, R. G., Wilson, J. A., and Williams, J. C. (2009). Evaluation of a modified Fitts law brain-computer interface target acquisition task in able and motor disabled individuals. *J. Neural Eng.* 6:056002. doi: 10.1088/1741-2560/6/5/056002

Fetz, E. E., and Baker, M. A. (1973). Operantly conditioned patterns of precentral unit activity and correlated responses in adjacent cells and contralateral muscles. *J. Neurophysiol.* 36, 179–204.

Fetz, E. E., Perlmutter, S. I., Prut, Y., Seki, K., and Votaw, S. (2002). Roles of primate spinal interneurons in preparation and execution of voluntary hand movement. *Brain Res. Rev.* 40, 53–65. doi: 10.1016/S0165-0173(02)00188-1

Fitts, P. M. (1954). The information capacity of human motor system in controlling the ampltude of movement. *J. Exp. Psychol.* 47, 381–391. doi: 10.1037/h0055392

Fitzsimmons, N. A., Lebedev, M. A., Peikon, I. D., and Nicolelis, M. A. L. (2009). Extracting kinematic parameters for monkey bipedal walking from cortical neuronal ensemble activity. *Front. Integr. Neurosci.* 3:3. doi: 10.3389/neuro.07.003.2009

Flanders, M., and Soechting, J. F. (1992). Kinematics of typing: parallel control of the two hands. *J. Neurophysiol.* 67, 1264–1274.

Fraser, G. W., Chase, S. M., Whitford, A., and Schwartz, A. B. (2009). Control of a brain-computer interface without spike sorting. *J. Neural Eng.* 6:055004. doi: 10.1088/1741-2560/6/5/055004

Fu, Q. G., Flament, D., Coltz, J. D., and Ebner, T. J. (1995). Temporal encoding of movement kinematics in the discharge of primate primary motor and premotor neurons. *J. Neurophysiol.* 73, 836–854.

Ganguly, K., and Carmena, J. M. (2009). Emergence of a stable cortical map for neuroprosthetic control. *PLoS Biol.* 7:e1000153. doi: 10.1371/journal.pbio.1000153

Ganguly, K., Dimitrov, D. F., Wallis, J. D., and Carmena, J. M. (2011). Reversible large-scale modification of cortical networks during neuroprosthetic control. *Nat. Neurosci.* 14, 662–667. doi: 10.1038/nn.2797

Georgopoulos, A. P. (2014). Cell directional spread determines accuracy, precision, and length of the neuronal population vector. *Exp. Brain Res.* 232, 2391–2405. doi: 10.1007/s00221-014-3936-7

Georgopoulos, A. P., and Grillner, S. (1989). Visuomotor coordination in reaching and locomotion. *Science* 245, 1209–1210. doi: 10.1126/science.2675307

Gilja, V., Nuyujukian, P., Chestek, C. A., Cunningham, J. P., Yu, B. M., Fan, J. M., et al. (2012). A high-performance neural prosthesis enabled by control algorithm design. *Nat. Neurosci.* 15, 1752–1757. doi: 10.1038/nn.3265

Giszter, S. F., and Hart, C. B. (2013). Motor primitives and synergies in the spinal cord and after injury–the current state of play. *Ann. N. Y. Acad. Sci.* 1279, 114–126. doi: 10.1111/nyas.12065

Grafton, S. T., Arbib, M. A., Fadiga, L., and Rizzolatti, G. (1996). Localization of grasp representations in humans by positron emission tomography. 2. Observation compared with imaginations. *Exp. Brain Res.* 112, 103–111. doi: 10.1007/BF00227183

Grillner, S. (1985). Neurobiological bases of rhythmic motor acts in vertebrates. *Science* 228, 143–149. doi: 10.1126/science.3975635

Hager-Ross, C., and Schieber, M. H. (2000). Quantifying the independence of human finger movements: comparisons of digits, hands, and movement frequencies. *J. Neurosci.* 20, 8542–8550.

Hall, T. M., de Carvalho, F., and Jackson, A. (2014). A common structure underlies low-frequency cortical dynamics in movement, sleep, and sedation. *Neuron* 83, 1185–1199. doi: 10.1016/j.neuron.2014.07.022

Harris, C. M., and Wolpert, D. M. (1998). Signal-dependent noise determines motor planning. *Nature* 394, 780–784. doi: 10.1038/29528

Hochberg, L. R., Bacher, D., Jarosiewicz, B., Masse, N. Y., Simeral, J. D., Vogel, J., et al. (2012). Reach and grasp by people with tetraplegia using a neurally controlled robotic arm. *Nature* 485, 372–375. doi: 10.1038/nature11076

Hochberg, L. R., Serruya, M. D., Friehs, G. M., Mukand, J. A., Saleh, M., Caplan, A. H., et al. (2006). Neuronal ensemble control of prosthetic devices by a human with tetraplegia. *Nature* 442, 164–171. doi: 10.1038/nature04970

Homer, M. L., Nurmikko, A. V., Donoghue, J. P., and Hochberg, L. R. (2013). Sensors and decoding for intracortical brain computer interfaces. *Annu. Rev. Biomed. Eng.* 15, 383–405. doi: 10.1146/annurev-bioeng-071910-124640

Humphrey, D. R., and Reed, D. J. (1983). Separate cortical systems for control of joint movement and joint stiffness: reciprocal activation and coactivation of antagonist muscles. *Adv. Neurol.* 39, 347–372.

Humphrey, D. R., Schmidt, E. M., and Thompson, W. D. (1970). Predicting measures of motor performance from multiple cortical spike trains. *Science* 170, 758–762. doi: 10.1126/science.170.3959.758

Hutchinson, D. T. (2014). The quest for the bionic arm. *J. Am. Acad. Orthop. Surg.* 22, 346–351. doi: 10.5435/JAAOS-22-06-346

Ifft, P. J., Lebedev, M. A., and Nicolelis, M. A. L. (2011). Cortical correlates of fitts' law. *Front. Integr. Neurosci.* 5:85. doi: 10.3389/fnint.2011.00085

Jackson, A., Gee, V. J., Baker, S. N., and Lemon, R. N. (2003). Synchrony between neurons with similar muscle fields in monkey motor cortex. *Neuron* 38, 115–125. doi: 10.1016/S0896-6273(03)00162-4

Jagacinski, R. J., and Monk, D. M. (1985). Fitts' law in two dimensions with hand and head movements. *J. Mot. Behav.* 17, 77–95. doi: 10.1080/00222895.1985.10735338

Jarosiewicz, B., Chase, S. M., Fraser, G. W., Velliste, M., Kass, R. E., and Schwartz, A. B. (2008). Functional network reorganization during learning in a brain-computer interface paradigm. *Proc. Natl. Acad. Sci. U.S.A.* 105, 19486–19491. doi: 10.1073/pnas.0808113105

Jiang, B., Wang, R., Zhang, Q., Zhang, J., Zheng, X., and Zhao, T. (2011). A pilot study on two stage decoding strategies. *Proc. IEEE EMBS Conf.* 2011, 3700–3703. doi: 10.1109/iembs.2011.6090627

Johannes, M. S., Bigelow, J. D., Burck, J. M., Harshbarger, S. D., and Kozlowski, M. V (2011). An overview of the developmental process for the modular prosthetic limb. *Johns Hopkins APL Tech. Dig.* 30, 207–216.

Kahn, K., Schieber, M. H., Thakor, N. V., and Sarma, S., V (2011). Neuron selection for decoding dexterous finger movements. *Conf. Proc. IEEE Eng. Med. Biol. Soc.* 2011, 4605–4608. doi: 10.1109/IEMBS.2011.6091140

Kang, N., Shinohara, M., Zatsiorsky, V. M., and Latash, M. L. (2004). Learning multi-finger synergies: an uncontrolled manifold analysis. *Exp. Brain Res.* 157, 336–350. doi: 10.1007/s00221-004-1850-0

Kang, X., Sarma, S., Santaniello, S., Schieber, M. H., and Thakor, N. (2015). Task-independent cognitive state transition detection from cortical neurons during 3D reach-to-grasp movements. *IEEE Trans. Neural Syst. Rehabil. Eng.* 23, 676–682. doi: 10.1109/TNSRE.2015.2396495

Kaufman, M. T., Churchland, M. M., Ryu, S. I., and Shenoy, K. V (2014). Cortical activity in the null space: permitting preparation without movement. *Nat. Neurosci.* 17, 440–448. doi: 10.1038/nn.3643

Kemere, C., Santhanam, G., Yu, B. M., Afshar, A., Ryu, S. I., Meng, T. H., et al. (2008). Detecting neural-state transitions using hidden Markov models for motor cortical prostheses. *J. Neurophysiol.* 100, 2441–2452. doi: 10.1152/jn.00924.2007

Lassek, A. M. (1954). *The Pyramidal Tract: Its Status in Medicine*. Springfield, IL: Charles C. Thomas.

Latash, M. L., Scholz, J. P., Danion, F., and Schöner, G. (2002). Finger coordination during discrete and oscillatory force production tasks. *Exp. Brain Res.* 146, 419–432. doi: 10.1007/s00221-002-1196-4

Latash, M. L., Scholz, J. P., and Schöner, G. (2007). Toward a new theory of motor synergies. *Motor Control* 11, 276–308.

Law, A. J., Rivlis, G., and Schieber, M. H. (2014). Rapid acquisition of novel interface control by small ensembles of arbitrarily selected primary motor cortex neurons. *J. Neurophysiol.* 112, 1528–1548. doi: 10.1152/jn.00373.2013

Lebedev, M. A., Carmena, J. M., O'Doherty, J. E., Zacksenhouse, M., Henriquez, C. S., Principe, J. C., et al. (2005). Cortical ensemble adaptation to represent velocity of an artificial actuator controlled by a brain-machine interface. *J. Neurosci.* 25, 4681–4693. doi: 10.1523/JNEUROSCI.4088-04.2005

Lebedev, M. A., and Nicolelis, M. A. L. (2011). Toward a whole-body neuroprosthetic. *Prog. Brain Res.* 194, 47–60. doi: 10.1016/B978-0-444-53815-4.00018-2

Lee, D., Port, N. L., Kruse, W., and Georgopoulos, A. P. (1998). Variability and correlated noise in the discharge of neurons in motor and parietal areas of the primate cortex. *J. Neurosci.* 18, 1161–1170.

Li, Z., O'Doherty, J. E., Hanson, T. L., Lebedev, M. A., Henriquez, C. S., and Nicolelis, M. A. L. (2009). Unscented Kalman filter for brain-machine interfaces. *PLoS ONE* 4:e6243. doi: 10.1371/journal.pone.0006243

MacKenzie, I. S. (1992). Fitts' law as a research and design tool in human-computer interaction. *Hum. Comput. Interact.* 7, 91–139. doi: 10.1207/s15327051hci0701_3

Mahan, M. Y., and Georgopoulos, A. P. (2013). Motor directional tuning across brain areas: directional resonance and the role of inhibition for directional accuracy. *Front. Neural Circuits* 7:92. doi: 10.3389/fncir.2013.00092

Maier, M. A., Perlmutter, S. I., and Fetz, E. E. (1998). Response patterns and force relations of monkey spinal interneurons during active wrist movement. *J. Neurophysiol.* 80, 2495–2513.

Mason, C. R., Theverapperuma, L. S., Hendrix, C. M., and Ebner, T. J. (2004). Monkey hand postural synergies during reach-to-grasp in the absence of vision of the hand and object. *J. Neurophysiol.* 91, 2826–2837. doi: 10.1152/jn.00653.2003

Moran, D. W., and Schwartz, A. B. (1999). Motor cortical representation of speed and direction during reaching. *J. Neurophysiol.* 82, 2676–2692.

Moritz, C. T., Perlmutter, S. I., and Fetz, E. E. (2008). Direct control of paralysed muscles by cortical neurons. *Nature* 456, 639–642. doi: 10.1038/nature07418

Müller, K., Anderson, C. W., and Birch, G. E. (2003). Linear and nonlinear methods for brain-computer interfaces. *IEEE Trans. Neural Syst. Rehabil. Eng.* 11, 165–169. doi: 10.1109/TNSRE.2003.814484

Opris, I., Fuqua, J. L., Huettl, P. F., Gerhardt, G. A., Berger, T. W., Hampson, R. E., et al. (2012). Closing the loop in primate prefrontal cortex: inter-laminar processing. *Front. Neural Circuits* 6:88. doi: 10.3389/fncir.2012.00088

Opris, I., Santos, L., Gerhardt, G. A., Song, D., Berger, T. W., Hampson, R. E., et al. (2013). Prefrontal cortical microcircuits bind perception to executive control. *Sci. Rep.* 3:2285. doi: 10.1038/srep02285

Orsborn, A. L., Dangi, S., Moorman, H. G., and Carmena, J. M. (2012). Closed-loop decoder adaptation on intermediate time-scales facilitates rapid BMI performance improvements independent of decoder initialization conditions. *IEEE Trans. Neural Syst. Rehabil. Eng.* 20, 468–477. doi: 10.1109/TNSRE.2012.2185066

Pancrazio, J. J., and Peckham, P. H. (2009). Neuroprosthetic devices: how far are we from recovering movement in paralyzed patients? *Expert Rev. Neurother.* 9, 427–430. doi: 10.1586/ern.09.12

Pfurtscheller, G., and Neuper, C. (1997). Motor imagery activates primary sensorimotor area in humans. *Neurosci. Lett.* 239, 65–68. doi: 10.1016/S0304-3940(97)00889-6

Porro, C. A., Francescato, M. P., Cettolo, V., Diamond, M. E., Baraldi, P., Zuiani, C., et al. (1996). Primary motor and sensory cortex activation during motor performance and motor imagery: a functional magnetic resonance imaging study. *J. Neurosci.* 16, 7688–7698.

Resnik, L., Klinger, S. L., and Etter, K. (2013). The DEKA Arm: Its features, functionality, and evolution during the Veterans Affairs Study to optimize the DEKA Arm. *Prosthet. Orthot. Int.* 38, 492–504. doi: 10.1177/0309364613506913

Roh, J., Cheung, V. C. K., and Bizzi, E. (2011). Modules in the brain stem and spinal cord underlying motor behaviors. *J. Neurophysiol.* 106, 1363–1378. doi: 10.1152/jn.00842.2010

Rouse, A. G., and Schieber, M. H. (2014). "Location then object representations sequentially predominate in the widely distributed activation of the primary motor cortex during reach to grasp," in *Society for Neuroscience Annual Meeting* (Washington, DC).

Sadtler, P. T., Quick, K. M., Golub, M. D., Chase, S. M., Ryu, S. I., Tyler-Kabara, E. C., et al. (2014). Neural constraints on learning. *Nature* 512, 423–426. doi: 10.1038/nature13665

Santello, M., Flanders, M., and Soechting, J. F. (1998). Postural hand synergies for tool use. *J. Neurosci.* 18, 10105–10115.

Santos, L., Opris, I., Hampson, R., Godwin, D. W., Gerhardt, G. A., and Deadwyler, S. (2014). Functional dynamics of primate cortico-striatal networks during volitional movements. *Front. Syst. Neurosci.* 8:27. doi: 10.3389/fnsys.2014.00027

Schieber, M. H. (2002). Training and synchrony in the motor system. *J. Neurosci.* 22, 5277–5281.

Schieber, M. H., and Rivlis, G. (2005). A spectrum from pure post-spike effects to synchrony effects in spike-triggered averages of electromyographic activity during skilled finger movements. *J. Neurophysiol.* 94, 3325–3341. doi: 10.1152/jn.00007.2005

Scholz, J. P., Reisman, D., and Schöner, G. (2001). Effects of varying task constraints on solutions to joint coordination in a sit-to-stand task. *Exp. Brain Res.* 141, 485–500. doi: 10.1007/s002210100878

Scholz, J. P., and Schöner, G. (1999). The uncontrolled manifold concept: identifying control variables for a functional task. *Exp. Brain Res.* 126, 289–306. doi: 10.1007/s002210050738

Seki, K., Perlmutter, S. I., and Fetz, E. E. (2003). Sensory input to primate spinal cord is presynaptically inhibited during voluntary movement. *Nat. Neurosci.* 6, 1309–1316. doi: 10.1038/nn1154

Serruya, M. D., Hatsopoulos, N. G., Paninski, L., Fellows, M. R., and Donoghue, J. P. (2002). Instant neural control of a movement signal. *Nature* 416, 141–142. doi: 10.1038/416141a

Shalit, U., Zinger, N., Joshua, M., and Prut, Y. (2012). Descending systems translate transient cortical commands into a sustained muscle activation signal. *Cereb. Cortex* 22, 1904–1914. doi: 10.1093/cercor/bhr267

Shanechi, M. M., Hu, R. C., Powers, M., Wornell, G. W., Brown, E. N., and Williams, Z. M. (2012). Neural population partitioning and a concurrent brain-machine interface for sequential motor function. *Nat. Neurosci.* 15, 1715–1722. doi: 10.1038/nn.3250

Shanechi, M. M., Orsborn, A., Moorman, H., Gowda, S., and Carmena, J. M. (2014). High-performance brain-machine interface enabled by an adaptive optimal feedback-controlled point process decoder. *Proc. IEEE EMBS Conf.* 36, 6493–6496. doi: 10.1109/embc.2014.6945115

Shik, M. L., and Orlovsky, G. N. (1976). Neurophysiology of locomotor automatism. *Physiol. Rev.* 56, 465–501.

Singhal, G., Aggarwal, V., Acharya, S., Aguayo, J., He, J., and Thakor, N. (2010). Ensemble fractional sensitivity: a quantitative approach to neuron selection for decoding motor tasks. *Comput. Intell. Neurosci.* 2010, 648202. doi: 10.1155/2010/648202

Slifkin, A. B., and Newell, K. M. (1999). Noise, information transmission, and force variability. *J. Exp. Psychol. Hum. Percept. Perform.* 25, 837–851. doi: 10.1037/0096-1523.25.3.837

Soechting, J. F., and Flanders, M. (1992). Organization of sequential typing movements. *J. Neurophysiol.* 67, 1275–1290.

Soechting, J. F., and Flanders, M. (1997). Flexibility and repeatability of finger movements during typing: analysis of multiple degrees of freedom. *J. Comput. Neurosci.* 4, 29–46. doi: 10.1023/A:1008812426305

Srinivasan, L., and da Silva, M. (2011). Breaking the fixed-arrival-time restriction in reaching movements of neural prosthetic devices. *IEEE Trans. Biomed. Eng.* 58, 1555–1564. doi: 10.1109/TBME.2010.2101599

Stein, P. S. G. (1978). Motor systems, with specific reference to the control of locomotion. *Annu. Rev. Neurosci.* 1, 61–81. doi: 10.1146/annurev.ne.01.030178.000425

Stieglitz, T., Rubehn, B., Henle, C., Kisban, S., Herwik, S., Ruther, P., et al. (2009). "Brain-computer interfaces: an overview of the hardware to record neural signals from the cortex," in *Progress in Brain Research*, eds J. Verhaagen, E. M. Hol, I. Huitenga, J. Wijholds, A. B. Bergen, G. J. Boer, and D. J. Swaab (Amsterdam: Elsevier), 297–315. doi: 10.1016/S0079-6123(09)17521-0

Taylor, D. M., Tillery, S. I. H., and Schwartz, A. B. (2002). Direct cortical control of 3D neuroprosthetic devices. *Science* 296, 1829–1832. doi: 10.1126/science.1070291

Tehovnik, E. J., Woods, L. C., and Slocum, W. M. (2013). Transfer of information by BMI. *Neuroscience* 255, 134–146. doi: 10.1016/j.neuroscience.2013.10.003

Thach, W. T. (1978). Correlation of neural discharge with pattern and force of muscular activity, joint position, and direction of intended next movement in motor cortex and cerebellum. *J. Neurophysiol.* 41, 654–676.

Tkach, D., Reimer, J., and Hatsopoulos, N. G. (2007). Congruent activity during action and action observation in motor cortex. *J. Neurosci.* 27, 13241–13250. doi: 10.1523/JNEUROSCI.2895-07.2007

Tseng, Y., Scholz, J. P., and Schöner, G. (2002). Goal-equivalent joint coordination in pointing: affect of vision and arm dominance. *Motor Control* 6, 183–204.

Tsianos, G. A., Goodner, J., and Loeb, G. E. (2014). Useful properties of spinal circuits for learning and performing planar reaches. *J. Neural Eng.* 11:056006. doi: 10.1088/1741-2560/11/5/056006

Velliste, M., McMorland, A. J. C., Diril, E., Clanton, S. T., and Schwartz, A. B. (2012). State-space control of prosthetic hand shape. *Conf. Proc. IEEE Eng. Med. Biol. Soc.* 2012, 964–967. doi: 10.1109/EMBC.2012.6346093

Velliste, M., Kennedy, S. D., Schwartz, A. B., Whitford, A. S., Sohn, J.-W., and McMorland, A. J. C. (2014). Motor cortical correlates of arm resting in the context of a reaching task and implications for prosthetic control. *J. Neurosci.* 34, 6011–6022. doi: 10.1523/JNEUROSCI.3520-13.2014

Velliste, M., Perel, S., Spalding, M. C., Whitford, A. S., and Schwartz, A. B. (2008). Cortical control of a prosthetic arm for self-feeding. *Nature* 453, 1098–1101. doi: 10.1038/nature06996

Vigneswaran, G., Philipp, R., Lemon, R. N., and Kraskov, A. (2013). M1 corticospinal mirror neurons and their role in movement suppression during action observation. *Curr. Biol.* 23, 236–243. doi: 10.1016/j.cub.2012.12.006

Vinjamuri, R., Weber, D. J., Mao, Z.-H., Collinger, J. L., Degenhart, A. D., Kelly, J. W., et al. (2011). Toward synergy-based brain-machine interfaces. *IEEE Trans. Inf. Technol. Biomed.* 15, 726–736. doi: 10.1109/TITB.2011.2160272

Williams, J. J., Rouse, A. G., Thongpang, S., Williams, J. C., and Moran, D. W. (2013). Differentiating closed-loop cortical intention from rest: building an asynchronous electrocorticographic BCI. *J. Neural Eng.* 10:046001. doi: 10.1088/1741-2560/10/4/046001

Wodlinger, B., Downey, J. E., Tyler-Kabara, E. C., Schwartz, A. B., Boninger, M. L., and Collinger, J. L. (2015). Ten-dimensional anthropomorphic arm control in a human brain-machine interface: difficulties, solutions, and limitations. *J. Neural Eng.* 12:016011. doi: 10.1088/1741-2560/12/1/016011

Wolpaw, J. R. (2010). Brain-computer interface research comes of age: traditional assumptions meet emerging realities. *J. Mot. Behav.* 42, 351–353. doi: 10.1080/00222895.2010.526471

Wu, W., Black, M. J., Gao, Y., Bienenstock, E., Serruya, M. D., Shaikhouni, A., et al. (2003). Neural decoding of cursor motion using a Kalman Filter. *Adv. Neural Inf. Process. Syst.* 133–140.

Xu, K., Wang, Y., Wang, Y., Wang, F., Hao, Y., Zhang, S., et al. (2013). Local-learning-based neuron selection for grasping gesture prediction in motor brain machine interfaces. *J. Neural Eng.* 10:026008. doi: 10.1088/1741-2560/10/2/026008

Zhang, Y., and Chase, S. M. (2013). A stabilized dual Kalman filter for adaptive tracking of brain-computer interface decoding parameters. *Conf. Proc. IEEE Eng. Med. Biol. Soc.* 2013, 7100–7103. doi: 10.1109/EMBC.2013.6611194

Zohary, E., Shadlen, M. N., and Newsome, W. T. (1994). Correlated neuronal discharge rate and its implications for psychophysical performance. *Nature* 370, 140–143. doi: 10.1038/370140a0

10

Adaptation to elastic loads and BMI robot controls during rat locomotion examined with point-process GLMs

Weiguo Song[1], *Iahn Cajigas*[2], *Emery N. Brown*[2,3,4] *and Simon F. Giszter*[1,5*]

[1] Department of Neurobiology and Anatomy, Drexel University College of Medicine, Drexel University, Philadelphia, PA, USA, [2] Brain and Cognitive Sciences, Massachusetts Institute of Technology, Cambridge, MA, USA, [3] Institute for Medical Engineering and Science, Massachusetts Institute of Technology, Cambridge, MA, USA, [4] Department of Anesthesia, Critical Care and Pain Medicine, Harvard Medical School, Massachusetts General Hospital, Boston, MA, USA, [5] School of Biomedical Engineering, Drexel University, Philadelphia, PA, USA

Edited by:
Mikhail Lebedev, Duke University, USA

Reviewed by:
Monzurul Alam, University of California, USA
Dean Robert Freestone, The University of Melbourne, Australia
Matthew D. Golub, Carnegie Mellon University, USA

***Correspondence:**
Simon F. Giszter, Department of Neurobiology and Anatomy, Drexel University College of Medicine, Drexel University, 2900 Queen Lane, Philadelphia, PA, USA
sgiszter@drexelmed.edu

Currently little is known about how a mechanically coupled BMI system's actions are integrated into ongoing body dynamics. We tested a locomotor task augmented with a BMI system driving a robot mechanically interacting with a rat under three conditions: control locomotion (BL), "simple elastic load" (E) and "BMI with elastic load" (BMI/E). The effect of the BMI was to allow compensation of the elastic load as a function of the neural drive. Neurons recorded here were close to one another in cortex, all within a 200 micron diameter horizontal distance of one another. The interactions of these close assemblies of neurons may differ from those among neurons at longer distances in BMI tasks and thus are important to explore. A point process generalized linear model (GLM), was used to examine connectivity at two different binning timescales (1 ms vs. 10 ms). We used GLM models to fit non-Poisson neural dynamics solely using other neurons' prior neural activity as covariates. Models at different timescales were compared based on Kolmogorov-Smirnov (KS) goodness-of-fit and parsimony. About 15% of cells with non-Poisson firing were well fitted with the neuron-to-neuron models alone. More such cells were fitted at the 1 ms binning than 10 ms. Positive connection parameters ("excitation" ~70%) exceeded negative parameters ("inhibition" ~30%). Significant connectivity changes in the GLM determined networks of well-fitted neurons occurred between the conditions. However, a common core of connections comprising at least ~15% of connections persisted between any two of the three conditions. Significantly almost twice as many connections were in common between the two load conditions (~27%), compared to between either load condition and the baseline. This local point process GLM identified neural correlation structure and the changes seen across task conditions in the rats in this neural subset may be intrinsic to cortex or due to feedback and input reorganization in adaptation.

Keywords: augmenting BMI, elastic field, point-process general linear model, exoskeleton robot model system, motor adaptation

Introduction

Brain Machine Interfaces (BMIs) hold the potential to provide functions to spinal-injured patients (Hochberg et al., 2006) or to augment normal motor functions in novel ways. The operation of BMIs depends on reliable neural decoding during ongoing behaviors and on a subject's adaptation of activity to achieve function across differing ongoing tasks. To date, most efforts in BMI have worked in mechanically isolated contexts and concentrated on highly-trained manipulation tasks of the forelimb (Chapin et al., 1999; Hochberg et al., 2006; Moritz et al., 2008; Velliste et al., 2008). They have largely neglected locomotion or its augmentation using invasive single unit methods, with notable exceptions (Fitzsimmons et al., 2009; Song et al., 2009; Manohar et al., 2012; Alam et al., 2014). Further, a future BMI application of lower limb control would likely require the user to manage on-line motor adaptations and integrate the lower limb BMI control with their whole body control.

The effect on neural modulation of BMI integration into the body scheme has not been thoroughly investigated. The stability of cortical neural responses remains controversial. Some data showed that cells can be functionally stable and BMI systems maintain performance across days with the same decoder (Serruya et al., 2003; Greenberg and Wilson, 2004; Chestek et al., 2007). However, significant neural plasticity was also reported in non-BMI force-field adaptation experiments and in BMI systems exposed to a given decoder across days (Li et al., 2001; Carmena et al., 2005; Jackson et al., 2006; Rokni et al., 2007; Zacksenhouse et al., 2007; Jarosiewicz et al., 2008; Ganguly and Carmena, 2009; Song and Giszter, 2011). Even when responses become fairly stable, and switching among BMI controls are achieved easily, for example after over-training, issues will remain in integrating and adapting the BMI controls to new tasks and mechanical contexts in activities of daily living. Conceivably, highly-trained BMI designs with complicated decoding algorithms may impede the use of the intrinsic plasticity of the brain to adapt and improve the BMI control in dynamic environments. Current efforts to develop adaptive decoders must balance their potential advantages against the potential for conflict with the user's own adaptation. An alternative strategy may be to provide simpler interfaces (Moritz et al., 2008), and allow the brain's plasticity and processing power to adapt and incorporate the novel actions.

Using a relatively simple interface strategy to generate a neural driven force from the robot, like Fetz and colleagues (Moritz et al., 2008), we examined the use of the BMI in this dynamic environment. Rats were exposed to three conditions during treadmill locomotion:(a) control, (b) simple elastic loading (E), and (c) BMI with elastic load (BMI/E) in which BMI lifting control was made available in parallel with the elastic load used in (b). Previously, we found that cells could modulate their firing patterns differently during each adaptation in different experimental conditions (Song and Giszter, 2011).

To understand the function of neuronal circuits and systems, it is essential to characterize the connections between individual neurons (Brown et al., 2004; Shigeyoshi, 2008; Stevenson and Körding, 2010) and their dynamics across tasks or condition changes. Correlations of cells relate to network connectivity and common inputs and processing. The cross-correlation, coherence and joint peri-stimulus time histogram (JPSTH) methods have been used for pairs of cells (Gerstein and Perkel, 1969; Jarvis and Mitra, 2001; Schneidman et al., 2006; Shigeyoshi, 2008). To characterize the strengths and any dynamics of the connections between neurons, variants of information based methods have been used in computational neuroscience for analyzing spiking neural systems (Strong et al., 1998). However, in many brain areas, each neuron receives input from a large population, and the generalized linear model (GLM) provides another framework to examine connectivity based on the point process representation of the spike trains (Brown et al., 2002; Truccolo et al., 2005; Acharya et al., 2008; Stevenson et al., 2008; Héliot et al., 2010). The GLM attempts to predict a neuron's firing patterns based on its own spikes and the spikes of other neurons, and on external inputs. By combining a KS statistical analysis for the goodness of fit in each model, it provides a powerful tool for neural network functional connectivity analysis (Brown et al., 2002; Truccolo et al., 2005; Acharya et al., 2008; Kositsky et al., 2009; Gerhard et al., 2011). By utilizing a point process framework and GLM, we examined the neural dynamics at the functional network level.

We examined "functional connectivity" which we here define as an analysis and estimation of how firing of each neuron appears to influence each other neuron in a given data set, given the data collected and included in the analysis, with such influences expressed in the most parsimonious way possible. This represents a compact description of firing pattern correlations and apparent influences on one another in the observed data. Because the neural activity is incompletely observed, it is necessarily limited in relation to anatomy and actual circuit structure. Results showed significant differences in network organization as estimated by the GLM analysis of functional connectivity under different conditions, with some fraction of "core connectivity" in the GLM models, and the observed firing pattern features, preserved across the trials.

Methods and Materials

Surgical Procedure and Neural Recording

Six adult Sprague-Dawley rats, weighing 250 $\sim$ 300 g, were used in these experiments. Care and treatment of the animals conformed to protocols approved by the University Laboratory Animal Resources and Institutional Animal Care and Use Committee of the College of Medicine of Drexel University. Methods are published in Song and Giszter (2011). The detailed procedures for pelvic and cortical implantations have also been described previously (Song and Giszter, 2011). For short, after anesthesia using KXA (63 mg/Kg Ketamine, 6 mg/Kg Xylazine, 0.05 mg/Kg Acepromazine), rats were implanted with a pelvic orthosis, which allowed a PHANTOM robot (Sensable Devices) to apply forces directly to the skeleton. Tetrode arrays, which consisted of 6 tetrodes positioned around the neck of an etched spear-shaped fine tungsten rod, were implanted stereotactically in the hindlimb / trunk area of the motor cortex (2.0 mm lateral of the midline, 1.6 mm caudal to bregma and 1.0–1.5 mm in depth). Recording sites of all electrodes in a rat were within from 50 to 200 microns of one another in the cortex using our probe design. Intracortical microstimulation of rat M1 in this recorded region generates hindlimb/trunk movements in all rats tested. At the end of the final recording session, strong electrolytic lesions were made and brain slices were cut in 40 μm sections to validate electrode placement. Neural data were recorded using a Cerebus system (Cyberkinetics, Inc. / Blackrock systems) after animals recovered from surgery. Neural signals were band-pass filtered (300–7.5 KHz) and digitized at a sampling frequency of 30 kHz. Spikes were detected online using thresholding. The detected spikes could be automatically classified on-line after setting the templates of each waveform. The on-line sorted spikes were used in a real time "BMI with elastic load" control. The controller and real-time OS code were custom laboratory written code (available on request). They implemented the algorithms in Equation (1) below, with the parameters noted there. The detected spike trains, as well as all the thresholded spike waveforms, were also saved for off-line analysis. Multiple single units were isolated off-line using Off-line Sorter (Plexon Neurotech Com.) after noise removal by cluster cutting method (Shoham et al., 2003). This analysis uses the offline sorted data. Up to 24 channels of neural activity at a time in a single array could be recorded, and 1 or 2 individual cells from most wires of the tetrodes could be recorded; around 15–38 well isolated single units were used in each trial.

Robot Controls and Training Protocols

The robotic system employed and the training protocol used have been described in detail previously (Song and Giszter, 2011). Briefly, different force fields (linear, non-linear, isotropic, anisotropic, piecewise discontinuities etc.) could be applied to the pelvis of the rat using our custom control software. This was achieved through an implanted orthosis, directly interacting with the skeleton using the orthosis attached robot. Robot control was updated at a frequency of 1 KHz, and these controls were synchronized and coupled with neural recordings. Neural data recorded could be used in the robot control scheme after a delay of under 3 ms from spike occurence. In elastic load trials (*abbrevation **E***), unidirectional (vertical forces only, i.e., radially anisotropic) elastic fields were used. Elastic loading (downward) fields F_e were applied in condition E by setting an equilibrium point on the horizontal equilibrium plane of the elastic field around 12.5 mm under the rat's normal pelvic height with a field stiffness of 44 N/m, which gives around 15% of the body weight. In trials termed here "BMI with elastic load" (abbrev. BMI/E), a neural driven lifting elastic force F_n was combined with the above simple elastic force F_e, and both forces were combined and applied simultaneously. The neural driven elastic force was calculated according to the equation

$$F_n = K_n \times N_{af} \times (X - X_{n0}), \tag{1}$$

where N_{af} was aggregate firing rate in the prior 100 ms window, $K_n = 80\ N/m$ was the stiffness, $X_{n0} = 55\,mm$ was the equilibrium point, and X the current vertical position of the pelvis with respect to the horizontal equilibrium plane. This gave the rat in BMI/E trials a means to offset the elastic load F_e using neural activity N_{af} to modulate an opposing force F_n. Experiments except where noted comprised one or more iterations of 3 conditions: 2 min of baseline (BL) with no loading, followed by 2 min of elastic load (E) in which the rat experienced F_e, and then 2 min of BMI + load (BMI/E) in which the rat had access to the BMI driven field F_n and could potentially offset F_e.

Rats were trained to walk on a treadmill at a speed ranging from 0.1 to 0.15 m/s depending on the normal preferred walking speed of individual rats. One daily experimental session used in analysis below was divided into three trials as described above: (i) the BL (baseline) trial, in which rats walked on treadmill without any force; (ii) the E (simple elastic load) trial; (iii) the BMI/E (BMI with elastic load) trial. Each session thus consisted of three 2-min trials of treadmill walking (~120 steps) with 5 min intervals of rest occurred between each trial.

Neural Network Functional Connectivity Analysis by Using GLM Model

We follow Stevenson et al. (2009) and Okatan et al. (2005) in defining functional connectivity: we seek to characterize how each neuron appears to influence each other neuron in the data sets in the most parsimonious way possible. The neural modulation of single cells that was observed during BMI usage and motor adaptation observed in our experimental paradigm was previously reported (Song and Giszter, 2011).

The procedure for functional connectivity analysis was as shown in **Figure 1**. Briefly, neural spiking activity is modeled as a point process which is completely characterized by its conditional intensity function (Daley and Vere-Jones, 2003) defined as

$$\lambda(t \mid H_t) = \lim_{\Delta \to 0} \frac{P(N(t+\Delta) - N(t) = 1 \mid H_t)}{\Delta} \tag{2}$$

where H_t is all the history information from 0 up to time t, and $N(t)$ is a counting process containing the sum of all the spikes up to time t. The conditional intensity function can be considered a generalization of the "rate" for a homogenous Poisson process. Under the restriction that $\lambda(t|H_t)\,\Delta$ follows a distribution in the exponential family, the GLM framework can be used to fit statistical models for the conditional intensity function (McCullagh and Nelder, 1989). Goodness of fit can be assessed by Kolmogorov-Smirnov test (KS-test) after the time rescaling theorem (Brown et al., 2002).

The conditional intensity function of the ith spiking neuron was modeled with the spiking history of neighbor cells either at a short timescale (1 ms, $L = 1$) or long timescale (10 ms, $L = 10$) as Equation (3),

$$\lambda_i(t_k \mid H_t) = \exp\left(\mu_i + \sum_{\substack{j=1 \\ j \neq i}}^{J} \beta_{ij} \cdot \Delta N_j(t_k)\right) \tag{3}$$

where J is the total number of neurons recorded in the current trial; μ_i is the baseline level of firing rate; $\Delta N_j(t_k) = N_j(t_k) - N_j(t_{k-L})$ is the number of spikes of the jth neuron between time t_{k-L} and t_k, $L = 1$ or 10 for the short and long timescale model respectively, and β_{ij} is the regression coefficient to be estimated representing the strength of effect between the firing of the jth

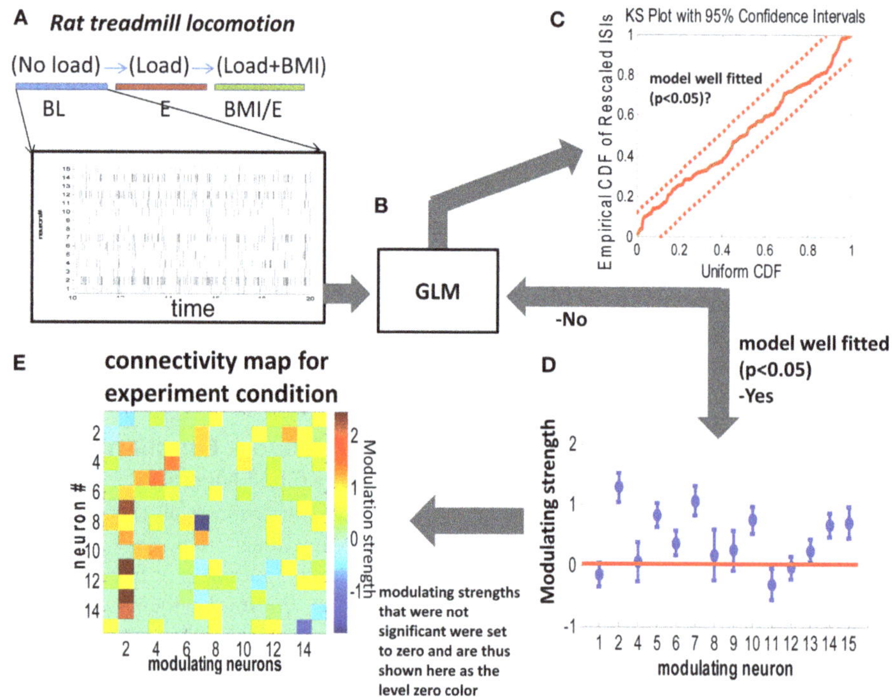

FIGURE 1 | Generalized linear model (GLM) based network connectivity analysis. (A,B) The conditional intensity function of each neuron was modeled with GLM by using a single step spiking history of the whole population of neurons over two different timescales (1 ms vs. 10 ms). **(C)** A Kolmogorov Smirnov (KS) criteria was used to test the goodness of fit of the model. According to the time rescaling theorem for point processes, the rescaled spike times under the true conditional intensity function would be independent, identically distributed, exponential random variables with unit rate. **(D)** For neurons which showed a significant nonzero contribution in the GLM model, the nonzero modeling strength was used to construct an element in the connectivity matrix (map) in **(E)**. Parameters whose confidence interval crossed zero (the horizontal red line) in **(D)** were deemed not significantly different from zero and were set to zero in the connectivity maps in **(E)**.

neuron in the short or long timescale and the current firing rate of the *i*th neuron. We term the β_{ij} as the functional connectivity coefficient of neuron *j* to neuron *i*. Note that with this definition, $\beta_{ij} \neq \beta_{ji}$ in general and both that both short and long timescale models have the same number of parameters. We define the functional connectivity map, $\boldsymbol{\beta}$, as the matrix containing β_{ij} in the *i*th row and *j*th column. The structure of $\boldsymbol{\beta}$ is one measure of the connections between neurons or a representation of the functional network between the neurons.

The activity of each neuron was modeled by its neighboring neurons' immediately preceding history within a 10 ms window (type A in Equation 3) and in a small number of test models by its own history (type B, self-history included - i.e., remove the $j \neq i$ constraint in Equation 3). The Type B model (with neural self history) was evaluated in 2 rats. Models with the self history inclusion on the timescales tested here differed little in their network neighbor interactions. They showed significant overlap of network connections with the similar networks identified and estimated without self history. However, they generally showed some reduction of external network connections (22% in BL, 11% in E, and 15% in BMI, when using 1 ms time bins) with increasing history parameters but also a decreasing quality metric (see below). Here we present data from the network models without self-history, consistent with our quality metric used (see below).

Statistical Methods

After GLM fitting (glmfit, MATLAB) for each neuron, a Kolmogorov-Smirnov (KS) test was applied to test the goodness of fitting. If the fitting was within the 95% confidence interval, we classified the neuron as well fitted. Then, the significant parameters that were nonzero ($p < 0.05$) were used to construct the functional connectivity map as in **Figure 1**.

In order to test the functional connectivity map changes between two conditions, and their significance, the functional connectivity map identified and estimated in each was converted to a binary functional connectivity matrix by setting the *significant* nonzero elements to one and the others to zero as in **Figure 4**. Connection density was defined as the percentage of significant connected links, in relation to the total possible links and used as a criterion for analysis and comparison of model structures and conditions. In a first pass analysis we modeled all recorded neurons as stationary Poisson processes to test for non-Poisson behavior. In a second pass analysis (type II models), we modeled those neurons whose firing was not fitted by a mean rate parameter, and thus non-Poisson by our test criterion used for model fit assessment (time rescaling theorem/Kolmogorov Smirnov tests with $p < 0.05$). Such cells could not be well-predicted simply by using a mean rate parameter (type I model) and were thus firing based on locomotion variables or one another. The number of such non-Poisson cells found differed in the data sets, varying based on binning. We found such "non-Poisson patterned" cells using both 1 ms and 10 ms binning. In total 573 neurons were analyzed. Cell numbers that were non-Poisson were as follows: 1 ms binning: 287 (BL), 328 (E), 303(BMI/E); 10 ms: 348 (BL), 368 (E), 361 (BMI/E). The first pass analysis was equivalent to an assumption of the possible presence of neither locomotion task information nor neural interaction information in the cell firing. Cells not fitted in this way would need a more complex fitting, which could further improve conditional intensity function fit and KS statistic if modeled correctly, using neural or locomotion variable effects. The second pass analysis we used examined neural interactions alone. Effectively, we assumed that the first pass Poisson fitted cells were unrelated to the motor tasks, and were simply noise sources in the cortical network, though potentially important predictors of other neural firing. We ignored the external covariate effects, focusing on neural correlation alone. We compared GLM model structures to capture the non-Poisson population of neurons at a short timescale using 1 ms binning and at a longer timescale using 10 ms binning based on the parsimonious selection of GLM fitting. We sought models that captured the most neurons with the best levels of individual neuron parameter parsimony. To assess this model quality we calculated a model parameter Q,

$$Q = n/N \tag{4}$$

where n is the percentage of neurons with non-Poisson firing that were well fitted using the model, N is the square root of the significant connection density (number of possible connections growing as the square of neurons recorded). High Q values indicate good parsimonious fitting of the (non-Poisson) activity in the network, and the sparsest possible connectivity description of firing. If two models had the same numbers of well-predicted neurons total in a data set but one fitting had higher Q (i.e., fewer connections/ parameters required) it was considered a better model form. If two models fitted different numbers of neurons in a data set, but the model fitting of larger number of neurons had a much lower Q this would indicate a more complex individual neural functional connectivity was necessary in the model to capture the greater number of neurons and achieve fitting. When the activity of each neuron was modeled from its neighboring simultaneous firing neurons, but not using self history and recursive self connections, the overall parsimony and Q value obtained was significantly lower, so we only present data using the history effects of neighbor neurons not self history (Equation 3).

From the binary functional connectivity matrix of significant parameters found using models with the best Q, we could then test the significance of functional connectivity maps changes. We did by using a binomial distribution test. That is, by assuming the probability of keeping or changing the original link had the same chance, then if the probability of the pattern of change observed was less than 0.05, then a significant change had occurred. In practice this statistical test was likely unnecessary, since we found that only about 15–27% of model connections persisted across different conditions in an animal. Nonparametric signed rank tests (signrank, MATLAB) were used to compare the significance of such individual changes and differences across sessions and rats. All the tests were set to a significance level of 0.05. All data analysis was performed using custom software written in MATLAB. A suite of refined and related MATLAB tools including these is freely available (Cajigas et al., 2012).

Results

In total 21 robot and BMI interaction sessions were collected in 6 normal rats that were implanted with multi-electrode recording probes. Rats performed treadmill locomotion in three conditions: (1) unloaded baseline (BL), (2) a robot driven elastic load condition (E) in which rats experienced a vertical elastic load, and (3) a robot driven elastic load and BMI condition (BMI/E), see **Figure 1A**. In the last condition the rat could in principle offset elastic load using neural activity. In BMI/E the recorded neural activity of the rat regulated the stiffness of a second "BMI elastic field." This could potentially be employed to offset the elastic load, as was described in Song and Giszter (2011). We have reported previously that rats do quite quickly begin to adjust and to offset the load (Song and Giszter, 2011). We sought to assess changes in functional connectivity as rats proceeded from BL to E to BMI/E conditions. In order to do this we compared functional connections in GLM fitted networks for the data (**Figures 1A–E**) in each successive test condition. We thus separately fitted each condition. 21 fitted networks were here obtained and compared for each condition (BL, E, and BMI/E) using GLM models. We tested fits of the GLM models at two different binning timescales: 1 ms and 10 ms. In total 573 neurons were analyzed in the 21 sessions. Cell numbers that were non-Poisson and supported network connection modeling were as follows: 1 ms binning: 287 (BL), 328 (E), 303 (BMI/E); 10 ms: 348 (BL), 368 (E), 361 (BMI/E). In addition to these sessions, in control experiments we tested repetitions of the baseline, and repetitions of the full sequence of tests in a rat, to assess the connection and network drift (gradual network functional connection changes within a condition), relative to the measures of change we saw between conditions.

Network Fitting Procedures and Network Characteristics

We first modeled each neuron in each task condition (BL, E, and BMI/E) by using a 1 step spiking history of the ensemble neurons using either short timescale (1 ms bin) or longer timescale (10 ms bin) steps. Type I models ignored interactions, simply fitting cells independently as point processes to discover non-Poisson pattern cells. Type II models used cell interactions. We found that about 60% of recorded cells were well fitted at the short timescale. However, the number of well-predicted non-Poisson firing cells was not high. About 15% of such non-Poisson pattern cells were well-predicted using the short timescale. Significantly less cells were well-predicted in the long timescale, matching the total cell fitting patterns. The numbers of total and non-Poisson firing pattern cells that were well fitted at each timescale were not significantly different between the three different adaptation conditions. We used a measure Q of fitting complexity to compare the models and binnings (see Methods). The numbers of cells that were well-predicted and the Q statistic in both the shorter timescale (1 ms) and longer timescale (10 ms) analyses are

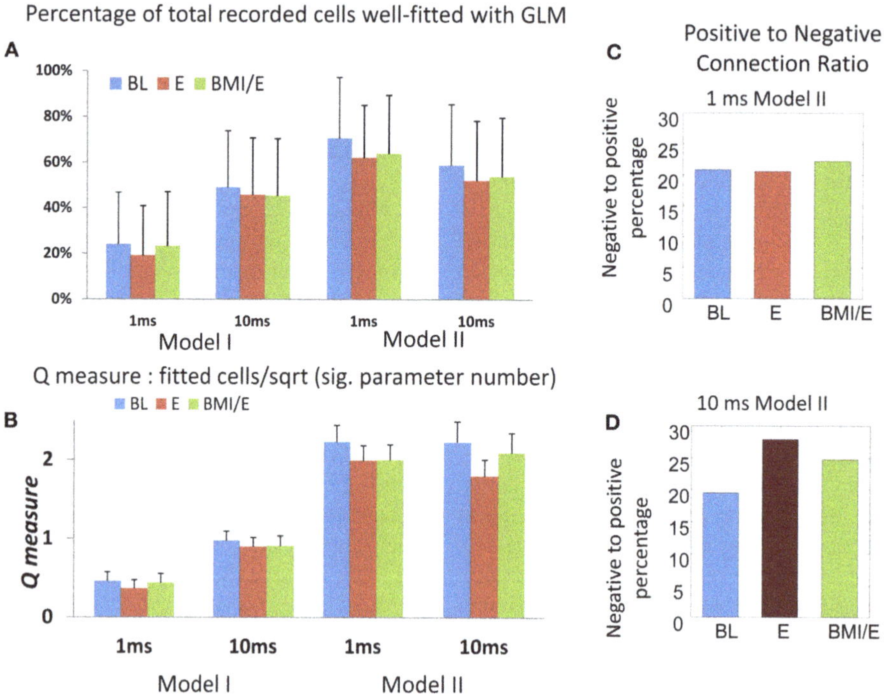

FIGURE 2 | Numbers of cells fitted with GLM model and Q-measure. **(A)** Percentage of total cells from the whole population ($n = 573$) fitted in each model and adaptation condition. The model II with 1 ms timescale had the highest capture of cells and best Q (indicated with the red dotted box). Note that despite good overall fits, only about 15% of neurons with firing interval statistics not captured by a mean rate parameter (non-Poisson firing) were well-predicted in the GLM networks here. More total and non-Poisson cells were fitted in the E condition than in the other two conditions (BL or BMI/E) at both short timescale (1 ms binning) and long timescale (10 ms binning). **(B)** The Q-measure. This was defined as the ratio of the percentage of neurons with non-Poisson firing that were well-predicted using the model, to the square root of the significant connection density required. Coupled with **(A)** the Q-measure analysis favors the type II models at the 1 ms binning scale. The error bars indicates mean ± S.E. **(C)** The percentage of significant negative parameters as a portion of significant positive modulation parameters in the 1 ms bin model II is shown in each task condition. **(D)** The percentage of significant negative parameters as a portion of significant positive modulation parameters in the 10 ms bin model II is shown in each task condition. The number of significant negative interactions was lower than positive ones in each network, while there was no significant difference between the different adaptation conditions for each model. Overall, in the 10 ms binned model II fits, the number of negatively modulating interactions increased. Abbrev. BL baseline, E elastic load, BMI/E brain machine interface and elastic load.

shown in **Figure 2**. The 10 ms binned fits were almost as good as the 1 ms model fits. Although a simple 1 step history linear filter is presented here, we also tested type I and type II models with basis function filters similar to Truccolo (Truccolo et al., 2010), and tested models with a 10 ms (five basis function) history in two rats. There was no significant improvement in the number of cells which could be well-predicted using KS-criteria, when compared to using the 1 ms binning used here. Thus, we kept the 1 step history window in our subsequent modeling. We present the analyses only for the simpler 1 ms bin and 10 ms history type II model. In the 1 ms bin short timescale, the GLM models captured the binary spike train behaviors, where temporal coding might feature, while the 10 ms bin long timescale GLM model corresponds more to rate coding. More cells could be well fitted using the short timescale models than with the long timescale models. This suggests that with 1 ms binning, the individual cells predicted (or "influenced") the short term information of the neighboring cells better (more) than was seen on the long timescale. Thus, the better-fitted functional connectivity network structures examined here using 1 ms binning likely represent short timescale processes.

We also examined the fitted networks' significant parameters to see if numbers of excitatory or inhibitory types of connections were dominant, and the average strengths of each type of connection. In each network, we found that the number of significant negative interactions ("inhibition") was lower than the number of positive ones ("excitation") constituting about on fifth on average (**Figures 2C,D**). When we compared these connection numbers for the models between experimental conditions, we found that there was no significant difference in the positive/negative parameter balances in models among the different task conditions. However, the number of negatively modulating interactions in the models using 10 ms binning and timescale were increased overall compared to 1 ms binning and timescale (**Figures 2C,D**).

Network Stability in Continuously Repeated Trials of a Condition, and Repetitions of Conditions after Delays and Condition Switches

In control trials, we found that in successive repetitions of the baseline conditions, the fitted networks showed some connection variability but that overall more than 30% of connections were preserved over the entire series of repetitions, and around 40% or more similarity was found between tests of networks adjacent in time (**Figure 3A**). Similarly, we found that networks fitted to repetitions of each condition after other interleaved conditions showed more connection similarity with each other (**Figure 3B**) than with the networks fitted to different conditions that were adjacent in time, and this difference was significant under an assumption of random variations (e.g., for data in **Figure 3B**, one-tailed t-test $p < 0.05$).

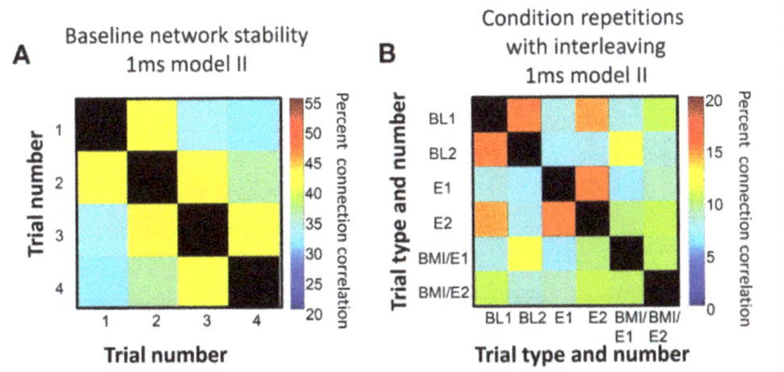

FIGURE 3 | Connection persistence within condition. (A) Repeated baseline recordings with 5 min pauses between them showed more than 30% of connections were preserved from the first to last recording. However, over the repetitions there was a slow drift in connection pattern. The matrix of percentage of common connections, and the color map scale are shown. On the diagonal, the black squares indicate 100% correlation (self to self). **(B)** Repetitions of the basic experiment used, with successive trials of BL, E, BMI/E in a rat. The matrix of common connection percentages is organized with BL1 and BL2 grouped, E1 and E2 grouped, and BMI/E1 and BMI/E2 grouped but these were separated in time in the experiment. The repetitions of each condition are generally more similar to one another than to other conditions. The level of within condition similarity is not consistent with random assortment of the matrix elements and their variance. On the diagonal, the black squares indicate 100% correlation (self to self). Note also that the color scale range in **A** and **B** differ.

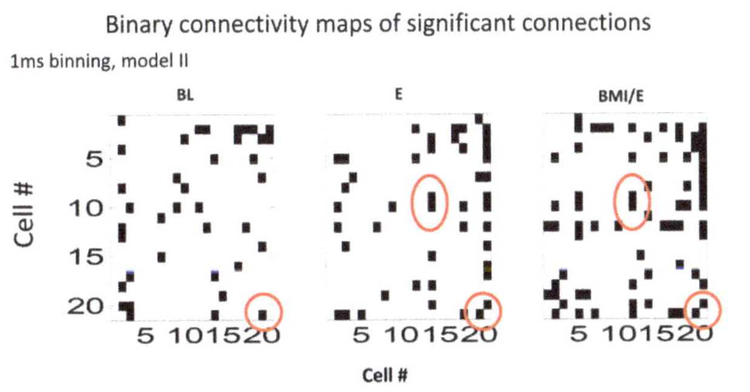

FIGURE 4 | Binary connectivity maps from the GLM fits in a typical session (from the same session as is shown in Figure 5). Significant connections are shown in black. The networks showed sparse connectivity. The connection density was higher for the 1 ms bin time scale that is shown (1 ms binning). Examples of a few connections found in common in the GLM fits in each condition, are circled in red. These show consistency in modeling of some connections across all the conditions. Abbrevations: BL, baseline; E, elastic load; BMI/E, brain machine interface and elastic load.

Network Changes across Different Adaptation Conditions

We next analyzed the model connectivity changes occuring between the three adaptation conditions when they followed in close succession in a complete experiment series. Our rationale was that although the numbers of cells, which could be well-predicted by either type I or type II GLM models were not significantly different among each adaptation task condition, the network structure might change or reorganize in these different contexts. Thus, we looked in detail at how the fitted network statistics changed in the transitions between the different task conditions, compared across conditions, and at the different binning timescales. Both the binary connection maps (**Figure 4**) and the functional connectivity strengths (**Figures 5, 6**) showed significant differences at the two different model timescales (1 ms, and 10 ms). These also differed among the three adaptation conditions tested (BL, E, and BMI/E). Some fraction of the connections persisted across different task conditions (**Figure 4**, circled examples). Connections that persisted in common between the three adaptation conditions remained correlated in strengths (**Figure 5** red points in each plot), however other patterns of functional connectivity often changed significantly. The binary functional connectivity maps showed distinct patterns depending on timescales analyzed, as seen in **Figure 4**. Generally, we found that in the longer 10 ms binned data most connections were unique and many fewer were shared with the other adaptation conditions (not shown). We therefore focused accordingly on the short time scale 1 ms binned models (1 ms Type II Models) see **Figures 4, 5**. We showed previously

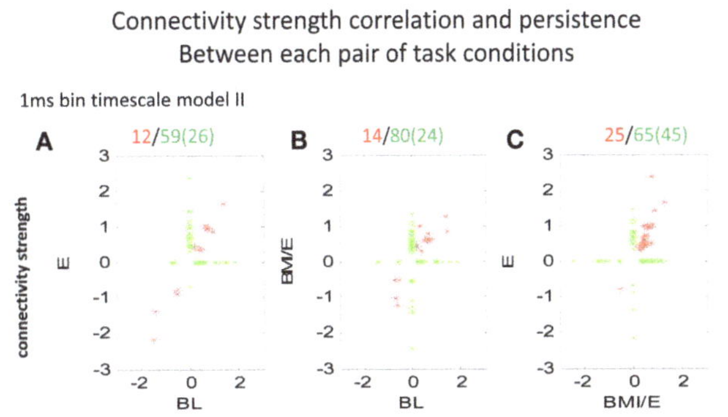

FIGURE 5 | Comparison of connectivity strengths between two conditions modeled at the 1 ms binned timescale. Each point marker in the figure denotes a significant parameter and connectivity strength from a pair of neurons, related between two conditions (**A** BL vs. E, **B** BL vs. BMI/E, and **C** E vs. BMI/E). The red markers denote that the connection between the neurons was significantly different from zero under both the two tested conditions, while the green marker denotes the connectivity of the neurons was only significantly different from zero under one condition (BL, E or BMI/E). The numbers in parentheses indicate number of cells on abscissa. Some of the network connectivity estimated with the GLM models shifted drastically, and much connectivity was unique to a given condition. However, there were also connections that persisted across conditions (red). These persistent connection strengths clearly also correlated. There were more connections in common between E and BMI/E in **C**, than in either **A** or in **B** when these were correlated to BL. Abbrevations: BL, baseline; E, elastic load; BMI/E, brain machine interface and elastic load.

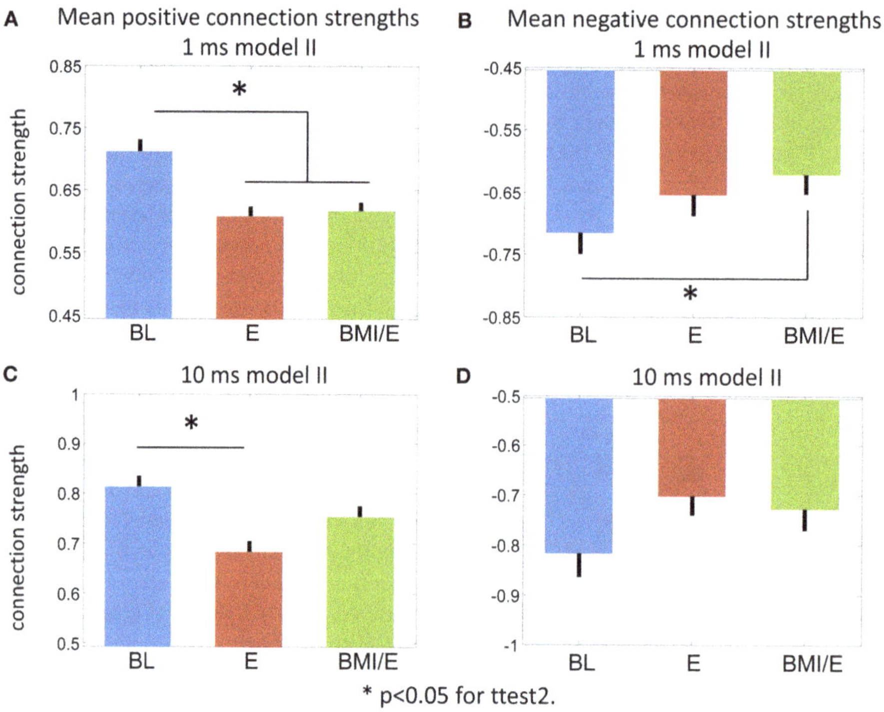

FIGURE 6 | Connection strength changes. (A,B) Model II 1 ms bin fitting. **(A)** Positive connections. **(B)** Negative connections. **(C,D)** Model II 10 ms bin fitting. **(C)** Positive connections. **(D)** Negative connections. * Significant difference in a two-tailed *t*-test, $p < 0.05$ (MATLAB ttest2).

that rats in BMI/E offset load while preserving more normal pelvic height compared to load alone (Song and Giszter, 2011). When rats experiencing applied loads in BMI/E were able to significantly offset these with the BMI, the network increased the number of connections during simple elastic load and BMI with elastic load conditions compared to baseline (e.g., see **Figures 4**, **5**). Further, significantly more of (almost double the number of) the connections persisted in the transition from Elastic load (E) to BMI (BMI/E) (~27% in **Figure 5C**) compared to those that seen were in common between Baseline and Elastic load (~16% in **Figure 5A**) or Baseline and BMI (~15% in **Figure 5B**). This statistically significant difference in common or shared functional connectivity was biased to positive connections between the two load conditions (**Figure 5C**, one red negative connection in common out of 25 total common), but instead included higher fractions of negative parameter connections when examining connections that were in common with baseline patterns of firing (**Figure 5A**, 4/12 negative, and **Figure 5B**, 4/14).

While the numbers of significant connections increased in the E and BMI/E conditions, the mean parameter strengths also altered. **Figure 6** shows the average positive and negative connection strengths tended in 1 ms and 10 ms models. In keeping with the other results the 10 ms binning results had weaker significance, only differing in positive connection strength between BL and BMI/E. In the 1 ms models, all connection strengths tended to decrease in the loading conditions compared to baseline. These changes were significant for the positive connections in both load conditions in the 1 ms models, and for negative connections compared to BMI/E.

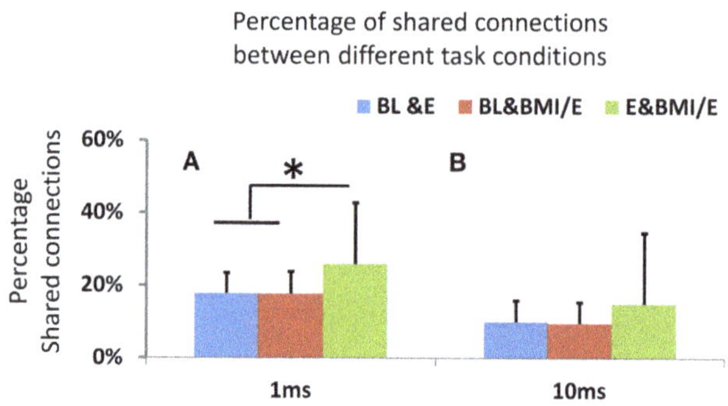

FIGURE 7 | (A) Shared connections between networks obtained in two conditions. On either 1 ms or 10 ms binned timescales, the networks showed significant differences in connectivity between two conditions (BL vs. E, BL vs. BMI/E and E vs. BMI/E) using binomial tests. However, with 1 ms binning there was a significantly higher percentage of shared connection between E and BMI/E than that between any other two conditions (BL vs. E and BL vs. BMI/E, indicated by *, two-tailed *t*-test, $p < 0.05$, MATLAB ttest2). **(B)** For the 10 ms binning there was no significant difference in the percentage of shared connection between any paired conditions, and percentages of shared connections were significantly lower than in the 1 ms binned GLM models.

By using functional connection density measures and the shared significant parameters as functional connectivity links or edges in a network graph, we compared the network structure changes. We found the number of common connections was significantly decreased in 10 ms timescale binned models compared to 1 ms binned (signed rank test, $p < 0.05$, MATLAB signrank), as in **Figure 7**. These differences held across baseline condition and elastic load condition as well as BMI with elastic load. All the networks built from the GLM models showed low numbers of shared connections (15–27%) and significant differences (assessed by signed rank tests, $p < 0.05$) between any two conditions. However, there were significantly higher percentages of shared connections between the two load adaptation conditions of E and BMI/E than between either of the load with baseline condition shared connections (BL vs. E and BL vs. BMI/E) (**Figure 7A**). The percentage of shared connections between any two compared conditions was also higher in 1 ms binning than in 10 ms binning **Figure 7B**. These differences among conditions could not be explained by drift over time in BL e.g., in **Figure 3A**. This suggests that the active cortical circuitry may in part share a similar common structure when rats adapt under simple elastic load and under BMI with elastic load, and may also indicate that apart from rate encoding (analyzing in long timescale), short term temporal coding (binary spike timing) might capture some information regarding these changes on a short timescale.

In conclusion, the fitted GLM model networks of cells here showed significantly different connection maps between each task condition potentially indicating significant changes in network dynamics with task conditions. A core of between 15 and 27% of network connections were in common between the individual conditions and over time, but this common core differed in extent between different task condition pairs, with baseline having less in common with the other two (loaded) conditions.

Discussion

Using the methods here we previously demonstrated that rats could adapt their locomotion under a simple elastic load and use a BMI to offset elastic load effectively (Song and Giszter, 2011). GLM methods allow us to move beyond our prior analyses of coarse firing rate in this paradigm, and to add point process assessments of functional connectivity. The differences in BMI adaptation compared to the simple load in this paradigm involve alterations in firing patterns and rate based correlation relationships among neurons, but not average firing rates compared with elastic loading (Song and Giszter, 2011). We previously also observed changes in the number of force-related neurons, their peak firing and burst activity timing in the step cycle (Song and Giszter, 2011). Here we focus on neuron-neuron interactions at the point process level among neurons all collected within a range of from 30 to 200 microns of each other in each rats, with the recording electrode sites around layer V of motor cortex. These spatially close neurons may potentially have different connectivity from spatially further separated neurons. As we have noted above the functional connectivity we uncovered here represents the most parsimonious account of apparent neural influences among one another based on the observed neurons and firing. Because not all neurons are observed the account is necessarily incomplete and may infer Granger type causal links where none exist in the complete biology. However, subject to these limitations the functional connectivity may give descriptive insights into aspects of network operation. By using a GLM approach here, our data analysis has shown some features of cortical network dynamics occuring at different timescales during these adaptation processes. The neural network in hindlimb/trunk cortex of rats as assessed here in a subset of well-predicted neurons was extensively reorganized in terms of GLM parameters during adaptation to different elastic load force fields applied in locomotion. The networks shared more common connections between elastic load and BMI with elastic load condition than between any other condition pairs. More of the functional network connections identified were preserved during transitions from elastic load (E) to BMI with elastic load (BMI/E) conditions, than from baseline (BL) to elastic load (E). However, only about 15% of the total population of non-Poisson firing cells were well-predicted by our models here, which were built without reference to the external covariates, and relied only on strong neural firing pattern interactions. Internal network functional connectivity and the network based firing predictions that are presented here thus represent an account of a small fraction of the patterned activity. The models thus also indicate a high degree of independence of much of the non-Poisson pattern firing cells from one another from the GLM modeling perspective, consistent with classical rate coding models and other frameworks (e.g., Sanger, 2010, 2011, 2014). Likely the strongest predictive relationships of the firing of the 85% of unfitted non-Poisson cells will be with external covariates and tuning to feedback or motor drive. Nonetheless, the internal relationships revealed here in well-predicted cells provide some insights into the adaptation processes and dynamics in augmenting BMIs (see Omar et al., 2011). Unfortunately, low firing rates for the GLM point process models preclude a confident analysis of the activity changes within a condition as was possible with other methods in Song and Giszter (2011). The relations of the local activity relations here to overall function of the network remain to be determined.

It should be noted that caution should be taken when interpreting the results from model dynamics and differences here. As noted, the model did not consider external covariates, which might have made a strong contribution to the models. This was especially likely during elastic load conditions, and some if not most of the non-Poisson firing pattern cells that were not well fitted with neural interactions alone can be expected to be captured with inclusion of these. Whether and how the sparse connections identified here are correlated with the overall network states across tasks still needed to be tested. On the other hand, as the model here used spiking history of the ensemble of recorded cells, any effects of the potential external covariates on the well-predicted subset of cells analyzed here might be captured by its being filtered and incorporated into the history effects of connected neighboring neurons in the ensemble. The lagged parameters of GLM models of cells here generally had a more significant effect on a current cells' firing than any immediate (1 ms) synchronization to other firing cells consistent with causal interactions but no proof of such. Similiarly, it should be made clear that the connections or functional connectivity maps constructed here were derived only from "apparent pattern" among neural spikes. There might be no anatomical connectivity representing the apparent connections in the cortical network.

The differences between open loop BMIs, BMIs with feedback, physically connected BMIs and differences between BMIs for proximal locomotion vs. distal reaching are not well understood (Acharya et al., 2008; Héliot et al., 2010). However, these different effects may become crucial as various feedback based BMIs are introduced and the range and scope of available BMI prosthetic devices increases (Moritz et al., 2008; Velliste et al., 2008; Fitzsimmons et al., 2009; Héliot et al., 2010; Song and Giszter, 2011). Recent studies showed that cells in the primary motor cortex demonstrated learning related plasticity during force field adaptation (Li et al., 2001). A stable relation between neural activity and behavior can clearly be established in well trained animals (Serruya et al., 2003; Greenberg and Wilson, 2004; Chestek et al., 2007). Moritz et al. demonstrated that individual cells can be rate modulated to control Functional Electrical Stimulation (Moritz et al., 2008). Variations of neural firing patterns in such differing adaptation processes are not well understood at this point. For example, patterns might differ between novel voluntary tasks and more vegetative "built-in" or evolutionarily older tasks, such as locomotion. The rats adapted to load (E) and adapted differently to load with BMI (BMI/E). The identified *functional* cortical network parameters, as identified from firing observed here, also clearly adapted, and reorganized differently between conditions. Previously we found the distribution of average firing rate from the whole population was not significantly different among conditions (Song and Giszter, 2011). The numbers of significantly connected cells here were not significantly different across conditions in these models either. However, the numbers of common connections over time were higher in BMI with elastic load than baseline, and the network connection density even decreased during elastic loading alone when the rat adapted from the first half trial to the second half trial. Zacksenhouse et al. showed that there are firing rate changes in the early sessions with other BMI experiments (Zacksenhouse et al., 2007), and we found here that 70–85% of the sparse network connections of well-predicted cells reorganized depending on the context. For elastic load locomotion, the connection density actually decreased here, while in the BMI with elastic load locomotion condition, the network as modeled kept the same connection density. Similar results were obtained examining more standard long timescale correlations of rate in our earlier study (Song and Giszter, 2011). These data might indicate that rats need a longer time to achieve a stable and perhaps more sparse network state during BMI/E adaptation and conditioning when they were tested in our experimental framework, compared to the simpler elastic loaded locomotion. This evolving relationship between cortical firing effects, network changes, and feedback and relationships with external covariates is an area of active investigation using this framework.

When animals adapt their locomotion to new environments, initially cortex becomes more activated and engaged. Engaging a BMI in this period appears to alter and at least briefly stabilize the changes involved in the adaptation of neural network structure. Despite the small role of cortex in the normal locomotion of rats, cortex can be engaged in a BMI augmenting locomotion during this adaptation. Our data thus supports the idea that activity normally involved in monitoring, or simply correlated with and not normally driving a behavior in an animal, can nonetheless be engaged through motor adaptation processes to drive behavior in a BMI. Neuron-neuron correlation metrics estimated here provide one set of measures on the changes in neural dynamics on short adaptation time scales that can be extended to high practice use of BMIs and load adaptation over time, to examine transitions from naive user of an augmenting BMI to an expert practiced user. Understanding the patterns of these adaptive changes better may be essential in order to provide prostheses that can integrate seamlessly with normal motor adaptations and feedback effects across the many contexts encountered in activities of daily living.

Acknowledgments

This work was supported by NIH NS54894 to SG, NIH 1F31NS058275-01A2 to IC, NIH DP1 OD003646 to EB and R01 GM104948 to EB.

References

Acharya, S., Tenore, F., Aggarwal, V., Etienne-Cummings, R., Schieber, M. H., and Thakor, N. V. (2008). Decoding individuated finger movements using volume-constrained neuronal ensembles in the M1 hand area. *IEEE Trans. Neural Syst. Rehabil. Eng.* 16, 15–23. doi: 10.1109/TNSRE.2007.916269

Alam, M., Chen, X., Zhang, Z., Li, Y., and He, J. (2014). A brain-machine-muscle interface for restoring hindlimb locomotion after complete spinal transection in rats. *PLoS ONE* 9:e103764. doi: 10.1371/journal.pone.0103764

Brown, E. N., Barbieri, R., Ventura, V., Kass, R. E., and Frank, L. M. (2002). The time-rescaling theorem and its application to neural spike train data analysis. *Neural Comput.* 14, 325–346. doi: 10.1162/08997660252741149

Brown, E. N., Kass, R. E., and Mitra, P. P. (2004). Multiple neural spike train data analysis: state-of-the-art and future challenges. *Nat. Neurosci.* 7, 456–461. doi: 10.1038/nn1228

Cajigas, I., Malik, W. Q., and Brown, E. N. (2012). nSTAT: open-source neural spike train analysis toolbox for Matlab. *J. Neurosci. Methods* 211, 245–264. doi: 10.1016/j.jneumeth.2012.08.009

Carmena, J. M., Lebedev, M. A., Henriquez, C. S., and Nicolelis, M. A. L. (2005). Stable ensemble performance with single-neuron variability during reaching movements in primates. *J. Neurosci.* 25, 10172–10176. doi: 10.1523/JNEUROSCI.2772-05.2005

Chapin, J. K., Markowitz, R. A., Moxon, K. A., and Nicolelis, M. A. L. (1999). Direct real-time control of a robot arm using signals derived from neuronal population recordings in motor cortex. *Nat. Neurosci.* 2, 664–670. doi: 10.1038/10223

Chestek, C. A., Batista, A. P., Santhanam, G., Yu, B. M., Afshar, A., Cunningham, J. P., et al. (2007). Single-neuron stability during repeated reaching in macaque premotor cortex. *J. Neurosci.* 27, 10742–10750. doi: 10.1523/JNEUROSCI.0959-07.2007

Daley, D., and Vere-Jones, D. (2003). *An Introduction to the Theory of Point Processes.* New York, NY: Springer-Verlag.

Fitzsimmons, N. A., Lebedev, M. A., Peikon, I. D., and Nicolelis, M. A. L. (2009). Extracting kinematic parameters for monkey bipedal walking from cortical neuronal ensemble activity. *Front. Integr. Neurosci.* 3, 1–19. doi: 10.3389/neuro.07.003.2009

Ganguly, K., and Carmena, J. M. (2009). Emergence of a stable cortical map for neuroprosthetic control. *PLoS Biol.* 7:e1000153. doi: 10.1371/journal.pbio.1000153

Gerhard, F., Pipa, G., Lima, B., Neuenschwander, S., and Gerstner, W. (2011). Extraction of network topology from multi-electrode recordings: is there a small-world effect? *Front. Comput. Neurosci.* 5:4. doi: 10.3389/fncom.2011.00004

Gerstein, G. L., and Perkel, D. H. (1969). Simultaneously recorded trains of action potentials: analysis and functional interpretation. *Science* 164, 828–830. doi: 10.1126/science.164.3881.828

Greenberg, P. A., and Wilson, F. A. W. (2004). Functional stability of dorsolateral prefrontal neurons. *J. Neurophysiol.* 92, 1042–1055. doi: 10.1152/jn.00062.2004

Héliot, R., Ganguly, K., Jimenez, J., and Carmena, J. M. (2010). Learning in closed-loop brain-machine interfaces: modeling and experimental validation. *IEEE Trans. Syst. Man Cybern. B Cybern.* 99, 1–11. doi: 10.1109/TSMCB.2009.2036931

Hochberg, L. R., Serruya, M. D., Friehs, G. M., Mukand, J. A., Saleh, M., Caplan, A. H., et al. (2006). Neuronal ensemble control of prosthetic devices by a human with tetraplegia. *Nature* 442, 164–171. doi: 10.1038/nature04970

Jackson, A., Mavoori, J., and Fetz, E. E. (2006). Long-term motor cortex plasticity induced by an electronic neural implant. *Nature* 444, 56–60. doi: 10.1038/nature05226

Jarosiewicz, B., Chase, S. M., Fraser, G. W., Velliste, M., Kass, R. E., and Schwartz, A. B. (2008). Functional network reorganization during learning in a brain-computer interface paradigm. *Proc. Natl. Acad. Sci. U.S.A.* 105, 19486–19491. doi: 10.1073/pnas.0808113105

Jarvis, M. R., and Mitra, P. P. (2001). Sampling properties of the spectrum and coherency in sequences of action potentials. *Neural Comput.* 13, 717–749. doi: 10.1162/089976601300014312

Kositsky, M., Chiappalone, M., Alford, S. T., and Mussa-Ivaldi, F. A. (2009). Brain-machine interactions for assessing the dynamics of neural systems. *Front. Neurorobot.* 3:1. doi: 10.3389/neuro.12.001.2009

Li, C. S., Padoa-Schioppa, C., and Bizzi, E. (2001). Neuronal correlates of motor performance and motor learning in the primary motor cortex of monkeys adapting to an external force field. *Neuron* 30, 594–607. doi: 10.1016/S0896-6273(01)00301-4

Manohar, A., Flint, R. D., Knudsen, E., and Moxon, K. A. (2012). Decoding hindlimb movement for a brain machine interface after a complete spinal transection. *PLoS ONE* 7:e52173. doi: 10.1371/journal.pone.0052173

McCullagh, P., and Nelder, J. (1989). *Generalized Linear Models, 2nd Edn.* Boca Raton, FL: Chapman and Hall/CRC. doi: 10.1007/978-1-4899-3242-6

Moritz, C. T., Perlmutter, S. I., and Fetz, E. E. (2008). Direct control of paralyzed muscles by cortical neurons. *Nature* 456, 639–642. doi: 10.1038/nature07418

Okatan, M., Wilson, M. A., and Brown, E. N. (2005). Analyzing functional connectivity using a network likelihood model of ensemble neural spiking activity. *Neural Comput.* 17, 1927–1961. doi: 10.1162/0899766054322973

Omar, C., Akce, A., Johnson, M., Bretl, T., Ma, R., Maclin, E., et al. (2011). A feedback information-theoretic approach to the design of brain-computer interfaces. *Int. J. Hum. Comput. Interact.* 27, 5–23. doi: 10.1080/10447318.2011.535749

Rokni, U., Richardson, A. G., Bizzi, E., and Seung, H. S. (2007). Motor learning with unstable neural representations. *Neuron* 54, 653–666. doi: 10.1016/j.neuron.2007.04.030

Sanger, T. D. (2010). Neuro-mechanical control using differential stochastic operators. *Conf. Proc. IEEE Eng. Med. Biol. Soc.* 2010, 4494–4497. doi: 10.1109/IEMBS.2010.5626029

Sanger, T. D. (2011). Distributed control of uncertain systems using superpositions of linear operators. *Neural Comput.* 23, 1911–1934. doi: 10.1162/NECO_a_00151

Sanger, T. D. (2014). Risk-Aware Control. *Neural Comput.* 26, 2669–2691. doi: 10.1162/NECO_a_00662

Schneidman, E., Berry, M. J. II, Segev, R., and Bialek, W. (2006). Weak pairwise correlations imply strongly correlated network states in a neural population. *Nature* 440, 1007–1012. doi: 10.1038/nature04701

Serruya, M., Hatsopoulos, N., Fellows, M., Paninshki, L., and Donoghue, J. P. (2003). Robustness of neuroprosthetic decoding algorithms. *Biol. Cybern.* 88, 219–228. doi: 10.1007/s00422-002-0374-6

Shigeyoshi, F. (2008). behavior-dependent short term assembly dynamics in the medial prefrontal cortex. *Nat. Neurosci.* 11, 823–833. doi: 10.1038/nn.2134

Shoham, S., Fellows, M. R., and Normann, R. A. (2003). Robust, automatic spike sorting using mixtures of multivariate t-distributions. *J. Neurosci. Methods* 127, 111–122. doi: 10.1016/S0165-0270(03)00120-1

Song, W. G., and Giszter, S. F. (2011). Adaptation to a cortex controlled robot attached at the pelvis and engaged during locomotion in rats. *J. Neurosci.* 31, 3110–3128. doi: 10.1523/JNEUROSCI.2335-10.2011

Song, W. G., Ramakrishnan, A., Udoekwere, U. I., and Giszter, S. F. (2009). Multiple types of movement-related information encoded in hindlimb/trunk cortex in rats and potentially available for brain–machine interface controls. *IEEE Trans. Biomed. Eng.* 56, 2712–2716. doi: 10.1109/TBME.2009.2026284

Stevenson, I. H., and Körding,. K. P. (2010). On the similarity of functional connectivity between neurons estimated across timescales *PLoS ONE* 5:e9206. doi: 10.1371/journal.pone.0009206

Stevenson, I. H., Rebesco, J. M., Hatsopoulos, N. G., Haga, Z., Miller, L. E., and Körding, K. P. (2009). Bayesian inference of functional connectivity and network structure from spikes. *IEEE Trans. Neural Syst. Rehabil. Eng.* 17, 203–213. doi: 10.1109/TNSRE.2008.2010471

Stevenson, I. H., Rebesco, J. M., Miller, L. E., and Körding, K. P. (2008). Inferring functional connections between neurons. *Curr. Opin. Neurobiol.* 18, 582–588. doi: 10.1016/j.conb.2008.11.005

Strong, S. P., Koberle, R., de Ruyter van Steveninck, R. R., and Bialek, W. (1998). Entropy and information in neural spike trains. *Phys. Rev. Lett.* 80, 197–200. doi: 10.1103/PhysRevLett.80.197

Truccolo, W., Eden, U. T., Fellows, M. R., Donoghue, J. P., and Brown, E. N. (2005). A point process framework for relating neural spiking activity to spiking history, neural ensemble, and extrinsic covariate effects. *J. Neurophysiol.* 93, 1074–1089. doi: 10.1152/jn.00697.2004

Truccolo, W., Hochberg, L. R., and Donoghue, J. P. (2010). Collective dynamics in human and monkey sensorimotor cortex: predicting single neuron spikes. *Nat. Neurosci.* 13, 105–111. doi: 10.1038/nn.2455

Velliste, M., Perel, S., Spalding, M. C., Whitford, A. S., and Schwartz, A. B. (2008). Cortical control of a prosthetic arm for self-feeding. *Nature* 453, 1098–1101. doi: 10.1038/nature06996

Zacksenhouse, M., Lebedev, M. A., Carmena, J. M., O'Doherty, J. E., Henriquez, C., and Necolelis, M. A. L. (2007). Cortical modulations increase in early sessions with brain-machine interface. *PLoS ONE* 7, 1–10. doi: 10.1371/journal.pone.0000619

11

Augmented brain function by coordinated reset stimulation with slowly varying sequences

Magteld Zeitler[1]* *and Peter A. Tass*[1,2,3]

[1] Research Center Jülich, Institute of Neuroscience and Medicine, Neuromodulation (INM-7), Jülich, Germany, [2] Department of Neurosurgery, Stanford University, Stanford, CA, USA, [3] Department of Neuromodulation, University of Cologne, Cologne, Germany

Edited by:
Mikhail Lebedev,
Duke University, USA

Reviewed by:
Theoden I. Netoff,
University of Minnesota, USA
Hayriye Cagnan,
University of Oxford, UK

***Correspondence:**
Magteld Zeitler,
Research Center Jülich, Institute of Neuroscience and Medicine, Neuromodulation (INM-7),
Wilhelm-Johnen-Straße, 52425 Jülich, Germany
m.zeitler@fz-juelich.de

Several brain disorders are characterized by abnormally strong neuronal synchrony. Coordinated Reset (CR) stimulation was developed to selectively counteract abnormal neuronal synchrony by desynchronization. For this, phase resetting stimuli are delivered to different subpopulations in a timely coordinated way. In neural networks with spike timing-dependent plasticity CR stimulation may eventually lead to an anti-kindling, i.e., an unlearning of abnormal synaptic connectivity and abnormal synchrony. The spatiotemporal sequence by which all stimulation sites are stimulated exactly once is called the stimulation site sequence, or briefly sequence. So far, in simulations, pre-clinical and clinical applications CR was applied either with fixed sequences or rapidly varying sequences (RVS). In this computational study we show that appropriate repetition of the sequence with occasional random switching to the next sequence may significantly improve the anti-kindling effect of CR. To this end, a sequence is applied many times before randomly switching to the next sequence. This new method is called SVS CR stimulation, i.e., CR with slowly varying sequences. In a neuronal network with strong short-range excitatory and weak long-range inhibitory dynamic couplings SVS CR stimulation turns out to be superior to CR stimulation with fixed sequences or RVS.

Keywords: coordinated reset, slowly varying sequences, desynchronization, spike timing-dependent plasticity, anti-kindling

Introduction

Abnormally strong neuronal synchronization characterizes several brain disorders, e.g., Parkinson's disease (Lenz et al., 1994; Nini et al., 1995; Hammond et al., 2007), epilepsy (Wong et al., 1986; Schomer and Lopes da Silva, 2010), and tinnitus (Ochi and Eggermont, 1997; Llinas et al., 1999; Weisz et al., 2005; Eggermont and Tass, 2015). Coordinated reset (CR) stimulation (Tass, 2003a,b) was developed in order to specifically counteract abnormal neuronal synchrony by desynchronization (Tass, 1999). CR stimulation means to deliver phase resetting stimuli at different times to different sub-populations involved in abnormal neuronal synchronization (Tass, 2003a,b). Computational studies showed that in neuronal populations with spike timing-dependent plasticity (STDP) (Gerstner et al., 1996; Markram et al., 1997; Bi and Poo, 1998; Feldman, 2000) CR stimulation has long-lasting, sustained effects (Tass and Majtanik, 2006; Hauptmann and Tass, 2007; Popovych and Tass, 2012). This is because

CR stimulation employs the multistability of neuronal networks with STDP (Tass and Majtanik, 2006; Hauptmann and Tass, 2007; Maistrenko et al., 2007; Popovych and Tass, 2012). CR-stimulation causes a desynchronization and in turn, due to STDP (Gerstner et al., 1996; Markram et al., 1997; Bi and Poo, 1998; Feldman, 2000), leads to a decrease of the mean synaptic weight. In this way, CR stimulation shifts the neuronal network from a pathological attractor with up-regulated synchrony and connectivity to a physiological attractor with down-regulated synchrony and connectivity (Tass and Majtanik, 2006; Hauptmann and Tass, 2007; Popovych and Tass, 2012). In this way CR applied induces an unlearning of the abnormal synaptic connectivity and abnormal neuronal synchrony, so that an anti-kindling is achieved (Tass and Majtanik, 2006).

Computational studies showed that anti-kindling can robustly be achieved in networks of spiking or bursting model neurons where the neurons interact via plastic excitatory and inhibitory synapses (Popovych and Tass, 2012; Tass and Popovych, 2012). These studies show also that anti-kindling occurs irrespective of whether CR stimulation is delivered to the somata or to excitatory or inhibitory synapses.

In accordance with these computational findings, long-lasting CR-induced desynchronization was achieved in pre-clinical as well as clinical studies with invasive and non-invasive stimulation modalities. Electrical CR stimulation induced long-lasting desynchronization in rat hippocampal slice rendered epileptic by magnesium withdrawal (Tass et al., 2009). Therapeutic long-lasting after-effects of electrical CR deep brain stimulation were observed in parkinsonian non-human primates (Tass et al., 2012b). Unilateral CR stimulation applied to the subthalamic nucleus (STN) of parkinsonian MPTP monkeys for only 2 h per day during 5 subsequent days caused significant sustained bilateral therapeutic after-effects for at least 30 days, while no after-effects were induced by standard permanent high-frequency deep brain stimulation (Tass et al., 2012b). By the same token, lasting after-effects of electrical CR stimulation of the STN were also verified in parkinsonian patients (Adamchic et al., 2014a). So far, non-invasive CR stimulation was realized with acoustic stimuli and applied to the treatment of chronic subjective tinnitus (Tass and Popovych, 2012; Tass et al., 2012a). In a proof of concept-study it was shown that acoustic CR stimulation causes a statistically and clinically significant and sustained reduction of tinnitus symptoms (Adamchic et al., 2012a,b; Tass et al., 2012a) along with a concomitant reduction of abnormal neuronal synchrony (Tass et al., 2012a; Adamchic et al., 2014b), abnormal effective connectivity (Silchenko et al., 2013) and abnormal cross-frequency coupling (Adamchic et al., 2014c) within a tinnitus-related network of brain areas.

We here set out to further improve the efficacy of CR stimulation by focusing on a key element of CR, the stimulation site sequence, i.e., the temporal sequence of activating the different stimulation sites exactly once, which in what follows will briefly be called *sequence*. Keeping the sequence constant for all stimulation cycles is optimal in neuronal networks without STDP, since it enables optimal desynchronization at minimal intensities (Tass, 2003a,b). The situation gets more sophisticated in the presence of STDP. In a network of phase oscillators with couplings subject to STDP the sequence was randomly varied from cycle to cycle in order to avoid reverberations which might possibly lead to the formation of sequence-related neuronal subclusters and/or to a delayed anti-kindling (Tass and Majtanik, 2006). However, in several computational studies addressing different aspects of CR a robust anti-kindling was achieved with CR stimulation with fixed sequence (Hauptmann and Tass, 2007, 2009; Tass and Hauptmann, 2007, 2009) as well as with sequences randomly varying form cycle to cycle (Tass and Majtanik, 2006; Tass and Hauptmann, 2006; Popovych and Tass, 2012; Tass and Popovych, 2012; Ebert et al., 2014). We denote CR stimulation with sequences randomly varied from cycle to cycle as *RVS CR stimulation*, i.e., CR with rapidly varying sequences, whereas CR stimulation with fixed sequence is called *FS CR stimulation*, i.e., CR stimulation with fixed sequence. Although some findings indicated that RVS CR might lead to a quicker anti-kindling (Tass and Majtanik, 2006), so far no systematic comparison or deeper analysis was performed. In pre-clinical and clinical studies mainly RVS CR stimulation was applied (Tass et al., 2012a,b; Adamchic et al., 2014c), while FS CR stimulation was used only in an *in vitro* experiment (Tass et al., 2009). The available results do not allow to judge whether RVS CR or FS CR stimulation or possibly another variant of CR might be superior.

In this study we investigate the efficacy of a new CR stimulation variant for which a sequence is repeated during n stimulation cycles in a row before randomly switching to the next sequence. This type of CR will be called *SVS-n CR stimulation*, where SVS stands for slowly varying sequences. We show that repetition with occasionally switching of the sequence may significantly improve the performance of CR stimulation, leading to a more robust and quicker anti-kindling. To this end, we use a neuronal network model with STDP as described in Section Materials and Methods. The impact of the RVS and the SVS-n CR stimulation are compared in Section Slowly Varying Sequences Boost CR Stimulation Effect. Finally, in Section Optimal Number of Different Sequences Used for SVS CR Stimulation we demonstrate that optimal anti-kindling requires both variation and substantial repetition of the sequence. In fact, a sequence has to be repeated sufficiently often, e.g., at least 25 times, before randomly switching to another sequence.

Materials and Methods

Conductance-Based Hodgkin-Huxley Model

The neural network used in this study consisted of N ($N = 200$) spiking conductance-based Hodgkin-Huxley neurons (Hodgkin and Huxley, 1952). The membrane potential V of each neuron i ($i = 1, \dots, N$) is characterized by Hansel et al. (1993), Popovych and Tass (2012):

$$C\frac{dV_i}{dt} = I_i - g_{Na}m_i^3 h_i (V_i - V_{Na}) - g_K n_i^4 (V_i - V_K) - g_l (V_i - V_l) + S_i + F_i. \quad (1)$$

C is the membrane capacitance, I_i the constant depolarizing current injected into neuron i, S_i is the current that represents synaptic input of the neurons within the network to neuron i and F_i is the current induced in neuron i by CR stimulation. Values used in this study are: $C = 1\ \mu\text{F/cm}^2$, maximum conductance per unit area for the sodium, potassium and leak currents, $g_{Na} = 120\ \text{mS/cm}^2$, $g_K = 36\ \text{mS/cm}^2$, $g_l = 0.3\ \text{mS/cm}^2$, with sodium reversal potential $V_{Na} = 50\,\text{mV}$, potassium reversal potential $V_K = -77\,\text{mV}$, leak reversal potential $V_l = -54.4\,\text{mV}$. For the equations of the time-varying gate variables m, h, and n see Hansel et al. (1993). The injected constant currents (I_i) are uniformly distributed random numbers ($I_i \in [I_0 - \varepsilon_I, I_0 + \varepsilon_I]$, in this study $I_0 = 11.0\ \mu\text{A/cm}^2$ and $\varepsilon_I = 0.45\ \mu\text{A/cm}^2$) and determine the intrinsic firing rate of the uncoupled neurons.

The coupling term S_i from Equation (1) (Popovych and Tass, 2012) contains a weighted ensemble average of all post-synaptic currents received by neuron i from the other neurons in the network and is given by:

$$S_i = N^{-1} \sum_{j=1}^{N} \left(V_{r,j} - V_i\right) c_{ij} \left|M_{ij}\right| s_j. \tag{2}$$

N is the number of neurons within the ensemble, $V_{r,j}$ is the reversal potential of the synaptic coupling (20 mV for excitatory and –40 mV for inhibitory coupling), and c_{ij} is the synaptic coupling strength from neuron j to neuron i. There are no neuronal self-connections within the network ($c_{ii} = 0\ \text{mS/cm}^2$). M_{ij} has the form of a Mexican hat (Wilson and Cowan, 1973; Dominguez et al., 2006; De la Rocha et al., 2008) and defines the strength and type of neuronal interaction: strong short-range excitatory $\left(M_{ij} > 0\right)$and weak long-range inhibitory interactions $\left(M_{ij} < 0\right)$. This spatial profile of coupling between neurons i and j is given by:

$$M_{ij} = \left(1 - d_{ij}^2/\sigma_1^2\right) \exp\left(-d_{ij}^2/(2\sigma_2^2)\right) \tag{3}$$

where $d_{ij} = d\left|i - j\right|$ is the distance between neurons i and j,

$$d = d_0/(N-1) \tag{4}$$

is the lattice distance between two neighboring neurons within the ensemble, d_0 is the length of the neuronal chain, $\sigma_1 = 3.5$, and $\sigma_2 = 2.0$ as used in Popovych and Tass (2012). To minimize boundary effects, the neurons form a ring, which implies that $d_{ij} = d \cdot min\left(\left|i-j\right|, N - \left|i-j\right|\right)$.

The synaptic variable s_j in Eqn. 2 is given by:

$$\frac{ds_j}{dt} = \frac{0.5(1-s_j)}{1 + exp\left[-\left(V_j - 5\right)/12\right]} - 2s_j. \tag{5}$$

Spike Timing-Dependent Plasticity

In general, synaptic coupling strengths change depending on the precise timing of pre- and post-synaptic spikes (Markram et al., 1997; Bi and Poo, 1998). In the present study all synaptic weights c_{ij} were considered to be dynamic variables dependent on the time difference (Δt_{ij}) between the onset of the post- and pre-synaptic spikes t_i, respectively t_j $\left(\Delta t_{ij} = t_i - t_j\right)$. According to the spike timing-dependent plasticity (STDP) rule (Bi and Poo, 1998) the change in synaptic weight is given by:

$$\Delta c_{ij} = \begin{cases} \beta_1 e^{\frac{-\Delta t_{ij}}{\gamma_1 \tau}}, \Delta t_{ij} \geq 0 \\ \beta_2 \frac{\Delta t_{ij}}{\tau} e^{\frac{\Delta t_{ij}}{\gamma_2 \tau}}, \Delta t_{ij} < 0 \end{cases} \tag{6}$$

See Popovych and Tass (2012), In our model we update the synaptic weights c_{ij} in an event-based manner by adding $\delta \cdot \Delta c_{ij}$ for excitatory connections and $-\delta \cdot \Delta c_{ij}$ for inhibitory connections with learning rate $\delta > 0$ every time a neuron spikes. To avoid an unbounded strengthening or weakening, the synaptic weights are restricted to the interval $c_{ij} \in [0, 1]\ \text{mS/cm}^2$ for excitatory synapses and $c_{ij} \in [0, c_{max}]\ \text{mS/cm}^2$ for inhibitory synapses with $c_{max} = 1$ unless stated otherwise. In this study the following values are used for the STDP parameters: $\beta_1 = 1$, $\beta_2 = 16$, $\gamma_1 = 0.12$, $\gamma_2 = 0.15$, $\tau = 14$ ms, and $\delta = 0.002$.

Due to STDP and the different intrinsic periods of the neurons, the synaptic weights change constantly. In this study the dynamics of the synaptic weights were investigated on a population level. The strength of the coupling within the neuronal population at time t is given by the synaptic weight averaged over the population:

$$C_{av}(t) = N^{-2} \sum_{i,j} sgn\left(M_{ij}\right) c_{ij}(t), \tag{7}$$

with M_{ij} as defined in Equation (3) and the sign-function sgn. The amount of synchronization of the neuronal activity within the ensemble is influenced by the synaptic weights and can be represented by the order parameter (Haken, 1983; Kuramoto, 1984)

$$R(t) = \left|N^{-1} \sum_j e^{i\varphi_j(t)}\right|, \tag{8}$$

Where $\varphi_j(t) = 2\pi(t - t_{j,m})/(t_{j,m+1} - t_{j,m})$ for $t_{j,m} \leq t < t_{j,m+1}$ is a linear approximation of the phase of neuron j between its mth and $(m+1)^{th}$ spikes at spiking times $t_{j,m}$ and $t_{j,m+1}$. The order parameter R measures the extent of phase synchronization in the neuronal ensemble and takes values between 0 (complete desynchronization) and 1 (perfect in-phase synchronization). For our data analysis the order parameter was averaged over the last 1.6 s of the CR-off period and will be denoted as average order parameter R_{av}.

Coordinated Reset Stimulation Algorithms

Coordinated Reset (CR) stimulation was delivered to the neuronal ensemble of N spiking Hodgkin-Huxley neurons. This was done sequentially via N_s equidistantly spaced stimulation sites (Tass, 2003a): one stimulation site was active during T_s/N_s, while the other stimulation sites were inactive during that period. After that another stimulation site was active during the next T_s/N_s period. All N_s stimulation sites were stimulated exactly once within one stimulation ON-cycle. Therefore, the duration of each ON-cycle is T_s. This spatiotemporal activation of stimulation sites is represented by the indicator functions $\rho_k(t)\,(k\epsilon\,\{1,\ldots,N\})$:

$$\rho_k(t) = \begin{cases} 1, & k^{th}\text{stimulation site is active at } t \\ 0, & \text{otherwise} \end{cases} \qquad (9)$$

The stimulation signals induced single brief excitatory post-synaptic currents. The evoked time-dependent normalized conductances of the post-synaptic membranes are represented by α-functions given by Popovych and Tass (2012):

$$G_{stim}(t) = \frac{t - t_k}{\tau_{stim}} e^{-(t-t_k)/\tau}, \quad t_k \le t \le t_{k+1}. \qquad (10)$$

Here $\tau_{stim} = T_s/(6N_s)$ denotes the time-to-peak of G_{stim}, and t_k is the onset of the kth activation of the stimulation site. The spatial spread of the induced excitatory post-synaptic currents in the network is defined by a quadratic spatial decay profile (see Popovych and Tass, 2012 for motivation) given as a function of the difference in index of neuron i and the index x_k of the neuron at stimulation site k:

$$D(i, x_k) = \frac{1}{1 + d^2(i - x_k)^2/\sigma_d^2}, \qquad (11)$$

with d the lattice distance between two neighboring neurons as defined in Equation (4) and $\sigma_d = 0.08d_0$ the spatial decay rate of the stimulation current.

The stimulation current from Equation (1) is given by:

$$F_i = [V_r - V_i(t)] \cdot K \sum_{k=1}^{N_s} D(i, x_k)\,\rho_k(t)\,G_{stim}(t), \qquad (12)$$

where $V_r = 20\,\text{mV}$ denotes the excitatory reverse potential, V_i the membrane potential of neuron i, K the stimulation intensity, and D, ρ, G are given by Equations (11), (10), and (9).

In this paper we study three different CR algorithms: RVS CR stimulation (Tass and Hauptmann, 2006; Tass and Majtanik, 2006; Popovych and Tass, 2012; Tass and Popovych, 2012), FS CR stimulation (Tass, 2003a,b; Hauptmann and Tass, 2007, 2009; Tass and Hauptmann, 2007, 2009), and our novel SVS CR stimulation. During one sequence each stimulation site is activated exactly once. There are $N_s!$ (in our study 4!=24) different sequences possible to stimulate N_s stimulation sites. In the RVS CR algorithm for each ON-cycle a new sequence was drawn randomly from the set of $N_s!$ possible sequences (see **Figure 1A**). For the slowly varying sequences CR algorithm (SVS-n) the sequence order is random and determined a priori in such a way that each sequence used, is consecutively repeated n times before another one is applied. For the SVS-4 CR stimulation signals as shown in **Figure 1B** one sequence was applied during the first n consecutive ON-cycles. After that the next sequence was applied during the next n consecutive ON-cycles, and so on (see **Figure 1B** for $n = 4$).

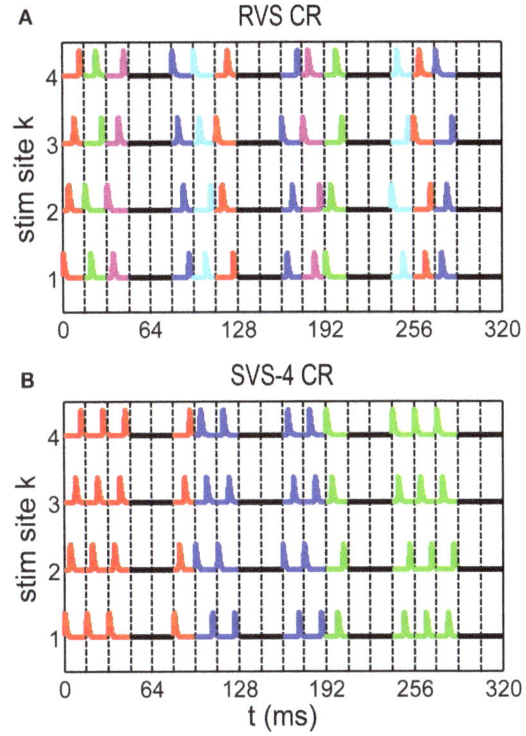

FIGURE 1 | Spatiotemporal stimulation signals of CR stimulation. (A) An example sequence order for the rapidly varying sequences (RVS) CR. **(B)** An example sequence order for the slowly varying sequence CR with every sequence repeated 4 times (SVS-4) before the next sequence is used. A change of color indicates a new sequence. Vertical dashed lines separate stimulation ON- and OFF cycles: three ON-cycles are followed by two OFF-cycles.

Simulation Details and Data Analysis

We ran simulations for different initial network conditions and different sequence orders. For each initial network condition the initial conditions of all N neurons were randomly drawn from uniform distributions ($n_i, m_i, h_i, s_i \in [0, 1]$; $V_i \in [-65, 5]\,mV$; $I_i \in [I_0 - \sigma_I, I_0 + \sigma_I]$). The initial synaptic weights c_{ij} between the neurons were drawn from a normal distribution ($c_{ij} \sim N(\mu = 0.5\mu A/cm^2, \sigma = 0.01\mu A/cm^2)$). After an initial equilibration phase of 2 s, STDP was included for the rest of the simulation. During the first 60 s with STDP the network was given the opportunity to rewire its connections without any influence from an external stimulation. At the end of this STDP-only period the network activity was highly synchronized and the CR simulation was applied for 64 s from $t = 0$ s on. During this CR-on period three stimulation ON-cycles alternated with two OFF-cycles as in the example stimulation signal shown in **Figure 1**. No stimulation was applied during the OFF-cycles. Each ON- and OFF-cycle lasted $T_s = 16$ ms. After 64 s the CR stimulation was stopped permanently and the 64 s lasting CR-off period started. After going through this procedure for one particular stimulation intensity, K, the procedure was repeated from $t = 0$ s on for the other K-values ($K \in \{0.10, 0.20, 0.30 \ldots, 0.60\}$). For each CR stimulation this whole process was repeated for eleven different initial network conditions and sequence orders. Besides the RVS CR stimulation also the SVS-100 CR stimulations were applied for eleven different combinations of initial conditions and sequence orders. Finally, the optimal number of different sequences used in the SVS CR stimulation was explored.

The resulting values of C_{av} (Equation 7) at $t = 128$ s and R_{av} (Equation 8) averaged over the last 1.6 s of the CR-off period) were plotted in boxplots (Tukey, 1977). In order to compare the results of different CR algorithms for a constant stimulation strength, K, the obtained boxplots are plotted next to each other, whereby the color represents which CR algorithm was used. Statistical significances of differences between the results of the different CR algorithms were determined by the one-sided Mann-Whitney test.

Results

Slowly Varying Sequences Boost CR stimulation Effect

To verify whether the SVS CR stimulation is more successful than the RVS CR stimulation, the effect of both CR algorithms on the average synaptic weight, C_{av}, as well as on the synchronization of neuronal activity R has to be investigated. Each measure will be explored first for the RVS and then for the SVS CR stimulation.

As visualized in **Figure 2A** the RVS CR stimulation causes a weakening of the average synaptic weight C_{av} during the CR-on period for all stimulation intensities K. At the end of the subsequent CR-off period, the average synaptic weight is still much weaker than before the CR stimulation was applied, except for the weakest stimulation intensity. **Figure 2B** then shows how the SVS CR stimulation, delivered to the same initial network, decreases the average synaptic weights even more and causes in general lower long-lasting C_{av}–values compared to the RVS CR stimulation. Since we are interested in the long-lasting effects of the CR stimulation period, we will concentrate on the values at the end of the CR-off for the remainder of this work.

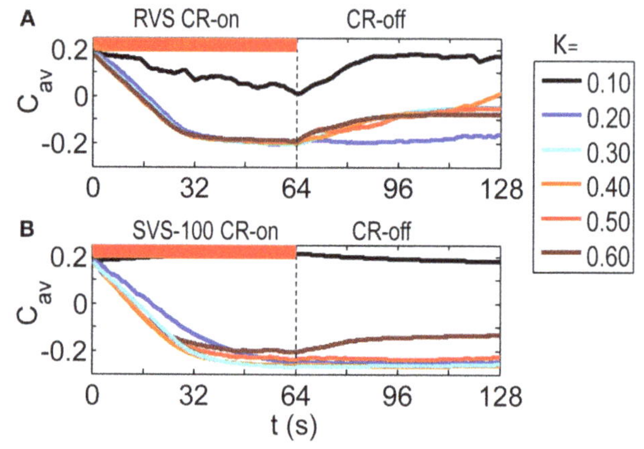

FIGURE 2 | Dynamics of the average synaptic weight, C_{av}, for different stimulation intensities, K. (A) Results of the RVS CR stimulation. **(B)** Results of the SVS-100 CR stimulation. The initial network is the same for all simulations. The sequence order used for each CR method is constant for all K-values. The CR-on period, represented by the red horizontal bar, starts at $t = 0$ s and is switched off at $t = 64$ s (dashed vertical line). During the subsequent 64 s CR-off period, no stimulation is delivered, and C_{av} evolves spontaneously. $c_{max} = 1$ for all simulations.

To investigate whether this observed improvement by the SVS CR stimulation is just a coincidence, we have also changed the sequence order or the initial network conditions. **Figure 3A** shows that by applying another RVS order to the same initial network or by applying the initial sequence order to a network with different initial conditions, different long-lasting C_{av}-values were obtained. Only for the weakest stimulation intensity, $K = 0.10$, the RVS algorithm caused similar long-lasting C_{av}-values. For other stimulation intensities, it suggests that the effect of the RVS CR stimulation depends on the sequence order used and on the initial network conditions. As follows from **Figure 3B**, the success of the SVS-100 CR stimulation depends less strongly on the exact sequence order and the initial network conditions and the SVS-100 CR stimulation results in a smaller C_{av}-value than the RVS CR stimulation, over a wide range of stimulation intensities K continuing the superiority of this method.

Robustness against variations of the sequence order and against initial network conditions is of crucial importance for the CR therapy. Therefore, all stimulations were repeated 11 times for different combinations of initial network conditions and sequence orders. The boxplots in **Figure 4A** show that the long-lasting effect of decreasing the average synaptic strength is significantly better for the SVS-100 than for the RVS CR stimulation over a wide range of stimulation intensities K (one-sided Mann-Whitney test, $p < 0.05$). Besides generating a better C_{av}-value, the SVS CR stimulation is also more robust against initial network conditions and sequence orders. The SVS-100 also induces a significant smaller R_{av} than the RVS CR stimulation (one-sided Mann-Whitney test $p < 0.01$), but for a smaller set of K-values as shown in **Figure 4B**. R_{av} is the value of the order parameter averaged over the last 1.6 s of the CR-off period.

To rule out false estimates of the time averaged order parameter R, we used different window lengths. False estimates could, for instance, be caused by low-frequency oscillations of R with periods exceeding the window length used for our averaging analysis. In our analysis of the order parameter R, presented in this paper, we averaged over the last 1.6 s of the 64 s during CR-off period. Averaging R over a quarter (=16 s) of the total CR-off period gave very similar results. Hence, we can consider our results to be sufficiently robust with respect to variations of the length of the time window used for our evaluation.

Simulations for SVS-25 CR stimulation during the 64 s lasting CR-on period gave similar results for C_{av} and R_{av} as the SVS-100 CR (results not shown), illustrating that 25 consecutive repetitions of each sequence are already enough to improve the CR effect.

From the standpoint of clinical applications it is important to understand the relationship between the acute effect achieved during stimulation and the after-effect observed after cessation of stimulation. To this end, we studied the relationship between the values of C_{av} and R_{av} at the end of the CR-on period ($t = 64$ s) and their values at the end of the CR-off period ($t = 128$ s) (**Figure 5**). The relation between C_{av} at $t = 64$ s and at $t = 128$ s

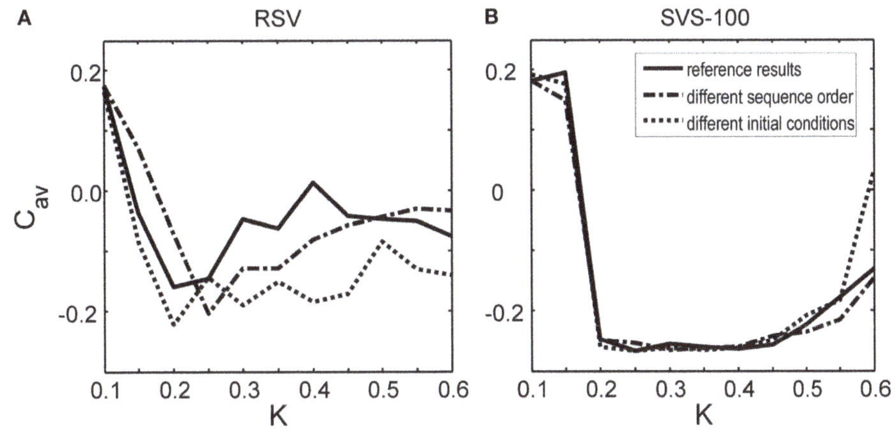

FIGURE 3 | Effect of the sequence order and of the initial network conditions on the average synaptic weight C_{av} at $t = 128$ s as a function of stimulation intensity K. (A) C_{av}-values at $t = 128$ s obtained by the RVS CR stimulation. **(B)** C_{av}-values at $t = 128$ s obtained by the SVS-100 CR stimulation. The $C_{av}(t = 128\,\text{s})$ values in **Figure 2** are the reference results and represented by the solid lines in this Figure. The dashed-dotted lines show the result for a simulation with the same initial network conditions as used to obtain the reference results but for another randomly chosen sequence order. The dotted lines represent the obtained C_{av}-values at $t = 128$ s for a simulation with the same sequence order as used to obtain the reference results, but for other initial network conditions.

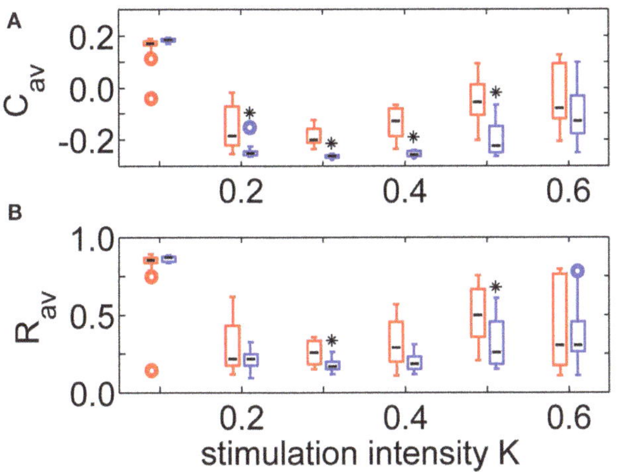

FIGURE 4 | Comparison of the anti-kindling effects at $t = 128$ s for the RVS and the SVS-100 CR stimulation. (A) Boxplots of the average synaptic strength, C_{av}, at $t = 128$ s as a function of the stimulation intensity, K, for the RVS and the SVS-100 CR stimulation. **(B)** Boxplots of the order parameter R averaged over the last 1.6 s, R_{av}, as a function of K for the RVS and the SVS-100 CR stimulation. The RVS CR results for the same K-values are shown in red and slightly shifted to the left and the SVS-100 results are shown in blue and slightly shifted to the right. The black lines within the boxes show the medians for each condition, the boxes the middle 50% and the whiskers below (above) the boxes the first (last, respectively) 25%. Outliers are defined as 1.5 times the length of the box below or above the box and represented by open circles. For each condition (K-value and type of CR) the simulations are repeated eleven times for different initial conditions of the network in combination with different sequence orders. One asterisk indicates a significantly lower C_{av} - or R_{av}-value compared to the values obtained by the RVS CR stimulation (one-sided Mann-Whitney test with $p < 0.05$).

is visualized in **Figure 5A**. In a first approximation, small values C_{av} and R_{av} at $t = 64$ s are required but not necessarily sufficient for small values of C_{av} and R_{av} at $t = 128$ s. Hence, with a certain probability a pronounced acute stimulation effect is associated with a good long-term outcome. In contrast, poor acute stimulation effects are not related to pronounced after-effects.

Optimal Number of Different Sequences Used for SVS CR Stimulation

In this section we analyze the impact of sequence changes on the dynamics of the average synaptic connectivity as assessed by C_{av}. To this end, first, we perform a CR stimulation with fixed sequence (FS CR) and compare it to CR stimulation epochs where the sequence is either changed once or at three equidistant times without changing the total duration of the CR-on period. This implies that the number of different sequences multiplied with the number of consecutive repetitions, n, is constant. Finally, the optimal number of different sequences used in the SVS CR stimulation was explored.

We analyzed the effect of *FS CR stimulation* for eleven different initial network conditions in combination with a different sequence for each network, respectively. **Figure 6A** clearly shows that for the FS CR stimulation (SVS-2400) with $K = 0.20$, the decrease of C_{av} strongly depends on which sequence is used. Pronounced long-lasting effects are achieved by some sequences, whereas no anti-kindling is observed for other sequences. Increasing the stimulation intensity to $K = 0.45$ improves the robustness of FS against the choice of the sequence used and the initial network conditions (**Figure 6B**). For $K = 0.45$ the average synaptic weight stabilizes at a small to intermediate value, depending on the sequence and the initial network conditions. The stabilization of C_{av} is more rapidly achieved at higher stimulation intensity K.

By using *two different sequences* instead of just one sequence, the first sequence may stabilize C_{av} at an intermediate value of C_{av} and, hence, lead to a sub-optimal outcome. However, at $t = 32$ s the second sequence takes over, and may further reduce C_{av} as

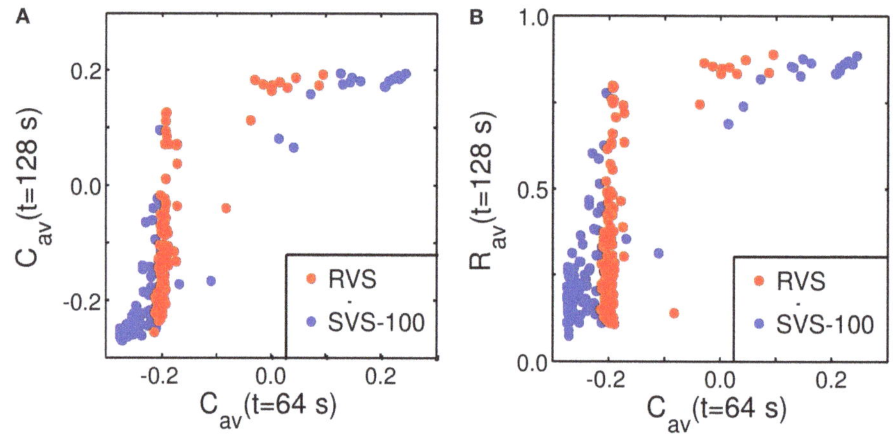

FIGURE 5 | Predictability of the anti-kindling effect by C_{av} at $t = 64$ s. (A) Relation between C_{av} at the end of the CR-on period ($t = 64$ s) and at the end of the CR-off period ($t = 128$ s). **(B)** Relation between C_{av} at the end of the CR-on period ($t = 64$ s) and R_{av} at the end of the CR-off period ($t = 128$ s). The C_{av}-values at $t = 64$ s are calculated and plotted against C_{av} or R_{av} at $t = 128$ s for each condition (initial network conditions, stimulation intensity, sequence order, $c_{max} = 1$) as used for **Figure 4**. Red circles represent the results of the RVS CR stimulation, blue circles of the SVS-100 CR stimulation. Note that the red circles are plotted on top of the blue circles.

shown by its kinks at $t = 32$ s (**Figure 6C** for $K = 0.20$ and SVS-1200), in particular, for the more effective stimulation intensity $K = 0.45$ (**Figure 6D**).

By the same token, the long-lasting effects on the mean synaptic connectivity C_{av} and the robustness of the stimulation further improve by using *four different sequences* (SVS-600, **Figure 6E** for $K = 0.20$ and **Figure 6F** for $K = 0.45$). Again, especially at higher stimulation intensity changes of the sequence may come with a stepwise-like further reduction of C_{av} showing up as kinks in the time course of C_{av} at times when sequences are changed ($t = 16$, 32, and 48 s).

Analogously, we further increase the number of different sequences used during one CR epoch. **Figure 7** shows the stimulation outcome in terms of synaptic connectivity C_{av} (**Figures 7A,C**) and order parameter R_{av} (**Figures 7B,D**) averaged over the last 1.6 s of the CR-off period for different stimulation intensities ($K = 0.20$ in **Figures 7A,B** and $K = 0.45$ in **Figures 7C,D**). The statistics obtained from a set of eleven simulations performed for different initial network conditions and sequence orders shows that the main part of the SVS-induced improvement of the CR effect is already achieved with four different sequences. Using more than four different sequences hardly leads to a further reduction of R_{av} and C_{av} and their variability.

Discussion

Our results show that the SVS CR stimulation leads to significantly weaker average synaptic weights than the RVS CR stimulation over a wide range of stimulation. Within this range the Inter-Quartile-Range (25th to 75th percentile) is smaller for the SVS CR approach compared to the RVS CR. This implies that the SVS CR approach is more robust against initial conditions of the network and against the order of the sequences than the RVS CR in this range. The differences between the results of the SVS with 25 and 100 consecutive repetitions of each sequence are in general not significant, although more repetitions tend to have a larger impact on the average synaptic weight (results not shown). A more significantly reduced average synaptic weight does not necessarily translate into more significantly reduced overall synchrony. In fact, for the SVS CR stimulation the network activity was significantly more desynchronized than for the RVS CR stimulation in a smaller range of stimulation intensities than for the weakening of the network connectivity.

Optimal anti-kindling is obtained at intermediate stimulation intensities (**Figures 3, 4**). This is in agreement with previous computational studies (e.g., Lysyansky et al., 2011a; Popovych and Tass, 2012; Ebert et al., 2014). On the one hand CR stimulation has to be of sufficient intensity to achieve phase resets of the different subpopulations, but on the other hand at high intensities the subpopulations are no longer separately stimulated. In the limiting case of very high intensities each stimulus affects nearly the whole neuronal population and causes an entrainment of the whole population which fosters synchronization rather than desynchronization. Our results are stable with respect to variations of model parameters, e.g., by doubling the maximum allowed inhibitory synaptic weight ($c_{max} = 2$ for inhibitory synapses, results not shown).

Our results show that optimal long-lasting desynchronization requires the right combination of appropriate repetition and occasional variation of sequences. In fact, SVS-CR stimulation is better than FS CR stimulation over a wide range of stimulation intensities. Furthermore, the optimal number of different sequences for the SVS CR stimulation is four or more. This implies that repetition alone, like in the case of FS CR simulation (Hauptmann and Tass, 2007, 2009; Tass and Hauptmann, 2007, 2009; Tass et al., 2009), is not the only ingredient for the improvement of CR stimulation. With insufficiently many different sequences in the SVS CR approach, the network can stabilize in a local minimum that is much larger than the global minimum C_{av}-value for a given stimulation intensity. In

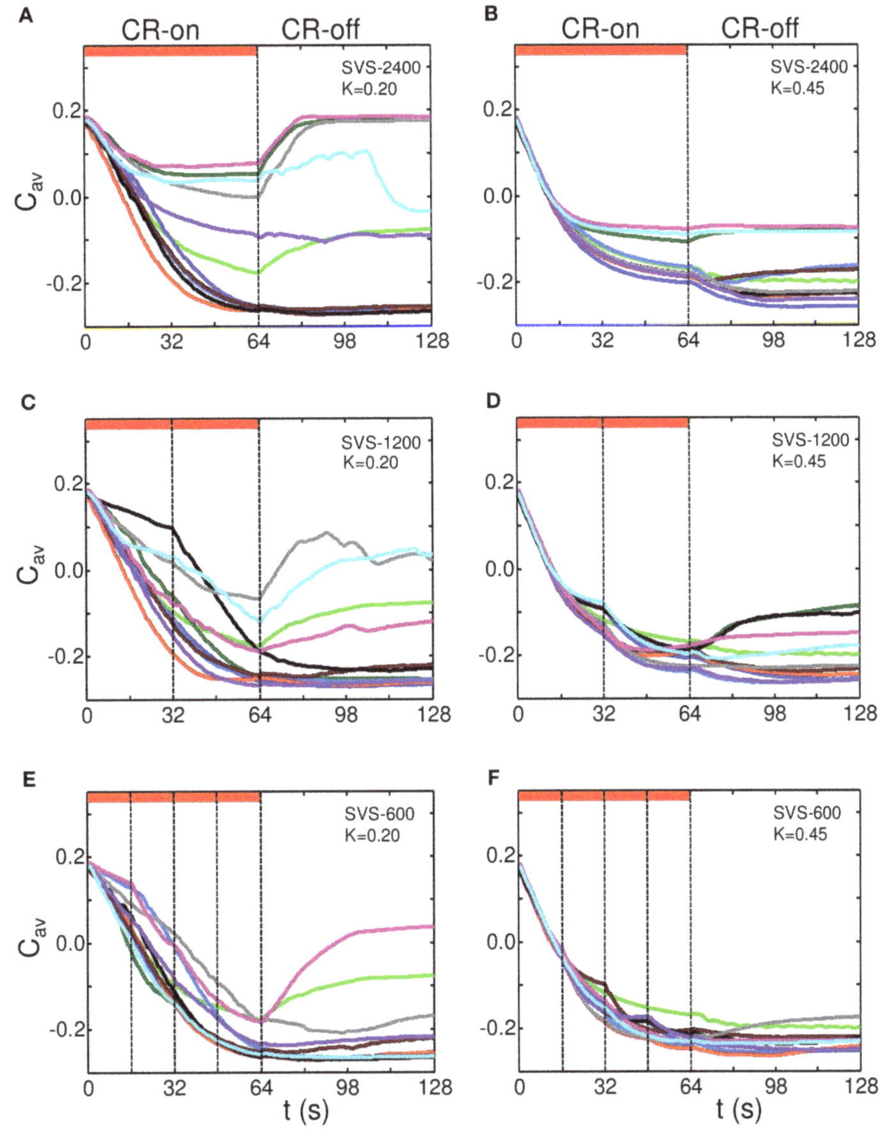

FIGURE 6 | Effect of switching the sequence during CR stimulation. In a series of simulations with different stimulation intensities ($K = 0.20$ in left panels and $K = 0.45$ in right panels) the sequence was either kept fixed [FS CR stimulation, **(A,B)**], randomly varied just once [in the middle of the stimulation period, at $t = 32$ s, **(C,D)**] or randomly varied at three equidistant times [at $t = 16$, 32, 48 s, **(E,F)**]. Simulations were performed for eleven different sequence orders and initial network conditions. Each panel shows the dynamics of C_{av} for each of the eleven simulations in a different color. FS CR stimulation **(A,B)**: Time course of C_{av} for eleven combinations of different initial network conditions and different sequence for SVS-2400, respectively, for $K = 0.20$ **(A)** and $K = 0.45$ **(B)**. Change of sequence in the middle of the stimulation epoch **(C,D)**: Two different sequences, each applied 1200 times in a row. Change of sequence at $t = 32$ s, with $K = 0.20$ **(C)** and $K = 0.45$ **(D)**. Sequence is changed three times at equidistant times ($t =$, 16, 32, and 48 s) during the stimulation epoch **(E,F)**: In each simulation four different sequences are applied 600 times in a row, so that after 16 s the next sequence randomly chosen, with $K = 0.20$ **(E)** and $K = 0.45$ **(F)**. The red horizontal bars represent CR-on periods. The vertical dashed-dotted lines indicate a change of sequence. $c_{max} = 1$ in all simulations.

case the sequence is replaced after many repetitions by another sequence and again after a large number of repetitions by another sequence, the network connectivity can stepwise decrease from one local minimum to another, in this way, approaching the global minimum for a given stimulation intensity. Using more than four different sequences in the SVS CR stimulation does not significantly improve the long-lasting anti-kindling effects compared to those obtained with just four different sequences. The different local minima correspond to different attractors of the network (see Popovych et al., 2015). In fact, in our model network a multitude of attractors with different amount of mean synaptic weight and neuronal synchrony coexist, covering the whole spectrum from minimal mean connectivity and synchrony up to strongly up-regulated mean connectivity and synchrony. Hence, our results indicate that SVS CR stimulation prevents the network from getting stuck in undesirable attractors (with

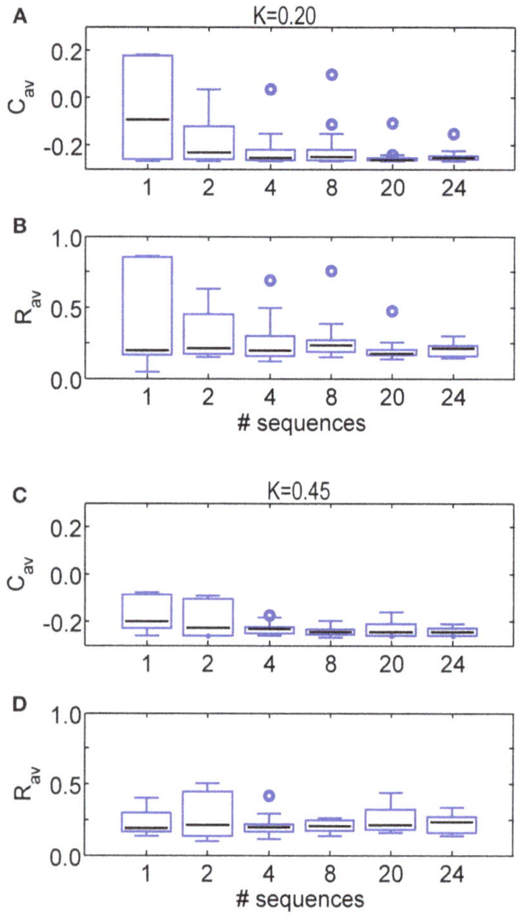

FIGURE 7 | Comparison of the anti-kindling effects for some numbers of different sequences applied during the SVS CR stimulation. (A) Boxplots of C_{av} at $t = 128$ s for different numbers of sequence changes used in the SVS CR stimulation with $K = 0.20$. **(B)** Boxplots of R_{av} at $t = 128$ s for some numbers of different sequences used in the SVS CR stimulation with $K = 0.20$. **(C)** As in **(A)** for $K = 0.45$. **(D)** As in **(B)** for $K = 0.45$. The black lines within the boxes show the medians for each condition, the boxes the middle 50% and the whiskers below (above) the boxes the first (last, respectively) 25%. Outliers are defined as 1.5 times the length of the box below or above the box and represented by open circles. For each condition (K-value and number of sequences) the simulations are repeated eleven times for different initial conditions of the network in combination with different sequence(s). The number of consecutive sequence repetitions was adjusted with respect to the number of different sequences so that the duration of the CR-on period is always 64 s for each simulation. For example if two different sequences are used, each of them is repeated 1200 times in a row, in case four different sequences are used, each of them is repeated 600 times.

intermediate mean connectivity and synchrony) in the course of the anti-kindling stimulation.

Another difference between the SVS-100 and the RVS CR stimulation is that for the SVS CR stimulation by definition in a suitably large time window each sequence is repeated exactly 100 times, but that for the RVS CR stimulation the number of (timely separated) repetitions of each sequence can vary within such a time window, since by definition the sequence of the RVS CR changes from ON-cycle to ON-cycle, where each sequence occurs with equal probability. For an infinitely long time window also for the RVS CR stimulation the different sequences will occur with equal probability. However, on the time scale of one completed series of sequences of the SVS-100 CR stimulation, i.e., for larger, but not infinitely large numbers of sequences, this may be different. Taking a permutation of all 2400 applied sequences (including the repeated sequences) of a SVS-100 CR stimulation generates a CR stimulation signal in which the different sequences occur randomly, but each still exactly 100 times. Simulations with this permutated CR stimulation signal show that C_{av} and R_{av}-values are similar to those obtained by the RVS CR stimulation although the spread is in general larger for the permutated than the random signal (results now shown). This suggests that a constant frequency with which each sequence occurs in a wider time window does not contribute to the success of the SVS CR stimulation, but that it is mainly determined by the consecutive repetitions of a sequence and the number of different sequences. This is actually supported by the fact that already four different sequences in the SVS CR stimulation are sufficient to induce a full-blown anti-kindling (see above).

Applying our SVS CR approach to DBS may be particularly rewarding, since with the same stimulation intensity as used for RVS CR or fixed sequence CR, SVS CR might lead to a better therapeutic outcome. Reducing the stimulation energy will likely lead to a reduction of the rate of side effects. RVS CR DBS was successfully applied at stimulation amplitudes (of the single stimulation pulses) similar to those of standard permanent high-frequency DBS (Adamchic et al., 2014a) as well as corresponding to a third of the amplitude used for standard permanent high-frequency DBS (Tass et al., 2012a). Accordingly, within that range of stimulation amplitudes SVS CR-DBS might be superior to RVS CR-DBS. However, given the intensity dependence of the anti-kindling effects (e.g., **Figure 4**), systematic dose finding studies for both types of CR-DBS are required to best exploit their actual clinical potential. By the same token, systematic dose finding studies should be conducted for acoustic CR stimulation for the treatment of tinnitus (Tass et al., 2012b) for SVS CR. As yet, acoustic RVS CR stimulation was delivered at only one stimulation intensity (i.e., loudness level), namely for just super threshold loudness. In the context of dose finding studies the results from **Figure 5** might be important, since they show that—at least in the model under study—acute effects (achieved during stimulation) are necessary but not sufficient for pronounced long-term desynchronization effects observed after cessation of stimulation.

In a previous computational study it was shown that FS CR stimulation may augment brain function by counteracting cerebral hypo-activity without promoting pathological neuronal synchrony (Lysyansky et al., 2011b). Accordingly, a forthcoming study might focus on the comparison of the potential of SVS CR for activating brain areas and protecting the brain from abnormal synchrony and kindling as opposed to both FS CR and RVS CR.

References

Adamchic, I., Hauptmann, C., Barnikol, U. B., Pawelcyk, N., Popovych, O. V., Barnikol, T., et al. (2014a). Coordinated Reset has lasting aftereffects in patients with Parkinson's Disease. *Mov. Disord.* 29, 1679–1684. doi: 10.1002/mds.25923

Adamchic, I., Langguth, B., Hauptmann, C., and Tass, P. A. (2012a). Psychometric evaluation of Visual Analog Scale for the assessment of chronic tinnitus. *Am. J. Audiol.* 2, 215–225. doi: 10.1044/1059-0889(2012/12-0010)

Adamchic, I., Langguth, B., Hauptmann, C., and Tass, P. A. (2014c). Abnormal brain activity and cross-frequency coupling in the tinnitus network. *Front. Neurosci.* 8:284. doi: 10.3389/fnins.2014.00284

Adamchic, I., Tass, P. A., Langguth, B., Hauptmann, C., Koller, M., Schecklmann, M., et al. (2012b). Linking the tinnitus questionnaire and the clinical global impression: which differences are clinically important? *Health Qual. Life Outcomes* 10:79. doi: 10.1186/1477-7525-10-79

Adamchic, I., Toth, T., Hauptmann, C., and Tass, P. A. (2014b). Reversing pathologically increased EEG power by acoustic CR neuromodulation. *Hum. Brain Mapp.* 35, 2099–2118. doi: 10.1002/hbm.22314

Bi, G., and Poo, M. (1998). Synaptic modifications in cultured hippocampal neurons: dependence on spike timing, synaptic strength, and postsynaptic cell type. *J. Neurosci.* 18, 10464–10472.

De la Rocha, J., Marchetti, C., Schiff, M., and Reyes, A. D. (2008). Linking the response properties of cells in auditory cortex with network architecture: cotuning versus lateral inhibition. *J. Neurosci.* 28, 9151–9163. doi: 10.1523/JNEUROSCI.1789-08.2008

Dominguez, M., Becker, S., Bruce, I., and Read, H. (2006). A spiking neuron model of cortical correlates of sensorineural hearing loss: spontaneous firing, synchrony, and tinnitus. *Neural. Comp.* 18, 2942–2958. doi: 10.1162/neco.2006.18.12.2942

Ebert, M., Hauptmann, C., and Tass, P. A. (2014). Coordinated reset stimulation in a large-scale model of the STN-GPe circuit. *Front. Comput. Neurosci.* 8:154. doi: 10.3389/fncom.2014.00154

Eggermont, J. J., and Tass, P. A. (2015). Maladaptive neural synchrony in tinnitus: origin and restoration. *Front. Neurol.* 6:29. doi: 10.3389/fneur.2015.00029

Feldman, D. E. (2000). Timing-based LTP and LTD at vertical inputs to layer II/III pyramidal cells in rat barrel cortex. *Neuron* 27, 45–56. doi: 10.1016/S0896-6273(00)00008-8

Gerstner, W., Kempter, R., Van Hemmen, J. L., and Wagner, H. (1996). A neuronal learning rule for sub-millisecond temporal coding. *Nature* 383, 76–78. doi: 10.1038/383076a0

Haken, H. (1983). *Advanced Synergetices.* Berlin: Springer.

Hammond, C., Bergman, H., and Brown, P. (2007). Pathological synchronization in parkinson's disease: networks, models and treatments. *Trends Neurosci.* 30, 357–364. doi: 10.1016/j.tins.2007.05.004

Hansel, D., Mato, G., and Meunier, C. (1993). Phase dynamics of weakly coupled Hodgkin-Huxley neurons. *Europhys. Lett.* 23, 367–372. doi: 10.1209/0295-5075/23/5/011

Hauptmann, C., and Tass, P. A. (2007). Therapeutic rewiring by means of desynchronizing brain stimulation. *Biosystems* 89, 173–181. doi: 10.1016/j.biosystems.2006.04.015

Hauptmann, C., and Tass, P. A. (2009). Cumulative and after-effects of short and weak coordinated reset stimulation—a modeling study. *J. Neural Eng.* 6:016004. doi: 10.1088/1741-2560/6/1/016004

Hodgkin, A., and Huxley, A. F. (1952). A quantitative description of membrane current and application to conduction and excitation. *J. Physiol.* 117, 500–544. doi: 10.1113/jphysiol.1952.sp004764

Kuramoto, Y. (1984). *Chemical Oscillations, Waves and Turbulence.* Berlin; Heidelberg; New York: Spinger.

Lenz, F. A., Kwan, H. C., Martin, R. L., Tasker, R. R., Dostrovsky, J. O., and Lenz, Y. E. (1994). Single unit analysis of the human ventral thalamic nuclear group. *Brain* 117, 531–543. doi: 10.1093/brain/117.3.531

Llinas, R. R., Ribary, U., Jeanmonod, D., Kronberg, E., and Mitra, P. P. (1999). Thalamocortical dysrhythmia: a neurological and neuropsychiatric syndrome characterized by magnetoencephalography. *Proc. Natl. Acad. Sci. U.S.A.* 96, 15222–15227. doi: 10.1073/pnas.96.26.15222

Lysyansky, B., Popovych, O. V., and Tass, P. A. (2011a). Desynchronizing anti-resonance effect of *m: n* ON-OFF coordinated reset stimulation. *J. Neural Eng.* 8:036019. doi: 10.1088/1741-2560/8/3/036019

Lysyansky, B., Popovych, O. V., and Tass, P. A. (2011b). Multi-frequency activation of neuronal networks by coordinated reset stimulation. *Interface Focus* 1, 75–85. doi: 10.1098/rsfs.2010.0010

Maistrenko, Y. L., Lysyansky, B., Hauptmann, C., Burylko, O., and Tass, P. A. (2007). Multistability in the Kuramoto model with synaptic plasticity. *Phys. Rev. E* 75:066207. doi: 10.1103/PhysRevE.75.066207

Markram, H., Lübke, J., Frotscher, M., and Sakmann, B. (1997). Regulation of synaptic efficacy by coincidence of postsynaptic Aps and EPSPs. *Science* 275, 213–215. doi: 10.1126/science.275.5297.213

Nini, A., Feingold, A., Slovin, H., and Bergman, I. (1995). Neurons in the globus pallidus do not show correlated activity in the normal monkey, but phase-locked oscillations appear in the MPTP model of Parkinsonsism. *J. Neurophysiol.* 74, 1800–1805.

Ochi, K., and Eggermont, J. J. (1997). Effects of quinine on neural activity in cat primary auditory cortex. *Hear. Res.* 105, 105–118. doi: 10.1016/S0378-5955(96)00201-8

Popovych, O., and Tass, P. A. (2012). Desynchronizing electrical and sensory coordinated reset modulation. *Front. Hum. Neurosci.* 6:58. doi: 10.3389/fnhum.2012.00058

Popovych, O., Xenakis, M., and Tass, P. A. (2015).The spacing principle for unlearning abnormal neuronal synchrony. *PLoS ONE* 10:e0117205. doi: 10.1371/journal.pone.0117205

Wong, R. K., Traub, R. D., and Miles, R. (1986). Cellular basis of neuronal synchrony in epilepsy. *Adv. Neurol.* 44, 583–592.

Schomer, D. L., and Lopes da Silva, F. H. (2010). *Niedermeyer's Electroencephalography. 6th Rev. Edn.* Philadelphia, PA: Lippincott Williams & Wilkins.

Silchenko, A. N., Adamchic, I., Hauptmann, C., and Tass, P. A. (2013). Impact of acoustic coordinated reset neuromodulation on effective connectivity in a neural network of phantom sound. *Neuroimage* 77, 133–147. doi: 10.1016/j.neuroimage.2013.03.013

Tass, P. A. (1999). *Phase Resetting in Medicine And Biology: Stochastic Modelling and Data Analysis.* Berlin: Springer.

Tass, P. A. (2003a). A model of desynchronizning deep brain stimulation with a demand-controlled coordinated reset of neural subpopulations. *Biol. Cybern.* 89, 81–88. doi: 10.1007/s00422-003-0425-7

Tass, P. A. (2003b). Desynchronization by means of a Coordinated Reset of neural sub-populations. *Prog. Theor. Phys. Suppl.* 150, 281–296. doi: 10.1143/PTPS.150.281

Tass, P. A., Adamchic, I., Freund, H. J., von Stackelberg, T., and Hauptmann, C. (2012b). Counteracting tinnitus by acoustic coordinated reset neuromodulation. *Restor. Neurol. Neurosci.* 30, 137–159. doi: 10.3233/RNN-2012-110218

Tass, P. A., and Hauptmann, C. (2006). Long-term anti-kindling effects induced by short-term, weak desynchronizing stimulation. *Nonl. Phen. Compl. Syst.* 9, 298–312.

Tass, P. A., and Hauptmann, C. (2007). Therapeutic modulation of synaptic connectivity with desynchronizing brain stimulation. *Int. J. Psychophysiol.* 64, 53–61. doi: 10.1016/j.ijpsycho.2006.07.013

Tass, P. A., and Hauptmann, C. (2009). Anti-kindling achieved by stimulation targeting slow synaptic dynamics. *Rest. Neurol. Neurosci.* 27, 589–609. doi: 10.3233/RNN-2009-0484

Tass, P. A., and Majtanik, M. (2006). Long-term anti-kindling effects of desynchronization brain stimulation: a theoretical study. *Biol. Cybern.* 94, 58–66. doi: 10.1007/s00422-005-0028-6

Tass, P. A., and Popovych, O. V. (2012). Unlearning tinnitus-related cerebral synchrony with acoustic coordinated reset stimulation—theoretical concept and modelling. *Biol. Cybern.* 106, 27–36. doi: 10.1007/s00422-012-0479-5

Tass, P. A., Qin, L., Hauptmann, C., Doveros, S., Bezard, E., Boraud, T., et al. (2012a). Coordinated reset neuromodulation has sustained effects in parkinsonian non-human primates. *Ann. Neurol.* 72, 816–820. doi: 10.1002/ana.23663

Tass, P. A., Silchenko, A. N., Barnikol, U., Hauptmann, C., and Speckmann, E. J. (2009). Long-lasting desynchronization in rat hippocampal slice induced by coordinated reset stimulation. *Phys. Rev. E* 80:011902. doi: 10.1103/PhysRevE.80.011902

Tukey, J. W. (1977). *Exploratory Data Analysis.* Reading; London: Addison-Wesley Publishing Company, Inc.

Weisz, N., Moratti, S., Meinzer, M., Dohrmann, K., and Elbert, T. (2005). Tinnitus perception and distress is related to abnormal spontaneous brain activity as measured by magnetoencephalography. *PLoS Med.* 2, 546–553. doi: 10.1371/journal.pmed.0020153

Wilson, H. R., and Cowan, J. D. (1973). A mathematical theory of the functional dynamics of cortical and thalamic nervous tissue. *Kybernetik* 13, 55–80. doi: 10.1007/BF00288786

12

Optimal feedback control successfully explains changes in neural modulations during experiments with brain-machine interfaces

Miri Benyamini and Miriam Zacksenhouse *

Brain-computer Interfaces for Rehabilitation Laboratory, Department of Mechanical Engineering, Technion - Israel Institute of Technology, Haifa, Israel

Edited by:
Manuel Fernando Casanova, University of Louisville, USA

Reviewed by:
Ferran Galán, Newcastle University, UK
Frédéric Crevecoeur, Queen's University, Canada
Yuki Ueyama, Research Institute of National Rehabilitation Center for Persons with Disabilities, Japan

***Correspondence:**
Miriam Zacksenhouse, Brain-computer interfaces for rehabilitation Laboratory, Department of Mechanical Engineering, Technion - Israel Institute of Technology, Haifa 32000, Israel
mermz@technion.ac.il

Recent experiments with brain-machine-interfaces (BMIs) indicate that the extent of neural modulations increased abruptly upon starting to operate the interface, and especially after the monkey stopped moving its hand. In contrast, neural modulations that are correlated with the kinematics of the movement remained relatively unchanged. Here we demonstrate that similar changes are produced by simulated neurons that encode the relevant signals generated by an optimal feedback controller during simulated BMI experiments. The optimal feedback controller relies on state estimation that integrates both visual and proprioceptive feedback with prior estimations from an internal model. The processing required for optimal state estimation and control were conducted in the state-space, and neural recording was simulated by modeling two populations of neurons that encode either only the estimated state or also the control signal. Spike counts were generated as realizations of doubly stochastic Poisson processes with linear tuning curves. The model successfully reconstructs the main features of the kinematics and neural activity during regular reaching movements. Most importantly, the activity of the simulated neurons successfully reproduces the observed changes in neural modulations upon switching to brain control. Further theoretical analysis and simulations indicate that increasing the process noise during normal reaching movement results in similar changes in neural modulations. Thus, we conclude that the observed changes in neural modulations during BMI experiments can be attributed to increasing process noise associated with the imperfect BMI filter, and, more directly, to the resulting increase in the variance of the encoded signals associated with state estimation and the required control signal.

Keywords: brain-machine interfaces, neural modulations, optimal feedback control, computational motor control, process noise

1. Introduction

Brain-Machine Interfaces (BMIs) have been developed to provide a direct communication link between the brain and external devices, bypassing the remaining, potentially injured neuro-muscular system (Nicolelis, 2001; Taylor et al., 2002; Lebedev et al., 2005). Additionally, BMIs provide a unique window into information representation and processing in the brain. In particular, it was observed that the extent of neural modulations (during BMI experiments reported in Carmena et al., 2003) increased abruptly upon starting to operate the interface, and especially after the monkey stopped moving its hand (Zacksenhouse et al., 2007). In contrast, neural modulations that are correlated with the movement kinematics remained relatively unchanged. Here we develop an optimal feedback control model (OFC) of BMI experiments to explain the observed changes in neural modulations and to investigate how they are related to changes in state estimation during brain control.

OFC was recently proposed as a viable model for motor control during reaching movements (Todorov and Jordan, 2002; Todorov, 2005; Shadmehr and Krakauer, 2008). While the term "optimal feedback control" emphasizes the optimality of the control gains given the cost function, the main component of interest here is optimal state estimation. This component is hypothesized to integrate visual and proprioceptive information with prior state estimation from an internal model to optimize the posterior state estimate (Miall and Wolpert, 1996; Wolpert and Ghahramani, 2000). The relative weights given to the sensory measurements versus the internal estimation depend on the relative variance of measurement and process noise, and, for linear systems corrupted by Gaussian noise, are determined by the Kalman filter (Schwartz, 2004; Stengel, 2012). The main hypothesis of this paper is that changes in process and measurement noise caused by the switch to brain control can explain the observed changes in neural modulations.

OFC is adopted here, instead of alternative computational motor control models, such as feedback error learning (Kawato et al., 1987), active inference (Friston et al., 2010, 2011) and distal teacher (Jordan and Rumelhart, 1992), for three main reasons. First, OFC does not require explicit specification of the desired trajectory of movement. While the desired trajectory can be assumed to follow the minimum jerk profile, its specification during brain control, when the initial stroke does not reach the target, is not straightforward. In contrast, OFC generates the trajectory implicitly, rather than following an externally specified trajectory. Secondly, the optimization inherent in OFC constrains the parameters of the state estimation filter and the control gains, so the model has fewer free parameters that need to be tuned. Thus, OFC provides a coherent and principled framework for investigating possible mechanisms underlying changes in neural modulations following the transition to brain control. Finally, OFC explicitly accounts for the variance of the process and measurement noise, which are assumed to change when switching to brain control, and thus is most appropriated for investigating how these mechanisms may contribute to the observed changes in neural modulations.

The processing required for optimal state estimation and control are conducted in the state-space. Neural recording is simulated by modeling two populations of neurons that encode the relevant signals, including either just the estimated state or also the resulting control signal. Thus, the approach presented here combines the dynamical perspective, which focuses on how the brain commands movements, with the representational perspective, which investigates what the neurons encode (Shenoy et al., 2013), by suggesting that they encode the signals that are relevant for the computations that underlie state estimation and control. The goal of this work is to investigate whether the resulting neural activity would produce the observed changes in neural modulations during BMI experiments.

The above OFC framework for investigating the changes in neural modulations during BMI experiments should be distinguished from recent applications of state estimation (Schwartz, 2004; Wu et al., 2006; Cunningham et al., 2011) and OFC (Shanechi et al., 2013a,b) to improve neural decoders for BMIs. BMI decoders estimate the state by integrating the observed neural activity, which is assumed to encode the state of the movement, with a presumed or learned model of reaching movement dynamics. Advanced models (Shanechi et al., 2013a,b) account for the effect of the control signal generated by the brain on the movement dynamics by modeling the sensory motor system in the brain as OFC. However, since the focus of such models is the BMI decoder, the brain is assumed to know the actual state of the movement via noise-free sensory measurements, thereby eliminating the need for state estimation. In contrast, our focus is on state estimation in the brain, which is assumed to integrate noisy visual and proprioception observations with an internal model of movement dynamics (Miall and Wolpert, 1996; Wolpert and Ghahramani, 2000), and how the changes in sensory and process noise affect those estimations and the resulting neural activity.

In summary, this work investigates the hypothesis that the observed changes in neural modulations following the transition to brain control can be explained in the context of OFC model of motor control. We hypothesize that neurons in cortical motor areas, and in particular in primary motor area, M1, and premotor dorsal, PMd, encode the relevant signals for OFC of reaching movements, i.e., the estimated state and the resulting control signal, as depicted in **Figure 1**. Thus, the observed changes in neural rate modulations are hypothesized to reflect corresponding changes in the variance of these signals. Furthermore, we hypothesize that the increase in the variance of the estimated state and control signal is due to the higher process noise during brain control caused by the imperfect BMI filter. These hypotheses are investigated in three levels: (i) simulations of pole control and brain control, and evaluation of the corresponding changes in neural modulations (Section 3.2), (ii) theoretical analysis of the effect of increasing process noise during pole control (Section 2.4), and (iii) simulations of the effect of increasing process noise on neural modulations during pole control (Section 3.3). Other aspects of the model are investigated in Sections 3.1, 3.4–3.6.

2. Materials and Methods

2.1. Experimental Methods

The proposed model is evaluated by comparing the different properties of the simulated neural activity to those observed during the BMI experiments described in Carmena et al. (2003). The BMI experiments were conducted with macaque monkeys whose goal was to move the cursor to randomly appearing

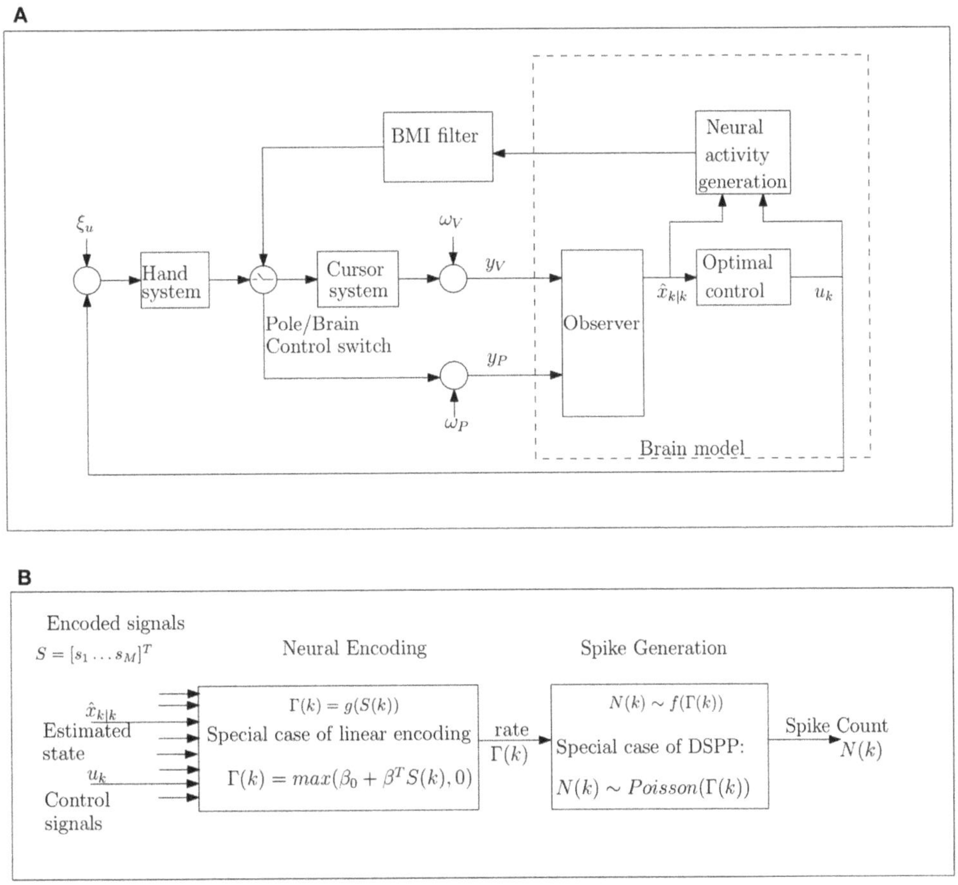

FIGURE 1 | Schematic model of movement control during BMI experiments under the hypothesis that the brain implements OFC (A), and detailed block diagram of neural activity generation (B). **(A)** The brain model receives noisy proprioceptive (y_P) and visual (y_C) measurements from the hand and cursor, corrupted by proprioceptive and visual measurement noise, ω_P and ω_V, respectively. These noisy measurements are integrated with prior predictions from the internal model to generate optimal state estimates $\hat{x}_{k|k}$ and control signal u_k, which are encoded by the neural activity. The control signal is corrupted by hand process noise ξ_u. The BMI filter is trained based on the neural activity in pole control and then used to move the cursor in brain control. **(B)** The cumulative bin rate, $\Gamma(k)$, at time step k, is modulated by the encoded signals $S = \left[s_1, \ \cdots \ , s_M\right]^T$ including the estimated state $\hat{x}_{k|k}$ and control signals u_k. The spike-count $N(k)$ is generated as a doubly stochastic Point process given the rate parameter $\Gamma(k)$. Here we consider the special case of linear encoding, where $\Gamma(k)$ is a linear combination of the encoded signals (including the estimated speed and the magnitude of the control signal), and doubly stochastic Poisson processes (DSPP), where the spike count $N(k)$ has a Poisson distribution with rate $\Gamma(k)$.

targets and hold the cursor on the target for 150 ms to accept a juice reward. Each experiment included three control modes: (i) pole control during which the monkey controlled the cursor using hand-held pole, (ii) brain control with hand movements (BCWHM), during which the cursor was controlled by the output of the BMI interface while the monkey continued moving the pole and (iii) brain control without hand movements (BCWOHM), during which the cursor was controlled by the BMI interface even though the monkey stopped moving the pole.

Neural activity was recorded from multiple brain area, but mostly from the primary motor area (M1) and the dorsal premotor area (PMd). The BMI interface binned the recorded spike trains in 100 ms bins, to generate the input to a linear filter. The linear BMI filter was trained with data recorded during the last 10 min of pole control, and held fixed during brain control.

2.2. Analysis Methods

2.2.1. Percent Overall Modulations

Spike-trains can be considered as realizations of point processes (Johnson, 1996). The number of spikes recorded in a bin, N, depends on the cumulative spike-rate during the bin, Γ (Zacksenhouse et al., 2007), which can be modulated by the encoded signals as outlined in **Figure 1B**. Since this dependence is stochastic, the variance of the spike-count $var(N)$ is higher than the variance of the cumulative spike-rate $var(\Gamma)$ (Zacksenhouse et al., 2007). While the variance of the spike-count can be measured directly, it is the variance of the cumulative spike-rate that captures the effect of the encoded signals on rate modulations. In order to quantify these rate modulations, the percent overall modulation (POM) is defined as Zacksenhouse et al. (2007)

$$POM = \frac{var[\Gamma]}{var[N]} \cdot 100\% \quad (1)$$

Since the variance of the bin-rate cannot be measured directly, the POM cannot be estimated without further assumptions. Consider first the simplest point process that can describe stochastic rate modulations, i.e., the doubly stochastic Poisson processes (DSPP), for which Snyder (1975), Zacksenhouse et al. (2007)

$$\begin{aligned} E(N_{DSPP}) &= E(\Gamma) \\ Var(N_{DSPP}) &= var(\Gamma) + E(\Gamma) \end{aligned} \quad (2)$$

In this case, the POM can be estimated form the mean and variance of the spike count as

$$\hat{POM}[N] = \frac{var[N] - E[N]}{var[N]} \cdot 100\% \quad (3)$$

where $\hat{POM}$ denotes the estimated POM. When applied to the analysis of spike trains recorded during BMI experiments, we assume that the movement is composed of an asynchronous sequence of reaching movements (Zacksenhouse et al., 2014) so the cumulative spike-rate and the binned spike-counts are stationary processes. Hence, the POM is estimated from Equation (3) using the temporal mean and variance rather than ensemble mean and variance.

In the general case of doubly stochastic Point processes (not necessarily Poisson distributed), the variance of the spike-counts can be decomposed into Churchland et al. (2011)

$$var(N) = var[E[N|\Gamma]] + E[var[N|\Gamma]] \quad (4)$$

The first term on the right reflects the variance of the cumulative spike-rate Γ, though is equal to it only for DSPPs. The second term can be interpreted as the Point process noise, since it contributes to the variance of the spike-counts even if Γ is constant. While this term equals the mean rate only for DSPPs, evidence suggests that in many cases it is proportional to the mean rate (Tolhurst et al., 1983; Geisler and Albrecht, 1995), i.e., $var[N|\Gamma] = \gamma E[N|\Gamma], (\gamma > 0)$ and hence $E[var[N|\Gamma]] = \gamma E[N]$. Hence, a revised definition of POM quantifies the ratio between the first term on the right, which reflects the variance of the cumulative spike-rate Γ, and the total variance in the spike counts

$$POM_{REV}(N) = \frac{var[E[N|\Gamma]]}{var(N)} \cdot 100\% \quad (5)$$

This can be related to the POM estimated by Equation (3) by inserting the expression for the point process noise in Equation (4) and Equation (5) to get

$$\hat{POM}_{REV}(N) = \frac{var[N] - \gamma E[N]}{var(N)} \cdot 100\% = (\gamma \hat{POM} - (1-\gamma)) \cdot 100\% \quad (6)$$

Thus, changes in the POM estimated by Equation (3) reflect proportional changes in the revised POM of Equation (5) up to a positive scaling and positive or negative offset. Having established this connection, the revised POM will not be used any further.

All the POM results described in Section 3 and shown in the Figures are $\hat{POM}$ (Equation 3), estimated from temporal statistics, while the theoretical analysis in Section 2.4 is based on the definition of POM in Equation (1).

2.2.2. Percent Kinematics Modulations

Numerous studies suggested that the neural activity can be related to the kinematics of the movement, including position, velocity and speed, via a linear model (Georgopoulos et al., 1986; Ashe and Georgopoulos, 1994; Moran and Schwartz, 1999; Todorov, 2000; Zacksenhouse and Nemets, 2008; Chang et al., 2014)

$$\begin{aligned} N(k) = &\sum_{l=-L_1}^{L_2} \omega_{p_{cx}}(l) p_{cx}(k+l) + \sum_{l=-L_1}^{L_2} \omega_{p_{cy}}(l) p_{cy}(k+l) \quad (7) \\ &+ \sum_{l=-L_1}^{L_2} \omega_{v_{cx}}(l) v_{cx}(k+l) + \sum_{l=-L_1}^{L_2} \omega_{v_{cy}}(l) v_{cy}(k+l) \\ &+ \sum_{l=-L_1}^{L_2} \omega_S(l) S_{pc}(k+l) + \omega_0 + \epsilon(k) \end{aligned}$$

where k is the index of the current bin, $N(k)$ is the binned spike count, p_{cx} and p_{cy} are the x and y components of the cursor position, v_{cx} and v_{cy} are the x and y components of the cursor velocity, $S_{pc} = \sqrt[2]{v_{cx}^2 + v_{cy}^2}$ is the cursor's speed, l is the relative lag, L_1 and L_2 are the number of preceding and succeeding lags, $\omega_{p_{cx}}$, $\omega_{p_{cy}}$, $\omega_{v_{cx}}$, $\omega_{v_{cy}}$ and ω_S are the corresponding regression weights, ω_0 is the bias parameters and $\epsilon(k)$ is the residual error.

The coefficient of determination of the spatio-temporal regression, R^2, describes the fraction of the variance in the binned spike-count that is linearly related to variations in the temporal profile of the kinematic signals in the surrounding temporal window. Expressed as a percentage, R^2 is referred to as the percent kinematic-related modulation, or PKM (Zacksenhouse et al., 2007).The PKM results reported here are computed with $L1 = L2 = 9$.

2.3. Modeling methods

The simplifying assumptions on which the proposed OFC model for BMI experiments is based are explicitly stated in Section 2.3.1. As depicted in **Figure 1A**, the model includes three main parts: (1) Hand and cursor model, (2) Brain model, and (3) BMI filter, as briefly explained in Sections 2.3.2–2.3.5, and detailed in Appendices A and B. Model parameters are detailed in Section 2.3.6, and the effect of process noise in pole control is investigated in Section 2.3.7.

2.3.1. Simplifying Assumptions

The goal of this work is to construct a simple model that can capture the observed abrupt changes in neural modulations following the transition to brain control, and to assess if those changes can be attributed to increasing process and measurement noise. Hence, within the framework of OFC (Todorov and Jordan, 2002; Todorov, 2005; Shadmehr and Krakauer, 2008) we made the following simplifying assumptions (SA):

SA1: Absolute delays are ignored, thought the relative time-shift between the command to the muscle and the force it produces is captured by a second order muscle model (Section 2.3.2). Thus, the model successfully reproduces the observed time-lag in the cross-correlation between the neural activity and the movement velocity (Lebedev et al., 2005) as detailed in Section 3.1. The effect of sensory delays on movement variability and bias can be accounted for by sensory noise, at least when the perturbations are not abrupt (Todorov and Jordan, 2002; Crevecoeur and Scott, 2013).

SA2: The process noise during pole control is assumed to be signal independent white Gaussian noise. This assumption is justified since the resulting velocity profile agrees well with the commonly observed minimum jerk velocity profile (Flash and Hogan, 1985). While evidence suggests that the variance of the process noise increases with the control signal (Harris and Wolpert, 1998; Wolpert and Ghahramani, 2000), this was not modeled in order to focus on the effect of brain control on process noise and neural modulations.

SA3: The internal forward model is assumed to be identical to the actual hand and cursor system in pole control. Adaptation to brain control is ignored since the focus is on the abrupt changes in neural modulations immediately after the transition to brain control. Adaptation is expected to be important in explaining the subsequent gradual decrease in neural modulations with BMI sessions (Zacksenhouse et al., 2007), and will be explored in future work.

SA4: Spike counts are generated as realization of doubly stochastic Poisson process with linear tuning curves (as detailed in Section 2.3.4) (Zacksenhouse and Nemets, 2008; Cunningham et al., 2011; Chang et al., 2014).

2.3.2. Simplified Hand and Cursor Model

Following Todorov (2005) the hand is modeled as a point mass driven by an over damped second order muscle model that responds to the control signal from the brain. An additional friction term is introduced to model the friction of the hand held pole, as described by Equation (A2) in Supplementary Material.

As in the BMI experiments (Carmena et al., 2003), the cursor position during brain control is generated by integrating the velocity predicted by the BMI interface and filtering it with a high pass filter (HPF) to remove low frequency drifts, as described by Equation (A7) in Supplementary Material. During pole control, the cursor position is determined in the same way, using the actual hand velocity instead of the predicted velocity.

The simulation is updated at 100 Hz, and the discrete dynamics of the combined system, including the hand, cursor and target along a single degree of freedom, can be expressed as (see Equation A10 in Supplementary Material)

$$x(k+1) = Ax(k) + B_u u(k) + B_{BMI} v_{BMI}(k) + \xi_p(k) \quad (8)$$

where x is the combined state (specified by Equation A9 in Supplementary Material), A, B_u, and B_{BMI} are the matrices describing the system dynamics, the effect of the control signal u generated by the optimal feedback controller implemented by the brain, and the integration of the velocity predictions v_{BMI} during brain control, respectively, as detailed in Equations (A11–A13 in Supplementary Material). The 2-degrees of freedom simulations are performed by evolving two independent systems for the x and y directions, respectively.

During normal simulations of pole and brain control, the process noise, ξ_p, stems only from the noise in the control signal ξ_u (Equation A3 in Supplementary Material), i.e., $\xi_p = B_u \xi_u$. Under assumption SA2, ξ_u is a white Gaussian noise, whose variance (note that in the single dimension case ξ_u is a scalar) is denoted by α_u^2. Hence the covariance matrix of the process noise can be expressed as

$$\Omega^p = \alpha_u^2 B_u B_u' \quad (9)$$

The position and velocity of the cursor are measured via visual (V) feedback, while the position and velocity of the hand are measured via proprioceptive (P) feedback. Both visual and proprioceptive measurements are assumed to be corrupted by zero mean white Gaussian measurement noise and the covariance matrix of the combined measurement is denoted by Ω^m.

2.3.3. Brain Model

Following current computational motor control theories, the brain is assumed to implement optimal state estimation and feedback control (Kuo, 1995; Wolpert et al., 1995; Todorov and Jordan, 2002). However, for simplicity, the computations are performed in the state space, rather than their neural representations. Neural recording is simulated by modeling neurons that encode the relevant signals including the estimated state and control signal (as detailed in Section 2.3.4). The brain model includes three parts as depicted in **Figure 1A** and further detailed in Appendix B (Supplementary Materials)(first two parts) and Section 2.3.4 (third part):

A: Observer that implements optimal state estimation by integrating the sensory feedback and internal model predictions. Under assumption (SA2), optimal estimation is achieved with Kalman filter (Wolpert et al., 1995; Stengel, 2012), as specified in Equation (B1 in Supplementary Material). During simulations of normal reaching movements (pole control) the internal model is assumed to be accurate and the Kalman filter is based on the actual covariance matrices of the process and measurements noise. By assumption (SA3), the same covariance matrices are also used for computing the Kalman filter when simulating brain control.

B: Optimal controller that, under assumption (SA2), reduces to Linear Quadratic Gaussian (LQG) controller (Stengel, 2012), as specified in Equations (B5–B8 in Supplementary Material). The controller gains were computed off-line to minimize a standard cost function that includes penalty for the control effort and for deviations from the target, as specified in Equations (B2–B4 in Supplementary Material) (Kuo, 1995; Wolpert et al., 1995; Todorov and Jordan, 2002).

C: Neural activity generator that converts the relevant signals i.e., the internally estimated cursor state and the control signal, into neural activity of a population of N_n simulated neurons using linear multi-variable tuning functions (as detailed in Section 2.3.4). This population of neurons simulates the population of neurons recorded during the BMI experiments, so their activity is used to train and drive the BMI filter during simulated pole and brain control, respectively, as detailed in 2.3.5. By assumption (SA4), spike-counts are generated as realizations of *doubly stochastic* Poisson processes.

2.3.4. Neural Activity Generator

Many studies (Georgopoulos et al., 1986; Moran and Schwartz, 1999) demonstrated that during reaching movements the neural activity is linearly correlated with several motor parameters, including hand position, velocity, speed and gripping force. One of the main hypotheses in this work is that the neurons encode the estimated state and control signal, and that the observed correlations with the above motor parameters result from this encoding. Since we are interested in the statistics of the binned spike-count (in bins of 100 ms), we generate the binned spike-counts directly (instead of simulating the spike-train, and then binning the data). As outlined in **Figure 1B**, the binned spike-counts of each neuron are generated as a realization of a DSPP (Johnson, 1996; Dayan and Abbott, 2001) whose cumulative rate Γ is a linear function of the encoded signals. Specifically, the cumulative spike-rate of neuron i during the k-th bin, $\Gamma^i(k)$, is given by

$$\Gamma^i(k) = max(\beta_{i,0} + \beta_i^T S(k), 0) \tag{10}$$

where $S(k)$ is the vector of encoded signals at time step k, $\beta_{i,0}$ is the bias of neuron $i = 1 \ldots N_n$ and β_i is the vector of its tuning weights.

Since the monkey is rewarded when the cursor is at the target, independent of the position of the hand, we assume that only the estimated cursor-state is encoded. Thus, the vector of encoded signals

$$S = \begin{bmatrix} \hat{p}_{cx} & \hat{p}_{cy} & \hat{v}_{cx} & \hat{v}_{cy} & \hat{S}_p & u_x & u_y & u_e \end{bmatrix}' \tag{11}$$

includes three 2-dimensional vectors: the estimated cursor position $\hat{p} = \begin{bmatrix} \hat{p}_{cx} & \hat{p}_{cy} \end{bmatrix}'$ velocity $\hat{v} = \begin{bmatrix} \hat{v}_{cx} & \hat{v}_{cy} \end{bmatrix}'$, and control signal $u = \begin{bmatrix} u_x & u_y \end{bmatrix}'$, and the magnitude of the last two (estimated speed $\hat{S}_p = ||\hat{v}||$ and control effort $u_e = ||u||$). The representation of the speed of movement in the neural activity, beyond the representation of the velocity vector, is well documented (Moran and Schwartz, 1999), and here we assume it reflects the encoding of the estimated speed $\hat{S}_p$. Similarity, we assume that the magnitude of the control signal u_e is also encoded.

The tuning weights β_i to the kinematic parameters (position, velocity and speed) were selected to obtain PKM levels similar to the PKM observed in the BMI experiments during pole control. Specifically, the tuning weights for each kinematic parameter were selected from a uniform distribution whose variance was proportional to the destined PKM associated with that kinematic parameter and inversely proportionally to its variance. The tuning weights for the control signal were also selected from a uniform distribution, but its variance was adjusted to get the proper time-shift in the cross-correlation between the neural activity and the velocity, which are described in Section 3.1. The tuning vectors for the position, velocity and control parameters define the respective, and in general different, preferred directions (PD) and modulation depths.

The literature on cortical motor units suggests that neurons in different areas in the brain encode different information.The activity of M1 neurons has been shown to correlate with both the kinematics, including velocity, speed and direction of movement (Georgopoulos et al., 1982; Ashe and Georgopoulos, 1994) and with the applied forces (Evarts, 1968; Ashe, 1997; Todorov, 2000). PMd neurons are modulated mainly by the direction and amplitude of the movement (Messier and Kalaska, 2000; Hendrix et al., 2009). In agreement with those studies, the activity of M1 units recorded during the BMI experiments considered here were shown to predict well hand position, velocity and gripping force (73, 66, and 83% of variance, respectively), while the activity of the recorded PMd units predicted well hand position and velocity (48 and 46% of variance, respectively), but not the gripping force (29% of variance) (Carmena et al., 2003). Considering the above evidence, we simulate the activity of two sub-populations of neurons encoding either: (i) only the estimated cursor state (position, velocity and speed), or (ii) both the estimated cursor state and the control signal (vector and magnitude). Based on the evidence in the literature, we expect that the behavior of simulated neurons in those two sub-populations would be similar to the behavior of recorded PMd and M1 units, respectively, and hence refer to them as PMd-like and M1-like neurons. Such similarities are demonstrated in Section 3.1, where the cross-correlations between the movement velocity and either the recorded or simulated neural activity are compared.

2.3.5. BMI Filter

As in the BMI experiments (Carmena et al., 2003), the velocity in simulated brain control was predicted from the simulated spike-counts by a linear multi-lag multi-variable BMI filter

$$v_{BMI}(k) = \theta_0 + \sum_{j=1}^{N_n} \sum_{l=-L}^{0} \theta_j(l) N_j(k+l) \tag{12}$$

where N_n is the number of simulated neurons, $L = 10$ the number of lags used for prediction and $N_j(k)$ the spike count of neuron j in bin k. The filter parameters θ_0 and $\theta_j(l)$, (where l is the index of the lag) were computed using truncated Singular Value Decomposition (Zacksenhouse et al., 2007). Two BMI filters were trained to reconstruct the velocity in x and y, respectively, using the last 10 min of simulated pole control.

The performance of the experimental BMI filter (similarly trained on the last 10 min of pole control) was assessed by testing its predictions on a different section of pole control and was quantified by a coefficient of correlation of $R(\hat{v}, v) = 0.755 \pm 0.02$. We expect that this imperfect performance is critical for generating the observed changes in neural modulations. Hence, this performance served as a benchmark for tuning the number of neurons and the process noise in the simulation to obtain a similar performance (as detailed in Section 2.3.6).

2.3.6. Model Parameters

Model parameters are detailed in **Table 1**. The basic parameters of the hand model, visual measurement noise and cost function were taken from Todorov (2005) as noted in **Table 1**. The basic hand model was extended with a friction term to model the friction of the hand held pole. The basic cost function was augmented to describe the requirement for holding the cursor on the target as described in Appendix B (Equations B2–B4 in Supplementary Material) using the same weight parameters. The reaching time t_f (in Supplementary Equation B3) is uniformly distributed between 1.7-2.2 s in pole control and 2.4-6 s in brain control.

As detailed in our simplifying assumption SA2, the process noise during pole control is assumed to be signal independent, and its magnitude is quantified by of α_u in Equation (9). Initial simulations revealed that the performance of the experimental BMI filter, quantified by $R(\hat{v}, v)$ (Section 2.3.5), is highly sensitive to the process noise during simulated pole control, as shown in **Figures 2A,B**. The magnitude of the process noise was normalized by the equivalent signal-independent process noise suggested in Todorov (2005), signal-independent process noise suggested in the process noise factor defined as $k_u = \frac{\alpha_u}{4.6N}$. **Figures 2A,C** also depicts the effect of the total number of simulated neurons N_n on $R(\hat{v}, v)$, while the ratio between the two populations of simulated neurons, the M1-like and PMd-like neurons, was kept constant (1:1). The results in **Figure 2** are based on 15 simulated sessions of 20 min pole control, each with a different, randomly selected targets, but all with the same set of neural tuning weights. In each session the coefficient of correlation between the actual and predicted velocity $R(\hat{v}, v)$ was computed from the first 10 min, while training was conducted on the last non-overlapping 10 min. Each data point and error bar (in (B-C)) depict the average and standard deviation of $R(\hat{v}, v)$ across the 15 sessions. **Figure 2** suggests that with $N_n = 50$ and $k_u = 0.1$ the average performance of the BMI filter trained on simulated activity is $R(\hat{v}, v) = 0.77$, close to the observed BMI filter performance. Hence, these are the default values used in all other standard simulations as indicated in **Table 1**.

While proprioceptive measurement noise has little effect on $R(\hat{v}, v)$ it has significant effect on the resulting changes in neural modulations. This effect is investigated in Section 3.5 and motivated the selection of a common 10-fold factor between the diagonal covariance matrices of the proprioceptive and visual measurements noise, as specified in **Table 1**. This proprioceptive noise factor, denoted by k_m, was used during simulations of pole control and BCWHM, while during simulations of BCWOHM it was increased to infinity to reflect the lack of relevant proprioception measurements in this mode.

2.3.7. Effect of Process Noise

Following our primary hypothesis that the observed changes in neural modulations can be explained in the framework OFC, we further hypothesize that these changes result from the higher process noise generated by the imperfect BMI filter that reconstructs the cursor velocity. This hypothesis is investigated both by simulations of noisy pole control, as outlined here, and by theoretical analysis in Section 2.4. Noisy pole control is simulated by using Equation (8) with the matrices associated with pole control (Equations A11–A13 in Supplementary Material), but with process noise that includes also the simulated effect of the BMI filter reconstruction error (as further explained in Appendix A2, Supplementary Material). Thus, instead of Equation (9) the covariance matrix of the process noise during noisy pole control simulations is

$$\Omega^{p}_{noisy} = \alpha_u^2 B_u B_u' + \alpha_{rec}^2 B_{BMI} B_{BMI}' \tag{13}$$

TABLE 1 | Model Parameters table.

Parameter	Description	Value	References
Δ	Discretization time of the hand model	0.01[s]	Todorov, 2005
m	Hand mass	1[kg]	Todorov, 2005
γ	Coefficient of friction	$7.7[\frac{kg}{s}]$	-
τ	Time constant of the muscle model	0.04[s]	Todorov, 2005
w_v	Velocity cost function weight	0.2	Todorov, 2005
w_f	Energy cost function weight	0.02	Todorov, 2005
t_f	Reaching time in pole control (range)	1.7 – 2.2[s]	Carmena et al., 2003
t_f	Reaching time in brain control (range)	2.4 – 6[s]	Carmena et al., 2003
σ^2_{Vp}	Variance of the visual (V) position measurement noise	$(0.01\text{m})^2$	Todorov, 2005
σ^2_{Vv}	Variance of the visual (V) velocity measurement noise	$(0.1\frac{m}{s})^2$	Todorov, 2005
σ^2_{Pp}	Variance of the proprioception (P) position measurement noise	$k_m(0.01\text{m})^2$	Section 2.3.6/3.5
σ^2_{Pv}	Variance of the proprioception (P) velocity measurement noise	$k_m(0.1\frac{m}{s})^2$	Section 2.3.6/3.5
k_m	Proprioception measurement noise factor	10	Section 2.3.6/3.5
α_u	Magnitude of the hand process noise	$k_u \cdot (4.6[N])$	Section 2.3.6
k_u	Hand process noise factor	0.1	Section 2.3.6
N_n	Number of neurons	50	Section 2.3.6
T	Bin size	0.1[s]	Carmena et al., 2003

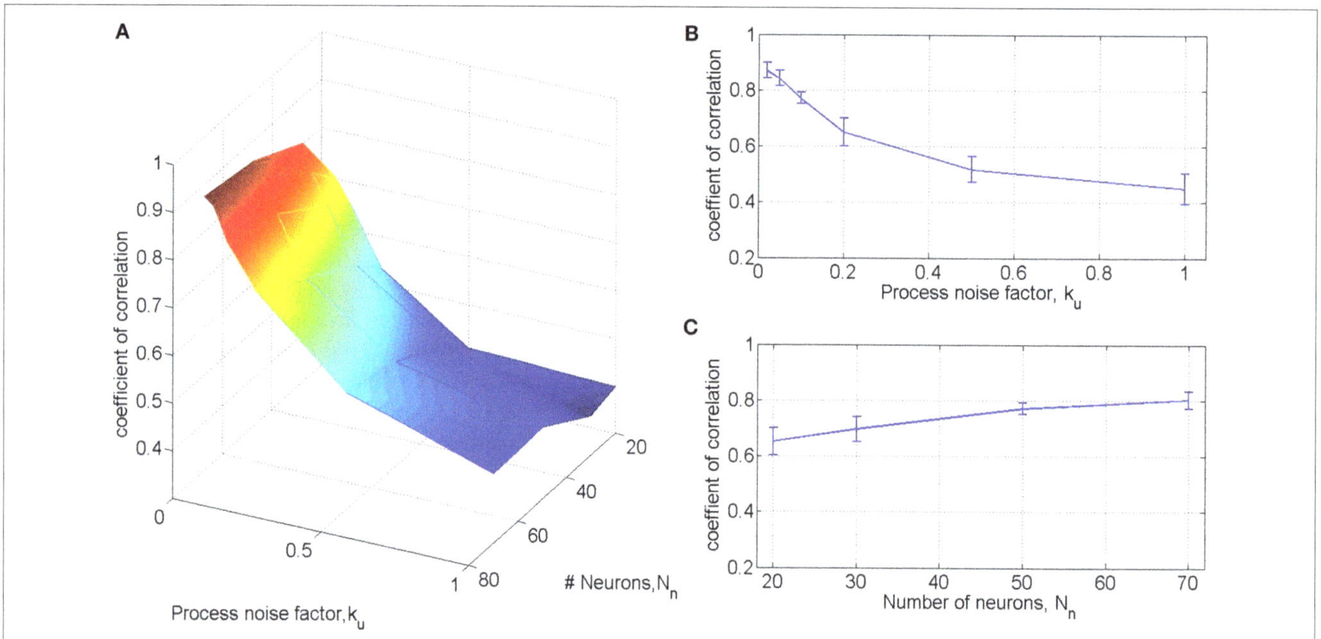

FIGURE 2 | BMI filter performance as a function of the number of neurons and the process noise factor. Results are based on 15 simulated sessions of 20 min pole control, each with a different, randomly selected targets, but all with the same set of neural tuning weights. In each session the BMI filter was trained on the last 10 min and its performance was quantified by the coefficient of correlation between the actual and predicted velocity in the first 10 min. Each data point and error bar (in **B,C**) depict the average and standard deviation of the coefficient of correlations across the 15 sessions for a specific process noise factor k_u and total number of neurons N_n. The effect of k_u is evaluated with $N_n = 50$ **(B)**, while the effect of N_n is evaluated with $k_u = 0.1$ **(C)**. A fixed 1:1 ratio is kept between the M1-like and PMd-like simulated neurons.

The first term represents the contribution of the noise in the control signal, and is the same as during regular pole control (Equation 9). The second term represents the additional noise introduced by the imperfect BMI filter, and its magnitude is quantified by α_{rec}. The effect of varying the magnitude α_{rec} on neural modulations is investigated in Section 3.4.

2.4. Theoretical Analysis of POM

As detailed in Section 2.3.7, we hypothesize that the observed changes in neural modulations following the transition to brain control result from the higher process noise introduced by the imperfect BMI filter. Here we investigate theoretically the effect of increasing process noise during simulations of normal reaching movements on POM defined theoretically in Equation (1), and show that under the assumptions of linear decoding and invariant internal model (see theoretical assumptions 1 and 2 below), the POM indeed increases with the process noise. The covariance matrix of the process noise, Ω^p, is assumed to increase from a nominal low level Ω^p_L to a high level Ω^p_H such that the difference $\Omega^p_H - \Omega^p_L$ is positive semi-definite (psd) (Horn and Johnson, 2012) and is denoted by $\Omega^p_H - \Omega^p_L \succcurlyeq 0$ or equivalently by $\Omega^p_H \succcurlyeq \Omega^p_L$. Note that this analysis is general and does not rely on the specific structures of Ω^p_L and Ω^p_H suggested by Equations (9, 13), respectively.

We make the following simplifying theoretical assumptions (TA):

TA1: The cumulative spike-rate Γ encodes a linear combination of the estimated state. Since the optimal control signal is proportional to the estimated state, this includes also the control signal. However, non-linear functions, and in particular the estimated speed $\hat{S}_p$ and the magnitude of the control effort u_e, which are included in Equation (11), are not considered here.

TA2: The internal model of the process noise does not change. This assumption follows directly from the simplifying assumption (SA3) that there is no adaptation to brain control.

Within the framework of state estimation and OFC, (TA1) implies that Γ can be expressed as the output of an extended linear system whose state $\tilde{x} = \begin{bmatrix} x_k & \hat{x}_{k|k} & 1 \end{bmatrix}^T$ includes both the actual and estimated states (of the hand and cursor). Following the details in Equations (C2–C5 in Supplementary Material), the extended system can be described as:

$$\tilde{x}_k = \tilde{A}_k \tilde{x}_{k-1} + \tilde{\xi}_k \qquad (14)$$
$$\Gamma_k = \tilde{H}_k \tilde{x}_k$$

where $\tilde{\xi}$ is the process noise of the extended system, which captures both the process noise of the actual system and the estimation error (Equation C4 in Supplementary Material). Since both are assumed to be white Gaussian noise, so is $\tilde{\xi}$, and its covariance matrix $E[\tilde{\xi}_i \tilde{\xi}_j] = \Omega^{\tilde{p}}_i \delta_{ij}$ is given by (see Equation C6 in Supplementary Material):

$$\Omega_k^{\tilde{p}} = \begin{bmatrix} \Omega_k^p & 0 & 0 \\ 0 & K_{k+1}H\Omega_k^p H^T K_{k+1}^T + K_{k+1}\Omega^m K_{k+1}^T & 0 \\ 0 & 0 & 0 \end{bmatrix} \quad (15)$$

Given (TA2), the Kalman gains K_k are optimized for the nominal system with the low process noise and are not updated to reflect the higher process noise.

Proposition: Let Γ_k^L and Γ_k^H be the outputs of two systems described by Equations (14,15) with the same parameters except for the process noise that is either Ω_L^p or Ω_H^p, respectively, where $\Omega_H^p \succcurlyeq \Omega_L^p$. Let POM^L and POM^H be the POM (Equation 1) of the resulting spike counts generated by DSPPs from Γ_k^L and Γ_k^H, respectively, then $POM^H \geq POM^L$.

Proof: Proposition C1 in Appendix C (Supplementary Material) proves that under the conditions of the proposition, the cumulative spike-rates Γ_k^L and Γ_k^H satisfy two conditions: (i) $E_m[\Gamma_k^L] = E_m[\Gamma_k^H]$ and (ii) $E_m[(\Gamma_k^H)^2] \geq E_m[(\Gamma_k^L)^2]$, where $E_m[\cdot]$ denotes ensemble average over different movements starting from the same distribution of initial conditions. Proposition C2 indicates that those two conditions assure that the POMs of the spike counts generated by DSPPs from Γ_k^L and Γ_k^H, i.e., POM^L and POM^H, respectively, satisfy $POM^H \geq POM^L$.

3. Results

The OFC model detailed in Section 2.3 was used to simulate 60 min sessions of BMI experiments equally divided into pole control, BCWHM and BCWOHM. Unless otherwise specified, new neural tuning weights and targets were randomly generated (as detailed in Sections 2.3.4 and 2.3.6) for each session. Since the performance of the BMI filter, quantified by $R(\hat{v}, v)$ (see Sections 2.3.5, 2.3.6), depends on the specific set of the neural tuning weights, only simulated sessions for which $R(\hat{v}, v)$ was between 0.65 and 0.85 were considered for further analysis (as further detailed in Section 3.2).

Simulated reaching movements under pole control resulted in an average speed profile that agrees well with the expected minimum jerk velocity profile (Flash and Hogan, 1985). Representative traces of the cursor during simulated pole control and BCWHM are shown in **Figure 3**. In order to facilitate comparison, the same sets of targets and desired reaching times were used. While in both phases the depicted traces reach the targets, they differ considerably, and are more variable in simulated BCWHM than in simulated pole control. In particular, the variance of the velocity (estimated over 2 min intervals) is significantly higher in simulated BCWHM than in simulated pole control (Wilcoxon rank sum test, $p < 0.0001$). This reproduces well the significant increase in the variance of the velocity from the experimental pole control to experimental BCWHM (Wilcoxon rank sum test, $p < 0.0002$).

The resulting cross correlations between the cursor velocity and neural activity generated during simulated pole control are investigated in Section 3.1 and compared with the cross-correlations derived from the BMI experiments. The main results regarding the changes in neural modulations are reported in Section 3.2. In Section 3.3 we investigate the effect of process noise on neural modulations during pole control, to support our hypothesis that increasing process noise introduced by the imperfect BMI filter contributes to the observed changes in neural modulations in brain control. Sections 3.4 and 3.5 evaluate the effect of the baseline measurement and process noise on estimated POM, respectively, and Section 3.6 investigates the effect of imperfect internal model. The $\hat{POM}$ results described in this section and shown in the Figures were estimated from temporal statistics as detailed in Section 2.2.1 using Equation (3).

3.1. Cross Correlation between Cursor Velocity and Neural Activity

The average cross correlations between the recorded cursor velocity and the recorded neural activity of either PMd

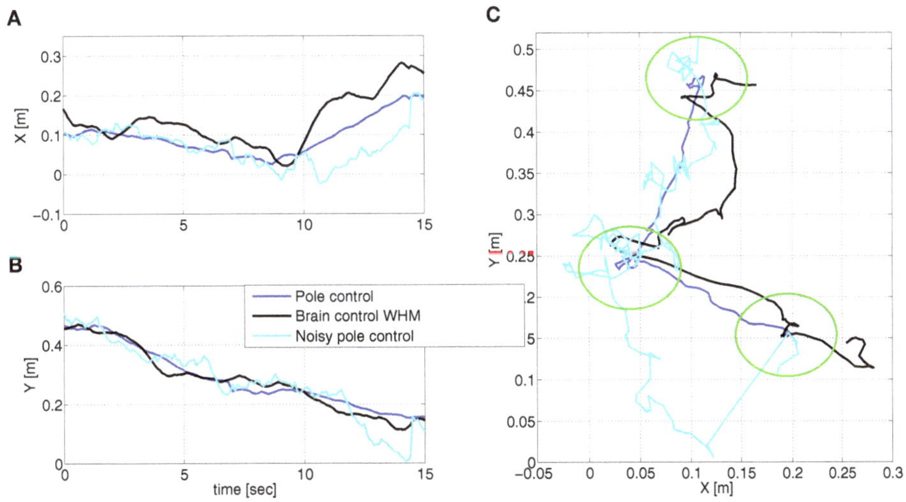

FIGURE 3 | Movement trajectories. Representative traces of the cursor during simulated pole control, brain control and noisy pole control (with $\alpha_{rec} = 0.035$). To facilitate comparison, the same set of targets (marked by green circles) and desired reaching times was used in these three simulations.

(**Figure 4A**) or M1 units (**Figure 4B**), demonstrate different temporal relationships. While there is no dominant time shift between the recorded neural activity of PMd neurons and the cursor velocity, the neural activity of M1 neurons clearly precede the velocity (Lebedev et al., 2005). The average cross correlations were computed by first calculating the cross-correlation for each unit from each non-overlapping 2-min interval, then averaging across units to get the ensemble-mean cross correlation, and finally averaging across intervals. Error bars depict the standard deviations of the ensemble-means across the non-overlapping 2-min intervals. Lags at which the cross correlation is significantly lower than the peak at either 0 s in (A) or −0.2 s in (B) are marked with open circles and stars, for significance level of $p = 0.05$ (standard) or $p = 0.005$ (Bonferroni corrected for 10 multiple comparisons), respectively (Wilcoxon rank sum test). It is evident that for M1 units, the peak at −0.2 s in **Figure 4B** is significantly higher than the cross-correlation at zero lag. In contrast, for PMd units, the cross-correlation at negative or positive lags are either significantly lower than the peak at 0 s or at least not significantly different (**Figure 4A**).

Similar temporal relationships are also observed in the simulations, depending on whether the simulated neurons encode only the estimated state or also the control signal. **Figure 4C** demonstrates that the activity of neurons that encode only the estimated state do not exhibit any dominant time shift with respect to the velocity, in agreement with the temporal relationship depicted by the recorded PMd units. As detailed in Section 2.3.4, this agreement is in line with the literature on PMd neural encoding (Messier and Kalaska, 2000; Hendrix et al., 2009), so we refer to these simulated neurons as PMd-like neurons.

In contrast, the activity of simulated neurons that encode both the estimated state and the control signal, precedes the simulated cursor velocity, as demonstrated in **Figure 4D**. In particular, the peak cross correlation at −0.2 s is significantly higher than the cross correlation at zero-lag.This is in agreement with the cross correlation depicted by the recorded M1 units. Given this agreement, and the literature on M1 neural encoding (Evarts, 1968; Kalaska et al., 1989; Todorov, 2000), we refer to these simulated neurons as M1-like neurons. The delay in the cursor velocity can be attributed to the effect of the muscles, which are modeled as a second order over-damped filter, and thus introduce a delay in the forces and eventually the movements that are generated in response to the control signal.

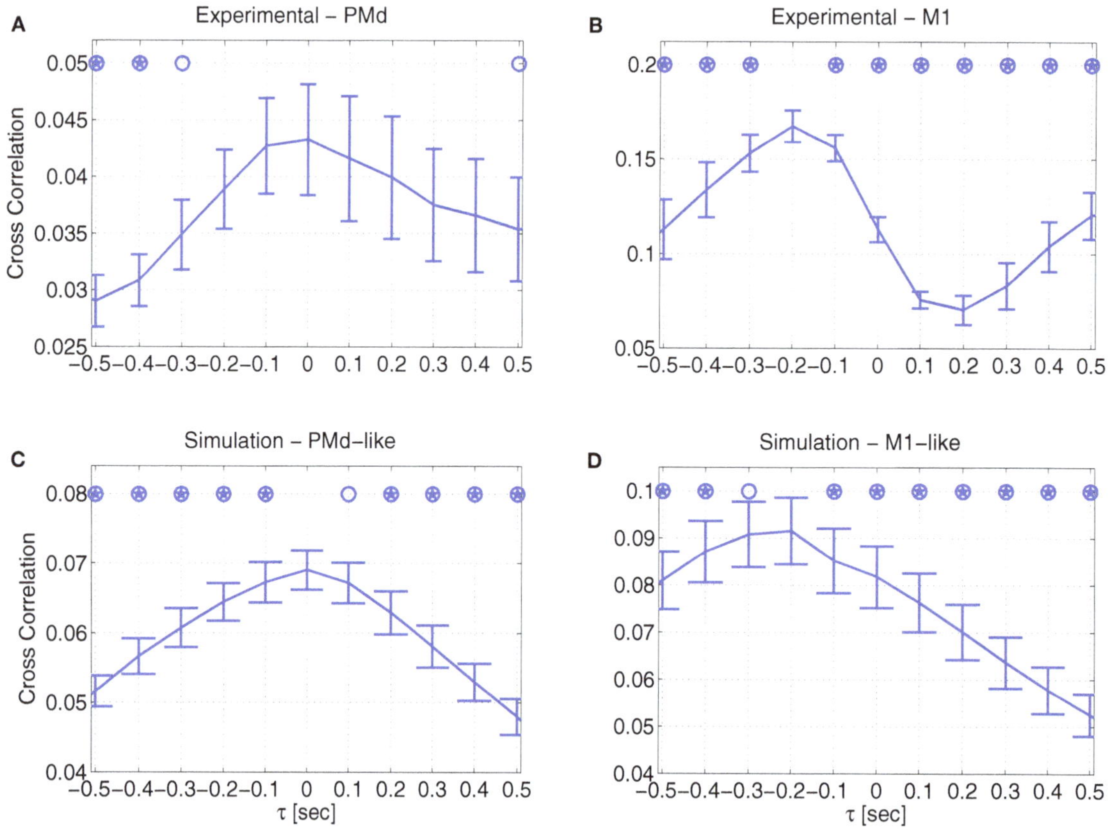

FIGURE 4 | Cross correlation between velocity and neural activity during pole control. Averaged cross correlation of: **(A)** recorded data from PMd units **(B)** recorded data from M1 units **(C)** simulated PMd-like neurons **(D)** simulated M1-like neurons. Error bars depict standard deviations across non-overlapping 2-min intervals. Open circles and stars indicate cross-correlations that are significantly lower than the peak at 0 s in **(A,C)**, and at −0.2 s at **(B,D)** with significance level of either $p = 0.05$ (standard) or $p = 0.005$ (Bonferroni corrected for 10 multiple comparisons), respectively.

3.2. Neural Modulations in Simulated Pole and Brain Control

Simulated neural activity generated by the model described in Section 2.3, based on the framework of OFC, successfully depicts the observed changes in neural modulations, as shown in **Figure 5**. **Figures 5A,B** depicts the results from a single session to facilitate direct comparison with the experimental results, while **Figures 5C,D** demonstrates the robustness of the results across a number of sessions with different sets of random tuning weights. As in Zacksenhouse et al. (2007), mean PÔM and PKM were computed by first estimating the PÔM and PKM from non-overlapping 2-min intervals of the binned spike-counts of individual neurons, then averaging across the relevant neurons to get the ensemble mean, and finally averaging across the 10 intervals of each control mode. Error bars in **Figures 5A,B** depict the standard deviations across the 10 intervals.

Figure 5 demonstrates that the PÔM estimated from a single simulated session increases significantly when switching to brain control, with no matching increase in PKM. Focusing first on the detailed results from a single session in **Figures 5A,B**, the ensemble-mean PÔM during simulated brain control is significantly higher than of ensemble-mean PÔM during simulated pole control (Wilcoxon rank sum test, $p = 0.001$ for both BCWHM and BCWOHM), while the ensemble mean PKM did not differ significantly ($p > 0.55$). This behavior is evident in the simulated neural activity of both PMd-like and M1-like simulated neurons. This reproduces well the significant increase in the ensemble mean PÔM from experimental pole control to BCWHM or BCWOHM (Wilcoxon rank sum test, $p < 0.008$), with no significant increase in the ensemble mean PKM ($p > 0.39$).

The robustness of the changes in neural modulations following the transition to brain control was investigated by simulating 100 sessions, each with a different set of tuning weights. Pole control was simulated first, while brain control was conducted only in the 78 sessions in which the performance of the BMI filter was within the constraint described above ($0.65 < R(\hat{v}, v) < 0.85$). The scatter plot in **Figure 5C** demonstrates that in these cases the PÔM in BCWHM and BCWOHM are significantly higher than the PÔM in pole control (Wilcoxon rank sum test, $p < 10^{-10}$). In contrast, the scatter plot in **Figure 5D** demonstrates that the PKM in BCWHM and BCWOHM are not significantly higher than the PKM in pole control ($p = 0.13$ and $p = 0.08$, respectively).

3.3. Effect of Process Noise on Neural Modulations

Our main hypothesis is that the higher PÔM in brain control, without matching increase in PKM, results from higher process noise introduced by the imperfect performance of the BMI filter.

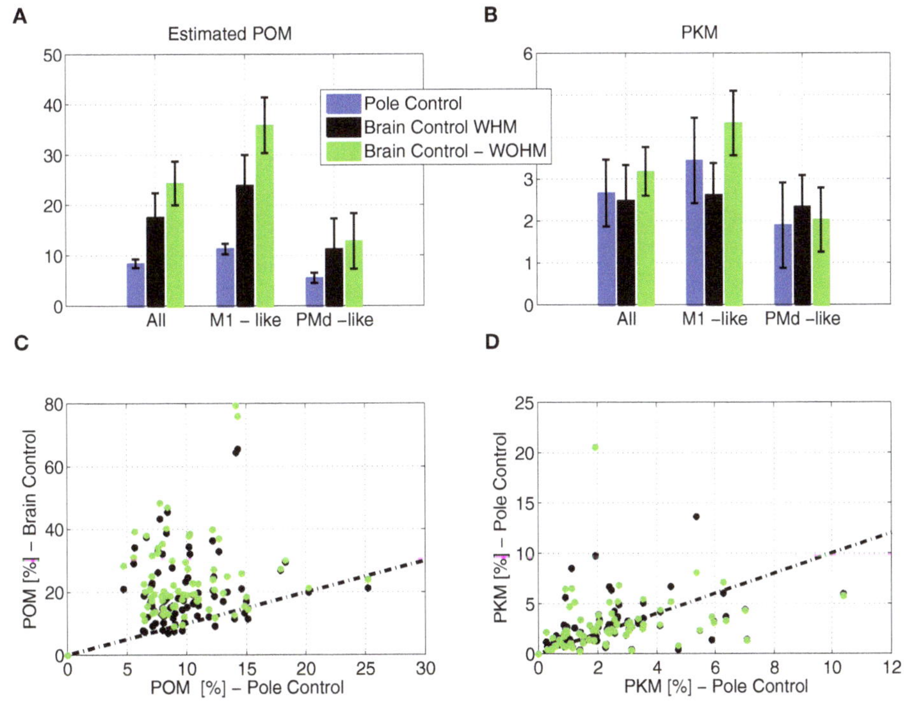

FIGURE 5 | Estimated POM and PKM of simulated neural activity. Estimated POM and PKM were computed by first estimating the POM and PKM of the binned spike-counts of individual neurons in 2-min intervals, and then averaging across the relevant neurons and across the 10 intervals of each control mode. Mean estimated POM **(A)** and PKM **(B)** across all neurons and across neurons that encode only the estimated state (PMd-like) or also the control signals (M1-like). Error bars depict the standard deviations across the 10 intervals. Scatter plot of estimated POM **(C)** and PKM **(D)** in brain vs. pole control for 78 out of 100 sessions (each with a different set of tuning weights) in which the performance of the BMI filter satisfied $0.65 < R(\hat{v}, v) < 0.85$. Dashed lines depict the identity relationship.

As detailed in Section 2.3.7, this hypothesis is investigated here by simulating noisy pole control in which the covariance of the process noise is characterized by Equation (13) instead of Equation (9). The additional term in Equation (13) describes the equivalent noise introduced by the imperfect BMI filter with magnitude that is quantified by α_{rec}. **Figure 3** demonstrates that indeed the cursor movements during noisy pole control (with $\alpha_{rec} = 0.035$) are more similar to those during brain control than those during pole control. In particular, the variance of the velocity in the simulated trajectories generated with $\alpha_{rec} = 0.0035$ was $88 \pm 7[(\frac{\text{cm}}{\text{sec}})^2]$, comparable with the variance of the velocity in the simulated trajectories during BCWHM ($75 \pm 29[(\frac{\text{cm}}{\text{sec}})^2]$), and significantly higher than the variance of the velocity in the simulated trajectories during pole control (Wilcoxon rank sum test, $p < 0.0001$).

The effects of α_{rec} on P$\hat{\text{O}}$M and PKM are depicted in **Figure 6** both when the internal model of the noise is not updated (in line with simplifying assumption SA3 that there is no adaptation) and when it is updated to match the actual process noise. All simulated sessions analyzed in **Figure 6** were performed with the same set of randomly selected targets and neural tuning weights. At each α_{rec}, the average P$\hat{\text{O}}$M and PKM and their standard deviations were computed from a singe simulated session as detailed in Section 3.2.

Figure 6 demonstrates that as the process noise increases, due to increasing α_{rec}, P$\hat{\text{O}}$M increases while PKM does not change or even decreases. This is evident by the high positive (> 0.99) and negative (< -0.96) cross correlations between α_{rec} and either P$\hat{\text{O}}$M or PKM, respectively. Furthermore, at all the noisy pole control cases analyzed in **Figure 6**, the P$\hat{\text{O}}$M was significantly higher than the P$\hat{\text{O}}$M with the standard process noise (i.e., with $\alpha_{rec} = 0$, Wilcoxon rank sum test, with Bonferroni corrected significance level of $p = 0.005$, corrected for the 10 multiple comparisons), as marked by stars in **Figure 6**. The effect is similar whether the internal model of the process noise is updated to match the actual process noise or not. The results shown in **Figure 6** are averaged P$\hat{\text{O}}$M and PKM across all the simulated neurons, but similar trends were also observed when averaging across PMd-like and M1-like simulated neurons separately.

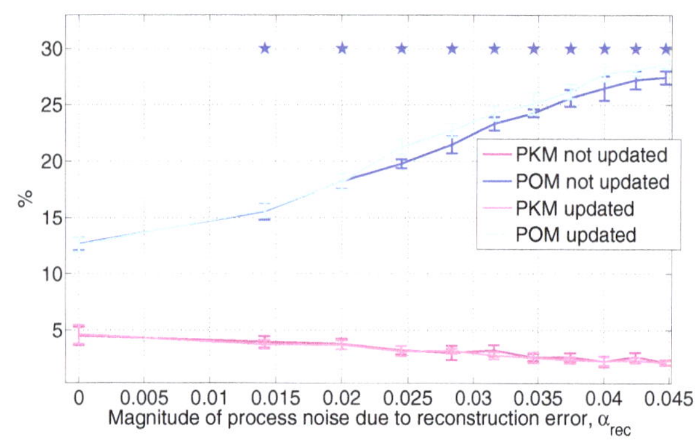

FIGURE 6 | Estimated POM and PKM during simulated noisy pole control. Noisy pole control includes both the baseline process noise due to the control signal, and an additional process noise, simulating the contribution of the BMI filter reconstruction error, as quantified by the magnitude of α_{rec} in Equation (13). At each α_{rec} and for each adaptation option (updated or not), the average estimated POM and PKM were computed from a single 20 min session of simulated pole control as detailed in the caption of **Figure 5**. Standard deviations were computed across the 10 2-min intervals and stars indicate the estimated POM (for not-updated case) that are significantly larger than the estimated POM at the standard process noise ($\alpha_{rec} = 0$) as determined by Wilcoxon rank sum test, with Bonferroni corrected significance level $p = 0.005$, corrected for 10 multiple comparisons. All sessions were performed with the same randomly selected targets and neural tuning weights.

3.4. Sensitivity to Baseline Measurement Noise

In this and the next section we investigate the sensitivity of P$\hat{\text{O}}$M to the baseline covariance matrices of the different sources of noise, i.e., the covariance matrices of the measurement and process noise during pole control. Since the internal model is assumed to be well-adapted for pole control, these are also the covariance matrices of the internal model of the noise. Each sensitivity analysis is conducted with 15 sessions simulated with the same set of neurons but different sets of targets. This is equivalent to simulating longer sessions, which improves the accuracy of the estimated POM. In particular, the mean P$\hat{\text{O}}$M across all the simulated neurons was estimated from each session and the average and standard deviations were computed across the 15 sessions.

The Kalman filter depends on the relative size of these covariance matrices, so the value of one of the elements can be kept constant. Furthermore, since we found that the P$\hat{\text{O}}$M is insensitive to the ratio between visual position and velocity measurements noise, we kept the diagonal covariance matrix of the visual measurement noise fixed and equals to the one suggested in Todorov (2005).

Focusing first on the sensitivity of P$\hat{\text{O}}$M to the baseline proprioceptive measurement noise, we found that the P$\hat{\text{O}}$M is insensitive to the proprioceptive position measurement noise. Hence, **Figure 7A** depicts only the effect of a common scaling factor between the covariance matrices of the visual and proprioceptive measurements noise, i.e., the effect of the proprioceptive measurement noise factor k_m in **Table 1**. **Figure 7A** indicates that the P$\hat{\text{O}}$M is sensitive to k_m only in BCWHM. When the covariance matrices of the proprioceptive and visual measurement noise are comparable ($0.5 < k_m < 2$), the P$\hat{\text{O}}$M in simulated BCWHM is significantly larger than the P$\hat{\text{O}}$M during the experimental BCWHM (Wilcoxon rank sum test, $p < 0.004$) and even larger than the P$\hat{\text{O}}$M in BCWOHM, in contrast with the observed relationship in the BMI experiments (Zacksenhouse et al., 2007). When the proprioceptive measurement noise is 10-fold larger than the visual measurement noise ($k_m = 10$), the P$\hat{\text{O}}$M in simulated BCWHM does not differ significantly from the P$\hat{\text{O}}$M during the experimental BCWHM and is lower than the P$\hat{\text{O}}$M in BCWOHM, as in the BMI experiments. Further increase in the the proprioceptive measurement noise has little effect on the P$\hat{\text{O}}$M even in BCWHM. These observations motivated the

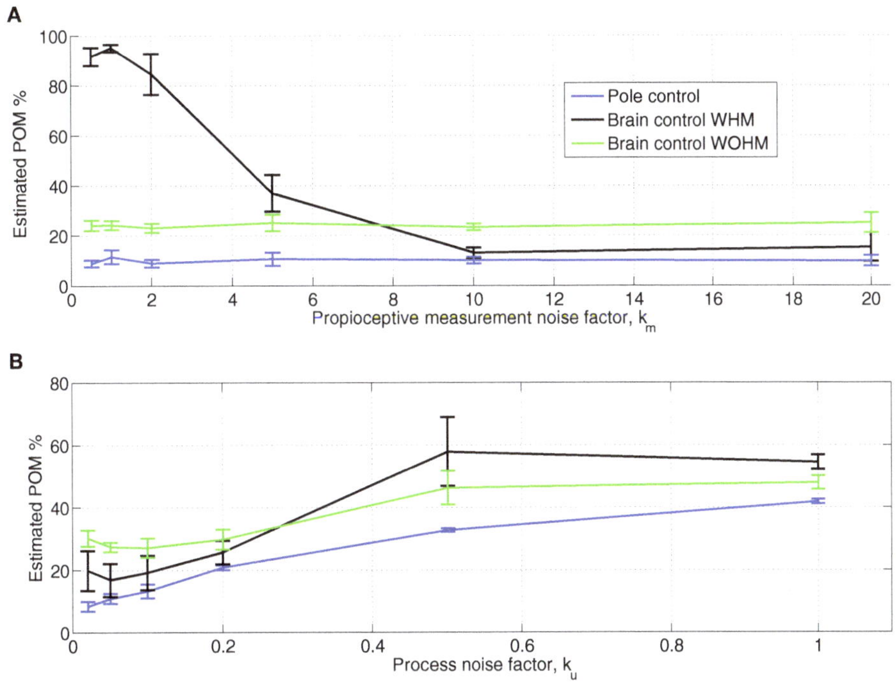

FIGURE 7 | Sensitivity of estimated POM to proprioceptive measurement noise (A) and magnitude of baseline process noise (B). The proprioceptive measurement noise factor k_m quantifies the ratio between the variance of the proprioceptive and the visual measurement noise (same factor for both position and velocity measurements). The process noise factor k_u quantifies the magnitude of hand process noise, as specified in **Table 1**. Each sensitivity analysis was conducted by simulating 15 sessions with the same set of neurons but different sets of targets. The mean estimated POM over the simulated neurons was computed for each session and the average and standard deviations across the 15 sessions are plotted.

selection of $k_m = 10$ as the default factor in all other simulations (**Table 1**).

The lack of sensitivity to proprioceptive measurement noise during pole control can be attributed to the perfect internal model and low baseline process noise, which cause state-estimation to be based mainly on the internal model. The high $\hat{POM}$ during BCWHM when the baseline proprioceptive and visual measurements noise are comparable can be attributed to the resulting similar Kalman gains for those two modalities. Due to the imperfect BMI filter, the estimation measurement error in brain control is high, and during BCWHM the proprioceptive measurement may differ from the visual measurement. When both modalities are given similar Kalman gains, the deviation between the proprioceptive and visual measurements contributes to higher variance in the resulting estimated state. Finally, during BCWOHM the proprioceptive measurement noise is increased to infinity to model the lack of relevant proprioceptive feedback in this mode, and hence the $\hat{POM}$ in this mode does not depend on the baseline proprioceptive measurement noise.

3.5. Sensitivity to Baseline Process Noise

During regular pole control, the covariance of the process noise is described by Equation (9) and its magnitude is quantified by α_u , or alternatively by the process noise factor k_u, as described in Section 2.3.6 and **Table 1**. As noted in Section 2.3.6 and **Figure 2**, adequate performance of the BMI filter in the simulated BMI sessions can be achieved with $k_u = 0.1$. Here we investigate the effect of k_u on $\hat{POM}$.

Figure 7B depicts the changes in the $\hat{POM}$ as a function of the process noise factor k_u. It is apparent that $\hat{POM}$ in brain control is always higher than $\hat{POM}$ in pole control, in agreement with the observed changes in the $\hat{POM}$ during the BMI experiments. However, for $k_u = 1$, the $\hat{POM}$ in each of control mode is too large compared with the experimentally observed $\hat{POM}$ (Wilcoxon rank sum test, $p < 0.002$ for each control mode). This further supports the selection of a smaller process noise factor, and in particular $k_u = 0.1$, made in section 2.3.6 based on the performance of the BMI filter. For this process noise, the relation between the $\hat{POM}$ in BCWHM versus BCWOHM agrees well with the experimental observations.

Figure 7B also shows that $\hat{POM}$ increases with the magnitude of the process noise. This is in agreement with the results described in Section 3.4, though in that section the magnitude of the process noise described by Equation (13) was manipulated by changing of α_{rec} instead of α_u (via k_u).

3.6. Internal Model Variations

The simulations presented so far were based on simplifying assumption SA3, so the internal model did not change due to transition to brain control. Since the monkey stopped moving its hand in BCWOHM, the internal model may change to account

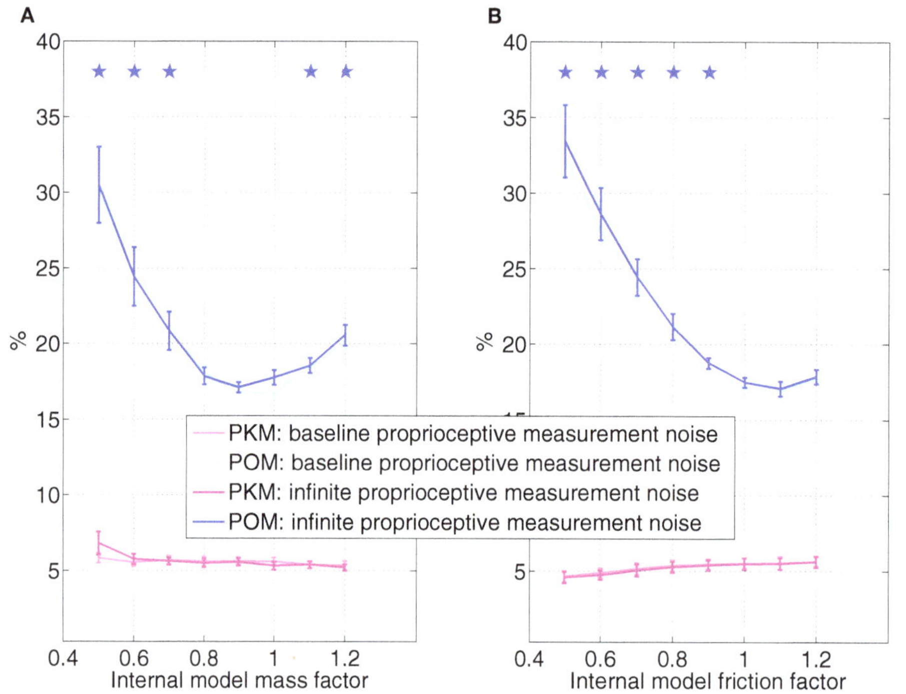

FIGURE 8 | Effect of internal model variations during pole control. The value of the mass **(A)** or the coefficient of friction **(B)** in the internal model is normalized to the value of the actual parameter. Simulations are conducted with either the baseline proprioceptive measurement noise characteristic of pole control or infinite proprioceptive measurement noise characteristic of BCWOHM. At each parameter value, and for each level of the proprioceptive measurement noise, the average estimated POM and PKM were computed from a single 20 min session of simulated pole control as detailed in the caption of **Figure 5**. Standard deviations were computed across the 10 2-min intervals and stars indicate estimated POMs that are significantly larger than the estimated POM at the nominal parameter (internal model factor = 1), as determined by Wilcoxon rank sum test with Bonferroni corrected significance level $p = 0.007$, corrected for 7 multiple comparisons. All sessions were performed with the same randomly selected targets and neural tuning weights.

for the lack of hand movements. **Figure 8** evaluates the effect of changing the parameters of the internal model, and in particular the mass (**Figure 8A**), or the coefficient of friction (**Figure 8B**), during pole control while keeping the external model the same. In both cases, the x-axis is the normalized parameter of the internal model (mass or coefficient of friction) relative to the nominal value of the parameter of the external model. The effect is evaluated both with the baseline proprioceptive measurement noise characteristic of pole control and BCWHM, and with infinite proprioceptive measurement noise characteristic of BCWOHM. All simulated sessions analyzed in **Figure 8** were performed with the same set of randomly selected targets and neural tuning weights, but not the same set used in other sections. At each parameter value, and for each level of the proprioceptive measurement noise, the average $\hat{\text{POM}}$ and PKM in **Figure 8** and their standard deviations were computed from a single simulated session as detailed in Section 3.2.

Figure 8 indicates that when the internal model deviates from the external model, the $\hat{\text{POM}}$ increases significantly, while the PKM does not change significantly or even decease over most of the range. Parameter values at which the $\hat{\text{POM}}$ (generated in simulations with infinite process noise) is significantly higher than the $\hat{\text{POM}}$ at the nominal parameter are marked by stars (Wilcoxon rank sum test with Bonferroni corrected significance level $p = 0.007$, corrected for 7 multiple comparisons). The effect of increasing the covariance matrix of the proprioceptive measurement noise to infinity, as in BCWOHM, is negligible. Hence, changes in the parameters of the internal model may further contribute the observed change in $\hat{\text{POM}}$ upon switching to brain control, and especially to BCWOHM.

4. Discussion

4.1. Modeling

The implemented OFC model successfully moves the hand and cursor in simulated pole control to reach randomly selected targets. Neural activity is generated to simulate neural recording and perform brain control. The simulated neurons are assumed to encode the signals that are relevant for OFC, i.e., the estimated state and the control signal, and spike-counts are generated as doubly stochastic Poisson processes. The model parameters were taken from the literature or selected to match the experimental observations. In particular, the magnitude of the process noise and the number of neurons were selected so the performance of the BMI filter trained on the simulated neural activity matches the performance of the BMI filter trained on the recorded neural activity. The resulting model successfully generates the main phenomena that it was developed to explain: the POM of the neural activity in brain control is higher than the POM in pole control with no matching increase in PKM.

OFC involves different computational tasks that can be mapped to different brain regions. In particular, it has been suggested (Shadmehr and Krakauer, 2008) that expected costs and rewards are evaluated by the basal ganglia, the forward model is implemented by the cerebellum, and the predicted sensory feedback is combined with the actual sensory feedback at the parietal cortex to estimate the state. Given the estimated state, the pre-motor and primary motor cortices are hypothesized to generate the control signals associated with visual and proprioceptive feedback, respectively. As mentioned above (Introduction and Section 2.3.3) the OFC is simulated in the state space, so all these computational tasks are included regardless of where they are implemented in the brain. In contrast, neural activity is generated to simulate neural recording from M1 and PMd only, since those are the main brain regions recorded in the BMI experiments considered here.

4.2. Neural Encoding

Neural encoding is an open and important research question. Common strategies to investigate this issue involve quantifying the correlation between the neural activity and different relevant signals, or assessing how well those signals can be predicted by the neural activity. However, those strategies are usually restricted to measurable signals. In particular, many studies investigated the correlation between the activity of cortical motor units and different kinematics and kinetics signals (Georgopoulos et al., 1984, 1986, 1992; Kalaska et al., 1989; Ashe and Georgopoulos, 1994; Ashe, 1997; Moran and Schwartz, 1999; Paninski et al., 2004; Kalaska, 2009). Since correlations do not imply causality, the observed correlations with any of the measurable signals do not imply that the neurons indeed encode these signals. Instead, the neurons may encode internal, hidden signals, which are also correlated with the measurable signals (Zacksenhouse et al., 2014) including, for example, muscle activation patterns (Todorov, 2000).

Here we suggest that cortical motor neurons encode signals that are relevant for performing state estimation and control, i.e., the estimated state and the control signal. Since these signals are internal signals generated by the brain, direct correlation cannot be evaluated. Nevertheless, during normal reaching movements, the actual movement should agree well with the estimated state, and thus the neural activity would appear to be correlated with the movement. However, in other conditions, and in particular during brain control, the estimated state may deviate from the measured state. This work suggests that the higher POM during brain control with no matching increase in PKM may arise from such deviations.

We noted that the neural activity recorded from M1 and PMd units exhibited different cross-correlations with the velocity. In particular, the average cross-correlations between the velocity and the recorded neural activity during pole control indicate that there is no time-shift between the neural activity of PMd units and the cursor velocity, while the neural activity of M1 neurons precedes the velocity. These temporal relationships are reproduced well by simulated neurons that encode only the estimated state or also the control signal, respectively. The time shift in the latter case can be ascribed to the delay in the response of the muscles. Hence, the different types of observed cross-correlations, with and without time shift, can be attributed to encoding different signals within the framework OFC, including and excluding the control signal, respectively. Encoding the control signal in M1 but not in PMd neurons agrees well with evidence that the activity of PMd neurons is modulated mainly by the direction and magnitude of movements while the activity of M1 neurons is correlated also with the forces (Evarts, 1968; Kalaska et al., 1989). Further support is provided by previous investigation of the BMI experiments considered here, which indicated that PMd neurons can predict well the position and velocity but not the force, while M1 neurons can predict well the force too (Carmena et al., 2003). While this specific distinction between M1 and PMd neurons may result from the specific sample of units recorded during the BMI experiments considered here, it is well reproduced by the simulated model based on OFC.

4.3. Process Noise

Our main hypothesis is that the observed increase in POM following the transition to brain control reflects increasing variance of the encoded signals due to higher process noise. The latter is assumed to occur in brain control due to the limited accuracy of the BMI filter. This hypothesis was proved theoretically and by simulations. Theoretical proof was limited to the case when the estimated process noise in the internal model is not updated, and the neurons encode linear combinations of the estimated state. The simulations demonstrate that increasing process noise during pole control results in higher POM even when neurons encode non-linear functions of the estimated state (e.g., speed and magnitude of the control signal) and regardless of whether the internal model is updated or not.

4.4. Implications for BMI

The proposed model attributes the increase in POM following the transition to brain control to the higher process noise introduced by the imperfect performance of the BMI filter. This suggests that the POM is a proxy for the performance of the BMI filter: High POM indicates that the BMI filter performs poorly while low POM indicates that the BMI filter performs well. As a proxy signal for the performance of the BMI filer, the POM could be used to adapt the BMI filter using reinforcement learning (DiGiovanna et al., 2009; Mahmoudi et al., 2013), especially in cases when an error signal cannot be determined (Bensmaia and Miller, 2014). Furthermore, the proposed model developed here, provides a framework for investigating this and other suggestion for improving BMIs. Finally, the proposed model can be used to investigate other changes that occur following the transition to brain control and in particular the changes in neural tuning (Lebedev et al., 2005).

4.5. Alternative Hypotheses

Our main hypothesis is that the observed changes in neural modulations following the transition to brain control are related to changes in the process and measurement noise induced by the transition, and in particular, the increase in process noise due to the imperfect BMI filter. OFC provides a coherent and concise framework for relating the changes in process and measurement noise to changes in the estimated state and control signals, and finally to changes in neural modulations. However, the key elements are state estimation and the encoding of the estimated state, so other models that include those components may produce similar results. In particular, state estimation and control may not be optimal, but only satisficing (Simon, 1956; Brown et al., 2004). The OFC framework was adopted here since optimization constrains the parameters of the estimation filter and the gains of the control law, resulting in fewer free parameters to be tuned, thus granting the resulting model higher credibility.

An alternative hypothesis that may contribute to the changes in neural modulations involve changes in the internal model. As was shown in Section 3.6, deviations between the internal model and the external system, and in particular deviations in the mass or the coefficient of friction, result in higher $\hat{\text{POM}}$ with no matching increase in PKM. Thus, changes in the internal model of the mass or coefficient of friction, may contribute to the increase in $\hat{\text{POM}}$ beyond what is attributed to the increase in process noise. Since the transition to BCWOHM involves stopping hand movements, it is conceivable that it is associated with a switch to a different internal model, with lower mass and coefficient of friction. However, the change in the internal model is not justified in the transition to BCWHM, when the monkey continues to make hand movements.

Alternative frameworks for explaining the changes in neural modulations may be provided by intermittent predictive control (Doeringer and Hogan, 1998; Gawthrop et al., 2011) and active inference (Friston et al., 2010, 2011). Intermittent predictive control alleviates the computational load of prediction that is necessary to address time delays (Doeringer and Hogan, 1998; Gawthrop et al., 2011). Due to the imperfect BMI filter, the transition to brain control is expected to result in more frequent updates of the predictor, and hence in higher variability in the predicted state. Since intermittent predictive control is based on OFC, this is an extension of the current model, and will be considered in future work. Indeed it could be argued that due to the inaccurate movements of the cursor during brain control, the monkey is making explorative movements to adapt to the new environment. While the explorative movements may contribute to higher POM, they are expected to also increase the PKM, in contrast with the observation.

In summary, we demonstrated that the observed changes in neural modulations following the transition to brain control can be successfully explained under the assumption that the neurons encode the estimated state and control signal. To be concrete we used the framework of OFC, but similar results are expected even if the controller is not optimal, as long as it relies on state estimation that deteriorates upon switching to brain control.

Acknowledgments

The BMI experiments were conducted at Nicolelis' lab, Duke University, and we thank MAL Nicolelis, J Carmena and M Lebedev for sharing the data. The research was supported by Fund C for research at the Technion's Autonomous Systems Program, under grant numbers 2018172. We thank Prof. Y. halevi for his suggestions on the theoretical analysis.

Supplementary Material

The Supplementary Material for this article can be found online at: http://journal.frontiersin.org/article/10.3389/fnsys.2015.00071/abstract

References

Ashe, J. (1997). Force and the motor cortex. *Behav. Brain Res.* 87, 255–269. doi: 10.1016/S0166-4328(97)00752-3

Ashe, J., and Georgopoulos, A. P. (1994). Movement parameters and neural activity in motor cortex and area 5. *Cereb. Cortex* 4, 590–600. doi: 10.1093/cercor/4.6.590

Bensmaia, S. J., and Miller, L. E. (2014). Restoring sensorimotor function through intracortical interfaces: progress and looming challenges. *Nat. Rev. Neurosci.* 15, 313–325. doi: 10.1038/nrn3724

Brown, E. N., Kass, R. E., and Mitra, P. P. (2004). Multiple neural spike train data analysis: state-of-the-art and future challenges. *Nat. Neurosci.* 7, 456–461. doi: 10.1038/nn1228

Carmena, J. M., Lebedev, M. A., Crist, R. E., O'Doherty, J. E., Santucci, D. M., Dimitrov, D. F., et al. (2003). Learning to control a brain-machine interface for reaching and grasping by primates. *PLoS Biol.* 1:E42. doi: 10.1371/journal.pbio.0000042

Chang, Y. H., Chen, M., Shanechi, M., Carmena, J. M., and Tomlin, C. (2014). "A design of neural decoder by reducing discrepancy between Manual Control (MC) and Brain Control (BC)," in *2014 European Control Conference (ECC)* (Strasbourg), 516–521.

Churchland, A. K., Kiani, R., Chaudhuri, R., Wang, X.-J., Pouget, A., and Shadlen, M. N. (2011). Variance as a signature of neural computations during decision making. *Neuron* 69, 818–831. doi: 10.1016/j.neuron.2010.12.037

Crevecoeur, F., and Scott, S. H. (2013). Priors engaged in long-latency responses to mechanical perturbations suggest a rapid update in state estimation. *PLoS Comput. Biol.* 9:e1003177. doi: 10.1371/journal.pcbi.1003177

Cunningham, J. P., Nuyujukian, P., Gilja, V., Chestek, C. A., Ryu, S. I., and Shenoy, K. V. (2011). A closed-loop human simulator for investigating the role of feedback control in brain-machine interfaces. *J. Neurophysiol.* 105, 1932–1949. doi: 10.1152/jn.00503.2010

Dayan, P., and Abbott, L. F. (2001). *Theoretical Neuroscience.* Cambridge, MA: MIT Press.

DiGiovanna, J., Mahmoudi, B., Fortes, J., Principe, J. C., and Sanchez, J. C. (2009). Coadaptive brain–machine interface via reinforcement learning. *Biomed. Eng. IEEE Trans.* 56, 54–64. doi: 10.1109/TBME.2008.926699

Doeringer, J. A., and Hogan, N. (1998). Intermittency in preplanned elbow movements persists in the absence of visual feedback. *J. Neurophysiol.* 80, 1787–1799.

Evarts, E. V. (1968). Relation of pyramidal tract activity to force exerted during voluntary movement. *J. Neurophysiol.* 31, 14–27.

Flash, T., and Hogan, N. (1985). The coordination of arm movements: an experimentally confirmed mathematical model. *J. Neurosci.* 5, 1688–1703.

Friston, K., Mattout, J., and Kilner, J. (2011). Action understanding and active inference. *Biol. Cybern.* 104, 137–160. doi: 10.1007/s00422-011-0424-z

Friston, K. J., Daunizeau, J., Kilner, J., and Kiebel, S. J. (2010). Action and behavior: a free-energy formulation. *Biol. Cybern.* 102, 227–260. doi: 10.1007/s00422-010-0364-z

Gawthrop, P., Loram, I., Lakie, M., and Gollee, H. (2011). Intermittent control: a computational theory of human control. *Biol. Cybern.* 104, 31–51. doi: 10.1007/s00422-010-0416-4

Geisler, W., and Albrecht, D. (1995). Bayesian analysis of identification performance in monkey visual cortex: nonlinear mechanisms and stimulus certainty. *Vis. Res.* 35, 2723–2730. doi: 10.1016/0042-6989(95)00029-Y

Georgopoulos, A., Caminiti, R., and Kalaska, J. (1984). Static spatial effects in motor cortex and area 5: quantitative relations in a two-dimensional space. *Exp. Brain Res.* 54, 446–454. doi: 10.1007/BF00235470

Georgopoulos, A. P., Ashe, J., Smyrnis, N., and Taira, M. (1992). The motor cortex and the coding of force. *Science* 256, 1692–1695. doi: 10.1126/science.256.5064.1692

Georgopoulos, A. P., Kalaska, J. F., Caminiti, R., and Massey, J. T. (1982). On the relations between the direction of two-dimensional arm movements and cell discharge in primate motor cortex. *J. Neurosci.* 2, 1527–1537.

Georgopoulos, A. P., Schwartz, A. B., and Kettner, R. E. (1986). Neuronal population coding of movement direction. *Science* 233, 1416–1419. doi: 10.1126/science.3749885

Harris, C. M., and Wolpert, D. M. (1998). Signal-dependent noise determines motor planning. *Nature* 394, 780–784. doi: 10.1038/29528

Hendrix, C. M., Mason, C. R., and Ebner, T. J. (2009). Signaling of grasp dimension and grasp force in dorsal premotor cortex and primary motor cortex neurons during reach to grasp in the monkey. *J. Neurophysiol.* 102, 132–145. doi: 10.1152/jn.00016.2009

Horn, R. A., and Johnson, C. R. (2012). *Matrix Analysis.* Cambridge, MA: Cambridge University Press. doi: 10.1017/CBO9781139020411

Johnson, D. H. (1996). Point process models of single-neuron discharges. *J. Comput. Neurosci.* 3, 275–299. doi: 10.1007/BF00161089

Jordan, M. I., and Rumelhart, D. E. (1992). Forward models: supervised learning with a Distal teacher. *Cogn. Sci.* 16, 307–354. doi: 10.1207/s15516709cog1603_1

Kalaska, J. F. (2009). "From intention to action: motor cortex and the control of reaching movements," in *Progress in Motor Control,* ed D. Sternad (Springer US), 139–178.

Kalaska, J. F., Cohen, D., Hyde, M. L., and Prud'Homme, M. (1989). A comparison of movement direction-related versus load direction-related activity in primate motor cortex, using a two-dimensional reaching task. *J. Neurosci.* 9, 2080–2102.

Kawato, M., Furukawa, K., and Suzuki, R. (1987). A hierarchical neural-network model for control and learning of voluntary movement. *Biol. Cybern.* 57, 169–185. doi: 10.1007/BF00364149

Kuo, A. D. (1995). An optimal control model for analyzing human postural balance. *Biomed. Eng. IEEE Trans.* 42, 87–101. doi: 10.1109/10.362914

Lebedev, M. A., Carmena, J. M., O'Doherty, J. E., Zacksenhouse, M., Henriquez, C. S., Principe, J. C., et al. (2005). Cortical ensemble adaptation to represent velocity of an artificial actuator controlled by a brain-machine interface. *J. Neurosci.* 25, 4681–4693. doi: 10.1523/JNEUROSCI.4088-04.2005

Mahmoudi, B., Pohlmeyer, E. A., Prins, N. W., Geng, S., and Sanchez, J. C. (2013). Towards autonomous neuroprosthetic control using hebbian reinforcement learning. *J. Neural Eng.* 10, 66005. doi: 10.1088/1741-2560/10/6/066005

Messier, J., and Kalaska, J. F. (2000). Covariation of primate dorsal premotor cell activity with direction and amplitude during a memorized-delay reaching task. *J. Neurophysiol.* 84, 152–165.

Miall, R., and Wolpert, D. M. (1996). Forward models for physiological motor control. *Neural Netw.* 9, 1265–1279. doi: 10.1016/S0893-6080(96)00035-4

Moran, D. W., and Schwartz, A. B. (1999). Motor cortical representation of speed and direction during reaching. *J. Neurophysiol.* 82, 2676–2692.

Nicolelis, M. A. (2001). Actions from thoughts. *Nature* 409, 403–407. doi: 10.1038/35053191

Paninski, L., Fellows, M. R., Hatsopoulos, N. G., and Donoghue, J. P. (2004). Spatiotemporal tuning of motor cortical neurons for hand position and velocity. *J. Neurophysiol.* 91, 515–532. doi: 10.1152/jn.00587.2002

Schwartz, A. B. (2004). Cortical neural prosthetics. *Annu. Rev. Neurosci.* 27, 487–507. doi: 10.1146/annurev.neuro.27.070203.144233

Shadmehr, R., and Krakauer, J. W. (2008). A computational neuroanatomy for motor control. *Exp. Brain Res.* 185, 359–381. doi: 10.1007/s00221-008-1280-5

Shanechi, M. M., Williams, Z. M., Wornell, G. W., Hu, R. C., Powers, M., and Brown, E. N. (2013a). A real-time brain-machine interface combining motor target and trajectory intent using an optimal feedback control design. *PLoS ONE* 8:e59049. doi: 10.1371/journal.pone.0059049

Shanechi, M. M., Wornell, G. W., Williams, Z. M., and Brown, E. N. (2013b). Feedback-controlled parallel point process filter for estimation of goal-directed movements from neural signals. *Neural Syst. Rehabil. Eng. IEEE Trans.* 21, 129–140. doi: 10.1109/TNSRE.2012.2221743

Shenoy, K. V., Sahani, M., and Churchland, M. M. (2013). Cortical control of arm movements: a dynamical systems perspective. *Annu. Rev. Neurosci.* 36, 337–359. doi: 10.1146/annurev-neuro-062111-150509

Simon, H. A. (1956). Rational choice and the structure of the environment. *Psychol. Rev.* 63, 129. doi: 10.1037/h0042769

Snyder, D. L. (1975). *Random Point Processes.* New York, NY: J. Willey & Sons.

Stengel, R. F. (2012). *Optimal Control and Estimation.* London: Courier Dover Publications.

Taylor, D. M., Tillery, S. I. H., and Schwartz, A. B. (2002). Direct cortical control of 3d neuroprosthetic devices. *Science* 296, 1829–1832. doi: 10.1126/science.1070291

Todorov, E. (2000). Direct cortical control of muscle activation in voluntary arm movements: a model. *Nat. Neurosci.* 3, 391–398. doi: 10.1038/73964

Todorov, E. (2005). Stochastic optimal control and estimation methods adapted to the noise characteristics of the sensorimotor system. *Neural Comput.* 17, 1084–1108. doi: 10.1162/0899766053491887

Todorov, E., and Jordan, M. I. (2002). Optimal feedback control as a theory of motor coordination. *Nat. Neurosci.* 5, 1226–1235. doi: 10.1038/nn963

Tolhurst, D. J., Movshon, J., and Dean, A. (1983). The statistical reliability of signals in single neurons in cat and monkey visual cortex. *Vis. Res.* 23, 775–785. doi: 10.1016/0042-6989(83)90200-6

Wolpert, D., Ghahramani, Z., and Jordan, M. (1995). Are arm trajectories planned in kinematic or dynamic coordinates? An adaptation study. *Exp. Brain Res.* 103, 460–470. doi: 10.1007/BF00241505

Wolpert, D. M., and Ghahramani, Z. (2000). Computational principles of movement neuroscience. *Nat. Neurosci.* 3, 1212–1217. doi: 10.1038/81497

Wu, W., Gao, Y., Bienenstock, E., Donoghue, J. P., and Black, M. J. (2006). Bayesian population decoding of motor cortical activity using a Kalman filter. *Neural Comput.* 18, 80–118. doi: 10.1162/089976606774841585

Zacksenhouse, M., Lebedev, M. A., Carmena, J. M., O'Doherty, J. E., Henriquez, C., and Nicolelis, M. a. L. (2007). Cortical modulations increase in early sessions with brain-machine interface. *PLoS ONE* 2:e619. doi: 10.1371/journal.pone.0000619

Zacksenhouse, M., Lebedev, M. A., and Nicolelis, M. A. L. (2014). Signal-independent timescale analysis (SITA) and its application for neural coding during reaching and walking. *Front. Comput. Neurosci.* 8:91. doi: 10.3389/fncom.2014.00091

Zacksenhouse, M., and Nemets, S. (2008). "Strategies for neural ensemble data analysis for brain-machine interface (BMI) applications," in *Methods Neural Ensemble Record*, 2nd Edition, Chapter 4, ed M. Nicolelis (Boca Raton, FL: CRC Press), 57–82. doi: 10.1201/9781420006414.ch4

13

Preserving cortico-striatal function: deep brain stimulation in Huntington's disease

Sean J. Nagel [1,2]*, *Andre G. Machado* [1,2], *John T. Gale* [1,3], *Darlene A. Lobel* [1,2] and *Mayur Pandya* [1,4]

[1] Cleveland Clinic, Neurologic Institute, Center for Neurological Restoration, Cleveland, Ohio, USA, [2] Department of Neurosurgery, Cleveland Clinic, Neurologic Institute, Cleveland, Ohio, USA, [3] Department of Neuroscience, Cleveland Clinic, Lerner Research Institute, Cleveland, Ohio, USA, [4] Department of Psychiatry, Cleveland Clinic, Neurologic Institute, Cleveland, Ohio, USA

Edited by:
Mikhail Lebedev, Duke University, USA

Reviewed by:
Adolfo Ramirez-Zamora, Albany Medical College, USA
Jonathan Miller, University Hospitals Case Medical Center, USA
Christopher Tolleson, Vanderbilt University, USA

***Correspondence:**
Sean J. Nagel, Cleveland Clinic, Neurologic Institute, Center for Neurological Restoration, 9500 Euclid Avenue – S3, Cleveland, Ohio, 44195 USA
nagels@ccf.org

Huntington's disease (HD) is an incurable neurodegenerative disease characterized by the triad of chorea, cognitive dysfunction and psychiatric disturbances. Since the discovery of the HD gene, the pathogenesis has been outlined, but to date a cure has not been found. Disease modifying therapies are needed desperately to improve function, alleviate suffering, and provide hope for symptomatic patients. Deep brain stimulation (DBS), a proven therapy for managing the symptoms of some neurodegenerative movement disorders, including Parkinson's disease, has been reported as a palliative treatment in select cases of HD with debilitating chorea with variable success. New insights into the mechanism of action of DBS suggest it may have the potential to circumvent other manifestations of HD including cognitive deterioration. Furthermore, because DBS is already widely used, reversible, and has a risk profile that is relatively low, new studies can be initiated. In this article we contend that new clinical trials be considered to test the effects of DBS for HD.

Keywords: deep brain stimulation, Huntington's disease, globus pallidus, striatum, cognition, chorea

Preserving Cortico-Striatal Function: Deep Brain Stimulation in Huntington's Disease

Few conditions in medicine present patients and their families the challenges of Huntington's disease (HD). Because it is a heritable disease, the majority of individuals at risk are exposed to a turbulent environment with a parent diagnosed with HD and faced with the reality of suffering a similar fate. At-risk patients have the option to learn if they have the disease and then must confront the sad truth that the disease will end in neurologic disability and premature death. For those who elect not to be tested, the specter of developing symptomatic HD still looms large. This in part contributes to the increased risk of suicide during early stages and engenders fear and desperation that perpetuates itself with time as families search for answers (Meiser and Dunn, 2000). This psychological burden, coupled with the absence of any promising interventions, contributes to low predictive testing rates and the potential to adopt overly optimistic beliefs about one's future, which at times may have undesirable consequences from a medical or economic standpoint (Oster et al., 2013).

It is estimated that 30,000 individuals in the United States alone have manifest symptoms of HD, with twice as many additional individuals yet to manifest symptoms. Extensive efforts on the part of researchers, emboldened by these unfortunate facts, identified the genetic basis of HD in the early 1990's. Since then, the effort to find a cure has accelerated, although to date only one therapeutic agent has been approved for clinical use. Physicians are therefore left to consider off-label uses of existing therapies. Deep brain stimulation (DBS) has been used in HD as a treatment for disabling chorea but targeted stimulation may be a potential consideration to palliate symptoms of HD.

Several longitudinal studies have contributed to the current understanding of the natural history of HD (Paulsen et al., 2008; Ross and Tabrizi, 2011; Ross et al., 2014). The mean age of onset is 40 with an additional 20 years of life expected after the disease manifests (Tabrizi et al., 2011). Onset is defined with the emergence of motor symptoms. Chorea—abrupt, random, involuntary movements—is the hallmark of HD. These movements often intensify before being replaced with voluntary motor deficits. The cognitive features of HD consist of executive dysfunction, visuospatial dysfunction, cognitive slowing, and loss of mental flexibility. Evidence suggests that cognitive dysfunction may parallel (or precede) the emergence of motor deficits (Paulsen and Long, 2014). The psychiatric manifestations vary widely, ranging from mood disturbances to obsessional anxiety and, rarely, psychosis. Furthermore, limbic dysfunction, in the setting of cognitive inflexibility and poor insight, contributes to a 'dysexecutive syndrome', characterized by perseveration, apathy, impulsivity and aggression. Non-pharmacologic interventions may be helpful in early stages but tend to become less effective as the disease progresses. Tetrabenazine is the only FDA-approved agent for the treatment of the chorea. Psychiatric symptoms are managed similarly to the general population. Cognitive symptoms are typically resistant to intervention. Biomarkers that correlate to disease stages have not yet been defined, although promising considerations in premanifest individuals have been identified (Paulsen et al., 2014).

Pathogenic Mechanisms of HD

HD exhibits autosomal dominant inheritance and is equally prevalent in men and woman. In those who inherit the mutation, a cytosine-adenosine-guanine (CAG) repeat expansion is added to the IT15 huntington (HTT) gene on the short arm of chromosome 4 (Raymond et al., 2011). Affected individuals with the mutated form have between 36 and 121 CAG repeats in the coding region that translate into a polyglutamine expansion. The age of onset of motor symptoms inversely correlates with the number of repeated sequences (Ross et al., 2014). In healthy persons, HTT encodes a protein (huntingtin) responsible for synaptic vesicular transit and other cellular functions that when absent leads to *in utero* death (Cepeda et al., 2007). For example, wild type huntingtin contributes to the cortical production of brain derived neurotrophic factor (BDNF) before the latter's downstream support of striatal neurons (Zuccato et al., 2010). In those with the mutation, glutamine residues accumulate and the mutant HTT protein disrupts cellular signals and homeostasis decades before symptoms emerge. The mutation is detectable in nervous tissue diffusely; however, the disease is uniquely characterized by its expression in the medium spiny neurons (MSNs) found in the caudate, putamen and cortical pyramidal cells. The eventual death of these MSNs is the pathological hallmark of the structural damage demonstrated in HD (Georgiou-Karistianis et al., 2013). The precise cascade of events that leads to neurodegeneration is still largely unknown (Raymond et al., 2011).

MSNs account for 90% of all neurons in the striatum and are its only output source (Murer et al., 2002). There are two subtypes of MSNs that are differentiated by the peptides co-expressed; the receptor subtypes and the target to which they project. These GABAergic MSNs exert their effect via a direct or indirect pathway. MSNs in the indirect pathway (striaopallidal, D2 receptors) project to the external segment of the globus pallidus (GPe) and subthalamic nucleus (Cepeda et al., 2007). These indirect pathway neurons are the first cell population to succumb in HD and are implicated in the hyperkinesia that heralds the onset of the disease. MSNs in the direct pathway (striatonigral, D1 receptors) project to the internal segment of the globus pallidus (GPi) and the substantia nigra pars reticulatea (SNr; Cepeda et al., 2007). Degeneration of direct pathway MSNs, and the resulting loss of substance P, may contribute to late stage motor features characterized by impaired voluntary movement (Raymond et al., 2011). This transition from hyperkinesia to akinesia during the natural history of the disease may confound the results of interventions aimed at arresting or controlling chorea.

Impaired dopamine homeostasis is another consequence of the mutation that contributes to the impaired information processing from cortical inputs to the striatum (André et al., 2010). Dopaminergic neurons projecting from the substantia nigra pars compacta, and to a lesser degree the ventral tegmental area (VTA), to the dorsal striatum regulate glutamate sensitivity as well (dorsal circuit). Indirect pathway MSNs express D2 receptors whereas D1 receptors are more abundant in direct pathway MSNs. Degeneration of these nigrostriatal dopaminergic neurons are observed in HD and may contribute to late onset akinesia (André et al., 2010; Raymond et al., 2011). Conversely, presynaptic hyperactivation of the nigrostiatal pathway may elicit the characteristic chorea of early stage disease (André et al., 2010). Agents affecting dopamine (DA) transmission are used to modulate HD symptoms with some effect. DA may facilitate the "upstate" or depolarized state that enables encoding of specific motor tasks routed by the corticostriatal pathway (Murer et al., 2002).

The primary inputs to the MSNs are glutamatergic projections from the neocortex. Cortical neuron death is also observed in HD, especially in layers III, V and VI. The cell death is profound enough to be observed on gross pathological specimens and predates the onset of motor symptoms. One hypothesis is that excitotoxicity at the cortico-striatal synapses underpins HD (Cepeda et al., 2007). This is supported by evidence that increased release of glutamate from cortical projections, together with reduced uptake from the synaptic cleft by glial cells and enhanced striatal sensitivity to glutamate contributes to an amplified affect (Wójtowicz et al., 2013). In mouse models of HD, down-regulation of GLT1 has been demonstrated (Liévens et al., 2001). GLT1, a sodium-dependent glutamate transporter, ordinarily serves to remove extracellular glutamate and limit excitotoxicity. This down-regulation, together with NMDA-R hypersensitivity, increases intracellular calcium and induces an apoptotic cascade in HD.

Aspiny cholinergic, fast spiking, interneurons that co-express parvoalbumin are the main inhibitory neurons within the striatum (Russo et al., 2013). Theses interneurons are typically preserved until the late stages of the disease and are at least partly responsible for information processing and integration in the normal striatum (Raymond et al., 2011). Although, the death of the interneurons lags behind the MSNs, the dystonia that is especially pronounced in early onset and juvenile HD may be related to interneuron death (Reiner et al., 2013).

Abnormal Electrophysiology in HD

Under normal conditions, the ventral, dorsolateral (motor) and dorsomedial (associative) striatum are both activated simultaneously during specific task learning (Williams and Eskandar, 2006; Gale et al., 2014; Thorn and Graybiel, 2014). As a behavior becomes habitual, the association between striatal components decouples and the ventral (Gale et al., 2014) and motor striatum emerges while the activity of the associative striatum, now redundant, recedes (Williams and Eskandar, 2006; Thorn and Graybiel, 2014). In the ventral striatum, the learning related facilitation of activity is thought to represent the increased expectation of reward for the execution of specific stimulus-motor behaviors (Gale et al., 2014). Thus, under normal conditions, it is thought that the ventral striatum provides the motivation to engage in reward obtaining behaviors. In HD, the depressive and limbic symptoms may be related to motivational changes brought on by dysfunction of striatal MSNs and/or dopamine de-innervation (via dopamine cell loss of the SNpc and VTA). In the dorsal striatum, once a task is learned, the specific motor sequences or chunks are organized within the basal ganglia as a concatenation of neuronal activity played out in the direct and indirect pathway. Co-activation of these pathways facilitates the desired movement by suppressing unwanted movements (indirect) and expressing the specific motor chunk (direct pathway) (Jin et al., 2014). Near limitless combinations of nested oscillating frequencies are able to associate with these specified action sequences. Normally, when an action is queued, an assembly of neurons transitions to the upstate, enabling the asynchronous, specified action to emerge (Stern et al., 1998). However, in HD, the bidirectional cortico-striatal network is no longer able to precisely orchestrate action as nested frequencies uncouple (Miller et al., 2011). Together with the thalamocortical network, which helps set the membrane potential of the MSNs, the system becomes deregulated. As redundancies in the system also dissociate, the behavior chunk fails.

This high degree of coordination needed to facilitate a desired movement is evident when studied on a smaller scale. In mouse models of HD, widespread electrophysiologic dysfunction at the neuronal level is observed. The MSNs demonstrate a depolarized resting membrane potential. This induces hyper-excitability of the depolarization dependent NMDA receptor in response to glutamate. The overactive cells create an energy sink that may lead to cellular death (Rebec et al., 2006). Similar findings are noted in cortical pyramidal cells. As the disease progresses, the overactive cortico-striatal pathway eventually becomes less active and cortical synaptic inputs are lost (Cepeda et al., 2003).

Normalizing large-scale nested oscillations or stabilizing more localized dysfunctional units in HD is challenging. To achieve this, establishing how fundamental frequencies within the striatum evolve throughout the course of HD will be paramount. Recordings from the dorsal striatum in one study of freely moving normal rats demonstrated LFPs in the 1–30 Hz range with a relatively isolated peak at 50–55 Hz (Masimore et al., 2004). Still, LFPs in HD patients have not been well characterized (Estrada-Sánchez and Rebec, 2013). Once known, an attempt to tune the local frequency with electrical stimulation (ES) to regulate function may be possible.

In HD, re-entrainment of the striatum through ES of both the direct and indirect pathway, may repair learning deficits or reduce the rate of loss of existing habitual circuits. ES may also be able to partially restore the energy imbalance by reducing the hyper-excitable state, consequently preserving cortical inputs. Interestingly, in some animal models of HD, the cortex assumes a hyper-excitable state only after the disease has progressed. This finding contrasts with the observations in MSNs but may mark an identifiable time point for intervention (Cummings et al., 2009).

Deep Brain Stimulation for HD

There are several reports describing the use of DBS in HD when debilitating chorea predominates in the presence of atrophy and structural changes. We must be cautious in the interpretation of these studies based on the heterogeneity (**Table 1**). The target most often selected was GPi and DBS was primarily offered to control medically refractory chorea in most cases; although the progression to hypokinesia later in the disease can sometimes complicate interventions (Reiner, 2004). Although cognition was either not addressed or mentioned only in brief, these studies serve as a starting point for the next generation of DBS therapies for HD.

In one of the earliest published reports, bilateral GPi leads were implanted in a patient with pharmacologically-refractory HD chorea (Moro et al., 2004). 40 Hz stimulation improved the chorea and dystonia in this patient. The effect was enhanced at higher frequencies (130 Hz) but this exacerbated the bradykinesia, corroborating findings in other studies. Positron Emission Tomography (PET) studies in this patient also demonstrated increased cerebral blood flow in the supplementary motor area, anterior cingulate cortex and sensorimotor cortex with "ON" stimulation only. It is unclear what, if any, cognitive gains may have been facilitated by DBS. In the wake of the success treating this initial patient, others followed, publishing their findings after bilateral GPi DBS for HD

TABLE 1 | Summary of published deep brain stimulation reports for HD.

	Target(s)	*N*	Ages(s) at surgery (years)	Approximate disease duration prior to DBS (years)	CAG repeat length(s)
Moro et al. (2004)	GPi	1	43	8	-
Hebb et al. (2006)	GPi	1	41	13	47
Biolsi et al. (2008)	GPi	1	60	10	44
Fasano et al. (2008)	GPi	1	72	17	-
Ligot et al. (2011)	GPe	5	41–60	2–5	41–53
Kang et al. (2011)	GPi	2	57	10	42
			50	5	41
Groiss et al. (2011)	GPi	1	65	-	-
Spielberger et al. (2012)	GPi	1	30	9	58
Cislaghi et al. (2013)*	GPi	1	27	12	74
Huys et al. (2013)	GPi	1	40	3	-
Velez-Lago et al. (2013)	GPi	2	34	7	60
			25	6	68
Gonzalez et al. (2014)	GPi	7	30–78	3–8	40–50
Gruber et al. (2014)	STN and GPi	1	41	9	49
Beste et al. (2014)	GPe	2	57	-	42
			32		53

**Westphal variant; (-) indicates data was not found or reported.*

with mixed, but generally favorable, results (Hebb et al., 2006; Spielberger et al., 2012).

Biolsi et al. described a patient with bilateral GPi DBS implantation for chorea, which also had moderate subcortical cognitive dysfunction at the time of surgery (Biolsi et al., 2008). Four years later, the cognitive dysfunction remained stable and the patient was still able to perform complicated motor tasks. DBS in this case reduced the chorea and may have been neuroprotective, although his disease progression had been noted to be slow even prior to DBS. In another case, bilateral GPi DBS was performed which demonstrated global progressive cognitive decline on serial testing. He, like others, developed bradykinesia after DBS that prevented stable ambulation (Fasano et al., 2008). In two other patients who underwent bilateral GPi, chorea was improved at 2 years but cognitive decline continued, suggesting DBS was unable to halt progression of cognitive dysfunction (Kang et al., 2011).

Another report of two patients who underwent DBS of the GPi as a palliative treatment for disabling motor symptoms was recently published (Velez-Lago et al., 2013). In one patient, for whom chorea was the predominate symptom, DBS reduced a chorea subscore on the Unified HD Rating Scale. In the second patient, DBS was offered as a treatment of generalized, non-fixed dystonia. This failed to improve her dystonia, and the devices were eventually turned off. Although GPi DBS is a well-established treatment for primary generalized dystonia, the dystonic symptoms in HD are unique and appear to reflect the loss of direct pathway striatal neurons in advanced disease.

In the largest published series to date, seven patients with refractory chorea were treated with bilateral GPi DBS between 2008 and 2010 (Gonzalez et al., 2014). Similar to the other studies, chorea improved on average 60% at 1 year but a favorable improvement on the total motor score was not observed (Gonzalez et al., 2014). Importantly, DBS did not alleviate dystonia; while deactivation of stimulation reactivated chorea, indicating that, as for other movement disorders, the effects on motor symptoms depend on continuous stimulation.

Gruber et al. implanted a patient using simultaneous STN and GPi DBS in an attempt to recalibrate the direct and indirect pathways. This strategy minimized the bradykinesia observed following GPi stimulation alone (Gonzalez et al., 2014). Not surprisingly, when STN was used alone, chorea was not sustainably improved (Gruber et al., 2014).

Because of its role in error processing control, the GPe is another potential target for DBS in patients with HD exhibiting cognitive dysfunction. Error processing control, a measure of negative feedback that updates a behavioral action in real time, is believed to underlie early executive dysfunction in HD (Smith et al., 2000). Temel et al. tested DBS of the globus pallidus externus in a transgenic rat model of HD to evaluate the effect on motor and cognitive function (Temel et al., 2006). Cognitive function was measured by performance on a choice reaction time test. Transgenic rats will prematurely release a lever associated with a food reward compared to controls. This indicates that transgenic rats are unable to suppress the unwanted response. In both wild type rats and transgenic rats, DBS improved performance on the choice reaction time test relative to preoperative testing. Although the number of animals tested was small, this study suggests DBS restores unwanted response inhibition in the indirect pathway-–a necessary precursor for executing learned behavior in the co-activation model.

In part, based on these results, Ligot et al. proposed that inhibitory stimulation of GPe would suppress thalamocortical hyperactivity-induced hyperkinesia as well as influence cognitive and behavioral symptoms (Ligot et al., 2011). To study this effect, the investigators used PET imaging to

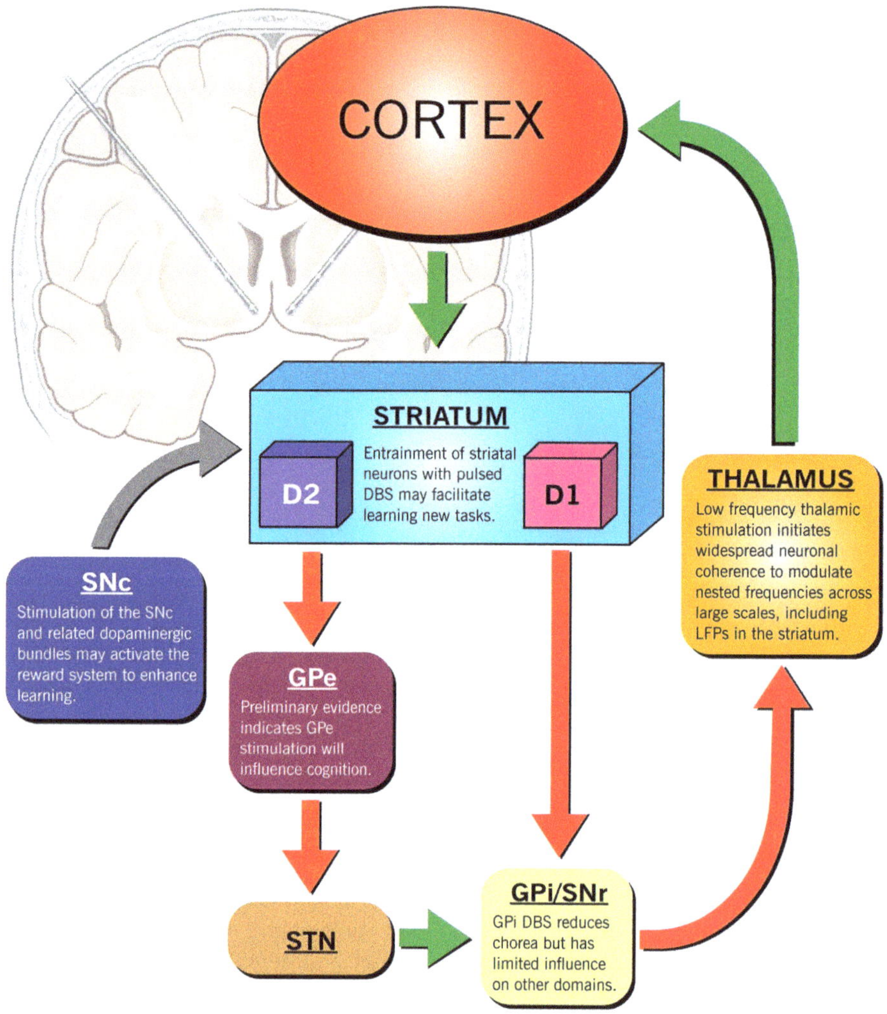

FIGURE 1 | Therapeutic targets for deep brain stimulation in HD. The scale of the response could be modulated by using different stimulation paradigms in addition to the location of the lead(s). For example, increasing dopaminergic activity through SNc stimulation may improve non-specific striatal processing that governs learning. Similarly, thalamic stimulation at low frequencies may modulate multiple nested frequencies simultaneously to re-establish a normal frequency spectrum. High frequency, triggered focal, pulsed stimulation of the striatum paired to a specific task could augment learning of specific skills by boosting event sequencing.

compare 15 control subjects with 5 HD patients implanted with stimulation electrodes in GPe. In the resting state, cortico-subcortical regional cerebral blood flow is reduced in HD with the stimulator off. In keeping with the basal ganglia thalamocortical circuit model, GPe stimulation modulated connectivity and further reduced regional cerebral blood flow in the basal ganglia, cortical structures and the default mode network (Ligot et al., 2011). These findings lead to the conclusion that stimulation of GPe may benefit patients with HD. In a recently completed prospective pilot study, intended to test both GPe and GPi stimulation using a crossover design, DBS of GPe in two patients with HD seemed to restore error processing control, although this effect was washed out when the system was turned off (Beste et al., 2014). Based on these studies and current models of learning, it is our impression, that GPe DBS warrants continued study as a potentially therapeutic target in HD.

Deep Brain Stimulation for HD: Future Directions

The effects of HD lead to cortical disassociation where new behaviors and motor tasks are no longer acquired and existing concatenations that subserve simple and complex skills are decoupled. While the current results of DBS in HD patients may seem disappointing at first, a great deal has been learned. Earlier human studies are primarily aimed at evaluating safety of a novel therapy. The current stage of knowledge seems to support that GPi and GPe DBS may or may not improve motor symptoms but, in general, effects of stimulation were not deleterious. With safety largely established, new studies can be initiated including controlled trials. New therapies could be aimed at realigning cortical and subcortical structures or reinforce existing pathways, particularly when neural compensation is most responsive (Papoutsi et al., 2014). Cognitive biomarkers that can be detected during the prodromal stages and followed during disease progression, such as working memory, psychomotor speed, reaction to negative emotions, and executive functioning, may be most promising (Dumas et al., 2013).

It is our opinion that DBS may hold promise in preserving brain function in patients with HD to maintain independence and reduce suffering. However, because the phenotypic expression of HD is heterogeneous, DBS may only benefit a select group of patients. Determining this subset is paramount to the success of any intervention. Fortunately, recent large-scale longitudinal studies (such as PREDICT-HD) that have identified specific functional imaging signals indicating early neuronal dysfunction in HD have exposed this window of opportunity. Targeted ES, early in the course of disease may be able to overcome limitations via several mechanisms including: (1) regulation of dopamine homeostasis, (2) focal inhibition or (3) activation of local brain regions, (4) task specific, triggered closed-loop stimulation or (5) diffuse modulation of multiple pathways with low frequency stimulation (**Figure 1**). Deciding when to initiate a disease modifying therapy in HD is challenging. Intervention in the prodromal stage exposes an individual to risk when they may be able to live and work independently for many more years. Similarly, initiating therapy after significant cell death, a precursor to end-stage disease, may be futile. The ethical considerations in delivering neuromodulation should therefore be taken very seriously before such an intervention is delivered to a desperate population (Ford and Kubu, 2006).

The question remains open on whether DBS may have any effect in slowing disease progression in HD. To date DBS has not demonstrated neuroprotection for motor decline in other degenerative conditions (Lilleeng et al., 2014). We believe HD may be unique to PD in the ability to identify gene positive individuals prodromally and closely predict the age of motor symptom onset, early in the course of cortico-striatal dysfunction. Furthermore, even if unable to change the trajectory of a terminal disease such as HD, the ability to successfully improve functional capacity and, in turn, optimism (especially early in the disease process), would have a substantial impact on quality of life at an individual level, and the potential for positive economic consequences at a societal level.

Author Contributions

Conception (SN, AM, MP); Drafting and/or revision (SN, AM, JG, DL, MP); Final approval (SN, AM, JG, DL, MP); Agreement to accountability (SN, AM, JG, DL, MP).

References

André, V. M., Cepeda, C., and Levine, M. S. (2010). Dopamine and glutamate in Huntington's disease: a balancing act. *CNS Neurosci. Ther.* 16, 163–178. doi: 10.1111/j.1755-5949.2010.00134.x

Beste, C., Mückschel, M., Elben, S., Hartmann, C. J., McIntyre, C. C., Saft, C., et al. (2014). Behavioral and neurophysiological evidence for the enhancement of cognitive control under dorsal pallidal deep brain stimulation in Huntington's disease. *Brain Struct. Funct.*. doi: 10.1007/s00429-014-0805-x. [Epub ahead of print].

Biolsi, B., Cif, L., El Fertit, H., Robles, S. G., and Coubes, P. (2008). Long-term follow-up of huntington disease treated by bilateral deep brain stimulation of the internal globus pallidus. *J. Neurosurg.* 109, 130–132. doi: 10.3171/jns/2008/109/7/0130

Cepeda, C., Hurst, R. S., Calvert, C. R., Hernández-Echeagaray, E., Nguyen, O. K., Jocoy, E., et al. (2003). Transient and progressive electrophysiological alterations in the corticostriatal pathway in a mouse model of Huntington's disease. *J. Neurosci.* 23, 961–969.

Cepeda, C., Wu, N., André, V. M., Cummings, D. M., and Levine, M. S. (2007). The corticostriatal pathway in Huntington's disease. *Prog. Neurobiol.* 81, 253–271. doi: 10.1016/j.pneurobio.2006.11.001

Cislaghi, G., Capiluppi, E., Saleh, C., Romano, L., Servello, D., Mariani, C., et al. (2013). Bilateral globus pallidus stimulation in westphal variant of huntington disease. *Neuromodulation* doi: 10.1111/ner.12098. [Epub ahead of print].

Cummings, D. M., Andre, V. M., Uzgil, B. O., Gee, S. M., Fisher, Y. E., Cepeda, C., et al. (2009). Alterations in cortical excitation and inhibition in genetic mouse models of Huntington's disease. *J. Neurosci.* 29, 10371–10386. doi: 10.1523/JNEUROSCI.1592-09.2009

Dumas, E. M., van den Bogaard, S., Middelkoop, H., and Roos, R. (2013). A review of cognition in Huntington's disease. *Front. Biosci. (Schol. Ed).* 5, 1–18. doi: 10.2741/S355

Estrada-Sánchez, A. M., and Rebec, G. V. (2013). Role of cerebral cortex in the neuropathology of Huntington's disease. *Front. Neural Circuits* 7:19. doi: 10.3389/fncir.2013.00019

Fasano, A., Mazzone, P., Piano, C., Quaranta, D., Soleti, F., and Bentivoglio, A. R. (2008). GPi-DBS in Huntington's disease: results on motor function and cognition in a 72-year-old case. *Mov. Disord.* 23, 1289–1292. doi: 10.1002/mds.22116

Ford, P. J., and Kubu, C. S. (2006). Stimulating debate: ethics in a multidisciplinary functional neurosurgery committee. *J. Med. Ethics* 32, 106–109. doi: 10.1136/jme.200x.013151

Gale, J. T., Shields, D. C., Ishizawa, Y., and Eskandar, E. N. (2014). Reward prediction and reinforcement by the nucleus accumbens during learning. *Front. Behav. Neurosci.* 8:114. doi: 10.3389/fnbeh.2014.00114

Georgiou-Karistianis, N., Scahill, R., Tabrizi, S. J., Squitieri, F., and Aylward, E. (2013). Structural MRI in Huntington's disease and recommendations for its potential use in clinical trials. *Neurosci. Biobehav. Rev.* 37, 480–490. doi: 10.1016/j.neubiorev.2013.01.022

Gonzalez, V., Cif, L., Biolsi, B., Garcia-Ptacek, S., Seychelles, A., Sanrey, E., et al. (2014). Deep brain stimulation for Huntington's disease: long-term results of a prospective open-label study. *J. Neurosurg.* 121, 114–122. doi: 10.3171/2014.2.JNS131722

Groiss, S. J., Elben, S., Reck, C., Voges, J., Wojtecki, L., and Schnitzler, A. (2011). Local field potential oscillations of the globus pallidus in Huntington's disease. *Mov. Disord.* 26, 2577–2578. doi: 10.1002/mds.23914

Gruber, D., Kuhn, A., Schoenecker, T., Kopp, U., Kivi, A., Huebl, J., et al. (2014). Quadruple deep brain stimulation in Huntington's disease, targeting pallidum and subthalamic nucleus: case report and review of the literature. *J. Neural Transm.* 121, 1303–1312. doi: 10.1007/s00702-014-1201-7

Hebb, M. O., Garcia, R., Gaudet, P., and Mendez, I. M. (2006). Bilateral stimulation of the globus pallidus internus to treat choreathetosis in Huntington's disease: technical case report. *Neurosurgery* 58:E383. doi: 10.1227/01.neu.0000195068.19801.18

Huys, D., Bartsch, C., Poppe, P., Lenartz, D., Huff, W., Prütting, J., et al. (2013). Management and outcome of pallidal deep brain stimulation in severe Huntington's disease. *Fortschr. Neurol. Psychiatr.* 81, 202–205. doi: 10.1055/s-0033-1335097

Jin, X., Tecuapetla, F., and Costa, R. M. (2014). Basal ganglia subcircuits distinctively encode the parsing and concatenation of action sequences. *Nat. Neurosci.* 17, 423–430. doi: 10.1038/nn.3632

Kang, G. A., Heath, S., Rothlind, J., and Starr, P. A. (2011). Long-term follow-up of pallidal deep brain stimulation in two cases of Huntington's disease. *J. Neurol. Neurosurg. Psychiatry* 82, 272–277. doi: 10.1136/jnnp.2009.202903

Liévens, J., Woodman, B., Mahal, A., Spasic-Boscovic, O., Samuel, D., Kerkerian-Le Goff, L., et al. (2001). Impaired glutamate uptake in the R6 Huntington's disease transgenic mice. *Neurobiol. Dis.* 8, 807–821. doi: 10.1006/nbdi.2001.0430

Ligot, N., Krystkowiak, P., Simonin, C., Goldman, S., Peigneux, P., Van Naemen, J., et al. (2011). External globus pallidus stimulation modulates brain connectivity in Huntington's disease. *J. Cereb. Blood Flow Metab.* 31, 41–46. doi: 10.1038/jcbfm.2010.186

Lilleeng, B., Brønnick, K., Toft, M., Dietrichs, E., and Larsen, J. P. (2014). Progression and survival in Parkinson's disease with subthalamic nucleus stimulation. *Acta Neurol. Scand.* 130, 292–298. doi: 10.1111/ane.12224

Masimore, B., Kakalios, J., and Redish, A. (2004). Measuring fundamental frequencies in local field potentials. *J. Neurosci. Methods* 138, 97–105. doi: 10.1016/j.jneumeth.2004.03.014

Meiser, B., and Dunn, S. (2000). Psychological impact of genetic testing for Huntington's disease: an update of the literature. *J. Neurol. Neurosurg. Psychiatry* 69, 574–578. doi: 10.1136/jnnp.69.5.574

Miller, B. R., Walker, A. G., Barton, S. J., and Rebec, G. V. (2011). Dysregulated neuronal activity patterns implicate corticostriatal circuit dysfunction in multiple rodent models of Huntington's disease. *Front. Syst. Neurosci.* 5:26. doi: 10.3389/fnsys.2011.00026

Moro, E., Lang, A. E., Strafella, A. P., Poon, Y. W., Arango, P. M., Dagher, A., et al. (2004). Bilateral globus pallidus stimulation for Huntington's disease. *Ann. Neurol.* 56, 290–294. doi: 10.1002/ana.20183

Murer, M. G., Tseng, K. Y., Kasanetz, F., Belluscio, M., and Riquelme, L. A. (2002). Brain oscillations, medium spiny neurons and dopamine. *Cell. Mol. Neurobiol.* 22, 611–632. doi: 10.1023/A:1021840504342

Oster, E., Shoulson, I., and Dorsey, R. E. (2013). Optimal expectations and limited medical testing: evidence from huntington disease. *Am. Econ. Rev.* 103, 804–830. doi: 10.1257/aer.103.2.804

Papoutsi, M., Labuschagne, I., Tabrizi, S. J., and Stout, J. C. (2014). The cognitive burden in Huntington's disease: pathology, phenotype and mechanisms of compensation. *Mov. Disord.* 29, 673–683. doi: 10.1002/mds.25864

Paulsen, J. S., Langbehn, D. R., Stout, J. C., Aylward, E., Ross, C. A., Nance, M., et al. (2008). Detection of Huntington's disease decades before diagnosis: the predict-HD study. *J. Neurol. Neurosurg. Psychiatry* 79, 874–880. doi: 10.1136/jnnp.2007.128728

Paulsen, J. S., and Long, J. D. (2014). Onset of Huntington's disease: can it be purely cognitive? *Mov. Disord.* 29, 1342–1350. doi: 10.1002/mds.25997

Paulsen, J. S., Long, J. D., Johnson, H. J., Aylward, E. H., Ross, C. A., Williams, J. K., et al. (2014). Clinical and biomarker changes in premanifest huntington disease show trial feasibility: a decade of the PREDICT-HD study. *Front. Aging Neurosci.* 6:78. doi: 10.3389/fnagi.2014.00078

Raymond, L. A., André, V. M., Cepeda, C., Gladding, C. M., Milnerwood, A. J., and Levine, M. S. (2011). Pathophysiology of Huntington's disease: time-dependent alterations in synaptic and receptor function. *Neuroscience* 198, 252–273. doi: 10.1016/j.neuroscience.2011.08.052

Rebec, G., Conroy, S., and Barton, S. (2006). Hyperactive striatal neurons in symptomatic Huntington R6/2 mice: variations with behavioral state and repeated ascorbate treatment. *Neuroscience* 137, 327–336. doi: 10.1016/j.neuroscience.2005.08.062

Reiner, A. (2004). Can lesions of GPe correct HD deficits? *Exp. Neurol.* 186, 1–5. doi: 10.1016/j.expneurol.2003.11.002

Reiner, A., Shelby, E., Wang, H., Demarch, Z., Deng, Y., Guley, N. H., et al. (2013). Striatal parvalbuminergic neurons are lost in Huntington's disease: implications for dystonia. *Mov. Disord.* 28, 1691–1699. doi: 10.1002/mds.25624

Ross, C. A., Aylward, E. H., Wild, E. J., Langbehn, D. R., Long, J. D., Warner, J. H., et al. (2014). Huntington disease: natural history, biomarkers and prospects for therapeutics. *Nat. Rev. Neurol.* 10, 204–216. doi: 10.1038/nrneurol.2014.24

Ross, C. A., and Tabrizi, S. J. (2011). Huntington's disease: from molecular pathogenesis to clinical treatment. *Lancet Neurol.* 10, 83–98. doi: 10.1016/S1474-4422(10)70245-3

Russo, G., Nieus, T. R., Maggi, S., and Taverna, S. (2013). Dynamics of action potential firing in electrically connected striatal fast-spiking interneurons. *Front. Cell. Neurosci.* 7:209. doi: 10.3389/fncel.2013.00209

Smith, M. A., Brandt, J., and Shadmehr, R. (2000). Motor disorder in Huntington's disease begins as a dysfunction in error feedback control. *Nature* 403, 544–549. doi: 10.1038/35000576

Spielberger, S., Hotter, A., Wolf, E., Eisner, W., Müller, J., Poewe, W., et al. (2012). Deep brain stimulation in Huntington's disease: a 4-year follow-up case report. *Mov. Disord.* 27, 806–807. doi: 10.1002/mds.24959

Stern, E. A., Jaeger, D., and Wilson, C. J. (1998). Membrane potential synchrony of simultaneously recorded striatal spiny neurons *in vivo*. *Nature* 394, 475–478. doi: 10.1038/28848

Tabrizi, S. J., Scahill, R. I., Durr, A., Roos, R. A., Leavitt, B. R., Jones, R., et al. (2011). Biological and clinical changes in premanifest and early stage Huntington's disease in the TRACK-HD study: the 12-month longitudinal analysis. *Lancet Neurol.* 10, 31–42. doi: 10.1016/s1474-4422(10)70276-3

Temel, Y., Cao, C., Vlamings, R., Blokland, A., Ozen, H., Steinbusch, H. W., et al. (2006). Motor and cognitive improvement by deep brain stimulation in a transgenic rat model of Huntington's disease. *Neurosci. Lett.* 406, 138–141. doi: 10.1016/j.neulet.2006.07.036

Thorn, C. A., and Graybiel, A. M. (2014). Differential entrainment and learning-related dynamics of spike and local field potential activity in the sensorimotor and associative striatum. *J. Neurosci.* 34, 2845–2859. doi: 10.1523/JNEUROSCI.1782-13.2014

Velez-Lago, F. M., Thompson, A., Oyama, G., Hardwick, A., Sporrer, J. M., Zeilman, P., et al. (2013). Differential and better response to deep brain stimulation of chorea compared to dystonia in Huntington's disease. *Stereotact. Funct. Neurosurg.* 91, 129–133. doi: 10.1159/000341070

Williams, Z. M., and Eskandar, E. N. (2006). Selective enhancement of associative learning by microstimulation of the anterior caudate. *Nat. Neurosci.* 9, 562–568. doi: 10.1038/nn1662

Wójtowicz, A. M., Dvorzhak, A., Semtner, M., and Grantyn, R. (2013). Reduced tonic inhibition in striatal output neurons from huntington mice due to loss of astrocytic GABA release through GAT-3. *Front. Neural Circuits* 7:188. doi: 10.3389/fncir.2013.00188

Zuccato, C., Valenza, M., and Cattaneo, E. (2010). Molecular mechanisms and potential therapeutical targets in Huntington's disease. *Physiol. Rev.* 90, 905–981. doi: 10.1152/physrev.00041.2009

14

Future think: cautiously optimistic about brain augmentation using tissue engineering and machine interface

E. Paul Zehr [1, 2, 3, 4, 5, 6*]

[1] *Rehabilitation Neuroscience Laboratory, University Victoria, Victoria, BC, Canada,* [2] *Human Discovery Science, International Collaboration on Repair Discoveries, Vancouver, BC, Canada,* [3] *Centre for Biomedical Research, University of Victoria, Victoria, BC, Canada,* [4] *Division of Medical Sciences, University of Victoria, BC, Canada,* [5] *School of Exercise Science, Physical, and Health Education, University of Victoria, Victoria, BC, Canada,* [6] *Zanshin Consulting, Inc., Victoria, BC, Canada*

Keywords: rehabilitation, enhancement, transhumanism, stem cell, engraftment, brain machine, neuroprosthetics, Asimov

"There is no sensible way in which we must take the possibility of misuse into account before determining that something is an enhancement." —John Harris in "Enhancing Evolution" (Harris, 2007)

"I need to wire the armor directly into my brain. Extremis could do that... I need to be the suit... I need to grow new connections" —Tony Stark talking about integration with the Iron Man armor in the graphic novel "Extremis" by Warren Ellis (Ellis, 2007)

Edited by:
Mikhail Lebedev,
Duke University, USA

Reviewed by:
Philip Kennedy,
Neural Signals Inc., USA
Roni Hogri,
Medical University of Vienna, Austria
Marios Kyriazis,
ELPIs Foundation for Indefinite Lifespans, UK

Correspondence:
E. Paul Zehr,
pzehr@uvic.ca

Introduction

Augmentation of brain function can imply restoration of function lost due to pathology or injury. On the other hand, techniques, approaches, and technologies used for brain augmentation in restoration can also amplify the range of human abilities in those without pathology. For example, non-invasive brain stimulation using transcranial magnetic stimulation (TMS) was originally applied for investigative and diagnostic purposes in neurological injury (Nollet et al., 2003). While TMS continues to be used in brain mapping and restoration of functional output (Romero et al., 2011; Bestmann and Krakauer, 2015), recent clinical applications in otherwise "healthy people" are widening. These include enhancing attention and vigilance (Nelson et al., 2014), motor learning (Cantarero et al., 2015) and various methods to "...improve attention, perception, memory and other forms of cognition..." (Clark and Parasuraman, 2014).

Technological augmentation of so-called "normal" human function moves us away from the functional limitations of our species and closer to "super" human function (Zehr, 2015), as with suggestions found in the transhumanist literature (Mcnamee and Edwards, 2006). Future applications of emerging technology can continue to shift us from our subspecies of *homo sapiens sapiens* to the transformative *homo sapiens technologicus*—a species that uses, fuses and integrates technology to enhance its own function (Zehr, 2011, 2015).

While there are many related approaches, this opinion article explores brain augmentation using approaches delimited to internally implanted biological enhancements (e.g. tissue engineering), and internal/external technological hardware [e.g., brain machine interface (BMI)].

Tissue Engineering and Stem Cell Chimeras

The pace of discoveries in the field of tissue engineering in regenerative medicine applications continues to accelerate (Leach et al., 2010; Elliott Donaghue et al., 2014). In 2013, Xiaoning Han and colleagues in the laboratories of Steven Goldman and Maiken Nedergaard at the University of Rochester Medical Center published a paper examining the possibility of augmenting neural processing ability of one species by surgically transplanting cells from the brain of another "more advanced" species (Han et al., 2013).

This research team was concerned with "biocompatability" in the mouse brain with certain evolutionary adaptations in human astroglial cells which are much larger with more complex structure than those found in the mouse. These astrocytes, which don't produce electric signals like neurons, are considered critical as physiological support and protection for the processing neurons, particularly in calcium signaling. This signaling is crucial for overall brain activity and human astrocytes operate threefold faster than those found in the mouse.

This generated the question: what would happen if you grafted human glial progenitor cells—the stem cells in the brain that would normally become astrocytes—into the forebrain of immunosuppressed mice? For how long would human cells survive in the mouse brain, and, critically, would the human astrocytes offer any behavioral advantage to the mice hosting the implanted cells?

Han and colleagues discovered that, in the mouse hippocampus, human glial cells thrived, and propagated calcium signals at the rate usually found in the human brain. Moreover, there was strengthened signal transmission between neurons (that is, long-term potentiation underlying learning and memory formation).

Critically, the functioning transplanted stem cells augmented behavior in the mice, including maze learning, fear conditioning, and enhanced ability to identify and find new objects in the murine habitat. The augmented chimeric mice with engrafted human glial cells essentially had improved all-around performance and this study represented an important test that cross-species grafting techniques could be a useful way to modify and augment (and examine in pathology) brain function.

Later, Martha Windrem and colleagues from the same laboratories, used an expanded protocol to examine the long term effects of engrafting human glial progenitor cells into the forebrains of neonatal mice (Windrem et al., 2014). Quite dramatically, there was a steady fall in murine cells coincident with an in increase in human cell content in the mouse brain. This proportional shift was so strong that after 1 year the glial progenitor cells found in the mouse forebrain populations were almost entirely of human origin.

That implanted human cells "outcompeted" and eventually replaced and "infected" the initial host mouse cells was an unexpected outcome. Windrem et al. "were surprised to note that the forebrains of these animals were often composed primarily of human glia and their progenitors" (Windrem et al., 2014).

External Technological Hardware and Augmentation with Brain Machine Interface

The interface of physiology and engineering represented by brain computer or brain machine interface has a history of success in non-human and human applications for restoration of function (Lebedev and Nicolelis, 2006; Wang et al., 2010; Shih et al., 2012). This tremendous success raises new questions. For example, is it possible to attach a biological brain to an external circuit and establish a functional connection for learning? This question was addressed by Theodore Berger and colleagues who showed that an input/output (stimulation and recording) neuroprosthetic interface enhanced memory function subserved by the rodent hippocampus and could overcome memory deficits mimicking natural damage (Berger et al., 2011). This approach was extended to restoration of cognitive decision making using a neuroprosthetic interfaced into the prefrontal cortex in the rhesus monkey (Hampson et al., 2012).

Simeon Bamford and colleagues established a proof of principle for direct applications of brain-machine neuroprosthetics in motor learning using cerebellar motor control and learning circuitry as the model (Prueckl et al., 2011; Bamford et al., 2012). They envisaged engineering scenarios that could meet the challenge required for truly integrated neuroprosthetics—a closed loop system. Such a system would be able to send to and receive from the brain inputs and processing to control devices that supplement the functionality of the brain itself (Bamford et al., 2012).

Cerebellar circuits are essential to classical conditioning of the eye-blink reflex (Cheron et al., 2013). In this protocol a conditioned stimulus (CS; a neutral stimulus like a sound) is paired with an unconditioned stimulus (US; e.g., an airpuff to the eye to evoke a blink reflex).

Initially only the US causes the blink reflex but over time the CS can evoke the blink in the absence of the US. Bamford and colleagues used the known input and output properties of the cerebellum to guide the development of a prototype chip fabricated as a microcircuit. Real data from anaestethized animals were used calibration and training. The circuit could be "conditioned in a manner very similar to that of a real intact cerebellum" thus establishing partial brain function replication using BMI (Bamford et al., 2012).

Herreros and colleagues successfully connected to the brain of an anesthetized rat as a "step toward the development of neuro-prostheses that could recover lost learning functions in animals and, in the longer term, humans" (Herreros et al., 2014). Most recently, this approach was used effectively in interfacing with the rodent brain for testing closed loop motor learning in real time (Hogri et al., 2015). These data lay the groundwork for refining future neuroprosthetics as well as creating a useful system for testing motor learning theories.

Miguel Pais-Vieira and colleagues, part of the Nicolelis and Lebedev groups, demonstrated that brain-machine interface concepts could be extended to brain-to-brain interfaces for shared information processing (Pais-Vieira et al., 2013). In this compelling research, two rats had electrode arrays implanted into the sensorimotor areas. One rat served as an "encoder" of sensorimotor information during performance of either a tactile or visual task. The cortical activity generated in the brain of the "encoder rat" was monitored and then relayed to a second "receiving" or "decoder" rat, located in a distant laboratory.

The brain of the "decoder rat" was electrically stimulated through the implanted electrode array based on the timing and pattern of activity received from the "encoder rat." The behavior of the "decoder rat" was directed by this activity and subsequently made similar task choices as did the "encoder rat." Thus, the distant "decoder rat" was taught by the neural traffic generated by the initial activity of the "encoder rat" and relayed by the direct brain-to-brain coupling afforded in this novel "artificial communication channel" (Pais-Vieira et al., 2013). This shows that rats linked through brain-to-brain electrode arrays could learn complex, cooperative, goal-directed behaviors.

A related human test of brain-to-brain interaction was conducted by Grau et al. (2014). They used non-invasive methodologies of electroencephalography (EEG) for signal detection at the "source" brain (essentially the "encoder" rat above) and TMS for transmission to the "receiver" brain (the "decoder" rat analog of Pias-Vieira et al.) to establish that direct communication between the brains of conscious humans was possible. This study focused only on transmission of simple language but heralds the future arrival of more complex communication.

Conclusion—Optimism Balanced with Some Cautious Forethought

Stem cell technologies continue to show promise and have the most imminent restorative applications in neurodegenerative disorders such as Alzheimer's disease, Parkinson's disease, and stroke. Critically, tissue engineering may help bootstrap this field while techniques for parallel non-invasive brain monitoring develop. While considerable progress continues, immune response and acute inflammation with implantations and microelectrode insertions into the brain present limitations on long-term viability of some approaches (Richter et al., 2011; Fernandez et al., 2014; Groothuis et al., 2014).

Applications of stem cell technologies in augmenting the "normal" range of human brain function await discovery. Possible avenues discoveries of superior cell function in specialized systems in other animals that may see implantation in humans to augment functions unrelated to processing speed. Assuming improvements in achieving robust and behaviorally-relevant interfaces allowing facile access to discrete input and output pathways, proven, and nascent BMI methodologies have implications for restoration of brain function on a large scale. As the dovetailing of stem cell technology and brain machine interface continues, I suggest we must also pay attention to the issues of security and ethics.

As for security, connecting a machine so the human operator can access the functional capacity of the machine also allows the machine access to the functional capacity of the human. In 1942 the scientist and science fiction writer Isaac Asimov presaged these concerns when describing artificial intelligence and robotics.

In his influential 1942 short story "Runaround," (later found in the book "I, Robot" ;Asimov, 1950) Asimov laid down his "Three Laws of Robotics" which aimed to protect the sanctity of human life. However, such concerns may be rendered moot if future neural interfaces function indistinguishably from the user since it enacts part of the control system that manifests as the will of the user. This means it may actually be impossible to separate between the actions of the neural interface and that of its wearer.

Assuming such convergence, this places a higher order of responsibility on such "augmented" users. I've reworked Asimov's Three Laws below to apply to the complexities of machine-brain-machine interfaces.

An augmented user with a neural interface:

- may not injure a human being or, through inaction, allow a human being to come to harm (Law 1);
- must protect its own existence as long as such protection does not conflict with Law 1 (Law 2).

In fact, this yields Two Laws, since Asimov's declaration (original Law 2) that a robot "must obey order given to it by human beings" is irrelevant. In this future look, the user is the interface and the term human being applies to all and related subspecies (e.g., *homo sapiens sapiens* and *homo sapiens technologicus*; Zehr, 2015).

As for ethical considerations, this sets the stage for complete fusion between trans-species biology and neuroengineering. This will bring us to real life artificial-human brain hybrids and increased applications to enhance and augment innate function rather than simply recover lost function. This includes the extension of the concept of brain augmentation to include the "global brain" suggested by Kyriazis (2015). Future applications to augmentation of otherwise healthy and intact brain function may well be in "the new wave of human enhancement" (Harris, 2007).

Yet, the issue of brain augmentation should proceed with appropriate caution in neurologically intact "normally functioning" people. The comment of Rudolf Jaenisch—in the context of the human gene editing controversy (Baltimore et al., 2015; Cyranoski, 2015; Vogel, 2015)—that "We need some principled agreement that we want to enhance humans in this way or we don't" (Wade, 2015) has resonance here.

Using the examples of brain augmentation discussed above, what other intact cellular interactions in the brain are disrupted by the effect of transpecies implants? What changes in brain structure and function may arise from long-term neuroprosthetic interface? What are the implications for what we now accept as "normal human behavior" and functional capacity?

Especially we need to establish what societal boundaries—if any—we will place on multi-species transplants and what does this mean for the concept of species itself? Many of the related ethical and moral issues are addressed elsewhere in more detail (Clark, 2014; Clark and Parasuraman, 2014; Kennedy, 2014; Hildt, 2015). Along the way forward it remains for us as scientists, engineers, and future users of brain augmentation methodologies to proceed with conviction and purpose, but also with suitable care and caution. Establishing the context for conviction, care and caution must also include dialogue with all members of our society including the general lay public.

Acknowledgments

I wish to thank those reviewers who provided excellent suggestions for improving this paper.

References

Asimov, I. (1950). *I, Robot.* New York, NY: DoubleDay

Baltimore, B. D., Berg, P., Botchan, M., Carroll, D., Charo, R. A., Church, G., et al. (2015). A prudent path forward for genomic engineering and germline gene modification. *Science* 348, 36–38. doi: 10.1126/science.aab1028

Bamford, S. A., Hogri, R., Giovannucci, A., Taub, A. H., Herreros, I., Verschure, P. F. M. J., et al. (2012). A VLSI field-programmable mixed-signal array to perform neural signal processing and neural modeling in a prosthetic system. *IEEE Trans. Neural Syst. Rehabil. Eng.* 20, 455–467. doi: 10.1109/TNSRE.2012.2187933

Berger, T., W., Robert, E. H., Dong, S., Anushka, G., Vasilis, Z. M., and Sam, A. D. (2011). A cortical neural prosthesis for restoring and enhancing memory. *J. Neural Eng.* 8, 046017. doi: 10.1088/1741-2560/8/4/046017

Bestmann, S., and Krakauer, J. (2015). The uses and interpretations of the motor-evoked potential for understanding behaviour. *Exp. Brain Res.* 233, 679–689. doi: 10.1007/s00221-014-4183-7

Cantarero, G., Spampinato, D., Reis, J., Ajagbe, L., Thompson, T., Kulkarni, K., et al. (2015). Cerebellar direct current stimulation enhances on-line motor skill acquisition through an effect on accuracy. *J. Neurosci.* 35, 3285–3290. doi: 10.1523/JNEUROSCI.2885-14.2015

Cheron, G., Dan, B., and Márquez-Ruiz, J. (2013). Translational approach to behavioral learning: lessons from cerebellar plasticity. *Neural Plast.* 2013:853654. doi: 10.1155/2013/853654

Clark, V. P. (2014). The ethical, moral and pragmatic rationale for brain augmentation. *Front. Syst. Neurosci.* 8:130. doi: 10.3389/fnsys.2014.00130

Clark, V. P., and Parasuraman, R. (2014). Neuroenhancement: enhancing brain and mind in health and in disease. *Neuroimage* 85, 889–894. doi: 10.1016/j.neuroimage.2013.08.071

Cyranoski, D. (2015). Ethics of embryo editing divides scientists. *Nature (London)* 519, 272–272. doi: 10.1038/519272a

Elliott Donaghue, I., Tam, R., Sefton, M. V., and Shoichet, M. S. (2014). Cell and biomolecule delivery for tissue repair and regeneration in the central nervous system. *J. Control. Release* 190, 219–227. doi: 10.1016/j.jconrel.2014.05.040

Ellis, W. (2007). *Invincible Iron Man: Extremis.* New York, NY: Marvel Comics.

Fernandez, E., Greger, B., House, P. A., Aranda, I., Botella, C., Albisua, J., et al. (2014). Acute human brain responses to intracortical microelectrode arrays: challenges and future prospects. *Front. Neuroeng.* 7:24. doi: 10.3389/fneng.2014.00024

Grau, C., Ginhoux, R., Riera, A., Nguyen, T. L., Chauvat, H., Berg, M., et al. (2014). Conscious brain-to-brain communication in humans using non-invasive technologies. *PLoS ONE* 9:e105225. doi: 10.1371/journal.pone.0105225

Groothuis, J., Ramsey, N. F., Ramakers, G. M. J., and Van Der Plasse, G. (2014). Physiological challenges for intracortical electrodes. *Brain Stimulation* 7, 1–6. doi: 10.1016/j.brs.2013.07.001

Hampson, R. E., Greg, A. G., Vasilis, M., Dong, S., Ioan, O., Lucas, S., et al. (2012). Facilitation and restoration of cognitive function in primate prefrontal cortex by a neuroprosthesis that utilizes minicolumn-specific neural firing. *J. Neural Eng.* 9:056012. doi: 10.1088/1741-2560/9/5/056012

Han, X., Chen, M., Wang, F., Windrem, M., Wang, S., Shanz, S., et al. (2013). Forebrain engraftment by human glial progenitor cells enhances synaptic plasticity and learning in adult mice. *Cell Stem Cell* 12, 342–353. doi: 10.1016/j.stem.2012.12.015

Harris, J. (2007). *Enhancing Evolution: the Ethical Case for Making Better People.* Princeton, NJ: Princeton University Press.

Herreros, I., Giovannucci, A., Taub, A. H., Hogri, R., Magal, A., Bamford, S., et al. (2014). A cerebellar neuroprosthetic system: computational architecture and *in vivo* test. *Front. Bioeng. Biotechnol.* 2:14. doi: 10.3389/fbioe.2014.00014

Hildt, E. (2015). What will this do to me and my brain? Ethical issues in brain-to-brain interfacing. *Front. Syst. Neurosci.* 9:17. doi: 10.3389/fnsys.2015.00017

Hogri, R., Bamford, S. A., Taub, A. H., Magal, A., Giudice, P. D., and Mintz, M. (2015). A neuro-inspired model-based closed-loop neuroprosthesis for the substitution of a cerebellar learning function in anesthetized rats. *Sci. Rep.* 5:8451. doi: 10.1038/srep08451

Kennedy, P. (2014). Brain-machine interfaces as a challenge to the 'moment of singularity'. *Front. Syst. Neurosci.* 8:213. doi: 10.3389/fnsys.2014.00213

Kyriazis, M. (2015). Systems neuroscience in focus: from the human brain to the global brain? *Front. Syst. Neurosci.* 9:7. doi: 10.3389/fnsys.2015.00007

Leach, J. B., Achyuta, A. K. H., and Murthy, S. K. (2010). Bridging the divide between neuroprosthetic design, tissue engineering and neurobiology. *Front. Neuroeng.* 2:18. doi: 10.3389/neuro.16.018.2009

Lebedev, M. A., and Nicolelis, M.A. L. (2006). Brain-machine interfaces: past, present and future. *Trends Neurosci.* 29, 536–546. doi: 10.1016/j.tins.2006.07.004

Mcnamee, M. J., and Edwards, S. D. (2006). Transhumanism, medical technology and slippery slopes. *J. Med. Ethics* 32, 513–518. doi: 10.1136/jme.2005.013789

Nelson, J. T., Mckinley, R. A., Golob, E. J., Warm, J. S., and Parasuraman, R. (2014). Enhancing vigilance in operators with prefrontal cortex transcranial direct current stimulation (tDCS). *Neuroimage* 85, Pt 3, 909–917. doi: 10.1016/j.neuroimage.2012.11.061

Nollet, H., Van Ham, L., Deprez, P., and Vanderstraeten, G. (2003). Transcranial magnetic stimulation: review of the technique, basic principles and applications. *Vet. J.* 166, 28–42. doi: 10.1016/S1090-0233(03)00025-X

Pais-Vieira, M., Lebedev, M., Kunicki, C., Wang, J., and Nicolelis, M. A. L. (2013). A brain-to-brain interface for real-time sharing of sensorimotor information. *Sci. Rep.* 3:1319. doi: 10.1038/srep01319

Prueckl, R., Taub, A. H., Herreros, I., Hogri, R., Magal, A., Bamford, S. A., et al. (2011). "Behavioral rehabilitation of the eye closure reflex in senescent rats using a real-time biosignal acquisition system," in *Engineering in Medicine and Biology Society, EMBC, 2011 Annual International Conference of the IEEE.* (Boston, MA).

Richter, A., Kruse, C., Moser, A., Hofmann, U. G., and Danner, S. (2011). Cellular modulation of polymeric device surfaces: promise of adult stem cells for neuroprosthetics. *Front. Neurosci.* 5:114. doi: 10.3389/fnins.2011.00114

Romero, J. R., Ramirez, D. M., Aglio, L. S., and Gugino, L. D. (2011). Brain mapping using transcranial magnetic stimulation. *Neurosurg. Clin. N.Am.* 22, 141–152. doi: 10.1016/j.nec.2010.11.002

Shih, J. J., Krusienski, D. J., and Wolpaw, J. R. (2012). Brain-computer interfaces in medicine. *Mayo Clin. Proc.* 87, 268–279. doi: 10.1016/j.mayocp.2011.12.008

Vogel, G. (2015). Embryo engineering alarm. *Science* 347:1301. doi: 10.1126/science.347.6228.1301

Wade, N. (2015, March 19). Scientists seek ban on method of editing the human genome. *New York Times.*

Wang, W., Collinger, J. L., Perez, M. A., Tyler-Kabara, E. C., Cohen, L. G., Birbaumer, N., et al. (2010). Neural interface technology for rehabilitation: exploiting and promoting neuroplasticity. *Phys. Med. Rehabil. Clin. N.Am.* 21, 157–178. doi: 10.1016/j.pmr.2009.07.003

Windrem, M. S., Schanz, S. J., Morrow, C., Munir, J., Chandler-Militello, D., Wang, S., et al. (2014). A competitive advantage by neonatally engrafted human glial progenitors yields mice whose brains are chimeric for human glia. *J. Neurosci.* 34, 16153–16161. doi: 10.1523/JNEUROSCI.1510-14.2014

Zehr, E. P. (2011). *Inventing Iron Man: the Possibility of a Human Machine.* Baltimore, MD: Johns Hopkins University Press.

Zehr, E. P. (2015). The potential transformation of our species by neural enhancement. *J. Mot. Behav.* 47, 73–78. doi: 10.1080/00222895.2014.916652

15

An integrated approach for the monitoring of brain and autonomic response of children with autism spectrum disorders during treatment by wearable technologies

Lucia Billeci[1, 2], Alessandro Tonacci[1], Gennaro Tartarisco[3], Antonio Narzisi[4], Simone Di Palma[5], Daniele Corda[6], Giovanni Baldus[6], Federico Cruciani[7], Salvatore M. Anzalone[8], Sara Calderoni[4], Giovanni Pioggia[3], Filippo Muratori[2, 4] and Michelangelo Study Group*

[1] Institute of Clinical Physiology, National Research Council of Italy, Pisa, Italy, [2] Department of Clinical and Experimental Medicine, University of Pisa, Pisa, Italy, [3] Institute of Applied Sciences and Intelligent Systems "Eduardo Caianiello", National Research Council of Italy, Messina, Italy, [4] Department of Developmental Neuroscience, IRCSS Stella Maris Foundation, Pisa, Italy, [5] Department of Information Engineering, University of Pisa, Pisa, Italy, [6] HelpyLife Technology, Oristano, Italy, [7] I+ srl, Florence, Italy, [8] Institute of Intelligent Systems and Robotics, University Pierre and Marie Curie, Paris, France

Edited by:
Mikhail Lebedev,
Duke University, USA

Reviewed by:
Andrea Caria,
University of Trento, Italy
Roberto Canitano,
University Hospital of Siena, Italy

Correspondence:
Lucia Billeci
lbilleci@fsm.unipi.it;
lucia.billeci@ifc.cnr.it

Autism Spectrum Disorders (ASD) are associated with physiological abnormalities, which are likely to contribute to the core symptoms of the condition. Wearable technologies can provide data in a semi-naturalistic setting, overcoming the limitations given by the constrained situations in which physiological signals are usually acquired. In this study an integrated system based on wearable technologies for the acquisition and analysis of neurophysiological and autonomic parameters during treatment is proposed and an application on five children with ASD is presented. Signals were acquired during a therapeutic session based on an imitation protocol in ASD children. Data were analyzed with the aim of extracting quantitative EEG (QEEG) features from EEG signals as well as heart rate and heart rate variability (HRV) from ECG. The system allowed evidencing changes in neurophysiological and autonomic response from the state of disengagement to the state of engagement of the children, evidencing a cognitive involvement in the children in the tasks proposed. The high grade of acceptability of the monitoring platform is promising for further development and implementation of the tool. In particular if the results of this feasibility study would be confirmed in a larger sample of subjects, the system proposed could be adopted in more naturalistic paradigms that allow real world stimuli to be incorporated into EEG/psychophysiological studies for the monitoring of the effect of the treatment and for the implementation of more individualized therapeutic programs.

Keywords: Autism Spectrum Disorders (ASD), quantitative EEG (QEEG), electrocardiogram (ECG), wearable sensors, monitoring, naturalistic, personalization, imitation

INTRODUCTION

Recent advances in neuroimaging and other less-invasive neurophysiological monitoring systems allow researchers to explore the relationship between neurophysiological signals, neurodevelopmental disorders and behavioral changes. In particular, atypical patterns of brain activity and connectivity have been documented in children with Autism Spectrum Disorders (ASD) and are the basis of impaired and atypical behaviors (Belmonte et al., 2004; Geschwind and Levitt, 2007; Coben et al., 2008; Cantor and Chabot, 2009).

Electroencephalography (EEG) is a non-invasive technique able to identify dysfunction in various brain regions in autistic individuals. EEG measurements can be investigated in the frequency domain, and it has been convincingly demonstrated that assessing specific frequencies can yield insights into the functional correlations between brain regions. The EEG patterns analysis in the frequency domain is known as Quantitative EEG (QEEG). Commonly QEEG has been used to capture electrical patterns at the scalp surface, which primarily reflect cortical electrical activity or "brainwaves" (Tong and Thakor, 2009). Recently, several studies have used QEEG as a tool for neurophysiological assessment of children with ASD during resting state condition or specific tasks (for a review see Billeci et al., 2013). Interestingly, QEEG measurements can provide a mean to establish treatment efficacy (Dawson et al., 2012). According to the above-mentioned evidence, QEEG provides sufficient sensitivity and specificity to be worthy of consideration for use in the diagnosis, treatment and outcome evaluation of neurodevelopmental disorders.

ASD are also characterized by altered autonomic function, which plays an important role in the regulation of behaviors during social interaction. Physiological parameters and vital signs including heart rate, systolic and diastolic pressure, pulse rate, skin conductance, body temperature, and fingertip temperature can be used as cues of autonomic functions. In particular, heart rate variability (HRV) is a well-recognized method to assess the cardiac autonomic balance of the autonomic nervous system (Goldberger, 1999; Friedman, 2007). Although a few parameters, such as the HRV, are influenced by physical activity, nevertheless they have been increasingly used to measure the activity of the autonomic nervous system and to study neurophysiological responses in naturalistic settings (Goodwin et al., 2006). Other studies have shown an extremely high autonomic arousal in individuals with ASD even though they appeared to be outwardly calm (Hirstein et al., 2001; Hoch et al., 2010; Ming et al., 2011).

One of the limitations of the physiological parameters' assessment protocol is the artificial setting in which signals are usually acquired, which may or may not be closely related with naturally occurring stimuli. Therefore, these protocols induce both systematic and non-systematic biases to the experimental outcome eluding the actual nature of the data. Furthermore, they do not allow an ecological assessment and monitoring during treatment or even at home.

The recording of physiological signals [such as electroecephalogram (EEG) or electrocardioram (ECG)] during treatment in a semi-naturalistic setting may reveal important cues about the engagement, the arousal and emotional state and can support clinicians during therapeutic sessions in the implementation of the most appropriate personalized treatment plan.

The study of engagement is particularly relevant in ASD as deficits in this field (that is when the child is not able to share his/her attention to the other) emerge very early, in the second half of the first year of life, leading to reduced engagement with social stimuli, and subsequently reduced opportunities for social learning (Dawson et al., 1998; Mundy and Neal, 2000; Chevallier et al., 2012). These early deficits may thus have cascading effects on social communication development in successive years. In order to contrast these cascading effects evidence-based models (i.e., Early Start Denver Model) suggest building therapeutic tasks around specific engagement skills (i.e., imitation or joint attention) as core of the intervention (Billeci et al., 2016; Bono et al., 2016). During these tasks in which there is a social interaction with a therapist, it is possible to explore the response to social engagement and emotion regulation in response to social disengagement (that is when the child is not involved in social attention). In particular in the last years some studies have been performed, which provide evidences that physiological signals could constitute an important marker of social functioning and well-being that differentiate between engagement and disengagement during social interactions or treatment sessions (Patriquin et al., 2013; Di Palma et al., 2016; Shahrestani et al., 2016).

It is important to underline that monitoring physiological parameters during therapeutic sessions or during daily basis routines is definitely more challenging than monitoring the same parameters under controlled conditions. It is mandatory for example that the equipment should not interfere with the activities performed by the children during the treatment session. Wearable systems and wireless technologies can overcome this problem allowing monitoring subjects in an unobtrusive way (Varshney, 2005, 2006; Yilmaz et al., 2010).

The present study aims at describing and discussing the implementation of a wearable technology system that can be used during naturalistic interactions between a child and a clinician during a treatment session for the monitoring of brain and autonomic response. A preliminary application in a sample of children with ASD is presented. This work has been carried out within the framework of MICHELANGELO, a project funded by the European Commission (FP7- ICT-288241) (http://www.michelangelo-project.eu/).

The combined analysis of QEEG and ECG signals in semi-naturalistic settings enables simultaneous examination of neurophysiological and physiological correlates while the child is engaged in socio-emotive interactions. This system is able to provide (i) ecologically synchronized quantitative measurements of brain signals, and (ii) autonomic responses not measurable with traditional research methods within a natural environment. For this purpose, wearable technologies for EEG and ECG have been used, which are suitable for young children with ASD. The system proposed will allow a reliable indication of brain activity and autonomic status in a naturalistic setting contributing toward the implementation of more individualized and effective treatment for children with ASD.

MATERIALS AND METHODS

Participants and Paradigm

The system was tested with five children with ASD (all males, age range = 6–8 years, mean age = 7.2 ± 0.83 years) (**Table 1**). The study was approved by the IRCSS Stella Maris Foundation's Ethical Committee and all the parents signed a written consent form to participate.

The ASD diagnosis was formulated according to the DSM-5 criteria (APA, 2013) and confirmed by the Autism Diagnostic Observation Schedule-2 (ADOS-2, Lord et al., 2012) and the Autism Diagnostic Interview-Revised (ADI-R, Lord et al., 1994).

The ADOS-2 diagnostic algorithm also provides an algorithm for computing the comparison score (CS), a measure of the severity of autism-related symptoms. The CS ranges from 1 to 10, where 1 indicates minimal-to-no evidence of autism-related symptoms and 10 indicates a high level of impairment.

The adaptive behavior was assessed according to the Vineland Adaptive Behavior Scale-II (VABS-II, Sparrow et al., 2005). A multidisciplinary team—including a senior child psychiatrist, and two clinical child psychologists experienced in ASD—conducted the diagnostic assessment during a 5-day extensive evaluation. The Wechsler Intelligence Scales for Children-IV (WISC-IV) were used to assess the Full Scale Intelligence Quotient (FSIQ).

The children involved in the experiment were monitored during one therapy session in clinic with the integrated system. The semi-naturalistic experimental paradigm was based on imitation (IM) in the context of a play-based setting (**Figure 1**). Each session took about 15 min. During all the session the children remained seated on a chair playing at a table with the therapist in order to limit artifacts in the data acquired.

The IM phase is realized according to three different tasks in which the therapist asks to the child to imitate what she is doing. In task 1, the therapist uses blocks, play-doh, or sheets and markets in order to elicit functional imitation in the child; in task 2 the therapist suggests the child gestural and symbolic imitation; in task 3 the therapist elicits facial expressions in the child. Each task was repeated sever times in order to have several segments of the signals, which could be mediated to have more consistent results. During the experimental sessions data brain, autonomic and video data were recorded and analyzed in post-processing with the integrated platform described in the following paragraphs.

Design

General Overview

The overall architecture of the integrated system is shown in **Figure 2**. It mainly consists of three modules: the biosignal sensor unit, the video mobile unit, and a Central Unit (CU).

The main function of the biosignal sensor unit is the wearable and wireless acquisition of EEG and ECG signals while allowing the child to interact with the therapist. The unit is composed by the Enobio wireless device (STARLAB, Barcelona, Spain) for EEG recording (Cester et al., 2008) and by a wireless ECG chest belt (Solar et al., 2012).

The integrated system is also provided of data analysis toolboxes for the processing of the recorded video, EEG and ECG signals. The collected data can be loaded and queried for data visualization, segmentation, and feature extraction. The toolboxes are developed as a research tool in order to investigate physiological and behavioral parameters correlated with behaviors of the child during treatment sessions. The main components of the system are described in the following paragraphs (for details about EEG and ECG feature extraction see Supplementary Materials).

Biosignal Sensor Unit

Enobio offers a high degree of unobtrusiveness (easy to use, wearable, only 65 grams weight). Each active digital electrode with a transduction interface and electrode is able to acquire, digitize, and transmit the signal on site in order to reduce the environmental noise while recording data away from the lab or controlled environments.

The system continuously records EEG signals over 19 channels positioned according to the 10/10 standard scheme and two references (placed on the mastoid), at 500 Hz with a 16-bit accuracy. Enobio is equipped both with gel and dry electrodes. While gel electrodes provide a better contact with the skin and lower impedance, their positioning can be very long and uncomfortable for the child. In this setting dry electrodes are chosen as they offer a shorter and easier set-up time comparable with gel electrodes, which is particularly important with children with ASD. Several articles indeed show that dry electrodes can yield performance comparable to gel electrodes (Zander et al., 2011; Guger et al., 2012). Data from Enobio are recorded by a dedicated software (NIC, Neuroelectrics).

The chest belt for ECG acquisition is a wearable device designed by our group based on the Shimmer® (Burns et al., 2010) wireless base module, which is CE certified and validated prior to the present study in a group of healthy subjects (Solar et al., 2012).

The system is powered by a 3.6 V rechargeable battery, which allows up to 7 h of continuous monitoring per charge. The system sample frequency can be set from a minimum of 100 Hz up to a maximum of 500 Hz. The hardware module was tailored to be compliant with the common cardio-fitness Polar™ or Adidas™ chest straps in order to gain in ergonomics, to be lightweight and allow long-term monitoring. These straps are fully washable and integrate dry electrodes applied directly to the patient's skin for single-lead acquisitions.

Video Mobile Unit

The video mobile unit is made up by two environmental cameras with a frame rate of 25 fps and a resolution of 640 × 480 for video recording. The cameras are wired and synchronized with the system to contextualize the neurophysiological parameters with the behavior of the child. With the aim of building an exploitable research tool to investigate EEG signal, inexpensive webcam were used as video capture devices (Microsoft LifeCam HD-5000).

TABLE 1 | Participants characteristics.

Subjects	Age in years	Diagnosis	ADOS-2 Module	ADOS (CS)	WISC-IV-FSIQ	VABS-II Composite
Child 1	7	Autism Spectrum	2	6	117	75
Child 2	8	Autism Spectrum	3	6	98	76
Child 3	6	Autism Spectrum	3	7	97	85
Child 4	7	Autism Spectrum	3	5	84	76
Child 5	6	Autism Spectrum	3	6	123	85

CS, Comparison Score; WISC-FSIQ, Wechsler Intelligence Scale for Children—Full Scale Intelligence Quotient; VABS, Vineland Adaptive Behavior Scale.

Central Unit

The CU (OS: Win8, RAM: 4 GB, CPU: Intel Core i5-3450—3.1 GHz—4 core) is positioned in the monitoring room and enables researchers to monitor the child during therapy and the neurophysiological signals. The monitoring room is located next to the therapy's room allowing the Bluetooth data transmission from the biosignal sensor unit and the video mobile data recording. Raw data are real-time displayed within *four* windows (ECG, EEG, Videos) as shown in **Figure 3**.

The CU manages the connection between the monitoring interface and the set of biosignal sensors and video mobile units, in particular the CU is responsible for notifying the "Start Session" message to all the recording units (RUs) involved and initializing each new session. All the communication between the CU and the RUs is transmitted in a validated XML format v1.0. The application manages security and privacy, real-time streaming and data synchronization. In particular the synchronization among the different devices is guaranteed by the fact their applications run in the same system and are launched simultaneously by an application running on the CU.

After data collection, the data analysis toolboxes running in the CU are able to analyze and process the collected data off-line by combining different data as a whole data source.

Video Analysis Toolbox

The video analysis toolbox allows the labeling of the children's behaviors in the recorded session and is based on the Dante annotation tool (Cruciani et al., 2011) customized for the labeling of behaviors of children with ASD.

Some of the behavioral features extracted are considered as instantaneous features (i.e., gesture), while others represent a state of the subject that persists in time (i.e., engagement).

The video analysis tool provides a Graphical User Interface (GUI) (**Figure 4**) to re-play the video of a recorded session, while examining annotated data and the integration of EEG/ECG data.

A manual annotation grid, referring to the child and the therapist, allows behavioral analysis of the therapeutic session, as defined in the coding scheme.

The grid distinguishes between "States" and "Behaviors." States identify behavioral states of a subject that persist for a given duration in time, for example Engagement and Dis-Engagement. States are always considered as mutually exclusive. In contrast, Behaviors are always considered as instantaneous events, meaning that the corresponding event will have the same timestamp for Start Time and End Time.

The Video Analysis interface produces an "Event File," an. xls file containing the information about the annotated events (type of state/behavior, Start Time, End Time). Through the annotation of these events, each therapy session can be analyzed to provide contextual information on significant behaviors of the child, useful for exploratory analysis of EEG/ECG signal.

EEG Analysis Toolbox

EEG signals are first-pre-processed using EEGLAB Toolbox (Delorme and Makeig, 2004) to remove noise and artifacts. The recorded EEG signals are high passed at 0.5 Hz to get rid of noise from breathing and low passed at a cut-off frequency of 70 Hz to get rid of the high frequency noise. A Notch filter (45–55 Hz) is also applied to remove power line interference.

Ocular and muscular artifacts are first removed by visual inspection. In particular blink artifacts are identified as segments of data having deflection >150 μV, while ocular flutters, or muscle movement artifacts as segments having deflections of 50 μV relative to baseline. Segments containing these artifacts are excluded from the following analyses. In addition bad channels are removed using the "channel statistics" tool of EEGLAB. On the basis of these statistics "bad" channels were considered as the ones that had distributions of potential values that were further away from a Gaussian distribution than other scalp channels, and they were remove from further analysis.

After artifacts removal baseline signal is removed form data acquired during the task.

After-pre-processing, EEG data are imported in a home-made Matlab analysis toolbox for QEEG analysis.

First, the Power Spectral Density (PSD) is evaluated by transforming the signal from the time domain to the frequency domain using the Welch method (Welch, 1967). Then the absolute and the relative power of each band (delta: 1–4 Hz, theta: 4–7 Hz, alpha: 8–13 Hz, beta: 14–29 Hz, and gamma: 30–70 Hz) are computed for each electrode. Relative powers are usually more reliable than absolute powers because they show less variability among different subjects and they are less affected by artifacts (Duffy, 1986). Inter-hemispheric asymmetry is computed by the Brain Symmetry Index (BSI) (van Putten et al., 2004). The BSI is calculated within each EEG band considering the total power in each region (frontal, temporal, central, parietal, and occipital) of the left and right hemisphere (sum of the electrodes).

The connectivity between brain regions is estimated with the calculation of coherence, which gives an estimation of the

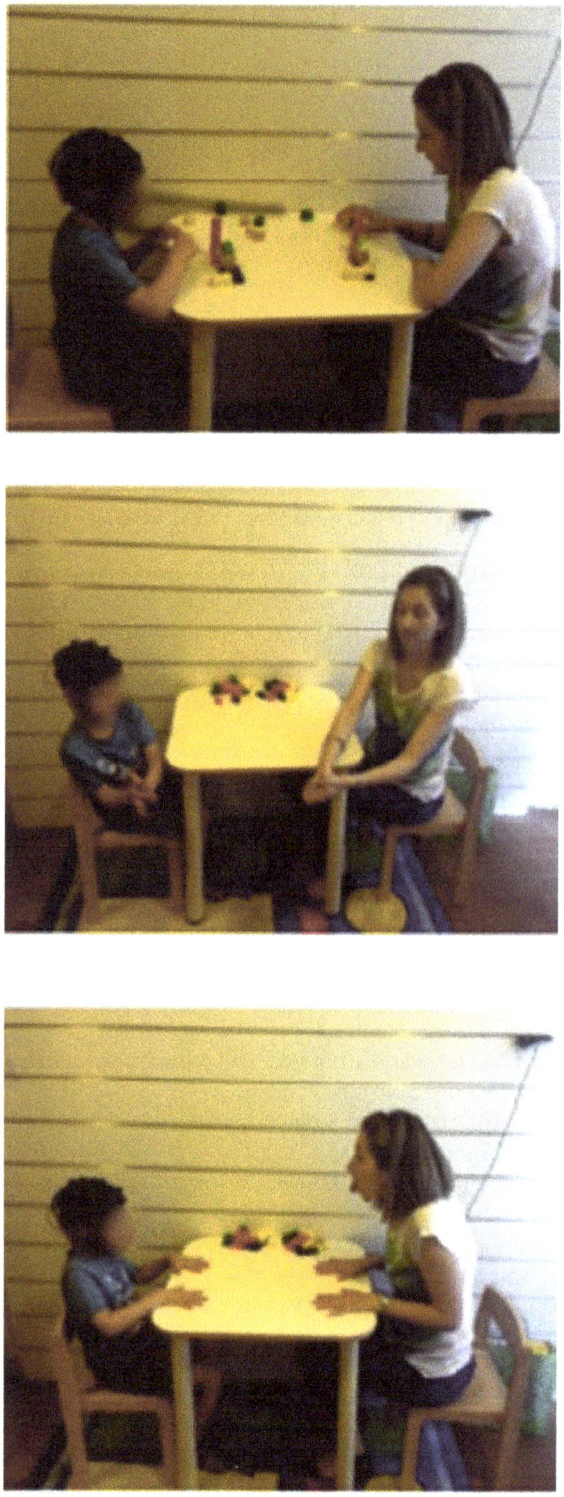

FIGURE 1 | Experimental paradigm.

linear correlation between two signals collected at two different scalp points as a function of frequency (Otnes and Enochson, 1972). Coherence is calculated for each pair of electrodes in each frequency band.

ECG Analysis Toolbox

ECG signals are pre-processed through a stepwise filtering process aimed at removing typical ECG artifacts and interferences. In particular, the baseline wander due to body movements and respiration artifacts are removed using a cubic spline 3rd order interpolation between the fiducial isoelectric points of the ECG (Jane et al., 1992). The power line interference and muscular noise are removed using an IIR (infinite impulse response) notch filter at 50 Hz and an IIR low pass filter at 40 Hz. In the final step of the pre-processing phase the Pan-Tompkins method is applied to detect the QRS complexes (Pan and Tompkins, 1985). The tachogram and the HRV are extracted according to the International Guidelines of HRV (Task Force of the European Society of Cardiology the North American Society of Pacing Electrophysiology, 1996). The tachogram is a vector whose elements represent the beat-to-beat interval between *two* adjacent R peaks in the ECG allowing the definition of useful features for a further quantitative analysis. At this step the tachogram signal might not be suitable yet for a proper features extraction due to the presence of possible residual movement artifacts and outliers, which can be easily detected by visual inspection. Artifact are visually identified and removed. In order to prevent the signal from excessive shortening, the user should operate a careful artifacts selection choosing the interval to remove as tight as possible. Outliers are replaced by division or summation. Division is applied when the outlier is determined by a failure to detect an R-peak while summation while it is caused by faulty detections of *two* or more peaks within a period representing the R-R interval.

After pre-processing significant features, which could give an indication of the engagement of the child during the therapy are extracted from the ECG signal. In particular the Heart Rate (HR), the Root Mean Square of the Successive Differences (RMSSD), and the Respiratory Sinus Arrhythmia (RSA) are selected. The HR measures the number of poundings of the heart occurring in a specific lapse of time and it is typically expressed as beats per minute (bpm). The RMSSD, indicator of vagal activity, was chosen as a time domain measure of the HRV. The RSA refers to the periodic fluctuations in HR that are linked to breathing. RSA is largely determined by vagal influences on the heart, providing a noninvasive index of parasympathetic activity, social functioning, and cognitive performances (Patriquin et al., 2013, 2014). The RSA component from tachogram signal is extracted using the Empirical Model Decomposition (EMD) (Balocchi et al., 2004).

Data Collection and Measurement Definition

Data were collected using the technological platform described above during a therapeutic session of each participant included in this study. The Biosignal Sensor Unit and the Video Mobile Unit were connected to the CU and a new acquisition session was recorded for each child. The EEG data were acquired using Enobio at 500 Hz while for ECG signals a sampling frequency of 200 Hz was chosen to avoid too much noise and to optimize data transfer.

Data collected were analyzed in post-processing. Each recording session was first imported in the "Video analysis toolbox" and then coded by clinicians who reviewed the videos to define the events of interest. In particular, in this study we focused on the alternation of the "States," i.e., the Engagement and the Disengagement, during the therapeutic session.

Two coders were trained to use the coding system, by observing and coding videos of children with ASD, who were not included in the study. The 1 month training period enabled the coders to become familiar with the meaning of the features, to identify them correctly, and to acquire ability in coding procedures. The coders were required to achieve a satisfactory level of agreement between them (Cohen's Kappa $\geq$0.70) and with two expert clinicians (AN and SC) for each Event behavior (imitation) and for each State behaviors (Engagement and Disengagement).

The tolerance window regarding time discrepancy between coding was set at 1 s for event behaviors and at 3 s for state behaviors. The coding recorded outside these windows was reported as a coding error and was considered a disagreement. Intercoder agreement was calculated for each item, and the values of k were $\geq$0.70.

The mean Intercoder reliability showed satisfactory agreement ($k = 0.81$). In order to verify the ongoing agreement, 25% of the collection of sequences were coded by both coders.

The mean Intercoder agreement calculated on these sequences was $k = 0.84$, and the values of k were ≥ 0.70. In all cases of discordance between coders, the expert coders advice was used.

For a definition of a baseline, both for EEG and ECG, signals were acquired for about 3 min before the beginning of the task.

The Event File containing the information about coding was used to extract EEG and ECG segments in order to link different physiological patterns with different states of the children.

For the EEG analysis, data acquired were divided in "Engagement" and "Disengagement" states using the information contained in the Event File. First the segments were imported in the EEGLAB Toolbox and pre-processed. The baseline signal was removed from the two state signals. The cleaned segments were then imported in the QEEG analysis GUI to extract features of interest. The proportion of data retained after cleaning was not different between Engagement and Disengagement phases (Engagement: 7.34%, Disengagement: 7.85%). Finally, features extracted for each segment type of each type of State were averaged.

For the purpose of data reduction, *four* EEG lead-groupings were considered to compute coherence (Coben et al., 2008; Machado et al., 2015; see Supplementary Materials).

ECG data were imported in the ECG analysis GUI and after pre-processing relevant features were extracted. The tool generates plots, which show the trend of the features over time, and also stores data for a further numerical analysis. To evaluate how the therapeutic stimuli influence the cardiac activity, physiological events were defined for each feature when the parameter undergoes or exceeds established values. A crucial step lies in the definition of thresholds, which denote the occurrence of a physiological event related to the feature of interest. Reference values were customized for each child at each acquisition since environmental, subjective, and current emotional states could heavily affect the HR baseline.

The values for "higher HR" and "lower HR" were respectively calculated by the 90th and the 5th percentile of the baseline signal. The event of "lower RMSSD" referred to values undergoing the 20 ms threshold and denoted more effective participation from the child (Althaus et al., 1999). The threshold for "lower RSA" ranged in an interval from 6.3 to 6.5 $\ln(ms^2)$ (Porges et al., 2013).

For each State the mean and the standard deviation of the feature extracted as well as the percentage of physiological events detected were recorded. The percentage of physiological events was evaluated as the ratio of occurrences of the events to the total engagement time The approach described allowed to evaluate, both with a visual and a quantitative method, the physiological response of the child to the stimuli received with distinct reference to the different phases identified during the treatment.

Data Analysis

A preliminary statistical analysis was performed to evaluate differences in the features extracted between Engagement and Disengagement. Statistical analyses were performed in SPSS (SPSS Inc., Chicago, IL, USA). The Shapiro-Wilk test was applied to test the normality of the variables. For normal distributed variables a paired-samples t-test was applied, while for nonparametric variables a Wilcoxon-test was adopted. Results were considered significant for $p < 0.05$.

RESULTS

Feasibility Evaluation

The children did not show sensory-motor and/or behavioral issues in wearing the devices and completing all the tasks, administered within a friendly, and supportive environment without any difficulties or constraints.

We used labeled data generated through Manual Annotation to validate the system. In particular, the synchronization between Video and the other signals was crucial, since the video was the reference for the validation process. However, the required constraints on synchronization were not particularly strict considering that:

- the Video footage, which is the reference, has a frame rate considerably smaller compared to the EEG sample rate (25 vs. 500 Hz);
- even in behavioral annotation performed by a trained psychologist, a lag of 1 s is acceptable.

Therefore, the residual synchronization error due to the latency time between the data sampling and the reception by the synchronized machine is marginal considering that, whatever is the instant annotated as the start of the State, we considered the whole duration of the State for the analysis.

The synchronization tests have been performed by inserting a spike in the signal and comparing the video timestamp with the sensor data timestamps. The resultant accuracy with this setup is in the order of tenths of second, which is acceptable for our purpose.

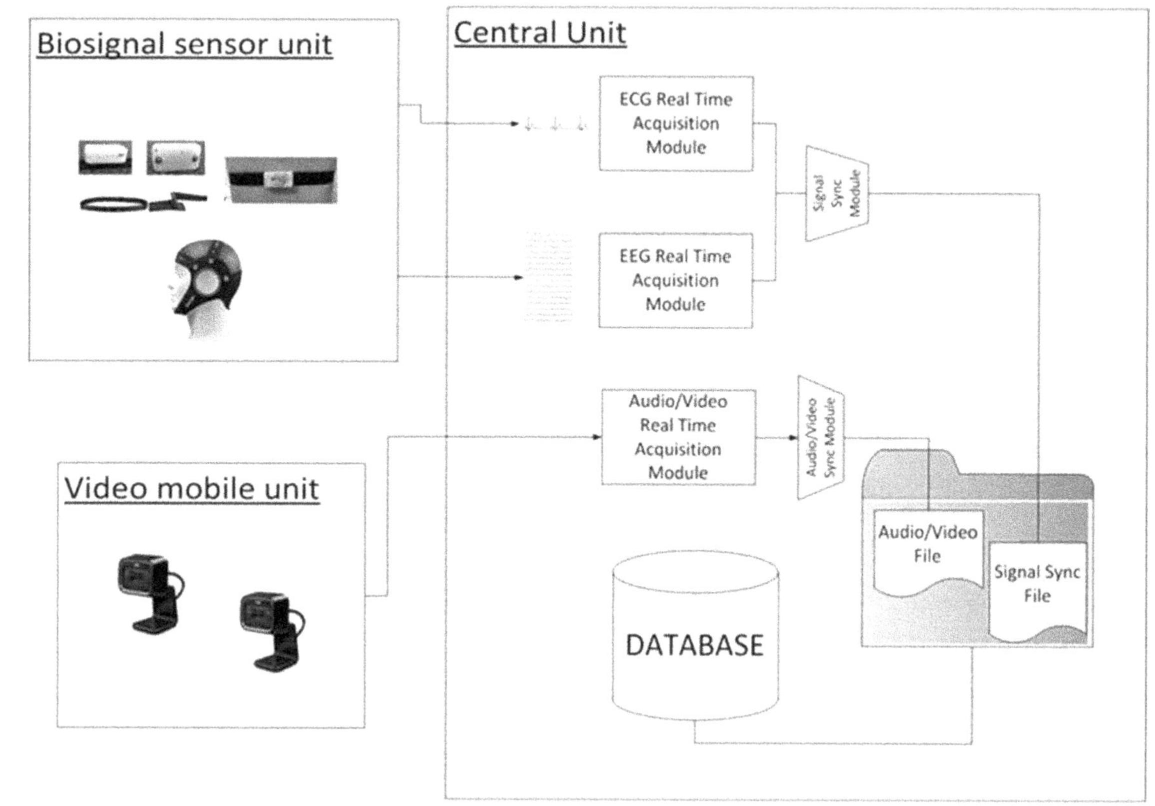

FIGURE 2 | Architecture overview.

EEG Results

Although each child showed his own individual pattern of brain activity and connectivity, all the children displayed visible changes of EEG pattern between the Engagement and Disengagement phases. Some of these changes were common among all the children and are summarized hereafter.

Figure 5 shows the location of the electrodes with statistically significant differences in PSD between Engagement and Disengagement phases.

Almost all the children displayed a significant relative power increase in most of the brain regions during the Engagement (**Figure 5**). At a group level analysis all the children showed significant power increase in frontal regions in delta band ($p = 0.04$). All but one child (Subject 3) also exhibited power increase in parietal regions in beta band ($p = 0.04$) and in occipital areas in theta, alpha, beta and gamma bands ($p = 0.04$). In Subject 3 there was not a significantly change in the PSD between Engagement and Disengagement in these frequency bands.

In the Engagement a transition from leftward to rightward asymmetry could be observed for almost all the frequency bands over the parietal areas. In particular this shift was significant in alpha and beta bands ($p = 0.04$). There was also a significant transition from rightward to leftward asymmetry in temporal areas in gamma band ($p = 0.04$).

Figure 6 shows statistically significant difference in coherence (coherence Engagement–coherence Disengagement) at the different cortical regions, in the different frequency bands.

A widespread increase of coherence was observed in almost all subjects during the Engagement in particular in theta, alpha and beta bands (**Figure 6**). The group level analysis revealed a significant increased in intrahemispheric coherence in posterior right and left areas in theta, alpha and beta bands ($p = 0.04$). Interhemispheric coherence increased at a central level in alpha and beta bands ($p = 0.04$) and at posterior level in beta band ($p = 0.04$). Although not significant at a group level analysis, it is possible to observe an increase of coherence in anterior regions in alpha band in almost all the subjects.

ECG Results

The system proved that the cardiac activity is strongly influenced by social engagement states and the ECG patterns turned out to be subjected to similar changes in the five subjects in response to changed psychological conditions. **Figure 7** shows example of plots of the HR, RMSSD, and RSA trends over time during acquisition intervals for Subjects 1 and 3, corresponding to the Engagement and Disengagement phases. Markers locate physiological events according to the thresholds previously described. The ECG analysis showed a clear correlation between

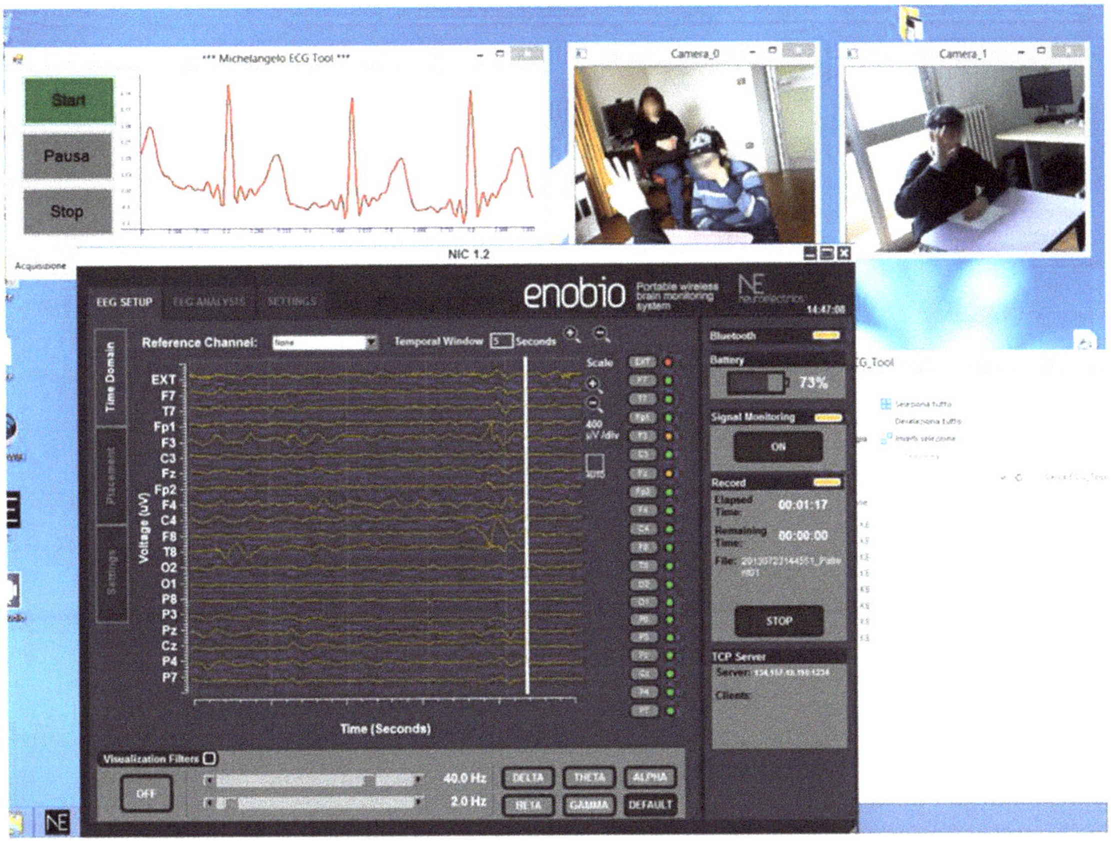

FIGURE 3 | Real-time acquisition of two camera video, ECG signal, and EEG signal during a therapeutic session.

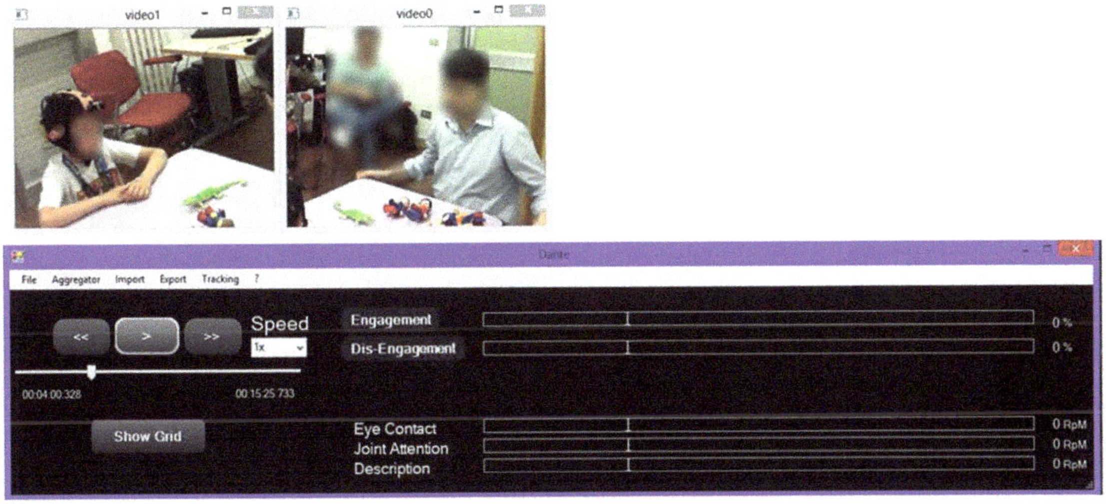

FIGURE 4 | Graphical User Interface for re-play and annotation of the recorded video session.

the detection of physiological events and the child's degree of involvement in the therapy. The plots reveal a greater presence of physiological events of "higher HR" and "lower HRV" and "lower RSA" in the Engagement as compared with the Disengagement. It was also evident that subjects displayed a remarkable RSA suppression compared with basal values in the Engagement. Furthermore, "lower HR" values turned out to be more frequent during the Disengagement.

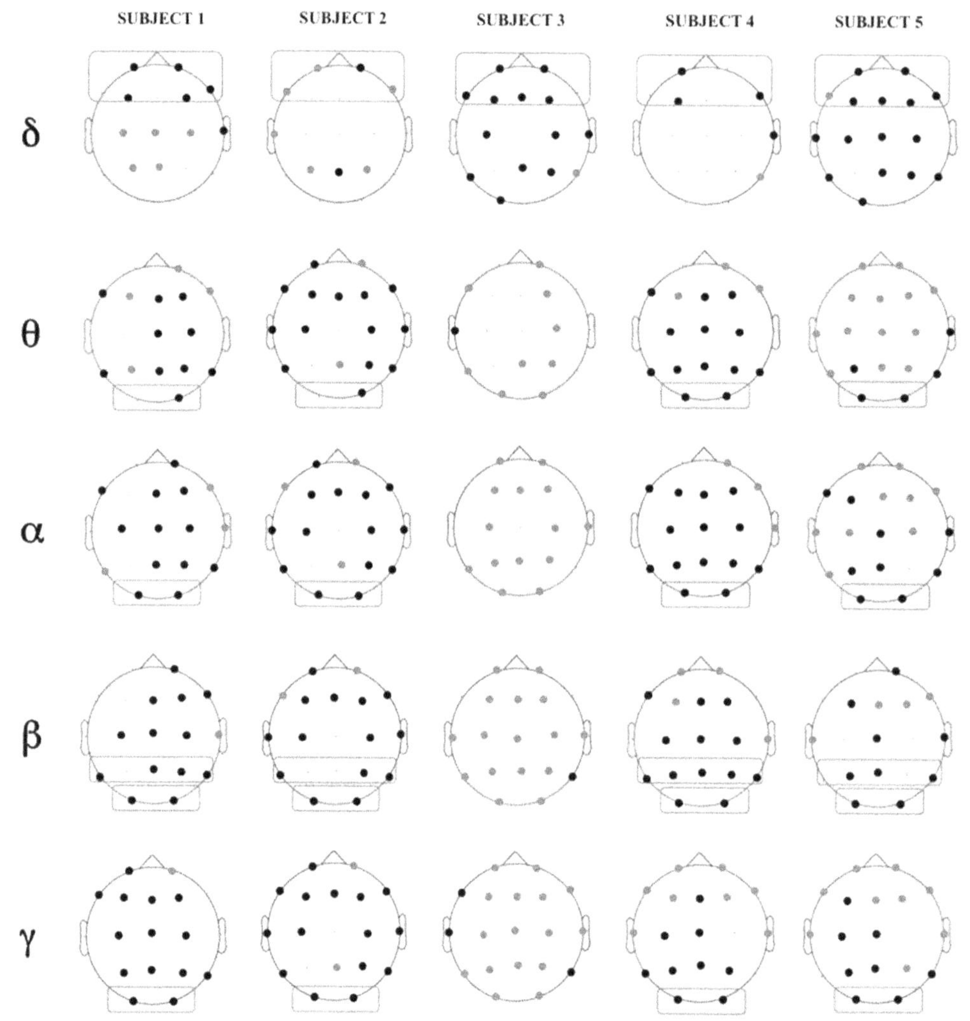

FIGURE 5 | Location of electrodes with significant differences in relative power in Engagement vs. Disengagement phase for each subject in each frequency band: black dots represent location of increase, gray dots location of decrease. Boxes represent brain regions with significant increase in relative power at a group level analysis.

Table 2 shows that children displayed an increased mean HR and a slightly significant greater percent number of "higher HR" physiological events during the Engagement compared to the Disengagement, excluding Subject 5 ($p = 0.07$). The mean RMSSD and mean RSA generally decreased during Engagement: therefore, the percent number of "lower HRV" and "lower RSA" events was significantly increased ($p = 0.04$ and $p = 0.005$ respectively).

DISCUSSION

The aim of this study was to develop and test innovative technologies to overcome some limitations of the present applications of physiological assessment in ASD (Bölte et al., 2016), including the artificial and constrained situations in which data are acquired and the need of a special compliance from the subjects, which prevented an ecological assessment so far.

This preliminary work represents an initial step to study the social cognition from an interactor point of view, based on the assumption that there is something fundamentally different when we are actively engaged with others in real-time social interaction as compared to when we merely observe them (Pfeiffer et al., 2012). The main contribution of this approach is that, if validated in a larger sample of subjects, would allow for more naturalistic paradigms that allow real world stimuli to be incorporated into EEG/psychophysiological studies.

In this pilot study, we have presented a paradigm for the acquisition of neurophysiological and physiological signals in a semi-naturalistic setting where children can interact with the examiner and play with different objects. Particular efforts have been provided to customize the ECG hardware, to integrate the videos, the ECG and the EEG units and to realize a user-friendly toolbox for data analysis.

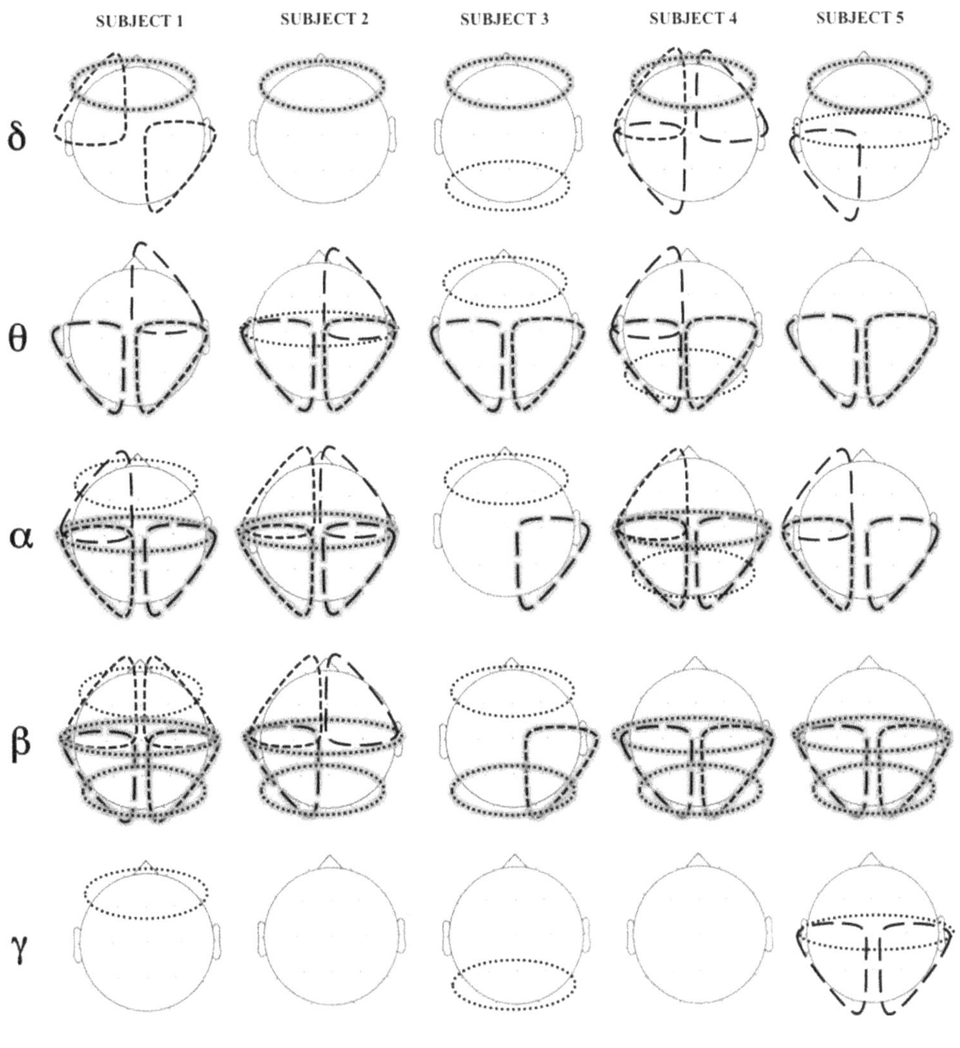

FIGURE 6 | Areas of significant increase in coherence in Engagement vs. Disengagement phase for each subject in each frequency band. Long dashed lines represent transversal coherence while short dashed lines represent short coherence. Shaded areas represent regions of significant increase at a group level analysis.

The wireless EEG cap and the chest strap containing the ECG demonstrated how unobtrusive tools can be suitable for young children and can be used with semi-naturalistic paradigms. This study confirmed our previous results about the feasibility of the application of wearable sensors and wireless technologies in young subjects with neuropsychiatric disorders (Billeci et al., 2015). The interaction with the examiner rather than with a screen like in most EEG paradigms, is another very important feature of this study, and allows recreating a more real situation with social interactions and cues. In this paradigm, we can assume that the signals acquired from the brain and the autonomic system are much more similar to what is generated while the child interacts in common life situations. This setting, relatively simple to be implemented, can be considered as one step toward a more behaviorally-driven analysis of neurophysiological activity.

The acquisition of physiological signals during treatment could provide important cues about the response of the child, which is commonly just observed from a behavioral point of view by clinicians. This can be extremely important to objectivize the effect of the treatment and to implement more effective therapies.

In particular, literature shows the importance of the QEEG technique for assessing brain connectivity and for the development of an individualized treatment program (Billeci et al., 2013). Previous QEEG studies showed how autistic children have differences in power spectra, coherence, and symmetry measures with respect to controls (Cantor and Chabot, 2009). This is true both when signals are acquired in a resting condition, with open or closed eyes, and when specific tasks are performed (Cantor and Chabot, 2009). Furthermore, it has been observed that it is possible to link a specific pattern of brain activation, characterized by specific features, to certain specific behaviors.

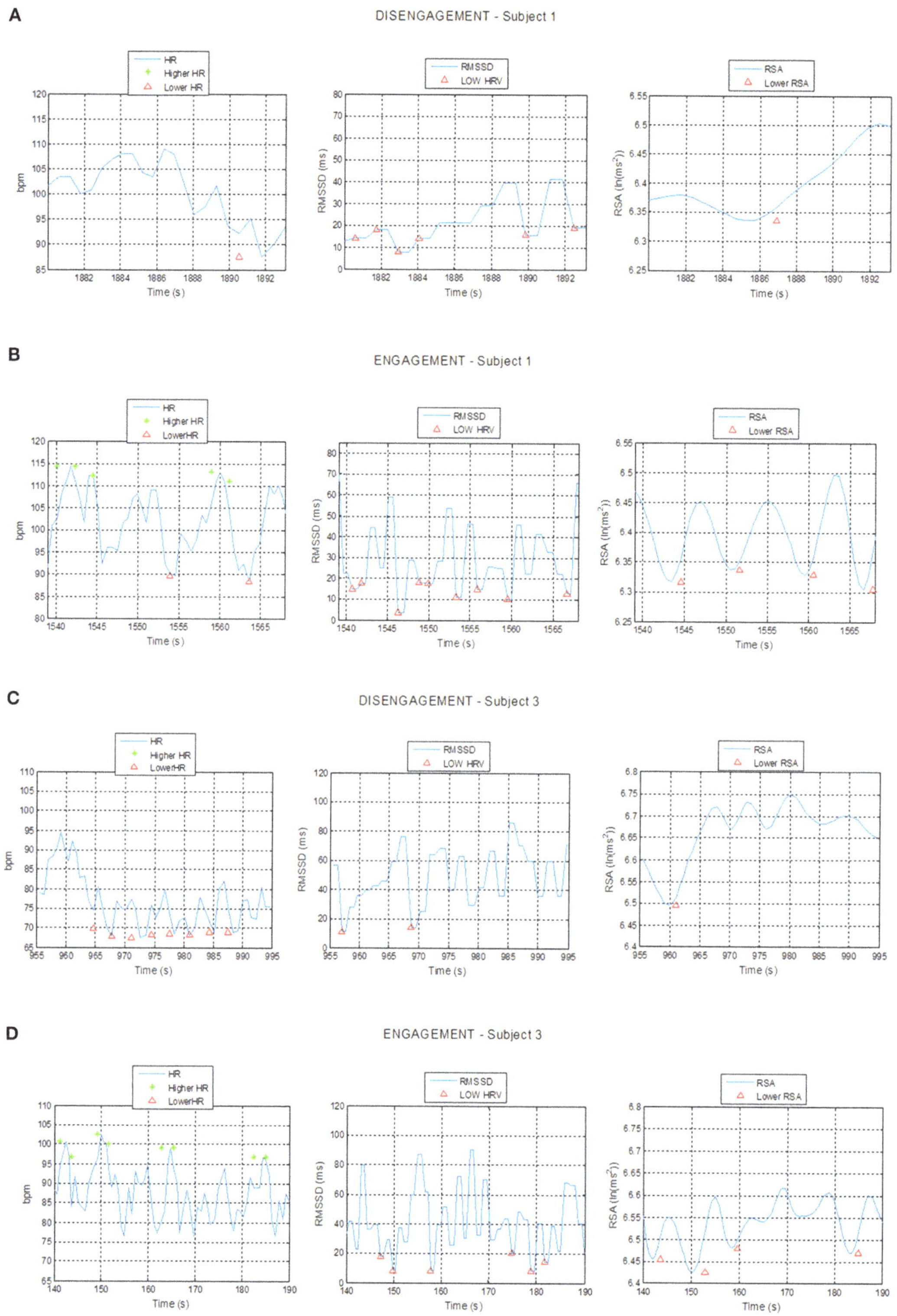

FIGURE 7 | Plot of Heart Rate (HR), Root Mean Square of the Successive Differences (RMSSD), and Respiratory Sinus Arrhythmia (RSA) trends during Disengagement (A,C) and Engagement (B,D) for Subject 1 and 3 with detection of physiological events: star markers represent HR value exceeding the high HR threshold while triangular markers represent HR, RMSSD, or RSA values undergoing the low HR, low RMSSD, and low RSA thresholds respectively.

TABLE 2 | Mean, Standard Deviation (SD), and percent number of physiological events for HR (bps), RMSSD (ms), and RSA (ln(ms²)) values during Engagement and Disengagement.

Subjects	Feature	Disengagement		Engagement	
		Mean ± SD	%Physiological events	Mean ± SD	%Physiological events
Subject 1	HR	104.33 ± 3.21	15.8	104.68 ± 3.11	16.80
	RMSSD	36.22 ± 5.65	45.16	28.78 ± 5.53	47.64
	RSA	6.36 ± 0.05	3.22	6.36 ± 0.03	6.65
Subject 2	HR	97.64 ± 9.61	9.09	100.03 ± 9.29	16.63
	RMSSD	38.94 ± 14.12	42.13	44.69 ± 8.24	44.24
	RSA	6.44 ± 0.10	2.72	6.35 ± 0.25	4.47
Subject 3	HR	82.43 ± 2.93	3.43	85.26 ± 5.45	6.24
	RMSSD	48.41 ± 13.40	9.79	42.24 ± 8.79	13.4
	RSA	6.59 ± 0.03	7.90	6.57 ± 0.05	9.50
Subject 4	HR	92.58 ± 1.20	10.15	80.33 ± 0.41	15.20
	RMSSD	46.17 ± 2.35	10.35	30.60 ± 4.21	13.54
	RSA	6.45 ± 0.32	1.05	6.62 ± 0.26	5.04
Subject 5	HR	108.23 ± 0.23	66.65	95.39 ± 1.31	13.52
	RMSSD	17.15 ± 4.58	26.47	44.25 ± 3.53	66.54
	RSA	6.32 ± 0.12	1.01	6.47 ± 0.11	4.70

Physiological events: higher HR, lower RMSSD, and lower RSA.

In this study, we showed that with this approach is possible to measure changes in the EEG pattern during treatment elicited by interaction of the child with the therapist. An increase in relative power in Engagement compared with Disengagement emerged in the group analysis. The increase in frontal delta during cognitive tasks has been previously linked to perceptual switching of objects (Okada et al., 2009), an ability which is elicited during the imitation tasks with cubes during the imitation protocol. Occipital activity is mainly due to visual stimuli during the imitation task linked to tactile components (gamma and beta activity) (Bauer et al., 2009) and auditory component (alpha and theta) (Gladwin and de Jong, 2005). The activation of beta band within parietal regions has been linked to planning and execution of movement, although its functional role is still matter of debate (Zaepffel et al., 2013).

Interestingly, we also observed a general increase in coherence during Engagement. EEG coherence, being the covariance of spectral activity at two electrode sites, is a measure for the synchrony of neuronal activity and thus can be used as an indicator of effective cortical connectivity. Coherence mainly increased in theta, alpha and beta bands both intra- and inter-hemispheres. The increased coherence in these bands may reveal the increase of attention control during the participation in the cognitive task (Sacchet et al., 2015). Interestingly the level of coherence in frontal-parietal region in alpha band has been linked to different performances in an imitation task (Van der Helden et al., 2010). Moreover, several studies have shown a positive correlation between coherence in theta, alpha and beta and task associated with motor processing and execution (von Stein et al., 1999; Sauseng et al., 2005; Wheaton et al., 2005; Rilk et al., 2011).

A modification in asymmetry during Engagement was also observed. Previous studies have shown altered asymmetry in ASD brain both structurally and functionally. In particular, left-side prevalence in alpha and beta bands was found compared with controls both in visual and non-visual areas at rest. Right asymmetry in alpha and beta bands has been previously associated with discrimination of speech prosody (Kujala et al., 2005), processing gaze direction in face perception (Senju et al., 2005), and sustained visual attention (Stroganova et al., 2007). On the contrary, left temporal asymmetry in gamma band has been associated with language processing (Kojima et al., 2013) and an atypical asymmetry (rightward) of gamma band has been observed in ASD at rest (Maxwell et al., 2015). It seems from this study that the pattern of asymmetry shifts to the typical pattern during the Engagement phase.

It is worth noting that only two of the five subjects exhibit mu desynchronization during the imitation tasks, which could suggest a deficit in the mirror neuron system at least in some of the subjects enrolled in the study (MNS, Oberman et al., 2005). Given that all the children were able to perform the task is it possible that increase in alpha and beta coherence rather than mu desynchronization is a more reliable predictor of good performance in vasomotor tasks as suggested by Rilk et al. (2011).

ECG analysis confirmed previous findings and demonstrated that the system developed is able to detect ASD children's level of engagement (Park et al., 2013).

Some studies have shown that mental effort causes an increase in physiological arousal as measured for example by HR (Lundberg and Frankenhaeuser, 1980; Peters et al., 1998). Thus, subjective perception of mental effort may reflect changes in arousal during performance of attentive tasks. Precedent studies demonstrated how decreased RMSSD (Nagendra et al., 2015) and RSA (Overbeek et al., 2014) represented meaningful indicators for a positive response to attention demanding stimuli and is positively associated with cognitive function, including better processing speed, working memory, learning, and receptive language skills.

The ECG features could represent a valid marker to evaluate the engagement and the social interaction of the child in real time (Moore et al., 2009).

Importantly, besides showing some common pattern of modification in physiological parameters in the enrolled subjects, the implemented protocols allowed to evidence some inter-individual differences fostering the application of this platform for a personalization of the therapeutic protocol. In particular, as regards EEG it is clearly evident that Subject 3 did not showed significant differences between Engagement and Disengagement in many cortical areas. The clinical profile of this subject shows that he has an important concentration deficit and this can explain why, despite from the behavioral observation he seemed to be engaged in the tasks proposed by the therapist as the other subjects, his brain activated differently. In addition the desynchronization of the MNS is not observed in all the subjects. If the possibility of using the proposed system for characterizing the physiological profile of specific endophenotype of ASD would be confirmed in a larger sample, it would be very useful to guide the therapist, representing a step forward in the implementation of individual therapeutic programs in ASD.

Some important issues emerged from this study that suggest future developments. First of all, the need of a standardized, objective and clear distinction of the different behaviors of each task promotes rigorous segmentation of the signals. In the future annotation of the video could be done not only with manual markers but also with automatic or semi-automatic action recognition from the video recording.

Moreover, real-time feature extraction algorithms could be implemented, which provide the therapist a feedback about the status of the child. In this way the therapist could decide to potentiate some tasks of the therapy that cause a particular engagement of the child or, on the contrary, change the therapy if the child appears to be disengaged, stressed or not interested by the task proposed.

Overall, the system presented in this study was proven to be suitable for a similar clinical scenario. The children highly accepted the monitoring platform, as demonstrated by the low dropout rate in the study and by the fact that the children included in the study did not express any discomfort/annoyance at the system. Thus, the high grade of acceptability of the monitoring platform is promising for further development and implementation of the tool. Furthermore, the smart sensorized system allowed a reliable psychophysiological characterization of the children enrolled. Such evidence fosters the applicability of the system proposed in a clinical setting, where it could be used as a smart monitoring tool to support the clinicians during the treatment. In the future the proposed system could supply useful feedback to the therapist in the treatment of ASD and even in other neurodevelopmental disabilities.

Further data collections will be needed to confirm these preliminary results. At first, larger studies would be useful to generalize the findings of this feasibility pilot study and to obtain a clearer picture of the parameters examined in ASD children. Then, when confirmed on larger cohorts, the psychophysiological characterization of the children with ASD related to different behaviors will possibly allow to personalize the treatment and to longitudinally verify the treatment effect through objective measures of brain and autonomic function of children with ASD. In conclusion, this kind of evaluation holds promise for future developments in instrumental evaluations of ASD.

Limitations

Some limitations need to be considered when interpreting the results. A first limitation is the small sample size. The study was designed as a feasibility study, thus only a small number of patients was recruited to test the applicability of the technology and the methodology.

The findings of the study need to be replicated with larger sample to prove the efficacy of the approach and the transferability in a clinical scenario. Larger sample will also allow for the evaluation of how different could be the physiological response of subgroups of children with ASD.

Another limitation is the absence of a control group, which prevents to discuss the nature of brain and autonomic response specific to ASD. In the future the comparison with a control group of age-matched children with typically development will allow to evaluate not only how different is the pattern between Engagement and Disengagement phases in ASD but also how this patterns are different from a typical pattern of response.

Finally another possible limitation is that we did not control for effects of physical movement. However, in our protocol the children were seated in a chair throughout the interaction and thus relatively restrained in their physical activity. As regards ECG, Porges et al. (2007) found that low intensity motor movements did not influence RSA or HRV in school-age children, so that movement were unlikely to have had a major impact on our results. As regards EEG we have removed muscular artifacts however visual inspection to is subjected to human error. In the future surface electromyography sensors could be used to control for children' muscular artifacts.

AUTHOR CONTRIBUTIONS

LB developed EEG algorithms and analyzed data, participated in the development of the study design, contributed in the discussion and interpretation of the results, in writing and approving the paper. AT participated in the acquisition analysis of data, contributed in the discussion and interpretation of the result, in writing and approving the paper. GT developed the ECG algorithms and contributed in writing and approving the paper. AN performed therapies and coding of videos, participated in the development of the study design, and contributed in writing and approving the paper. SP analyzed

ECG data and contributed in writing and approving the paper. DC developed the ECG communication protocol and approved the paper. GB developed the ECG software data and approved the paper. FC participated in the development of the study design, developed the video toolbox and approved the paper. SA participated in the development of technological platform and approved the paper. SC recruited the subjects and contributed in coding videos and in the discussion and interpretation of the result, in writing and approving the paper. GP participated in the development of the study design, was responsible of the technological protocol, and approved the paper. FM participated in the development of the study design, was responsible of recruitment and diagnosis of children and contributed in the discussion and approving the paper.

FUNDING

The research leading to this work has received funding from the European Union's Seventh Framework Programme (FP7-ICT-288241) Project MICHELANGELO: Patient-centric model for remote management, treatment, and rehabilitation of autistic children. SC was supported by the Ministry of Health, Italy and by Tuscany Region with the grant "GR-2010-2317873," and by Bando FAS Salute Sviluppo Toscana—ARIANNA Project.

ACKNOWLEDGMENTS

We would like to thank the children and the families that participated in the study.

REFERENCES

Althaus, M., Mulder, L. J. M., Mulder, G., Aarnoudse, C. C., and Minderaa, R. B. (1999). Cardiac adaptivity to attention-demanding tasks in children with a pervasive developmental disorder not otherwise specified (PDD-NOS). *Biol. Psychiatry* 46, 799–809. doi: 10.1016/S0006-3223(98)00374-6

American Psychiatric Association (APA) (2013). *Diagnostic and Statistical Manual of Mental Disorders, 5th Edn.* Washington, DC: American Psychiatric Association.

Balocchi, R., Menicucci, D., Santarcangelo, E., Sebastiani, L., Gemignani, A., Ghelarducci, B., et al. (2004). Deriving the respiratory sinus arrhytmia from the heartbeat time series using empirical mode decomposition. *Chaos Solitons Fractals* 20, 171–177. doi: 10.1016/S0960-0779(03)00441-7

Bauer, M., Oostenveld, R., and Fries, P. (2009). Tactile stimulation accelerates behavioral responses to visual stimuli through enhancement of occipital gamma-band activity. *Vision Res.* 49, 931–942. doi: 10.1016/j.visres.2009.03.014

Belmonte, M. K., Allen, G., Beckel-Mitchener, A., Boulanger, L. M., Carper, R. A., and Webb, S. J. (2004). Autism and abnormal development of brain connectivity. *J. Neurosci.* 24, 9228–9231. doi: 10.1523/JNEUROSCI.3340-04.2004

Billeci, L., Narzisi, A., Campatelli, G., Crifaci, G., Calderoni, S., Gagliano, A., et al. (2016). Disentangling the initiation from the response in joint attention: an eye-tracking study in toddlers with autism spectrum disorders. *Transl. Psychiatry* 6:e808. doi: 10.1038/tp.2016.75

Billeci, L., Sicca, F., Maharatna, K., Apicella, F., Narzisi, A., Campatelli, G., et al. (2013). On the application of quantitative EEG for characterizing autistic brain: a systematic review. *Front. Hum. Neurosci.* 7:442. doi: 10.3389/fnhum.2013.00442

Billeci, L., Tartarisco, G., Brunori, E., Crifaci, G., Scardigli, S., Balocchi, R., et al. (2015). The role of wearable sensors and wireless technologies for the assessment of heart rate variability in anorexia nervosa. *Eat. Weight Disord.* 20, 23–31. doi: 10.1007/s40519-014-0135-2

Bölte, S., Bartl-Pokorny, K. D., Jonsson, U., Berggren, S., Zhang, D., Kostrzewa, E., et al. (2016). How can clinicians detect and treat autism early? Methodological trends of technology use in research. *Acta Paediatr.* 105, 137–144. doi: 10.1111/apa.13243

Bono, V., Narzisi, A., Jouen, A. L., Tilmont, E., Hommel, S., Jamal, W., et al. (2016). GOLIAH: a gaming platform for home-based intervention in autism – principles and design. *Front. Psychiatry* 7:70. doi: 10.3389/fpsyt.2016.00070

Burns, A., Greene, B. R., McGrath, M. J., O'Shea, T. J., Kuris, B., Ayer, S. M., et al. (2010). SHIMMER^{TM} – A wireless sensor platform for noninvasive biomedical research. *IEEE Sens. J.* 10, 1527–1534. doi: 10.1109/JSEN.2010.2045498

Cantor, D. S., and Chabot, R. (2009). QEEG studies in the assessment and treatment of childhood disorders. *Clin. EEG Neurosci.* 40, 113–121. doi: 10.1177/155005940904000209

Cester, I., Dunne, S., Riera, A., and Ruffini, G. (2008). "ENOBIO: wearable, wireless, 4-channel electrophysiology recording system optimized for dry electrodes," in *International Workshop on Wearable Micro and Nanosystems for Personalised Health* (Valencia).

Chevallier, C., Kohls, G., Troiani, V., Brodkin, E. S., and Schultz, R. T. (2012). The social motivation theory of autism. *Trends Cogn. Sci.* 16, 231–239. doi: 10.1016/j.tics.2012.02.007

Coben, R., Clarke, A. R., Hudspeth, W., and Barry, R. J. (2008). EEG power and coherence in autistic spectrum disorder. *Clin. Neurophysiol.* 119, 1002–1009. doi: 10.1016/j.clinph.2008.01.013

Cruciani, F., Donnelly, M. P., Nugent, C. D., Parente, G., Paggetti, C., and Burns, W. (2011). "DANTE: a video based annotation tool for smart environments," in Sensor *Systems and Software*, Vol. 57. Lecture Notes of the Institute for Computer Sciences, Social Informatics and Telecommunications Engineering, eds G. Par and P. Morrow (Berlin; Heidelberg: Springer-Verlag), 179–188.

Dawson, G., Jones, E. J., Merkle, K., Venema, K., Lowy, R., Faja, S., et al. (2012). Early behavioral intervention is associated with normalized brain activity in young children with autism. *J. Am. Acad. Child Adolesc. Psychiatry* 51, 1150–1159. doi: 10.1016/j.jaac.2012.08.018

Dawson, G., Meltzoff, A. N., Osterling, J., Rinaldi, J., and Brown, E. (1998). Children with autism fail to orient to naturally occurring social stimuli. *J. Autism Dev. Disord.* 28, 479–485. doi: 10.1023/A:1026043926488

Delorme, A., and Makeig, S. (2004). EEGLAB: an open source toolbox for analysis of single-trial EEG dynamics. *J. Neurosci. Methods* 134, 9–21. doi: 10.1016/j.jneumeth.2003.10.009

Di Palma, S., Tonacci, A., Narzisi, A., Domenici, C., Pioggia, G., Muratori, F., et al. (2016). Monitoring of autonomic response to sociocognitive tasks during treatment in children with autism spectrum disorders by wearable technologies: A feasibility study. *Comput. Biol. Med.* pii:S0010-482530083-X. doi: 10.1016/j.compbiomed.2016.04.001

Duffy, F. H. (1986). *Topographic Mapping of Brain Electrical Activity.* Boston, MA: Butterworths.

Friedman, B. H. (2007). An autonomic flexibility–neurovisceral integration model of anxiety and cardiac vagal tone. *Biol. Psychol.* 74, 185–199. doi: 10.1016/j.biopsycho.2005.08.009

Geschwind, D. H., and Levitt, P. (2007). Autism spectrum disorders: developmental disconnection syndromes. *Curr. Opin. Neurobiol.* 17, 103–111. doi: 10.1016/j.conb.2007.01.009

Gladwin, T. E., and de Jong, R. (2005). Bursts of occipital theta and alpha amplitude preceding alternation and repetition trials in a task-switching experiment. *Biol. Psychol.* 68, 309–329. doi: 10.1016/j.biopsycho.2004.06.004

Goldberger, J. J. (1999). Sympathovagal balance: how should we measure it? *Am. J. Physiol.* 276, H1273–H1280.

Goodwin, M. S., Groden, J., Velicer, W. F., Lipsitt, L. P., Baron, M. G., Hofmann, S. G., et al. (2006). Cardiovascular arousal in individuals with autism. *Focus Autism Other Dev. Disabl.* 21, 100–123. doi: 10.1177/10883576060210020101

Guger, C., Krausz, G., Allison, B. Z., and Edlinger, G. (2012). Comparison of dry and gel based electrodes for p300 brain-computer interfaces. *Front. Neurosci.* 6:60. doi: 10.3389/fnins.2012.00060

Hirstein, W., Iversen, P., and Ramachandran, V. S. (2001). Autonomic responses of autistic children to people and objects. *Proc. Biol. Sci.* 268, 1883–1888. doi: 10.1098/rspb.2001.1724

Hoch, J., Moore, T., McComas, J., and Symons, F. J. (2010). Arousal and activity choice in autism: a single case assessment integrating autonomic and behavioral analysis. *J. Appl. Biobehav. Res.* 15, 119–133. doi: 10.1111/j.1751-9861.2010.00056.x

Jane, R., Laguna, P., Thakor, N. V., and Caminal, P. (1992). Adaptive baseline wander removal in the ECG: comparative analysis with cubic spline technique. *Proc. Comput. Cardiol.* 143–146. doi: 10.1109/CIC.1992.269426

Kojima, K., Brown, E. C., Rothermel, R., Carlson, A., Fuerst, D., Matsuzaki, N., et al. (2013). Clinical significance and developmental changes of auditory-language-related gamma activity. *Clin. Neurophysiol.* 124, 857–869. doi: 10.1016/j.clinph.2012.09.031

Kujala, T., Lepistö, T., Nieminen-von Wendt, T., Näätänen, P., and Näätänen, R. (2005). Neurophysiological evidence for cortical discrimination impairment of prosody in Asperger syndrome. *Neurosci. Lett.* 383, 260–265. doi: 10.1016/j.neulet.2005.04.048

Lord, C., Rutter, M., and Couteur, A. (1994). Autism diagnostic interview-revised: a revised version of a diagnostic interview for caregivers of individuals with possible pervasive developmental disorders. *J. Autism Dev. Disord.* 24, 659–685. doi: 10.1007/BF02172145

Lord, C., Rutter, M., Di Lavore, P. C., Risi, S., Gotham, K., and Bishop, S. L. (2012). *Autism and Diagnostic Observation Schedule, Second Edition (ADOS-2) Manual (Part I): Modules 1-4.* Torrance, CA: Western Psychological Services.

Lundberg, U., and Frankenhaeuser, M. (1980). Pituitary-adrenal and sympathetic-adrenal correlates of distress and effort. *J. Psychosom. Res.* 24, 125–130. doi: 10.1016/0022-3999(80)90033-1

Machado, C., Estévez, M., Leisman, G., Melillo, R., Rodríguez, R., DeFina, P., et al. (2015). QEEG spectral and coherence assessment of autistic children in three different experimental conditions. *J. Autism Dev. Disord.* 45, 406–424. doi: 10.1007/s10803-013-1909-5

Maxwell, C. R., Villalobos, M. E., Schultz, R. T., Herpertz-Dahlmann, B., Konrad, K., and Kohls, G. (2015). Atypical laterality of resting gamma oscillations in autism spectrum disorders. *J. Autism Dev. Disord.* 45, 292–297. doi: 10.1007/s10803-013-1842-7

Ming, X., Bain, J. M., Smith, D., Brimacombe, M., Gold von-Simson, G., and Axelrod, F. B. (2011). Assessing autonomic dysfunction symptoms in children: a pilot study. *J. Child Neurol.* 26, 420–427. doi: 10.1177/0883073810381921

Moore, G. A., Hill-Soderlund, A. L., Propper, C. B., Calkins, S. D., Mills-Koonce, W. R., and Cox, M. J. (2009). Mother-infant vagal regulation in the face-to-face still-face paradigm is moderated by maternal sensitivity. *Child Dev.* 80, 209–223. doi: 10.1111/j.1467-8624.2008.01255.x

Mundy, P., and Neal, R. A. (2000). "Neural plasticity, joint attention, and a transactional social-orienting model of autism" in *International Review of Research in Mental Retardation,* Vol. 23, ed R. C. Urbano (Salt Lake City, UT: Academic Press), 139–168.

Nagendra, H., Kumar, V., and Mukherjee, S. (2015). Cognitive behavior evaluation based on physiological parameters among young healthy subjects with yoga as intervention. *Comput. Math. Methods Med.* 2015, 821061. doi: 10.1155/2015/821061

Oberman, L. M., Hubbard, E. M., McCleery, J. P., Altschuler, E. L., Ramachandran, V. S., and Pineda, J. A. (2005). EEG evidence for mirror neuron dysfunction in autism spectrum disorders. *Brain Res. Cogn. Brain Res.* 24, 190–198. doi: 10.1016/j.cogbrainres.2005.01.014

Okada, M., Ono, Y., Iijima, Y., Ishiyama, A., and Kasai, N. (2009). Perceptual switching evokes frontal delta wave activity. *Int. J. Bioelectromagn.* 11, 120–122.

Otnes, R. K., and Enochson, L. D. (1972). *Digital Time Series Analysis.* New York, NY: Wiley.

Overbeek, T. J. M., van Boxtel, A., and Westerink, J. H. D. M. (2014). Respiratory sinus arrhythmia responses to cognitive tasks: effects of task factors and RSA indices. *Biol. Psychol.* 99, 1–14. doi: 10.1016/j.biopsycho.2014.02.006

Pan, J., and Tompkins, W. J. (1985). A real time QRS detection algorithm. *IEEE Trans. Biomed. Eng.* 32, 230–236. doi: 10.1109/TBME.1985.325532

Park, G., Van Bavel, J. J., Vasey, M. W., and Thayer, J. F. (2013). Cardiac vagal tone predicts attentional engagement to and disengagement from fearful faces. *Emotion* 13, 645–656. doi: 10.1037/a0032971

Patriquin, M. A., Lorenzi, J., Scarpa, A., and Bell, M. A. (2014). Developmental trajectories of respiratory sinus arrhythmia: associations with social responsiveness. *Dev. Psychobiol.* 56, 317–326. doi: 10.1002/dev.21100

Patriquin, M. A., Scarpa, A., Friedman, B. H., and Porges, S. W. (2013). Respiratory sinus arrhythmia: a marker for positive social functioning and receptive language skills in children with autism spectrum disorders. *Dev. Psychobiol.* 55, 101–112. doi: 10.1002/dev.21002

Peters, M. L., Godaert, G. L., Ballieux, R. E., van Vliet, M., Willemsen, J. J., Sweep, F. C., et al. (1998). Cardiovascular and endocrine responses to experimental stress: effects of mental effort and controllability. *Psychoneuroendocrinology* 23, 1–17. doi: 10.1016/S0306-4530(97)00082-6

Pfeiffer, U. J., Schilbach, L., Jording, M., Timmermans, B., Bente, G., and Vogeley, K. (2012). Eyes on the mind: investigating the influence of gaze dynamics on the perception of others in real-time social interaction. *Front. Psychol.* 3:537. doi: 10.3389/fpsyg.2012.00537

Porges, S. W., Heilman, K. J., Bazhenova, O. V., Bal, E., Doussard-Roosevelt, J. A., and Koledin, M. (2007). Does motor activity during psychophysiological paradigms confound the quantification and interpretation of heart rate and heart rate variability measures in young children? *Psychobiology* 49, 485–494. doi: 10.1002/dev.20228

Porges, S. W., Macellaio, M., Stanfill, S. D., McCue, K., Lewis, G. F., Harden, E. R., et al. (2013). Respiratory sinus arrhythmia and auditory processing in autism: Modifiable deficits of an integrated social engagement system? *Int. J. Psychophysiol.* 88, 261–270. doi: 10.1016/j.ijpsycho.2012.11.009

Rilk, A. J., Soekadar, S. R., Sauseng, P., and Plewnia, C. (2011). Alpha coherence predicts accuracy during a visuomotor tracking task. *Neuropsychologia* 49, 3704–3709. doi: 10.1016/j.neuropsychologia.2011.09.026

Sacchet, M. D., LaPlante, R. A., Wan, Q., Pritchett, D. L., Lee, A. K., Hämäläinen, M., et al. (2015). Attention drives synchronization of alpha and beta rhythms between right inferior frontal and primary sensory neocortex. *J. Neurosci.* 35, 2074–2082. doi: 10.1523/JNEUROSCI.1292-14.2015

Sauseng, P., Klimesch, W., Schabus, M., and Doppelmayr, M. (2005). Fronto-parietal EEG coherence in theta and upper alpha reflect central executive functions of working memory. *Int. J. Psychophysiol.* 57, 97–103. doi: 10.1016/j.ijpsycho.2005.03.018

Senju, A., Tojo, Y., Yaguchi, K., and Hasegawa, T. (2005). Deviant gaze processing in children with autism: an ERP study. *Neuropsychologia* 43, 1297–1306. doi: 10.1016/j.neuropsychologia.2004.12.002

Shahrestani, S., Stewart, E. M., Quintana, D. S., Hickie, I. B., and Guastella, A. J. (2016). Heart rate variability during social interactions in children with and without psychopathology: a meta-analysis. *J. Child Psychol. Psychiatry* 55, 981–989. doi: 10.1111/jcpp.12226

Solar, H., Fernández, E., Tartarisco, G., Pioggia, G., Cvetković, B., Kozina, S., et al. (2012). "A non invasive, wearable sensor platform for multi-parametric remote monitoring in CHF patients," in *Impact Analysis of Solutions for Chronic Disease Prevention and Management,* Vol. 7251. Lecture Notes in Computer Science, eds M. Donnelly, C. Paggetti, C. Nugent, and M. Mokhtari (Berlin; Heidelberg: Springer-Verlag), 140–147.

Sparrow, S. S., Cicchetti, V. D., and Balla, A. D. (2005). *Vineland Adaptive Behavior Scales, 2nd Edn.* Circle Pines, MN: American Guidance Service.

Stroganova, T. A., Nygren, G., Tsetlin, M. M., Posikera, I. N., Gillberg, C., Elam, M., et al. (2007). Abnormal EEG lateralization in boys with autism. *Clin. Neurophysiol.* 118, 1842–1854. doi: 10.1016/j.clinph.2007.05.005

Task Force of the European Society of Cardiology and the North American Society of Pacing and Electrophysiology (1996). Heart rate variability: standards of measurement, physiological interpretation and clinical use. *Circulation* 93, 1043–1065. doi: 10.1161/01.CIR.93.5.1043

Tong, S., and Thakor, N. V. (2009). *Quantitative EEG Analysis Methods and Clinical Applications.* Boston, MA: Artech House.

Van der Helden, J. V., Van Schie, H. T., and Rombouts, C. (2010). Observational learning of new movement sequences is reflected in frontoparietal coherence. *PLoS ONE* 5:e14482. doi: 10.1371/journal.pone.0014482 van Putten, M. J., Peters, J. M., Mulder, S. M., de Haas, J. A., Bruijninckx, C. M., and Tavy, D. L. (2004). A brain symmetry index (BSI) for online EEG monitoring in carotid endarterectomy. *Clin. Neurophysiol.* 115, 1189–1194. doi: 10.1016/j.clinph.2003.12.002

Varshney, U. (2005). Wireless networks for enhanced monitoring of patients. *Int. J. Healthcare Technol. Manage.* 6, 489–499. doi: 10.1504/IJHTM.2005.007009

Varshney, U. (2006). "Enhancing wireless patient monitoring by integrating stored and live patient information," in *Proceedings of 19th IEEE International Symposium on Computer-Based Medical Systems* (Washington, DC: IEEE Computer Society), 501–506.

von Stein, A., Rappelsberger, P., Sarnthein, J., and Petsche, H. (1999). Synchronization between temporal and parietal cortex during multimodal object processing in man. *Cereb. Cortex* 9, 137–150. doi: 10.1093/cercor/9.2.137

Welch, P. D. (1967). The use of fast Fourier transform for the estimation of power spectra: a method based on time averaging over short, modified periodograms. *IEEE Trans. Audio Electroacoust.* AU-15, 70–73. doi: 10.1109/TAU.1967.1161901

Wheaton, L. A., Nolte, G., Bohlhalter, S., Fridman, E., and Hallett, M. (2005). Synchronization of parietal and premotor areas during preparation and execution of praxis hand movements. *Clin. Neurophysiol.* 116, 1382–1390. doi: 10.1016/j.clinph.2005.01.008

Yilmaz, T., Foster, R., and Hao, Y. (2010). Detecting vital signs with wearable wireless sensors. *Sensors* 10, 10837–10862. doi: 10.3390/s101210837

Zaepffel, M., Trachel, R., Kilavik, B. E., and Brochier, T. (2013). Modulations of EEG beta powerduring planning and execution of grasping movements. *PLoS ONE* 8:e60060. doi: 10.1371/journal.pone.0060060

Zander, T. O., Lehne, M., Ihme, K., Jatzev, S., Correia, J., Kothe, C., et al. (2011). A dry EEG-system for scientific research and brain–computer interfaces. *Front. Neurosci.* 5:53. doi: 10.3389/fnins.2011.00053

16

The berlin brain-computer interface: progress beyond communication and control

Benjamin Blankertz [1,2], Laura Acqualagna [1], Sven Dähne [3], Stefan Haufe [2,3], Matthias Schultze-Kraft [1,2], Irene Sturm [1], Marija Uščumlic [1], Markus A. Wenzel [1], Gabriel Curio [2,4] and Klaus-Robert Müller [2,3,5]**

[1] Neurotechnology Group, Technische Universität Berlin, Berlin, Germany, [2] Bernstein Focus: Neurotechnology, Berlin, Germany, [3] Machine Learning Group, Technische Universität Berlin, Berlin, Germany, [4] Neurophysics Group, Department of Neurology, Campus Benjamin Franklin, Charité - University Medicine Berlin, Berlin, Germany, [5] Department of Brain and Cognitive Engineering, Korea University, Seoul, South Korea

Edited by:
Mikhail Lebedev, Duke University, USA

Reviewed by:
Surjo R. Soekadar, University Hospital of Tübingen, Germany
Sue Becker, McMaster University, Canada
Gert Cauwenberghs, University of California, San Diego, USA

***Correspondence:**
Benjamin Blankertz
benjamin.blankertz@tu-berlin.de
Klaus-Robert Müller
klaus-robert.mueller@tu-berlin.de

The combined effect of fundamental results about neurocognitive processes and advancements in decoding mental states from ongoing brain signals has brought forth a whole range of potential neurotechnological applications. In this article, we review our developments in this area and put them into perspective. These examples cover a wide range of maturity levels with respect to their applicability. While we assume we are still a long way away from integrating Brain-Computer Interface (BCI) technology in general interaction with computers, or from implementing neurotechnological measures in safety-critical workplaces, results have already now been obtained involving a BCI as research tool. In this article, we discuss the reasons why, in some of the prospective application domains, considerable effort is still required to make the systems ready to deal with the full complexity of the real world.

Keywords: Brain-Computer Interfacing (BCI), electroencephalography (EEG), covert user states, machine learning, mental workload, video quality, implicit information, cognitive neuroscience

1. INTRODUCTION

Since the discovery of electrical brain activity and the invention of the Electroencephalogram (EEG), by Hans Berger in 1924 (Berger, 1929), there have been many ideas and dreams about how to exploit this access to the center of human thoughts and emotions and the control of actions. Gray Walter developed the toposcope in 1951 which visualized rhythmic brain activity in 22 spatially laid out cathode ray tubes, each of which showing amplitude and phase in spiral displays (Walter and Shipton, 1951; Bladin, 2006). In the 1960s, realtime EEG was used in artistic performances (e.g., Lucier, 1965; Straebel and Thoben, 2014) and for neurofeedback training (Kamiya, 1969). The latter laid the foundation for possible clinical applications by neurofeedback (Sterman and Friar, 1972). This research led to the idea that human intentions could be transmitted directly from brain to computer (Vidal, 1973). By voluntarily acquiring certain mental states, the user of such a Brain-Computer Interface (BCI) could communicate or control a technical device while circumventing the need for any muscular activity (Dornhege et al., 2007; Wolpaw and Wolpaw, 2012). Clinical application has been the principal goal of BCI research for about four decades (Elbert et al., 1980; Kübler et al., 2005; Shih et al., 2012; Faller et al., 2014; Gallegos-Ayala et al., 2014; Hill et al., 2014; Morone et al., 2015; Soekadar et al., 2015).

In the last decade, the potential of *non*-medical applications of BCI technology has increasingly drawn renewed attention (Müller et al., 2008; Blankertz et al., 2010; van Erp et al., 2012). Two of the five application scenarios defined in the roadmap of brain/neural-computer interaction (BNCI Horizon 2020, 2015; Brunner et al., 2015), primarily target non-medical areas. The *enhance* scenario comprises applications that enhance human functions or user interactivity by adapting the device to their momentary mental state, for example, and by exploiting implicit information about the user's intention. The *research tool* scenario utilizes real-time analysis of neural signals to investigate and understand brain and cognitive functions.

In this review, we deliberately focus on certain developments that we discuss in some detail. We hope that this focused view on our own work will nevertheless be of use to the interested reader and still provide a broad account of the developments of BCI-enhanced neurotechnology. We leave aside a wide range of other relevant research, though it is no less important, pointing here exemplarily just at a few: One potentially interesting aspect for enhancing human-computer interaction is the possibility of predicting the subject confidence of participants (Graziano et al., 2015). Research on memory encoding processes is converging toward the feasibility of predicting the success of memorization by observing brain signals before and/or during encoding (Noh et al., 2014; Cohen et al., 2015). An elaboration of these techniques toward online prediction based on single-trial data would have interesting applications in adaptive learning software. A collective computer game was used to collect data sets from 523 participants in a single night who controlled an immersive art environment with the mental states of relaxation and concentration (Kovacevic et al., 2015).

2. OVERVIEW OF THE APPLICATIONS

Since our first review (Blankertz et al., 2010), 6 years have passed, bringing a wealth of novel developments. In this article, we review a selection of our research in this direction. Unlike in most medical applications, these approaches do not employ BCIs to let the user consciously transmit information to the computer. Instead, they use BCIs to infer covert user states and implicit information.

2.1. Types and Components of Brain Signals Being Exploited

Brain signals are either of the *exogenous* type, in which corresponding processes are elicited by external stimuli, or they are *endogenous*, originating from the participant independently of external events. Examples of endogenous brain signals include preparatory signals, such as the readiness potential (RP) and ongoing oscillations, like the alpha rhythm of the visual cortex. The exogenous signals that originate from the cortex can be roughly divided into those that are as being perception related, e.g., the visual evoked potential (VEP), the N1–P2 complex, and the steady-state visual evoked potential (SSVEP) or as being related to cognitive processes such as the P300 or the late positive component. The BCI applications that are reviewed here exploit all of these different types of brain signals—sometimes they are used in combination, sometimes just one alone.

2.2. Stratification of Use Cases

2.2.1. Type I: BCI as a Tool for Research

BCIs can provide an instantaneous estimate of the mental state and processing of an experimental subject. This possibility offers novel opportunities for (notably non-BCI-related) research. In Section 7, we show how closed-loop technology can be harnessed to study the relationship between preparatory signals (the RP) and corresponding actions—particularly the vetoing of such actions—and how it can thereby contribute to a fundamental question in cognitive neuroscience. The studies reviewed in Section 8 similarly target research questions in a different domain: the cognition and processing of music. In contrast to previous studies, it is not the real-time aspect that is exploited here, but rather the increased sensitivity to the methods that have been developed in BCI contexts. These algorithms enable a step forward in the analysis of music perception from fundamental studies with artificial and repeated stimuli toward investigating more natural behavior in music listening.

2.2.2. Type II: BCI as a Tool to Improve Devices, Interfaces, or Infrastructure

By providing brain-based measures while a participant is using a certain interface or product, or is interacting in a certain environment, one can assess and compare different variants and settings. A navigation system for a car may be tested and optimized with respect to how little it distracts the driver from the driving task as quantified by neural measures of workload or focused attention (Kohlmorgen et al., 2007; Blankertz et al., 2010). This is an example of an effect about which it is difficult to obtain reliable and unbiased measures through means such as questionnaires. The quantification of mental workload under real world conditions, however, is still a challenge for neurotechnologies. This ability would open an attractive range of applications. Section 5 presents some novel data analysis techniques that can be useful in this context. A workload index could also be employed to assess safety-critical aspects of infrastructure, such as harbors and bridges that require demanding maneuvers (Miklody et al., 2016).

An example of this application type in a quite different domain is given in Section 4. Visual perception of slight distortions in videos is probed and quantified as SSVEP amplitude, giving rise to a potential means of assessing the quality of video codecs. We contrast this approach with alternatives that employ cognitive event-related potential (ERP) components.

2.2.3. Type III: BCI as a Device to Enhance or Facilitate Human Actions

The direct control of computer applications with a BCI does not seem to be a realistic objective for healthy users. Yet some mileage could well be gained from using a BCI to obtain implicit information from a user during computer use. Added to the explicit information the computer obtains during an interaction, such implicit information should enable computers to understand human users better. We summarize studies dealing with various aspects of such implicit interactions in Section 6.

Section 3 explores the potential of BCI technology to provide information about an intended action before its execution. This potential is exemplified in the prediction of emergency braking when driving. A similar methodology is used in Section 7 as described above. But whereas the allter[PS1] use case exploits endogenous signals only, the prediction of emergency braking is based on a combination of different components, including perceptual and cognitive exogenous signals. For potential applications of the possibility of speeding up actions with BCIs, however, one needs to consider that this by-pass bears the risk of triggering actions on premature intentions and that it eliminates the possibility of vetoing the respective action in the last moment. This aspect is backed by the results reviewed in Section 7. The techniques for establishing a neural workload index, as mentioned above, may also be employed in a closed-loop fashion. Section 7 demonstrates such a type of application in the context of adapting working environments to the human factor.

2.3. Comparisons of the Categories of Use Cases

Type I. The use of BCIs as a tool for research is an easier case, in several ways. Experiments are conducted under laboratory conditions, complexity is often reduced to one variable of interest, standard EEG equipment with lengthy preparation times does not pose a serious problem, and it is not problematic if the system does not work for all participants. Still, specific requirements of a given use case can make the enterprise a challenge. In this category, the end users of the BCI are the researchers.

Type II. Using BCI technology in this way seems realistic in the medium term. The scenarios are often complex (e.g., driving a car), with mingled interactions between various perceptual and cognitive processes, calling for advanced decoding methods. On the other hand, there is no strict requirement for an easily deployable setup, the experimental conditions are somewhat controlled, and the experimental subjects can be selected according to the decodability of the given brain processes (provided that the selection criterion does not imply a bias with respect to the subject of investigation). Applications in this category mostly do not critically rely on the real-time aspect. In this case, the end users are the companies that develop the devices or interfaces, as well as the institutions that are responsible for the infrastructure.

Type III. BCI applications in this category are mostly rather far-reaching. The concepts are not yet ready for the dynamics and complexity of the real world, the measurement devices need to be easily deployable, yet also to provide robust signals, and the system should work preferably for anyone, as all human beings[PS3] are the end users in this category.

3. DETECTION OF EMERGENCY BRAKING INTENTION DURING DRIVING

This section summarizes two studies that investigate the possibility of predicting upcoming emergency braking from neural signals. The method makes use of exogenous ERPs related to perception and cognition in combination with an endogenous signal that indicates the preparation of a movement. We discuss potential benefits and caveats.

3.1. Context: Neurotechnology in the Context of Driving a Car

Neurotechnology can detect specific brain states before they reach consciousness and before they trigger behavioral actions (Section 7). Neuroergonomic approaches are therefore of interest for increasing our understanding of physiological aspects in time- and safety-critical applications, because a potentially dangerous situation may be detected before the user is aware of it and/or able to respond to it. In this section, we explore the feasibility and utility of this approach in driving a car. Kohlmorgen et al. (2007) and Dijksterhuis et al. (2013) study EEG correlates of mental workload during real-world and simulated driving, while (Kecklund and Åkerstedt, 1993; Papadelis et al., 2007; Schmidt et al., 2007, 2009; Gugler et al., 2010; Simon et al., 2011; Sonnleitner et al., 2012) study fatigue and attention during monotonous real-world driving. Reaction time in lane changing tasks has been investigated with EEG (Zhang et al., 2015a). Further studies demonstrate the detection of error and anticipatory potentials that could potentially be harnessed to increase driving safety (Khaliliardali et al., 2015; Zhang et al., 2015b). In emergency situations caused by obstacles on the road, drivers need to react quickly by braking. Such events lead to a cascade of mental responses from the perception and evaluation of the emergency-inducing stimulus to the activation of the lower limb muscles initiating the release of the gas pedal and the activation of the brake pedal. Due to the latencies inherent in motor responses, and due to the complexity of the required movement, the time spent between the stimulus and an effective deceleration of the vehicle can easily be on the order of 1 s, even if the decision to brake is made several hundred milliseconds earlier. This delay has led to attempts to retrieve the driver's braking intent earlier, which can be done by considering additional behavioral inputs such as gas pedal release, steering angle, foot position, and head movements (McCall and Trivedi, 2007; Trivedi and Cheng, 2007). Neuroergonomic approaches have the potential to prompt the user's decision even earlier—at the time of its very emergence—by tapping directly into the brain. This extra time might in principle either be used to prevent crashes through automatic braking, or to perform preparatory measures aimed at mitigating the impact of a crash through an automated response such as tightening the seat belts.

3.2. Two Studies on Predicting Emergency Braking

The first study to describe such a system was Haufe et al. (2011). In a driving simulator, $N = 18$ participants were instructed to follow a computer-controlled vehicle. The distance between vehicles was 20 m; the speed was 100 km/h. Occasionally (20–40 s inter-stimulus-interval, randomized), a rapid braking of the leading vehicle would induce an emergency braking situation. In order to avoid a crash, participants were required to perform immediate emergency braking in these situations. The onset of the lead vehicle's braking (and brake light flashing) is here referred to as the *stimulus*. The experiment comprised three blocks (45 min each) of driving with 10–15 min periods of rest in-between.

The authors measured myoelectric (EMG) activity using two bipolar electrodes located at the *M. tibialis anterior* and the knee of the right leg, as well as electroencephalography (EEG) from 64 scalp sites (nose reference). Behavioral and technical data—including brake and gas pedal deflections, the acceleration of the participant's vehicle, and the distance between vehicles—were also measured and synchronized with the physiological data. This yielded a multivariate, multi-modal time series from which the segments reflecting induced emergency situations and normal driving periods, respectively, were extracted.

Using univariate analysis, the authors discovered a characteristic event-related potential (ERP) signature preceding executed emergency braking in the EEG data. They then used multivariate machine learning to compare the predictive power (derived by distinguishing emergency braking from normal driving episodes) of a system utilizing all measurement modalities to systems either omitting EEG, EMG, or both. The study was later replicated with $N = 20$ subjects in a real car on a non-public test track (Haufe et al., 2014a).

Figure 1 depicts the event-related potentials that are characteristic of forced emergency braking. In both studies, a spatio-temporal ERP complex composed of the three overlapping subcomponents was observed: an early symmetric negative deflection in occipito-temporal areas, a negativity at central scalp sites, and a positive deflection in centro-parietal areas. The early occipital negativity is a visual-evoked potential (VEP) that can be attributed to low-level processing of the flashing of the brake light of the leading vehicle, which initiates the emergency situation. Higher-level processing of the importance of this flashing is reflected in the later centro-parietal positivity (P300). The late central negativity amounts to the readiness potential (RP), which reflects the motor preparation and execution related to pressing the brake pedal.

Figure 2 shows the detection accuracy of single-trial braking intention using a multivariate classifier as achieved on hold-out data and measured using the area under the curve (AUC) score. The classifier was evaluated at each stage of emergency braking between 0 and 1200 ms post-stimulus using data from the preceding 1500 ms. Without the EEG and EMG channels, the performance significantly dropped between approximately 200 and 1000 ms post-stimulus in both studies, indicating that EEG and EMG contain important information about the driver's intention that is not available in the combined remaining channels in the early stage of dealing with an emergency.

3.3. Conclusion and Outlook

Summarizing, Haufe et al. (2011) showed that EEG and EMG recordings reach the predictive accuracy of behavioral channels at earlier stages of the emergency situation. Their laboratory results were reproduced during real-world driving (Haufe et al., 2014a), demonstrating that well-designed simulator studies can be a useful proxy for real world studies. The results have also been confirmed under more diversified traffic conditions (Kim et al., 2014; Khaliliardali et al., 2015).

The robustness of our findings motivates the use of neuroergonomic approaches to driving assistance. Such a system may detect a driver's intention to brake before any of their actions become observable, and may thereby reduce the time after which appropriate action can be carried out. Haufe et al. (2011) evaluated a simplistic implementation of an online emergency braking detector in their simulation environment, and estimated that the time that can be saved by the system is around 130 ms. At 100 km/h, this amounts to a reduction of the braking

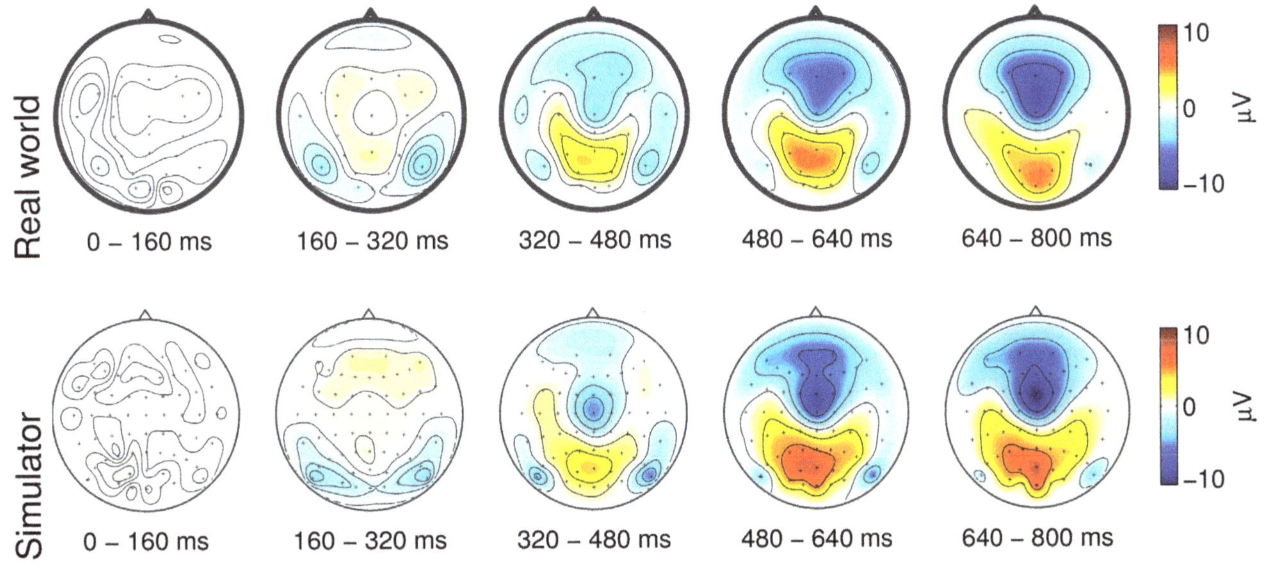

FIGURE 1 | Grand-average stimulus-aligned EEG responses to forced emergency braking during real-world (upper panel) and laboratory driving (lower panel). Potentials are visualized as topographical maps of grand-average ERPs in five temporal intervals. The stimulus onset ($t = 0$ ms) is the time of the brake lightbrake light flashing of the lead vehicle. Figure taken from Haufe et al. (2014a) with permission.

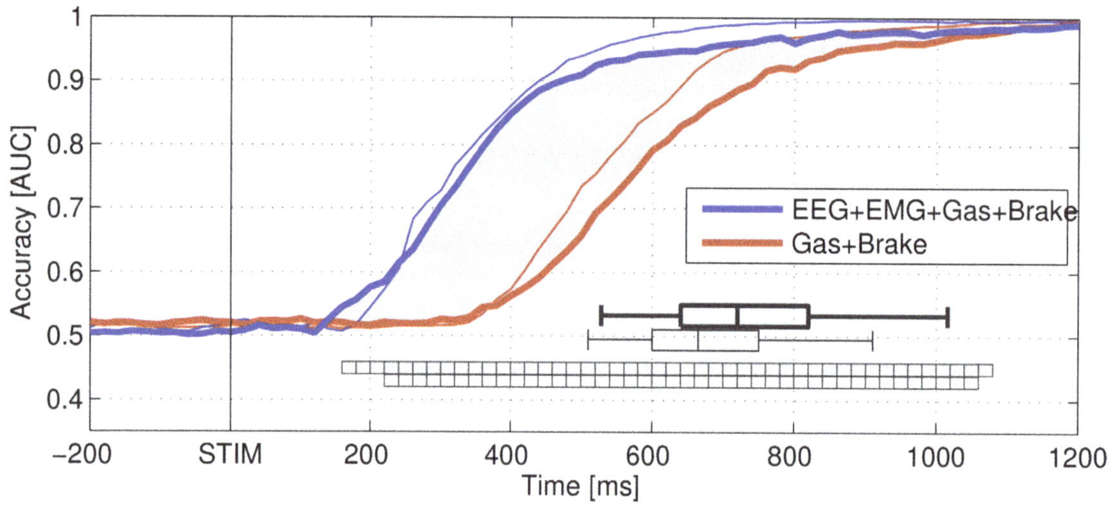

FIGURE 2 | Grand-average area under the curve (AUC) scores calculated from the outputs of linear classifiers that were optimized to distinguish normal driving intervals from stimulus-aligned target intervals representing different stages of emergency braking situations. STIM denotes the onset of braking (brake light flashing) of the lead vehicle. Thick lines represent the results of the real-world driving study (Haufe et al., 2014a), while thin lines represent results obtained in the driving simulator study of Haufe et al. (2011). The distribution of pooled braking response times in both datasets is indicated by box plots showing the 5th, 25th, 50th (median), 75th, and 95th percentiles. Classification was based on (spatio-) temporal features observed prior to the decision points. Performance of combinations of modalities. Blue: EEG+EMG+Gas+Brake (electrophysiological and behavioral channels). Red: Gas+Brake (only behavioral channels). The intervals, in which the inclusion of electrophysiological channels significantly improved classification accuracy are marked as square boxes (no filling for simulated driving, light gray filling for real-world driving). Figure taken from Haufe et al. (2014a) with permission.

distance by 3.66 m. With respect to practical implementation, another aspect has also to be considered. While anticipatory brain signals allow for an early prediction of an action, they do not necessarily reflect the final decision as shown in the study discussed in Section 7. In the presence of motor predictive brain signals, the participant may still change their mind and cancel the movement or act differently. In the scenario of emergency situations, this could be caused by the insight that under the given condition the avoidance of an obstruction might be a better option than braking.

4. EEG-BASED CLASSIFICATION OF VIDEO QUALITY PERCEPTION

By the virtue of a specific experimental paradigm, the watchers' SSVEP amplitudes were modulated by degradations in the quality of videos. Classification methods derived neural indices that correlated with the mean opinion scores (MOS) given by the participants in the standard behavioral assessment, giving rise to a new approach to video quality assessment.

4.1. Context: Brain-Guided Quality Assessment

As we elaborated in our first review (Blankertz et al., 2010), there is a good outlook for using neurotechnology in usability studies because it allows for an effortless continuous acquisition of usability parameters without requiring any action on the part of the user. It may also include aspects that are difficult to quantify objectively with conventional methods and access variables unknown to the test subjects themselves. In a similar vein, neurotechnology may prove useful for the quality assessment of such multi-media content (Moldovan et al., 2013; Antons et al., 2014). Such an approach may capitalize on neural correlates of perceptual or cognitive processes. The assessment of audio quality based on EEG was pioneered in Porbadnigk et al. (2010). Their results showed that the methodology taken from BCI research has the potential to detect changes in the brain signals of listeners, who were presented with audio signals that had quality degradations below the threshold of perception, (cf. also Antons et al., 2012; Porbadnigk et al., 2013). This demonstrated an increased sensitivity compared to behavioral measures, which was also found in studies on the visual domain (Porbadnigk et al., 2011). In this section, we review studies investigating the neurotechnology-based assessment of video quality with the aim of improving video codecs.

4.2. Studies on Neural Measures of Video Quality

For the transmission of video signals at today's high bit rates, video codecs usually employ high levels of compression, which might introduce distortions visible to the human eye. It is therefore desirable to measure the perceived distortions through the assessment of the visual quality of compressed video. This assessment is usually done through so-called mean opinion scores (MOS) that are obtained through questionnaires, in which participants are asked to rate the quality of a visual stimulus on a rating scale (ITU, 2002, 2008). These behavioral tests have many limitations, including large inter-subject variance and the requirement of a high number of participants to achieve statistical significance. The judgment of the participants can also be biased by several factors not related to the quality of the stimulus itself. In recent years, therefore, there has been increasing interest in investigating novel paradigms for video quality assessment through the direct measurement of neural activity via EEG (Hayashi et al., 2000; Babiloni et al., 2006; Arndt et al., 2011; Lindemann et al., 2011; Mustafa et al., 2012; Arndt et al., 2014; Kroupi et al., 2014).

The authors of Scholler et al. (2012) used an experimental design that capitalized on the ERP component P3 to quantify the perception of the human observer when being confronted with a change in video quality. As stimuli, they showed 8 s video clips based on a synthetic image of a textured checkerboard, which was deformed over time by simulating a swaying water surface on the top. The quality change was introduced by lossy compression, while its magnitude was controlled by the quantization parameter of the video coder. Participants had to acknowledge the perception of the quality change via button press. They found that quality changes elicited a P3 component that was positively correlated with the magnitude of the change, which could be classified on a single-trial basis using LDA. They report a single-trial classification with AUC-values close to 1 for the highest level of distortion in most subjects, referring only to trials correctly identified by the participants at the behavioral level. They also report, for three participants, an average 65% accuracy in classifying the trials in which the quality change was present but not detected by the subjects, advancing the hypothesis of higher sensitivity of the EEG compared to the behavioral response.

All the previously mentioned studies are based on the detection of the P3 component, which is a cognitive ERP not directly linked to sensory processing. Complementarily, we investigated a paradigm based on Steady-State Visual Evoked Potentials (SSVEPs) that reflect perceptual processes. The basic suitability of the SSVEP-based design for video quality assessment has been demonstrated (Norcia et al., 2014). Here, we review a systematic follow-up study (Acqualagna et al., 2015).

As stimuli, six gray-level natural images in six levels of degradation (corresponding to six compression rates) were used. The degradation levels were controlled by the quantization parameter, as in Scholler et al. (2012). The experiment comprised 51 videos in which all the textures in all the levels of degradation were displayed (**Figure 3**). The original and distorted textures were presented in alternating order with a stimulus onset asynchrony (SOA) of 333 ms (i.e., at a frequency of 3 Hz). The flickering effect of the sequence of quality changes caused the elicitation of SSVEPs in the occipital cortex, the amplitude of which increased with increased distortion levels.

In the first approach, single VEPs of the steady-state signal were classified using spatio-temporal features (Blankertz et al., 2011) applied to epochs without and with a time-lag of 160 ms (**Figure 4**, left). Single-trial classification achieved an average maximum AUC of 0.84 for the maximum distortion level. **Figure 4** (right) shows that the first three distortion levels (D1–D3), which were chosen to be below the threshold of perception, did not modulate the SSVEPs and classification stayed at chance level. Further on, classification performance linearly increases with the distortion level. AUC scores significantly linearly correlated with MOS-values for all the participants ($p < 0.01$).

The same trend was obtained for the classification of spectral features at 3 and 6 Hz (i.e., the frequencies of the EEG spectrum that showed the highest modulation). CSP filters were calculated on the training data between the epochs referred to the maximum distortion level (D6) and those referred to the original textures (D0). CSP filters were then applied on the test data for all distortion levels. Features consisted of the log-variance of the CSP filtered data. Epochs locked to the distorted textures (D1–D6) were classified vs. epochs locked to D0 using LDA, achieving the maximum average AUC of 0.74 for D6.

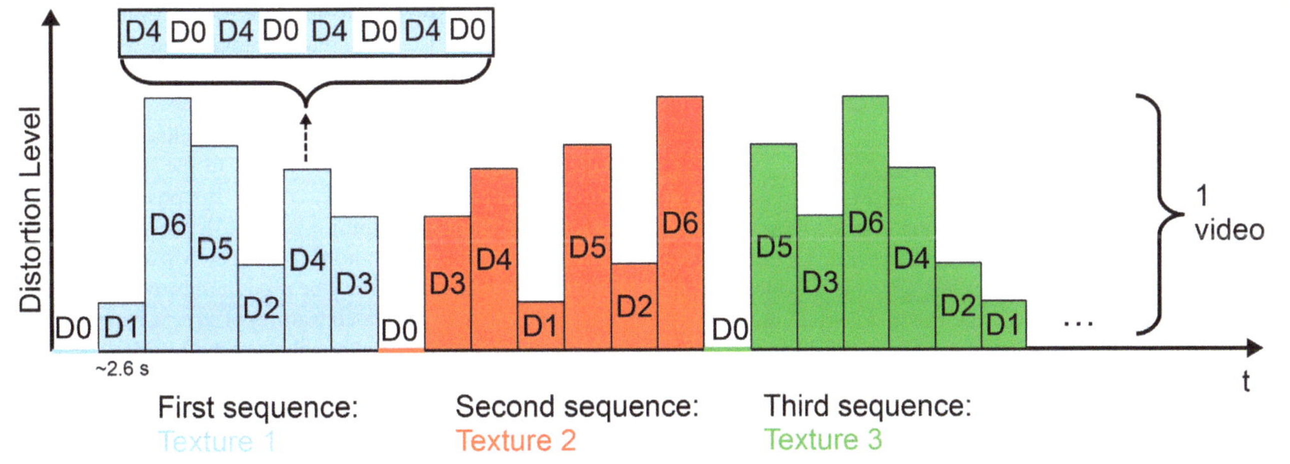

FIGURE 3 | SSVEP-based paradigm for video quality assessment. Each video comprised the six textures presented in all the levels of distortion (D1, ... , D6) in random order. Each texture was displayed distorted for 333 ms, followed by the undistorted form for 333 ms (D0) and the same succession was repeated four times for each level. Figure adapted from Acqualagna et al. (2015) with permission.

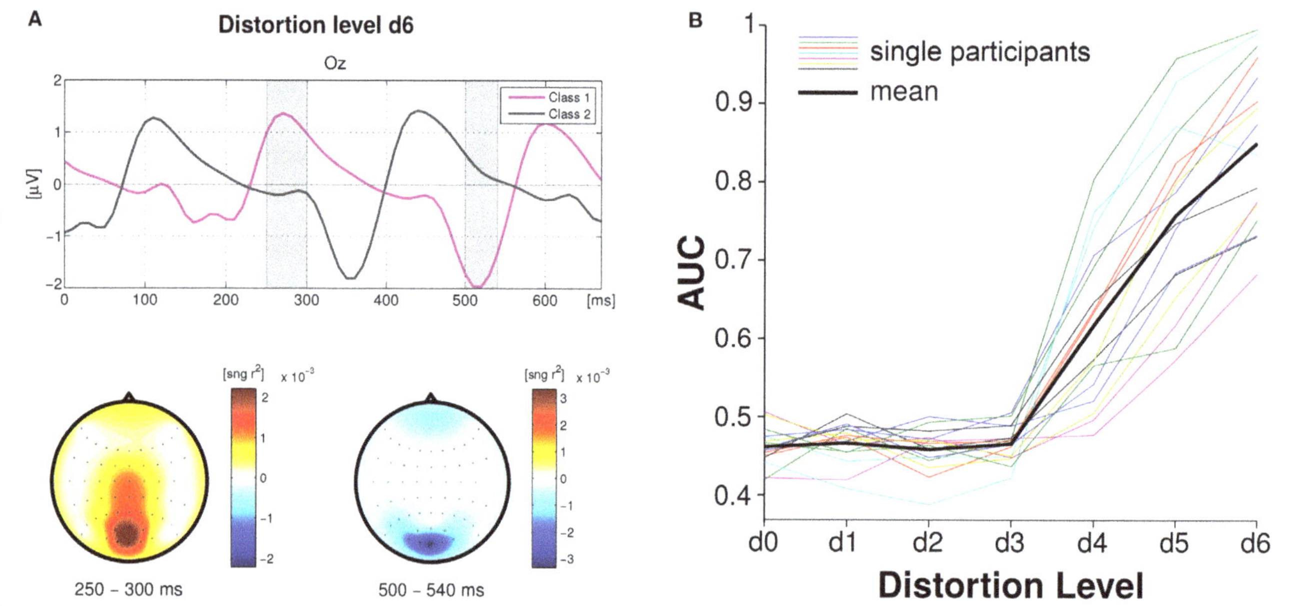

FIGURE 4 | Single-trial classification of VEPs based on spatio-temporal features. (A) Grand average brain activity over all participants at channel Oz, at maximum distortion level D6. The magenta line represents "Class 1" and the gray line "Class 2." Scalp plots underneath refer to the shaded areas in the time plot and display the magnitude of the $sign - r^2$ for each channel. **(B)** Classification performances using shrinkage LDA for all participants (colored lines) and mean (black thick line). Figure adapted from Acqualagna et al. (2015) with permission.

4.3. Concluding Remarks

Importantly, this study showed that an SSVEP-based paradigm allows a much quicker collection of trials than previous P3-based paradigms for quality assessment. The results of the neural assessment also correlated significantly with the MOS-values. The study thus demonstrated that an SSVEP-based video quality assessment can be considered a viable complement to behavioral-based assessments and a presumably faster alternative to methods based on the P3 component. For further details about the study and complementary analysis, please refer to Bosse et al. (2014, 2015) and Acqualagna et al. (2015). More generally, the results indicate the utility of the brain-based approach for usability testing and related quality assessment.

5. ADVANCED MONITORING OF WORKLOAD

This section reports methodological advancements in the context of brain-based mental state monitoring (Blankertz et al., 2010) and neuroergonomics (Mehta and Parasuraman, 2013). We take the estimation of the so-called operator workload as an application scenario, although the methodology is much more widely applicable. We explored estimates based on spectral features of endogenous brain rhythms that differ with respect to the label information required for training, including entirely unsupervised approaches. The explored estimators also differed with respect to the level at which the spectral features are extracted, thereby comparing traditional single-channel based approaches to approaches that employ recent advances in spatial filtering methods (Schultze-Kraft et al., 2016b).

5.1. Context: Neuroergonomics and Physiology of Operator Workload

Many work places with high levels of automation require human operators to perform monotonous but attention-demanding tasks, such as driving and air traffic control, or as in industrial contexts. In such work environments, the demand for high levels of alertness can lead to an overload of the human operator, which in turn can have critical consequences for health, safety, and efficiency. An assessment of the operator's workload (Gevins et al., 1995; Gevins and Smith, 2003) can be utilized to prevent overload and can lead to adaptive systems that automatically self-regulate the level of human-machine interaction (Pope et al., 1995; Prinzel et al., 2003; Parasuraman and Wilson, 2008). Another area of application is in training procedures, in which displaying the current workload level to the trainer as well as to the trainee her/himself is expected to facilitate learning or to make the alignment of difficulty levels to the trainee's progress more efficient (Borghini et al., 2016). This possibility has been explored for pilots (Borghini et al., 2013), air traffic controllers (Di Flumeri et al., 2015), and shipmasters (Miklody et al., 2016). The technique could similarly be used to improve infrastructure, by testing, for example, which features of streets, harbors, and the like require maneuvers that are likely to induce high workload.

The human EEG has been shown to provide reliable estimators of workload, based on the fact that changes in workload are associated with characteristic modulations in the power of oscillatory activity in particular frequency bands of the EEG (Buzsáki and Draguhn, 2004). The most prominent frequency bands with power changes related to workload are theta (4–7 Hz) and alpha (8–12 Hz). Theta power has been shown to be positively correlated with workload, most notably in frontal regions (Gevins et al., 1998; Smith et al., 2001; Holm et al., 2009), whereas alpha power is typically found to be negatively correlated with workload, in parietal regions in particular (Gevins and Smith, 2003; Holm et al., 2009). This effect cannot be expected in general, however, as these results refer to the visual modality only (see the discussion Section 9).

5.2. Study Comparing Methodologies for Estimating Workload

The experiment setup in Schultze-Kraft et al. (2016b) was designed to emulate an industrial working scenario in which an operator performs tasks requiring a continuous effort of visual and motor processing with alternating difficulty. Ten healthy male subjects, aged 26–40, participated in the experiments. Subjects were instructed to carry out a task on a 21-inch touch screen lying on a table in front of them (**Figure 5A**).

The task was designed as a computer game in which objects consisting of three vertically aligned screws (screw triplets) were falling from random positions at top of the screen and had to be caught in a bucket at the bottom of the screen. Subjects could move the bucket horizontally by sliding it with one of their index fingers. The coloring of the bucket could be adjusted by touching colored buttons that were positioned on either side of the screen. The catching task was further complicated by the constraint that the coloring of the bucket had to match the coloring of a screw triplet before catching it. Not catching a screw triplet was considered an error and so was catching a triplet with a color scheme that did not match the color scheme of the bucket. In the low workload condition (L), the interval between falling screw triples was constant, whereas in the high workload condition (H) the intervals were shorter and were randomly varied. The experiment was conducted in four runs, where each run lasted 24 min and consisted of alternating low and high workload blocks, with each block lasting 90 s. See **Figure 5B** for the experimental design.

In addition to 64-channel EEG, we also determined task performance (error rate) and measured the following peripheral physiological measures (PPM): respiratory frequency, cardiac frequency, and electrodermal response. See **Figures 5C–F** for the task-induced effects on error rate and PPMs. Switching from low to high workload induced consistent and significant increases in error rate and all PPMs.

In order to classify (or predict) workload levels, we compared six different predictive models. Three of them are based on spectral features at *channel-level*, whereas the other three used specific data-driven *spatial filters*. In the channel-level approaches, spectral features are computed for each recording

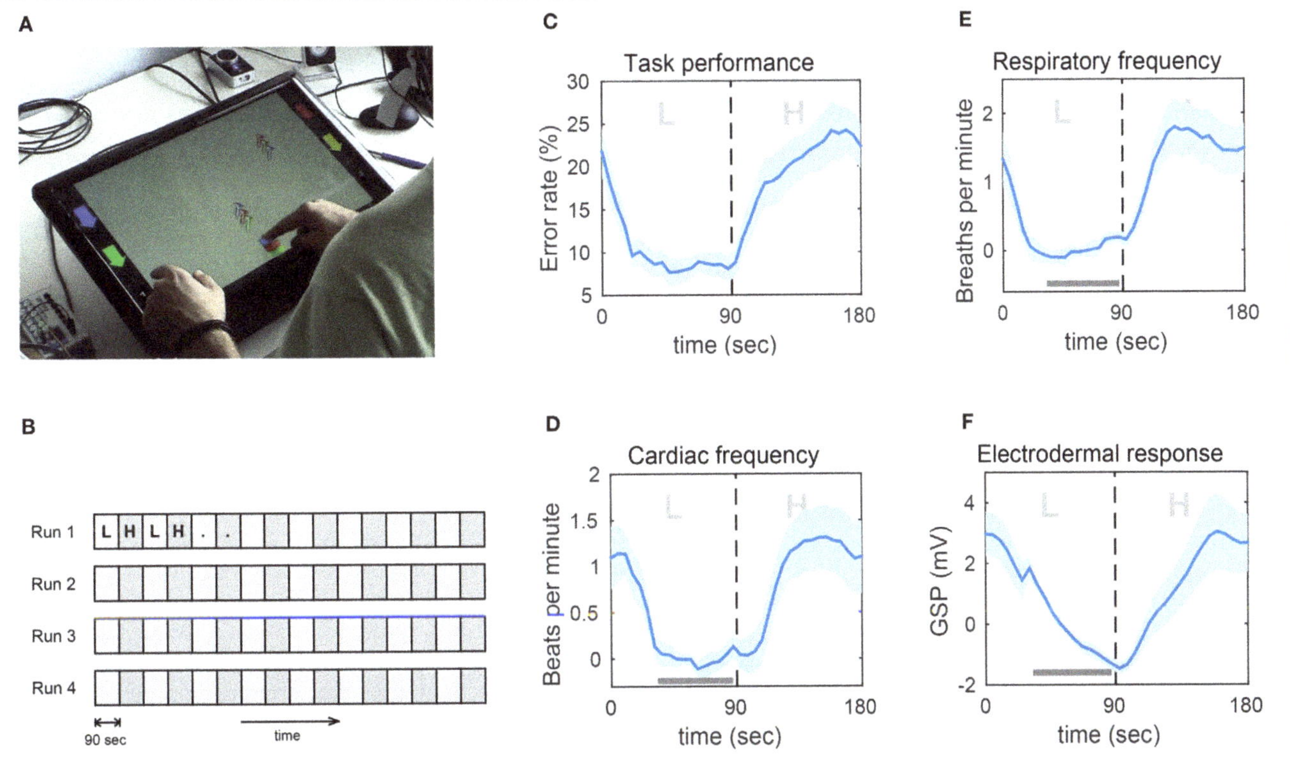

FIGURE 5 | Experimental task and impact of the experimental paradigm on task performance and peripheral physiological measures (PPM). (A) Snapshot from one of the experiments showing a subject playing the game on the touch screen. **(B)** Block structure of the experiment. Participants performed four runs of 24 min, each consisting of 90-s blocks of alternating low (*L*) and high (*H*) workload conditions. **(C)** Error rate. **(D)** Respiratory frequency in breaths per minute. **(E)** Cardiac frequency in beats per minute. **(F)** Electrodermal response in Galvanic skin potential. Shown are the grand averages of the mean over all L–H block pairs. The light blue shadings indicate the standard error of the mean. Due to large inter-subject differences in the average of the PPMs, the grand average and standard error were computed after subtracting the mean in the indicated bar. Thus, the plotted values represent changes from this baseline. Figure taken from Schultze-Kraft et al. (2016b) with permission.

channel separately. In the spatial-filter-level approaches, the data are first projected onto a set of optimized spatial filters. Spectral features are then computed based on the output of the spatial filters. Each of the channel-level and spatial-filter-level approaches fall into one out of three sub-categories, depending on the amount of information required by the approach. These sub-categories include (a) use of binary class labels (classification models, tag *cfy*), (b) use of a continuous error measure (regression models, tag *regr*), and (c) no use of a supervision signal at all (unsupervised models, tag *unsup*). In the classification models, spectral features were combined using regularized linear discriminant analysis (LDA) in combination with binary labels. In the regression models, spectral features were combined using regularized least-squares regression (LSR) in combination with the subject's error rate as a supervision signal. Finally, the output of the unsupervised models was simply the difference between theta and alpha features (Power diff). These three sub-categories represent a progression from (a) controlled laboratory conditions in which full label information is available to more realistic settings in which either (b) only a proxy-variable, such as the error rate is available, or (c) no external information about the variable of interest is available at all. This last scenario requires assumptions about the nature of the expected spectral changes in the EEG, which, in our case, is associated with workload (Gevins et al., 1998; Gevins and Smith, 2003; Holm et al., 2009).

Matching the level of additional information provided, we employed the following spatial filter methods. For the classification model, we used the Common Spatial Pattern (CSP) algorithm (Fukunaga, 1990; Koles, 1991; Blankertz et al., 2008) to train the spatial filters. For the regression model, we used the Source Power Co-modulation (SPoC) algorithm (Dähne et al., 2014a). For the unsupervised model, we used the canonical Source Power Co-modulation (cSPoC) algorithm (Dähne et al., 2014b). While CSP is a well-established method in the field of BCI, SPoC, and cSPoC represent recent advances in the development of spatial filtering methods. See Dähne et al. (2015) and Fazli et al. (2015) for further information on the background of these methods.

Figure 6A shows the mean classification accuracies for the six models, averaged across subjects. Both groups of models, with and without spatial filtering, show a decrease of performance with a decreasing amount of exploited label information. Between the groups, models using spatial filtering show a clear advantage that becomes greater the smaller the amount of label information that is available: 3.8% (CSP), 4.2% (SPoC), and 8.2% (cSPoC), compared to the respective channel-based method.

Given the modulation of PPMs by the workload condition (**Figures 5C,D**) and given that PPM features can be extracted from the data as an unsupervised signal, we assessed whether PPM features constitute an added value to the features extracted in the unsupervised models. We first of all found that the mean classification accuracy using only PPM features was 81.8% (**Figure 6B**, white bar). We then repeated the analysis with unsupervised models. This time, however, we augmented the EEG features with PPM features. This resulted in enhanced classification accuracies: a 3.6% increase for the channel-based (n.s.) and a significant increase of 4.3% for the spatial

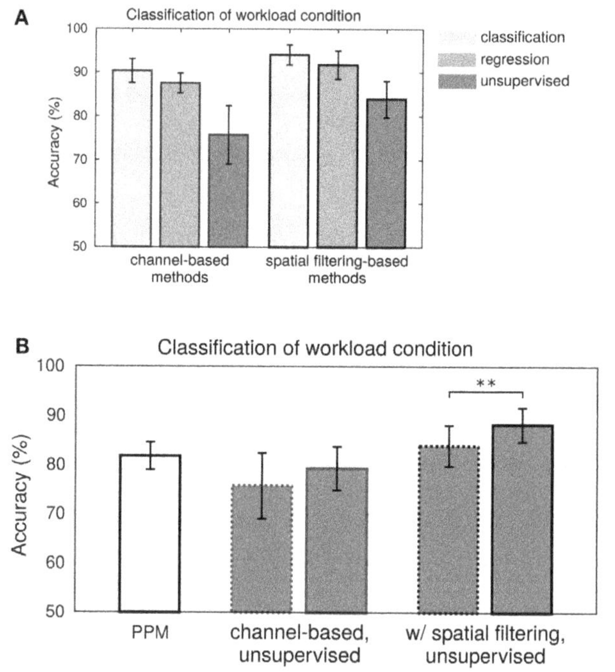

FIGURE 6 | Results. (A) Mean classification accuracy and standard error of the six models across subjects. **(B)** Added value of peripheral physiological measures. Mean classification accuracy and standard error across subjects when using only PPM features (white) and comparison to the two unsupervised predictive models before (dotted) and after (solid) augmenting with PPM features. Figure taken from Schultze-Kraft et al. (2016b) with permission. **Indicates a significance level of $p < 0.01$.

filtering-based method. Note that the unsupervised but PPM-augmented model outperformed the supervised channel-based model and even nearly equaled the performance of the supervised model, which used spatial filters. These results support the assumption that peripheral physiology can indeed provide an added value to the unsupervised model for the classification of workload.

Next to an increased signal-to-noise ratio, a further benefit of using spatial filtering methods is that they allow for the inspection and interpretation of spatial activation patterns, which are associated with the extracted signals (Haufe et al., 2014b). It is thus possible to verify that the signals extracted by the CSP, SPoC, and cSPoC filters were of cortical origin, as opposed to possibly stemming from ocular or other artifactual sources. For this purpose, we examined the spatial activation patterns that correspond to the components found using the three methods, as well as the corresponding power envelopes of the components' time series. **Figure 7** shows the activation patterns and corresponding power envelopes for one example subject. The activation patterns indicate that frontal theta activity and parietal/occipital alpha activity are the sources of workload modulated signals.

5.3. Conclusion and Outlook

In summary, we find that using established and, in particular, recently developed spatial filtering methods, it has become

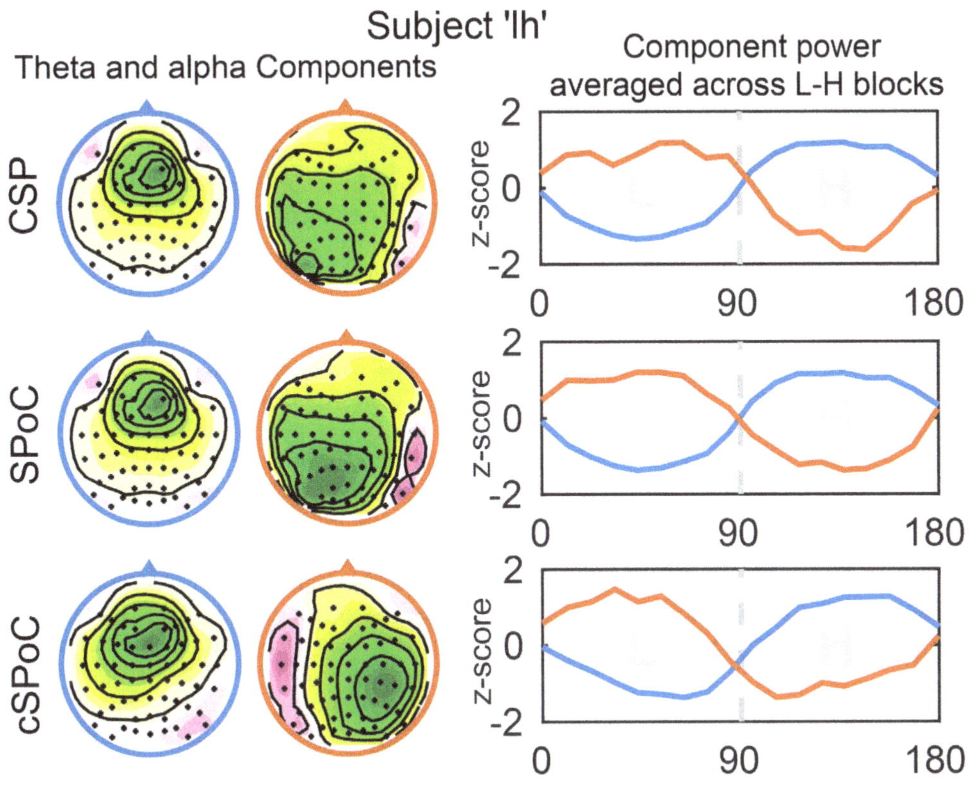

FIGURE 7 | Spatial activation patterns and power envelopes of components extracted by the three EEG spatial filtering methods. The shown activation patterns (scalp maps) and power envelopes correspond to the components with the highest value of the optimization criterion of the respective method. The left and middle column show the activation patterns of components obtained from the theta (blue) and alpha (red) bandpassed data, respectively. The color coding and sign of the activation patterns were adjusted to be consistent across methods, but are arbitrary otherwise. The power envelopes (right column) are color-coded accordingly (theta: blue; alpha: red), the x-axis shows time in seconds. Due to standardizing to *z*-scores, the amplitudes of the curves do not relate to discriminative power. Figure taken from Schultze-Kraft et al. (2016b) with permission.

possible to estimate an operator's workload based on brain signals and peripheral measures. Additionally, we would like to point out that we observed similarly promising results in a workload-related study (Naumann et al., 2016) in which subjects played the classical Tetris video game. In contrast to most workload-related studies, the task in Naumann et al. (2016) was not to classify workload into one of two categories (typically high vs. low workload). Instead, we aimed to predict the player's current game level, purely on the basis of spectral features from the brain. We employed the model outlined above (SPoC combined with regression) and we were able to predict the current gaming level with high precision (Naumann et al., 2016), results that are comparable with the findings presented in Schultze-Kraft et al. (2016b).

6. BRAIN-COMPUTER INTERFACES FOR HUMAN-COMPUTER INTERACTION

While intentional control of computer applications is the target of classic BCI research for patients, this approach does not seem promising for general users. Instead, it seems worthwhile to employ BCIs to infer implicit information during software usage and to use that information to augment the explicit interaction. In other words, to make the computer better at understanding the human user on the basis of soft skills. In view of this far-reaching goal, we have investigated several studies that pave the way.

6.1. Context: BCIs for General Human-Computer Interaction

The interaction with a complex interface might be facilitated if the system is able to exploit implicit information about the cognitive state of its user inferred from physiological signals. Measures from eye movement patterns, pupil size, electrodermal activity (EDA), facial electromyography (fEMG), and other peripheral physiological signals can provide insights into the user's mind with respect to relevance, attention, or intent (Oliveira et al., 2009; Hardoon and Pasupa, 2010; Cole et al., 2011a,b; Gwizdka and Cole, 2011; Haji Mirza et al., 2011; Hajimirza et al., 2012; Barral et al., 2015). However, electrophysiology may provide a more direct access to the cognition of the user in comparison to eye tracking or peripheral physiology (Zander and Kothe, 2011; Eugster et al., 2014; Ušćumlić and Blankertz, 2016; Wenzel et al., 2016).

Transferring the decoding results from the classic (fixed-gaze) BCI systems toward general human-computer interaction (HCI) applications, in which complex displays are explored in an unconstrained free-viewing manner, holds a number of challenges that we discuss in this section. These scenarios, which allow natural behavior, essentially require co-registration of eye-movements and EEG, since free viewing implies self-paced scene exploration. The emerging research on eye fixation-related potentials has shown that fixations on the object of search evoke EEG responses similar to the one evoked in the classical visual oddball paradigm with fixed gaze (Rämä and Baccino, 2010; Kamienkowski et al., 2012; Brouwer et al., 2013; Kaunitz et al., 2014), which motivated an expansion of potential BCI applications. The joint EEG and eye-tracking studies, such as those addressing active visual search of the target face in images of crowds (Kaunitz et al., 2014), or during navigation of 3D naturalistic environments (Jangraw et al., 2014), provide evidence for the feasibility of EEG-based intention decoding in realistic active visual search tasks. Both studies, however, impose certain constraints, either in terms of subjects' behavior (i.e., promoting longer fixations Kaunitz et al., 2014) or in terms of stimuli that prevent the overlap of target responses (Jangraw et al., 2014). Neither of these studies, moreover, address the system's performance with respect to the content of scenes, i.e., its semantic and spatial distribution, clutter, and temporal dynamic.

We conducted various experiments to approach these issues, taking as a guiding example the assessment of the relevance of the items on screen with regard to the user's task (e.g., information seeking). The goal is to obtain implicit information about the user's intention from the brain signals (as co-registered eye-tracker data) to supplement the explicit interaction with computer software via mouse and keyboard. Implicit relevance measures can be captured unobtrusively in the background and consume less time and effort in comparison to a laborious manual evaluation of the relevance of each item. In this transfer of BCI technology to realistic settings of human-computer interaction, we face a number of challenges that we address in the following section.

6.2. Variable Neural Latency in Dynamic Scenes

On the one hand, applications for information seeking and retrieval are nowadays characterized by rich and dynamic visual interfaces. Such interfaces inevitably engage different attentional and perceptual brain processes (e.g., covert attention and peripheral vision) to sample the relevant content of scenes through consecutive eye-fixations. On the other hand, information is typically provided as semantic concepts that are richer than a simple symbol or a plain word; they may be contained in data of different modalities (e.g., text, image, and video). While a semantic concept may be ambiguous or vague, its recognition may require integration of evidence over time. Typical examples of the latter case are action and behavior recognition, or the recognition of new content on a screen when transition visual effects are applied, as it is often the case in visual interfaces. Altogether, in real world applications the cognitive processing may vary in both duration and onset time with reference to fixations. Our recently published study (Ušćumlić and Blankertz, 2016), which was motivated by the non-stationarity of our natural visual environment, addressed the EEG correlates of visual recognition while participants overtly performed visual search in non-stationary scenes. Our research particularly concerned whether scene dynamics might intensify the temporal uncertainty of ERPs with reference to fixations, introducing an extra challenge for state-of-the-art EEG decoding methods. We designed three free-view visual search tasks mimicking the type of visual effects that may appear in real world human-computer visual interfaces. Alongside popping-up stimuli, two composite appearance styles based on fading-in, enlarging, and motion effects were considered (**Figure 8**). In the Pop-Up (PU) and Smooth Appearance (SA) conditions, stimuli appear at random but fixed positions on the screen. In the Motion Appearance (MA) condition, the constant stimuli motion causes the entire scene to continuously change (for details, see Ušćumlić and Blankertz, 2016). First, we investigated the performance of the state-of-the-art EEG decoding method *hierarchical discriminant components analysis (HDCA)* (Gerson et al., 2006) across different conditions. The results confirmed our concerns, indicating a drop in decoding performance when facing less certain timing of visual events (i.e., the appearance of new content in a scene) due to the transitional changes (cf. **Figure 9** upper panel). We showed, however, that the knowledge obtained from the paradigm characterized by less temporal uncertainty (i.e., popping-up stimuli) can be exploited to boost the EEG decoding performance in more challenging conditions. This is done by estimating posterior probabilities across different time lags with reference to fixation onset, using the classifier trained on popping-up condition, and by making the final decision based on a maximum of the estimated posteriors. The improved decoding performance, estimated in a 10-fold validation setting, is presented in **Figure 9** (lower panel), for fading-in and motion conditions, respectively.

6.3. Variable Neural Latency Due to Variable Saliency

In typical BCI experiments, different stimuli are flashed one-by-one (cf. **Figure 10A**) and the EEG is segmented in stimulus-aligned epochs that are used to predict the selected stimulus of interest (e.g., Treder et al., 2011). In regular software applications, several items are usually presented in parallel, rather than one-by-one. In this case, the saccades to the items, as measured with an eye tracker, can serve as time points of reference for the EEG segmentation (cf. **Figure 10B**). Using this approach, it is possible to estimate which items displayed on the screen are task-relevant and which are not (e.g., Brouwer et al., 2013; Kaunitz et al., 2014; Ušćumlić and Blankertz, 2016; Wenzel et al., 2016).

Pictograms and words shown in real software applications are usually diverse and feature different colors, shapes, and sizes. Saliency, which enables the recognition of relevant items, varies accordingly, such that recognition can happen either before the saccade (when the item is still in peripheral vision) or after the saccade to the item (when the item is in foveal vision; cf. **Figure 10C**). Accordingly, neural activity related to recognition can exhibit a temporal variability with respect to the saccades, which are used as time point of reference for the EEG

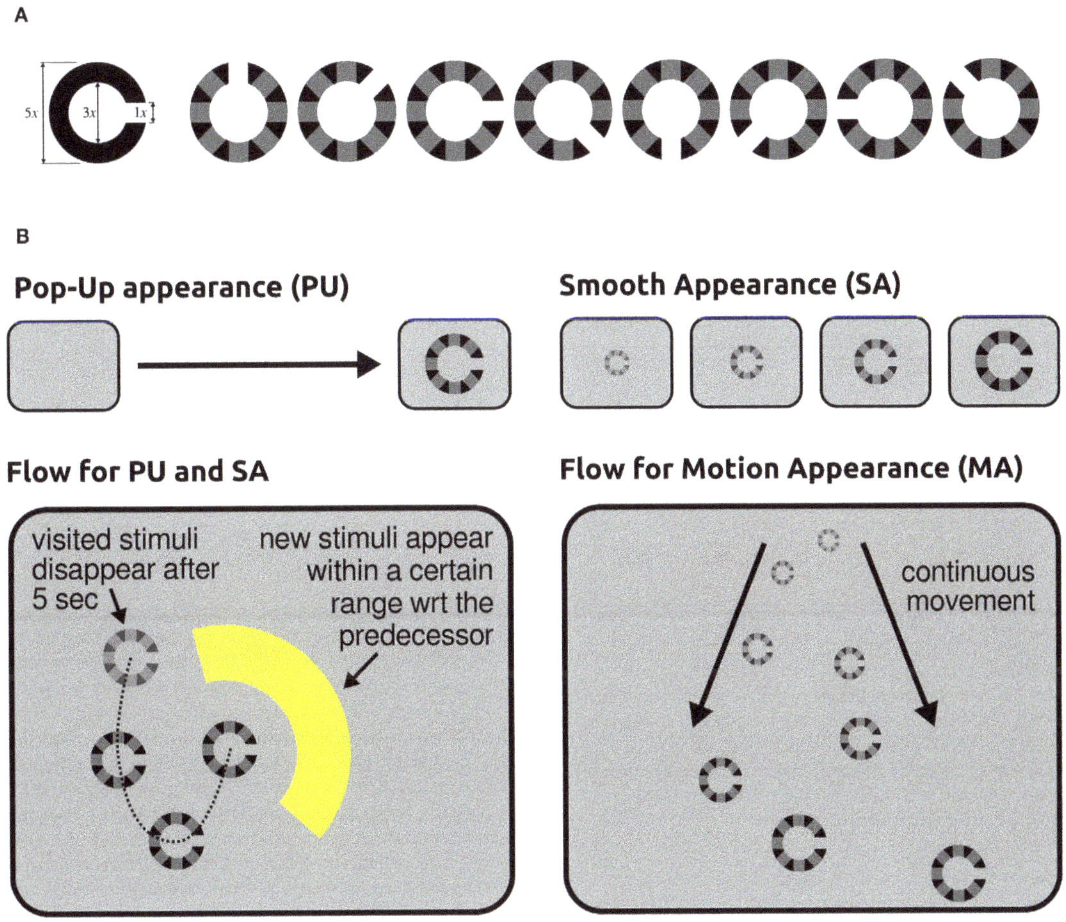

FIGURE 8 | (A) Left: A standard Landolt broken ring. **Right:** Eight modified Landolt rings that we used in our study. **(B)** Illustration of the stimuli presentation flow for different conditions. **Top-left:** In the PU condition, stimuli appear in one step. **Top-right:** Three intermediate steps of stimulus evolution in time are presented for the SA condition, followed by a completely revealed stimulus. **Bottom-right** The dashed line indicates the order of the appearance of stimuli in the PU and SA conditions. **Bottom-left** Several intermediate steps in the evolution of two successive stimuli are illustrated for the MA condition. The arrows indicate the direction of their continuous motion. This illustration is simplified, since multiple objects were present on the screen during the motion condition (MA). Stimuli are enlarged in comparison to the real screen dimensions. Figure taken from Uščumlić and Blankertz (2016) with permission.

segmentation. BCI prediction algorithms are not required to deal with this temporal variability because the stimulus onset serves as reference and the eyes are not moved in typical BCI experiments. An experiment with unrestricted eye gaze was performed in order to systematically investigate whether the algorithms can cope with this issue, which can be expected in realistic HCI settings (Wenzel et al., 2016). The participants were asked to find and count certain items that were presented in parallel on the screen and that were sometimes more and sometimes less salient. The continuous EEG data were segmented in epochs aligned to the (ends of the) saccades toward the items. Salient task-relevant items evoked an earlier neural response in comparison to less salient task-relevant items, presumably because recognition was possible already in peripheral vision. Nevertheless, even when the item saliency was mixed, a typical BCI prediction algorithm was suited to deal with the resulting temporal variability and was able to detect the task-relevant items in this search task.

6.4. Interference of Eye Movements with the EEG

EEG epochs used for the predictions in BCI experiments are usually set at several hundred milliseconds long in order to capture the P300 wave. But fixations often last only few hundred milliseconds and the subsequent saccade can occur during the same EEG epoch. This is problematic because eye movements can interfere with the EEG data. Yet, even when the eye movements were unrestricted, it was possible to capture neural signals related to recognition when the discriminative information was not (primarily) a result of eye movements (Wenzel et al., 2016). Interestingly, information from the two modalities of EEG and eye tracking were found to be complementary. An investigation of target detection with moving objects that require smooth-pursuit eye-movements showed no decrease of decoding performance if the timing of the event was known (Uščumlić et al., 2015).

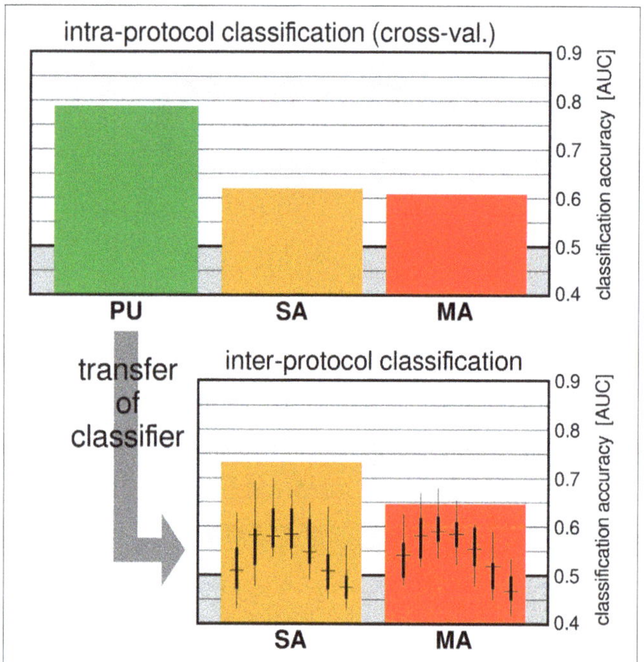

FIGURE 9 | Upper plot: Intra-protocol classification with an HDCA was cross-validated on the three conditions. **Lower plot:** For the inter-protocol classifier transfer, the HDCA was trained on the training data (PU condition) on a fixed time interval. The intermediate results of the testing datasets (conditions SA and MA), obtained for different positions of the sliding window (small boxplots), are combined to give the results indicated by the broad bars. Figure adapted from Ušćumlić and Blankertz (2016).

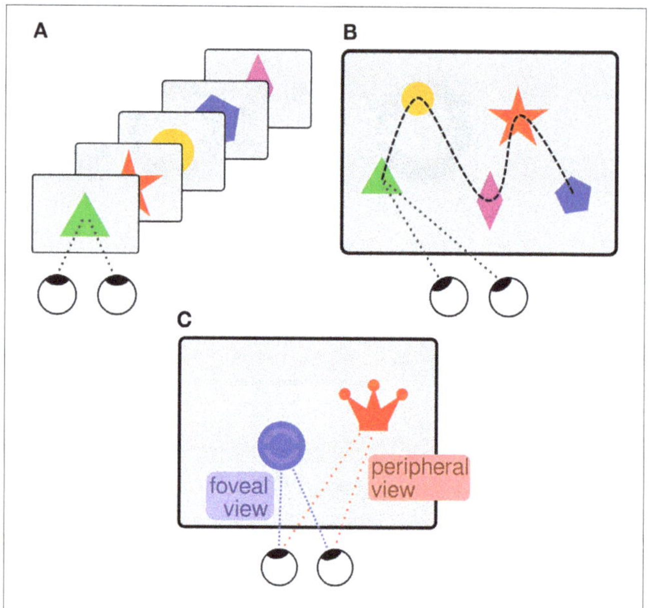

FIGURE 10 | (A) Sequential centered "BCI presentation." A simplified "mental typewriter" serves as example for an ERP-based BCI (cf. Treder et al., 2011). Different items (square, triangle, disc, pentagon) are flashed one-by-one, on the same spot on the screen. Each item stands for a (group of) letter(s). The subject selects a letter and silently counts the flashes of the corresponding item in order to direct their attention toward it. The selected (group of) letter(s) can be decoded from the EEG data using the flashes as time points of reference. **(B)** Item scanning in free-viewing. In an HCI scenario, words or pictograms (symbolized in the illustration) are displayed in parallel on the screen and are not flashed one-by-one. Items of particular interest for the user shall be decoded from the EEG data. The saccades (white arrow) to the items, as measured with an eye tracker, can serve as time points of reference for the EEG analysis. **(C)** The stimulus saliency may vary in HCI settings. An item of little saliency (here represented by a blue disc with indistinct interior) can only be recognized after a saccade when the item is in foveal vision. In contrast, a salient item (red crown) can be recognized already in peripheral vision, before a saccade toward it. A variable timing of recognition can therefore be expected with respect to the saccades, which are used as time points of reference for the EEG analysis.

6.5. Insufficient Accuracy in Single-Trials

EEG and eye tracking data can be informative about item relevance, but they are not sufficient for a reliable relevance estimate after a single fixation of an item. Brain-Computer Interfaces have to deal with a similar uncertainty and address this problem usually by combining predictions from several EEG epochs for class selection. The same strategy could be followed for the transfer to human-computer interaction. Practical applications should be designed such that evidence about user relevance is accumulated over time. This approach is favored naturally, because humans frequently move their eyes, which may result in a large number of saccade-aligned EEG epochs. For instance, when subjects scanned a mosaic of images that belonged to two classes, it was possible to reliably estimate, based on EEG and eye tracking data, which of the two classes of images was more relevant for the user, even if the predictions for the single images were not accurate. This strategy allowed the implicit resolution of ambiguities in an image web search (Golenia et al., 2015).

6.6. Conclusion and Outlook

Taken together, these results indicate the basic feasibility of exploiting implicit information through the use of BCI techniques for human-computer interaction. This holds also if the targets are not previously known stimuli, but rather semantically described categories consisting of a large variety of previously unseen stimuli (Acqualagna and Blankertz, 2015).

Apart from relevance, estimating the "depth of cognitive processing" would be useful in HCI when, for example, interfaces can adapt according to whether displayed information was adequately processed by the user or not. Recent work indicates that this variable can also be estimated sufficiently from the EEG (Nicolae et al., 2015a,b).

For a realistic perspective of using BCI technology in general human-computer interaction, the extraction of implicit information needs to be further improved, as in the context of, for example, more complex visual stimuli (Wenzel et al., 2015). Moreover, the co-registered acquisition of EEG and eye tracking data needs to be simplified to a deployable setup. We briefly discuss this aspect in a paragraph in the concluding Section 9.

7. BCI AS A RESEARCH TOOL IN COGNITIVE NEUROSCIENCE

Employing a BCI to obtain early predictions of motor intentions in a gaming scenario required participants to cancel self-initiated button presses upon seeing a stop signal. By virtue of this paradigm, conclusions about the deterministic coupling between preparatory brain signals and the corresponding motor actions could be drawn that have a number of important implications ranging from the debate over free will to ethical considerations about applications that potentially speed up human behavior.

7.1. Context: Preparatory Signals and Research Questions in Cognitive Neuroscience

The readiness potential (RP) is a slow, negative cortical potential that is observed over motor areas in the EEG and can start more than one second before voluntary, self-initiated movements (Kornhuber and Deecke, 1965). It gained particular fame in the work of Libet et al. (1983), who found that the conscious decision to move occurs several hundred milliseconds after the onset of the RP, thereby initiating a still-ongoing heated debate about free will (Libet, 1985). One particular question that has remained unanswered is whether a person can still exert a veto by inhibiting a voluntary movement after onset of the RP (Haynes, 2011). One possibility is that once that RP begins to build up the planned movement must occur and cannot be canceled (De Jong et al., 1990). Another possibility is that people can still exert a veto by canceling or altering the movement after the onset of the RP. If the latter is the case, a follow-up question is whether there exists a point of no return along the time course of the RP, after which people cannot stop the planned movement. In order to test this, we devised an experiment that required subjects to cancel a self-paced movement once an RP had been detected by a BCI in real time.

7.2. Study on the Coupling of Preparatory Signals and Corresponding Actions

The experimental task was designed as a "duel" between the subject and the computer. Subjects ($N = 10$) were confronted with a floor-mounted button and a light presented on a computer screen. If the subject pressed the button while the light on the screen was green, they would win a point. If they pressed the button after the computer had turned the light red (stop signal), they would lose a point. The experiment had three consecutive stages. In stage I, stop signals were elicited at random onset times. The EEG data from stage I were then used to train a classifier to predict upcoming movements. In stages II and III, movement predictions were made in real time by the BCI with the aim of turning on the stop signal in time to interrupt the subject's movement. EEG signals were continuously classified by the Berlin Brain-Computer Interface toolbox (https://github.com/bbci/bbci_public) in order to control the stop signal. Additionally, EMG was recorded from the calf muscle of the moving foot in order to determine the time of movement onset. For details on experimental procedures, please refer to Schultze-Kraft et al. (2016a).

Each trial could end in one of four possible ways (**Figure 11A**): In "missed button press" trials subjects, won a point when they pressed the button while the light was green, whereas in "predicted button press" trials, they lost a point when they pressed the button after the stop signal had been turned on. Another possibility is that the BCI indicated an RP, elicited a stop signal, and the subject started to move (as indicated by EMG activity), but canceled the movement early enough ("aborted button press" trials). In the last case, the stop signal was elicited, but the participant showed no overt sign of movement. This trial type is ambiguous because it could either result from a prepared movement being terminated at an early stage ("early cancelation") or it could reflect false positive detections by the classifier ("false alarm").

We first of all examined the efficiency of the BCI predictor to detect RPs and elicit stop signals in real time. **Figure 11B** shows that while during stage I (random predictions), roughly 2 out of 3 trials were "missed button press" trials, during stages II and III only 1 out of 3 button presses were missed. Furthermore, predicted or aborted button press trials occurred very rarely during stage I, while during stages II and III they occurred in roughly 20 and 15% of trials, respectively. "Early cancelation/false alarm" trials occurred at comparable rates in all three stages.

Next, we assessed how the timing of stop signals was related to movement onsets (as assessed by EMG). The distribution of stop signals in "predicted button press" trials (**Figure 12A**, red, top panel) shows that the vast majority of stop signals occurred after EMG onset. Since the movement was completed by pressing the button, the stop signal presumably came too late for a veto. Stop signals in "aborted button press" trials (**Figure 12A**, green, middle panel) occurred earlier (starting around 200 ms before EMG). Thus, when stop signals were presented at late stages of movement, preparation subjects could not stop themselves from beginning to move, even though they could abort the movement, once started. There was a gradual transition between stop signal times in which movements could be aborted and those in which they could not be aborted (**Figure 12A**, bottom panel).

It is interesting that there were rarely any cases in which subjects moved despite seeing stop signals earlier than 200 ms before EMG, even though RP onset occurred more than 1000 ms before EMG onset. We therefore examined the timing of predictions in "silent trials," which occurred in 40% of trials during stages II and III. Here, when the BCI predicted a movement, the time was silently recorded, but the stop signal was not turned on and the trial continued until the button was pressed. As a detailed investigation of those silent trials shows (cf., Schultze-Kraft et al., 2016a), although a majority of predictions also in silent trials occurred around movement onset, many silent predictions occurred more than 200 ms before movement onset. The fact that these early predictions were absent for predicted button press trials or aborted button press trials suggests that the BCI was indeed able to predict movements at such early stages and that subjects were caught early enough to cancel their decision without any overt sign of movement.

In order to further investigate this assumption and assert whether predictions in the ambiguous trial type were early cancelations or false alarms, we looked for the occurrence of event-related desynchronization (ERD) in these ambiguous trials at the time of prediction. ERD occurs before and during movements in particular frequency bands in the EEG and has been shown to have a different generator in the brain than the

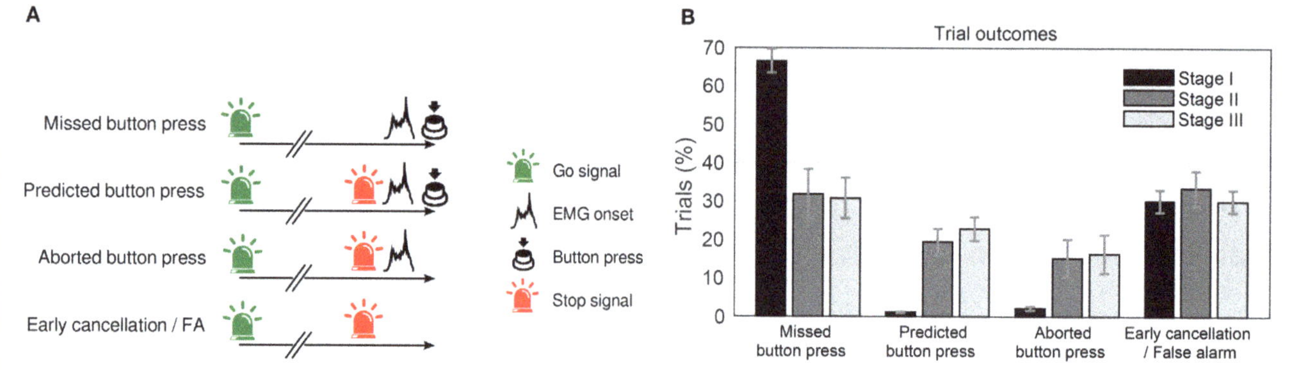

FIGURE 11 | (A) Possible trial outcomes during the experiment. See text for details. **(B)** Percentage of trial outcomes across stages for the four trial categories (as in panel **(A)**). All trial categories in one stage (bars of same color) add up to 100%. Shown is the average across subjects (error bars = SEM). Figure taken from Schultze-Kraft et al. (2016a) with permission.

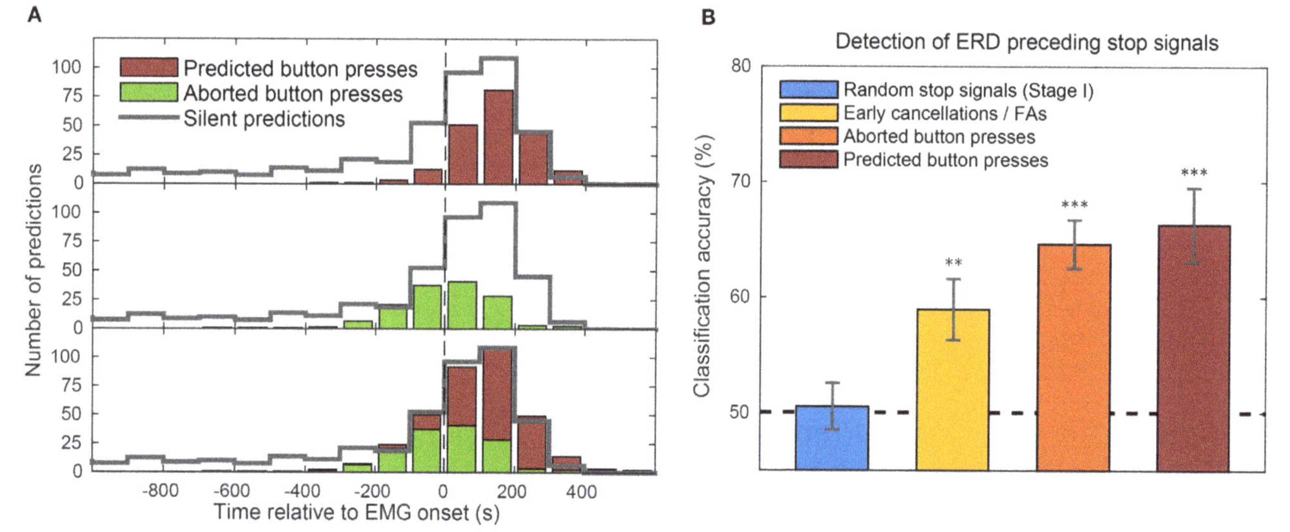

FIGURE 12 | (A) Distribution of BCI predictions time-locked to EMG onset (vertical line). The three panels show the distribution of stop signal timings in predicted button press trials (top, red) and in aborted button press trials (middle, green). The bottom panel (red and green) shows their joint distribution. The gray distribution superimposed as outline in all three panels shows the stop signal distribution in silent trials, adjusted to account for the imbalanced probability of a trial being silent (40%) or not (60%). All bins comprised intervals of 100 ms and counts were pooled across stages II and III of all subjects. **(B)** Accuracies of a classifier trained to detect an impending movement based on event-related desynchronization (ERD) occurring before stop signals. Bars show the mean accuracies of subjects (error bars = SEM) for four different trial types. Figure taken from Schultze-Kraft et al. (2016a) with permission. Significance above chance level is indicated by $^{**}p < 0.01$ and $^{***}p < 0.0001$.

RP, therefore making ERD an index for motor preparation that is independent of the RP (Pfurtscheller and Aranibar, 1979; Bai et al., 2006). The analyses revealed that ERD was detected in ambiguous trials, but not in the random stop signal trials from stage I (**Figure 12B**). Thus, at least a subset of ambiguous trials had likely already reached movement preparation and were not false alarms, but rather early cancelations.

7.3. Conclusion

Our findings suggest that subjects were able to cancel self-initiated movements, even after onset of the readiness potential. If a stop signal is elicited before a *point of no return* around 200 ms before movement onset, subjects are able to veto the prepared movement, while subjects cannot avoid moving when a stop signal occurs after that time point. Note, however, that the point of no return can be expected to vary from trial to trial, and that it might be impossible to determine when the point of no return has passed in single trials. This has the important implication that no critical actions should be triggered in this way, because the speed-up comes at the price of losing the opportunity to reevaluate the situation and possibly veto the action.

BCI technology offers the unique possibility of intervening in an experimental paradigm based on the momentary mental state (including intention and decision processes) of the test subject. This intriguing opportunity opens the potential for employing real-time BCIs as a research tool. While this perspective was mentioned already in the BNCI Roadmap (BNCI Horizon 2020, 2015), the presented study (Schultze-Kraft et al., 2016a) is, to the best of our knowledge, its first realization. The key point in our study is the capability of allowing for instantaneous feedback of motor intentions to subjects in real time (Blankertz et al., 2006; Salvaris and Haggard, 2014), thereby extending the important line of experimental work on the nature of predictive brain activity preceding self-initiated movements (Haggard and Eimer, 1999). This novel approach allowed us to elucidate a fundamental question in cognitive neuroscience, thereby demonstrating the potential of a Brain-Computer Interface as a powerful research tool.

8. ANALYZING NATURAL MUSIC LISTENING

In this section, we show how BCI technology can be applied to the study of the processing of music. In particular, we propose a regression-based method that enables the extraction of cortical responses to note onsets in music from the continuous EEG. The extracted continuous brain responses are used to assess the brain-stimulus synchronization with a measure called Cortico-Acoustic Correlation (CACor). Several examples show the application of CACor in a range of analysis scenarios related to music perception.

8.1. Context: Neural Processes in Real World Experiences

Brain states during real-word experiences have attracted growing research interest in the past decade (Hasson, 2004; Hasson et al., 2010; Dmochowski et al., 2012; Hasson and Honey, 2012; Gaebler et al., 2014); Listening to music is one example of an ongoing real world experience that relies on structured auditory input that can be subject to many forms of audio signal analysis. At the same time, listening to music is one of the richest human experiences (Altenmüller and Schlaug, 2013) encompassing sensory, sensorimotor, cognitive, affective, and memory-related processes. Studying how brain dynamics underlying perceptual and cognitive processes unfold along the structure of a naturalistic music stimulus has therefore been recognized as a fruitful approach for deepening the understanding of the transformation of sensory input into human experience (Alluri et al., 2012, 2013; Sturm et al., 2014; Jäncke et al., 2015).

In the music domain, linear classification methods have, beyond measures of discriminability, provided knowledge about the neural representations of complex musical sounds (Schaefer et al., 2011; Treder et al., 2014). Unsupervised ICA-based approaches identified common features in the EEG of music listeners (Cong et al., 2012, 2013; Thompson, 2013). The results support the idea that the waveform envelope (which contains information about the timing of note onsets) is reflected in EEG and therefore provides a good starting point for linking music signals and brain signals. Likewise, in the domain of speech processing, cortical onset responses that reflect changes in the waveform envelope (termed Envelope Following Responses or EFRs), have been a target of interest for a long time (Purcell et al., 2004; Aiken and Picton, 2006, 2008).

8.2. Two Studies Investigating Continuous Listening Experience

Here, we review a novel approach that utilizes the relationship of the EEG signal to the audio waveform envelope in an analysis framework that is applicable in any experimental setting in which EEG recordings and stimulus waveforms are available. As shown schematically in **Figure 13** Linear Ridge Regression with the audio power slope as a target function is used to extract continuous cortical onset responses from the EEG signal of the music listener. Note that regression with the audio power *slope* capitalizes on the brain's sensitivity to change and represents a further refinement of previous EFR-related methods. Two examples of EEG projections and the respective power slope are given in **Figure 14**. Based on the extracted EEG projections, a measure of brain-stimulus synchronization called Cortico-Acoustic correlation (CACor) is developed (for details of the method see Sturm et al., 2015a; Sturm, 2016). We demonstrate

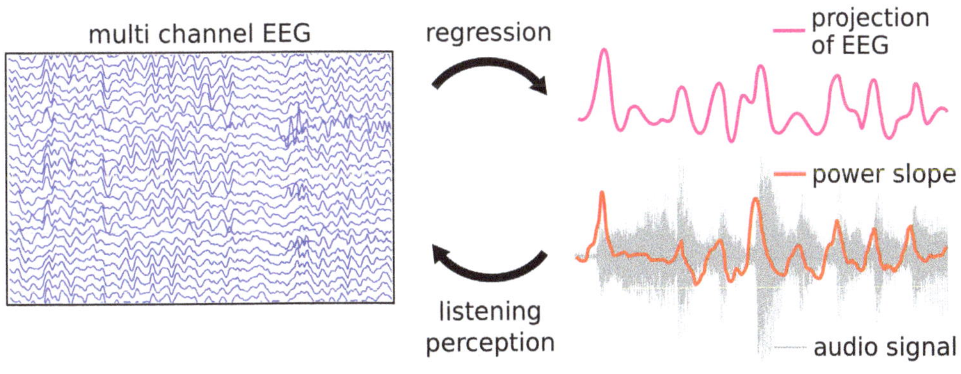

FIGURE 13 | Regression approach for extracting neural correlates of music perception. The perception of sound is reflected in the brain signals, the power slope of the sound waves being a crucial factor. Linear Ridge Regression is applied to the temporally embedded multichannel EEG signal using the audio power slope as a target function. This results in a spatio-temporal filter (regression weight matrix) that can be applied to new data. It reduces the multichannel EEG to a one-dimensional projection that can subsequently be examined with respect to Cortico-Acoustic correlation (CACor).

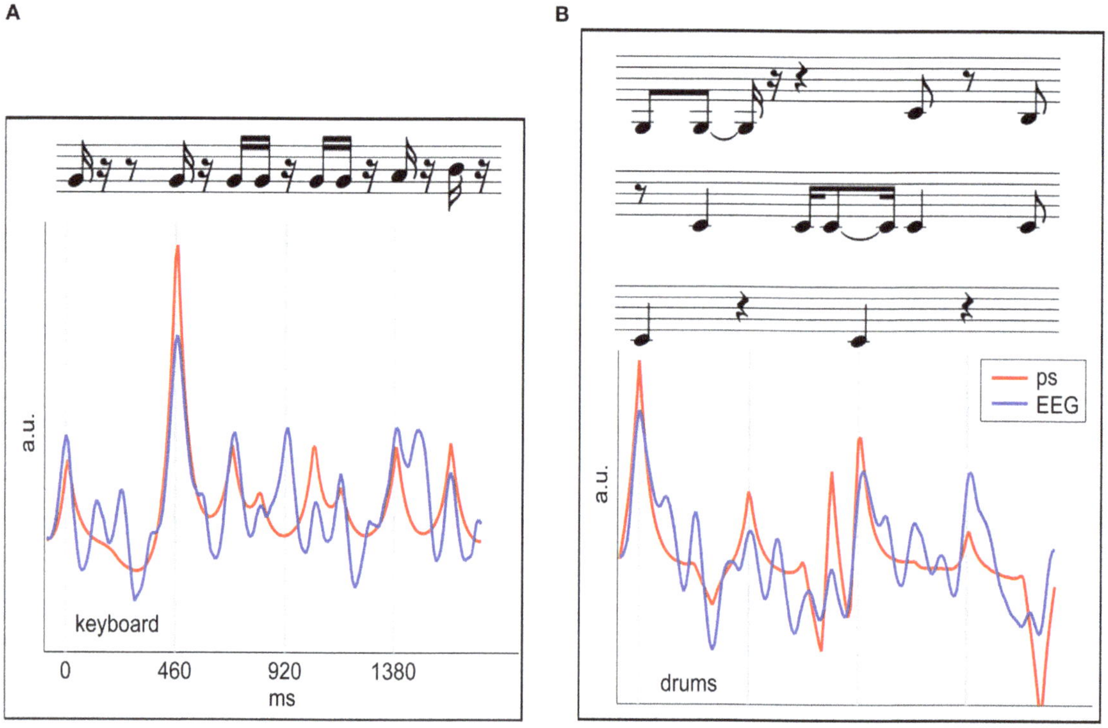

FIGURE 14 | EEG projections reflecting cortical responses to note onsets. The two examples of keyboard **(A)** and bass **(B)** show segments of an extracted EEG projection (blue) for a single stimulus presentation and a single subject and the respective audio power slope (red). Note that in the optimization procedure a time lag between stimulus and brain response is integrated in the spatio-temporal filter, and that, consequently, the EEG projections shown here are not delayed with respect to the audio power slope. Figure adapted from Sturm et al. (2015b).

that CACor can be applied for investigating brain-stimulus synchronization in experimental settings related to different aspects of music perception (Sturm et al., 2015b). We also provide examples of how CACor can be employed in the complementary analysis of EEG signals, behavioral measures, and audio signal analysis (Sturm et al., 2015a).

In a first study that explored the perception of naturalistic music, nine subjects passively listened to auditory stimuli from various sound categories, including full-length romantic piano pieces as well as simple tone sequences and natural (non-music) soundscapes (Sturm et al., 2015a). In a separate behavioral experiment, continuous ratings of the perceived tension in the same stimuli were obtained from an independent listener group. The regression approach (**Figure 13**) reduced the 61-channel EEG to one-time course optimally reflecting note onsets. The EEG projection was utilized to determine the Cortico-Acoustic Correlation (CACor). Significant CACor was detected in the individual listener's EEG signals of single presentations of full-length complex naturalistic music stimuli. The reliability of the occurrence of significant CACor in the group of participants differed among stimuli. It co-varied with the stimuli's average magnitudes of sharpness, spectral centroid, and rhythmic complexity. In particular, the subset of stimuli effecting a consistently strong CACor in the EEG participants (indicated by a high CACor score in **Figure 15**) also produced strongly coordinated tension ratings in the (independent) group of participants of the behavioral experiment. This relation between CACor and behavioral measures provides a first tentative link between neurophysiological responses to low-level acoustic events and the more cognitive-affective experience of tension in music. It is a first step toward bridging the gap between behavioral studies related to the perception of complex music and electrophysiological studies that use simplified musical stimulus material. If CACor scores are viewed as a measure of neural reliability, our findings add an interesting novel aspect to previous findings in which between-subject reliability of neural processing of naturalistic audiovisual stimuli indicates arousing and threatening passages (Dmochowski et al., 2012) and predicts the behavioral responses of large audiences (Dmochowski et al., 2014). Within this scope, our results indicate a more global, but very specific link between neural reliability and music stimulus features that might be useful for predicting listener behavior in the future.

In a second EEG study, music clips representing "rudimentary music" were presented to 11 subjects (Sturm et al., 2015b). These clips featured three instruments (keyboard, drums, and bass) playing repetitive music sound patterns, either in an ensemble version (resembling minimalistic electro-pop) or in the corresponding three solo versions (for details on stimuli and paradigm see also Treder et al., 2014). In the ensemble presentations, subjects were instructed to focus on just one of the instruments during each clip. For each instrument, a Linear

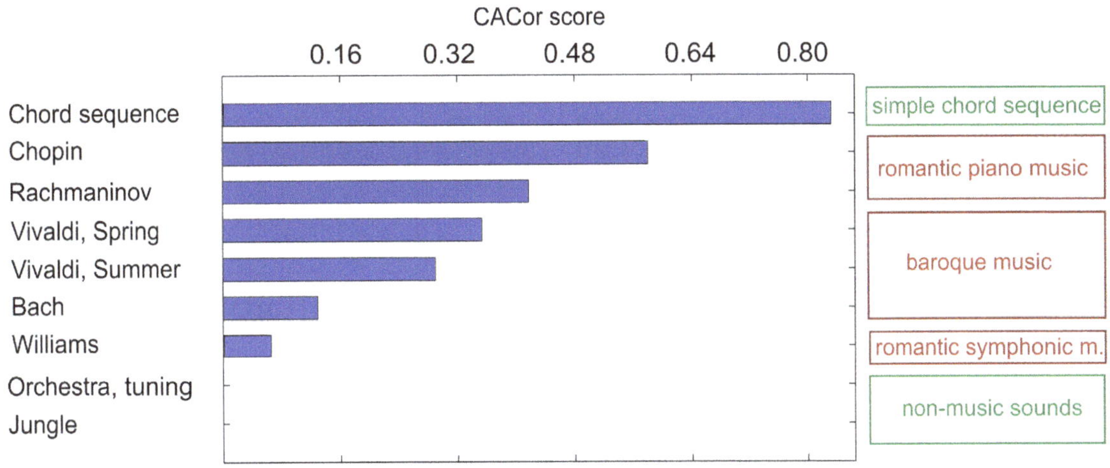

FIGURE 15 | The CACor score profile for the set of nine stimuli can be interpreted as a measure of reliability of the occurrence of significant CACor that can be compared across stimuli. The distribution of CACor scores for the set of nine stimuli is significantly correlated ($r = 0.9, p = 0.005$) with the distribution of coordination scores (not shown here) that quantify how strongly coordinated behavioral responses a stimulus produces (for details on the calculation of CACor and coordination scores see Sturm et al. (2015a)). The description on the right suggests that stimuli from the same category have similar CACor measures. Figure adapted from Sturm et al. (2015a) with permission.

Ridge Regression model was trained that extracted the EEG projection that represented the sequence of note onsets in the audio signal of the respective solo voice in an optimal way. In a second step, these instrument-specific filters were applied to EEG recorded during the ensemble presentations. CACor of the extracted EEG projections and the solo version of the music clip were assessed in order to probe whether a neural representation of the solo parts is present that is congruent to the natural ability of the subjects to perceive the single instrument's "voices" within the ensemble. Our results showed that the reflection of the melody instrument keyboard in the EEG exceeds that of the other instruments by far, suggesting a high-voice superiority effect in the neural representation of note onsets. The results further indicate that focusing attention on a particular instrument can enhance this reflection. We conclude that, in principle, the neural representation of tone onsets at the level of early auditory ERPs can parallel the perceptual segregation of ensemble music.

8.3. Conclusion and Outlook

In summary, the machine learning based multivariate methods for EEG analysis obviates the need to present a high number of stimulus repetitions, thereby paving the avenue for studying the physiological effect of long, complex stimuli, such as full-length pieces of natural music. The approach can provide a neural representation that parallels the separate streams a listener perceives in multi-voiced music. The proposed method therefore represents a promising tool for investigating auditory stream segregation in naturalistic listening scenarios. While the investigations discussed in this section do not require the real-time capability of BCI technology, closely related research may profit from the techniques presented here. EEG-enhanced assistive listening technology aims at recognizing cortical responses to the sound envelope as a promising way to determine the attended speech stream in complex listening situations (Ding and Simon, 2012; O'Sullivan et al., 2015; Akram et al., 2016). Through this, the function of hearing aids/auditory prostheses may be adapted in a situation-dependent manner (Mirkovic et al., 2015; O'Sullivan et al., 2015).

9. DISCUSSION

Most of the work on applications of BCI technology beyond communication and control is based on fundamental studies in cognitive science, psychophysics, and neuroscience. The results have been achieved in experimental studies that were confined to carefully controlled situations that limit fluctuating factors of natural tasks and behavior in order to exclude confounding variables. This is a reasonable approach for a rigorous investigation of fundamental concepts. In order to pave the way for incorporating neurotechnology into real-life applications, however, there needs to be a paradigm shift toward allowing more complex scenarios in neurocognitive studies. In this respect, it is important to note that increased noise (e.g., movement artifacts) is just one of the problems being faced.

To illustrate a more severe kind of challenge, we take the example of monitoring cognitive workload. There is a wealth of literature on the fundamental aspects of this topic, and a reliable system for real-time estimation of the current level of the user's workload would have useful applications in many areas. Studies have shown that the power of parietal alpha activity is negatively correlated with cognitive workload in visual tasks (Gevins and Smith, 2003; Holm et al., 2009). But in a complex scenario with a continuously changing visual background (such as driving a car), the alpha rhythm might be completely blocked already, such that no further decrease due to additional workload can be detected (Kohlmorgen et al., 2007). Other studies have shown that the parietal alpha amplitude *increases* with workload in non-visual tasks (Legewie et al., 1969; Galin et al., 1978; Markand, 1990), presumably as a cause of inhibition in order to focus resources to the relevant neural processes (Klimesch et al., 1999). In a natural task of high workload, the demands can change between the modalities. There might be phases when retrieving experience from memory or motor programs is critical, while in other phases the focus is on the analysis of the visual scene. The expected effect on parietal alpha is then reversed, such that this feature might be difficult to exploit in a natural task context.

A related challenge in the transfer to more complex scenarios is the sensitivity vs. specificity trade-off. Fundamental studies with confined settings have repeatedly demonstrated the high sensitivity of EEG for retrieving certain aspects of perception or cognition. Potential applications of neurotechnology often refer to this fact, e.g., when promising higher precision compared to behavioral measures. The effects found in the EEG, however, are often not very specific; the interpretation of the effect is only valid under the highly constrained experimental setting. In situations of more complex scenes or tasks there might be other factors, unrelated to the variable of interest, that can cause either the same or a reversed effect, potentially annihilating the usability of the EEG-based measure that was previously found viable in a laboratory setting.

This review excluded the aspect of a deployable setup for acquiring the brain signals. For some of the discussed applications the usual EEG hardware is appropriate (BCI as research tool, Section 7), for others a less intrusive setup is desirable (Neurousability, Section 4), while still others critically depend on the future availability of truly deployable devices (HCI applications, Section 6). Developments in this directions are the recently developed, invisible (Nikulin et al., 2010), and easy to set up, gel-free EEG electrodes (Zander et al., 2011; Guger et al., 2012; Mullen et al., 2015). Electrodes can also be placed so that they are barely visible in the ear (Looney et al., 2014; Goverdovsky et al., 2016), on the ear (Norton et al., 2015), or, as printed electrode arrays, around the ears (Debener et al., 2015). In addition, miniaturized mobile EEG systems (De Vos et al., 2014; Stopczynski et al., 2014) and NIRS systems are presently being developed (Piper et al., 2014; Von Lühmann et al., 2015). New affordable eye trackers (Dalmaijer, 2014) and the increasing commercial interest in wearable physiological sensors, such as heart-rate sensors in smart watches or a glucose sensor in a contact lens ("Google Contact Lens"), likewise promise to be beneficial for further development.

The (potential) applications of BCI technology beyond communication and control presented here have different levels of maturity. BCIs are ready for use as research tools (Sections 7 and 8). Using BCI technology to access certain user variables based on neural signals within a development cycle in order to optimize devices and interfaces is within reach for some application areas (Section 4). For other fields of applications (Sections 5 and 6), we expect that intense and challenging research is still necessary to pave the way to actual applications. The studies reviewed in this article are just the beginning (resp. already the second step) in this enterprise, which will hopefully be interesting and attractive to many researchers.

AUTHOR CONTRIBUTIONS

BB made the concept of the review, wrote Abstract, Introduction, Overview, and Conclusion, and revised all sections. SH wrote Section 3, LA Section 4, SD Section 5, MU, MW, and BB Section 6, MS Section 7, and IS Section 8. GC contributed to the research reviewed in Sections 3–5 and 8. KM contributed to the research reviewed in Section 4. All authors read, revised, and approved the manuscript.

FUNDING

This work was supported by a grant from the German Federal Ministry of Education and Research (BMBF) under contract No. 01GQ0850. Furthermore, some of the reviewed research has received funding from the European Union Seventh Framework Programme (FP7/2007-2013) under grant agreement No. 611570. SH was supported by a Marie Curie International Outgoing Fellowship (grant No. 625991) within the 7th European Community Framework Program. IS's work was supported by the Berlin School of Mind and Brain and by the Christiane-Nüsslein-Volhard Foundation. KM gratefully acknowledges funding by the Federal Ministry of Education and Research (BMBF) under the projects Adaptive BCI (FKZ 01GQ1115) and Berlin Big Data Center BBDC (01IS14013A), in part by the German Research Foundation (GRK 1589/1), and by the Brain Korea 21 Plus Program through the National Research Foundation of Korea funded by the Ministry of Education.

ACKNOWLEDGMENTS

We acknowledge inspiring and fruitful discussions with many researchers, with whom we discussed novel applications of BCI technology and advanced data analysis methods. Moreover, we would like to thank our coauthors for allowing us to use materials from former joint publications.

REFERENCES

Acqualagna, L., and Blankertz, B. (2015). "Neural correlates of relevant stimuli processing for brain computer interfaces," in *Engineering in Medicine and Biology Society (EMBC), 2015 37th Annual International Conference of the IEEE* (Milano: IEEE).

Acqualagna, L., Bosse, S., Porbadnigk, A. K., Curio, G., Müller, K.-R., Wiegand, T., et al. (2015). EEG-based classification of video quality perception using steady state visual evoked potentials (SSVEPs). *J. Neural Eng.* 12:026012. doi: 10.1088/1741-2560/12/2/026012

Aiken, S. J., and Picton, T. W. (2006). Envelope following responses to natural vowels. *Audiol. Neurotol.* 11, 213–232. doi: 10.1159/000092589

Aiken, S. J., and Picton, T. W. (2008). Human cortical responses to the speech envelope. *Ear Hear.* 29, 139–157. doi: 10.1097/AUD.0b013e31816453dc

Akram, S., Presacco, A., Simon, J. Z., Shamma, S. A., and Babadi, B. (2016). Robust decoding of selective auditory attention from MEG in a competing-speaker environment via state-space modeling. *Neuroimage* 124, 906–917. doi: 10.1016/j.neuroimage.2015.09.048

Alluri, V., Toiviainen, P., Jääskeläinen, I. P., Glerean, E., Sams, M., and Brattico, E. (2012). Large-scale brain networks emerge from dynamic processing of musical timbre, key and rhythm. *Neuroimage* 59, 3677–3689. doi: 10.1016/j.neuroimage.2011.11.019

Alluri, V., Toiviainen, P., Lund, T. E., Wallentin, M., Vuust, P., Nandi, A. K., et al. (2013). From Vivaldi to Beatles and back: predicting lateralized brain responses to music. *Neuroimage* 83, 627–636. doi: 10.1016/j.neuroimage.2013.06.064

Altenmüller, E., and Schlaug, G. (2013). Neurologic music therapy: the beneficial effects of music making on neurorehabilitation. *Acoust. Sci. Technol.* 34, 5–12. doi: 10.1250/ast.34.5

Antons, J.-N., Arndt, S., Schleicher, R., and Möller, S. (2014). "Brain activity correlates of quality of experience," in *Quality of Experience*, eds S. Möller and A. Raake (Berlin: Springer), 109–119.

Antons, J.-N., Schleicher, R., Arndt, S., Möller, S., Porbadnigk, A. K., and Curio, G. (2012). Analyzing speech quality perception using electroencephalography. *IEEE J. Sel. Top. Signal Process.* 6, 721–731. doi: 10.1109/JSTSP.2012.2191936

Arndt, S., Antons, J.-N., Schleicher, R., Moller, S., and Curio, G. (2014). Using electroencephalography to measure perceived video quality. *IEEE J. Sel. Top. Signal Process.* 8, 366–376. doi: 10.1109/JSTSP.2014.2313026

Arndt, S., Antons, J.-N., Schleicher, R., Möller, S., Scholler, S., and Curio, G. (2011). "A physiological approach to determine video quality," in *2011 IEEE International Symposium on Multimedia (ISM)* (IEEE), 518–523.

Babiloni, C., Vecchio, F., Bultrini, A., Romani, G. L., and Rossini, P. M. (2006). Pre-and poststimulus alpha rhythms are related to conscious visual perception: a high-resolution EEG study. *Cereb. Cortex* 16, 1690–1700. doi: 10.1093/cercor/bhj104

Bai, O., Vorbach, S., Hallett, M., and Floeter, M. K. (2006). Movement-related cortical potentials in primary lateral sclerosis. *Ann. Neurol.* 59, 682–690. doi: 10.1002/ana.20803

Barral, O., Eugster, M. J., Ruotsalo, T., Spapé, M. M., Kosunen, I., Ravaja, N., et al. (2015). "Exploring peripheral physiology as a predictor of perceived relevance in information retrieval," in *Proceedings of the 20th International Conference on Intelligent User Interfaces, IUI '15* (New York, NY: ACM), 389–399. doi: 10.1145/2678025.2701389

Berger, H. (1929). Über das elektroenkephalogramm des menschen. *Arch. Psychiatr. Nervenkr.* 87, 527–570. doi: 10.1007/BF01797193

Bladin, P. F. (2006). W. Grey Walter, pioneer in the electroencephalogram, robotics, cybernetics, artificial intelligence. *J. Clin. Neurosci.* 13, 170–177. doi: 10.1016/j.jocn.2005.04.010

Blankertz, B., Dornhege, G., Lemm, S., Krauledat, M., Curio, G., and Müller, K.-R. (2006). The Berlin Brain-Computer Interface: machine learning based detection of user specific brain states. *J. Univ. Comput. Sci.* 12, 581–607. doi: 10.3217/jucs-012-06-0581

Blankertz, B., Lemm, S., Treder, M. S., Haufe, S., and Müller, K.-R. (2011). Single-trial analysis and classification of ERP components - a tutorial. *Neuroimage* 56, 814–825. doi: 10.1016/j.neuroimage.2010.06.048

Blankertz, B., Tangermann, M., Vidaurre, C., Fazli, S., Sannelli, C., Haufe, S., et al. (2010). The Berlin Brain-Computer Interface: non-medical uses of BCI technology. *Front. Neurosci.* 4:198. doi: 10.3389/fnins.2010.00198

Blankertz, B., Tomioka, R., Lemm, S., Kawanabe, M., and Müller, K.-R. (2008). Optimizing spatial filters for robust EEG single-trial analysis. *IEEE Signal Process. Mag.* 25, 41–56. doi: 10.1109/MSP.2008.4408441

BNCI Horizon 2020 (2015). *Roadmap - The Future in Brain/Neural-Computer Interaction: Horizon 2020.* BNCI Horizon 2020.

Borghini, G., Arico, P., Astolfi, L., Toppi, J., Cincotti, F., Mattia, D., et al. (2013). "Frontal EEG theta changes assess the training improvements of novices in flight simulation tasks," in *Engineering in Medicine and Biology Society (EMBC), 2013 35th Annual International Conference of the IEEE* (Osaka: IEEE), 6619–6622.

Borghini, G., Aricò, P., Graziani, I., Salinari, S., Sun, Y., Taya, F., et al. (2016). Quantitative assessment of the training improvement in a motor-cognitive task by using EEG, ECG and EOG signals. *Brain Topogr.* 29, 149–161. doi: 10.1007/s10548-015-0425-7

Bosse, S., Acqualagna, L., Porbadnigk, A. K., Blankertz, B., Curio, G., Muller, K.-R., et al. (2014). "Neurally informed assessment of perceived natural texture image quality," in *2014 IEEE International Conference on Image Processing (ICIP)* (IEEE), 1987–1991.

Bosse, S., Acqualagna, L., Porbadnigk, A. K., Curio, G., Müller, K.-R., Blankertz, B., et al. (2015). "Neurophysiological assessment of perceived image quality using steady-state visual evoked potentials," in *SPIE Optical Engineering+ Applications*, ed A. G. Tescher (International Society for Optics and Photonics), 959914–959914.

Brouwer, A., Reuderink, B., Vincent, J., van Gerven, M., and van Erp, J. (2013). Distinguishing between target and nontarget fixations in a visual search task using fixation-related potentials. *J. Vis.* 13:17. doi: 10.1167/13.3.17

Brunner, C., Birbaumer, N., Blankertz, B., Guger, C., Kübler, A., Mattia, D., et al. (2015). BNCI Horizon 2020: towards a roadmap for the BCI community. *Brain Comput. Interf.* 2, 1–10. doi: 10.1080/2326263X.2015.1008956

Buzsáki, G., and Draguhn, A. (2004). Neuronal oscillations in cortical networks. *Science* 304, 1926–1929. doi: 10.1126/science.1099745

Cohen, N., Pell, L., Edelson, M. G., Ben-Yakov, A., Pine, A., and Dudai, Y. (2015). Peri-encoding predictors of memory encoding and consolidation. *Neurosci. Biobehav. Rev.* 50, 128–142. doi: 10.1016/j.neubiorev.2014.11.002

Cole, M. J., Gwizdka, J., and Belkin, N. J. (2011a). "Physiological data as metadata," in *SIGIR 2011 Workshop on Enriching Information Retrieval (ENIR 2011)* (Beijing).

Cole, M. J., Gwizdka, J., Liu, C., Bierig, R., Belkin, N. J., and Zhang, X. (2011b). Task and user effects on reading patterns in information search. *Interact. Comput.* 23, 346–362. doi: 10.1016/j.intcom.2011.04.007

Cong, F., Alluri, V., Nandi, A. K., Toiviainen, P., Fa, R., Abu-Jamous, B., et al. (2013). Linking brain responses to naturalistic music through analysis of ongoing EEG and stimulus features. *IEEE Trans. Multimedia* 15, 1060–1106. doi: 10.1109/TMM.2013.2253452

Cong, F., Phan, A. H., Zhao, Q., Nandi, A. K., Alluri, V., Toiviainen, P., et al. (2012). "Analysis of ongoing EEG elicited by natural music stimuli using nonnegative tensor factorization," in *Signal Processing Conference (EUSIPCO)*, 494–498.

Dähne, S., Bießman, F., Samek, W., Haufe, S., Goltz, D., Gundlach, C., et al. (2015). Multivariate machine learning methods for fusing functional multimodal neuroimaging data. *Proc. IEEE* 103, 1507–1530. doi: 10.1109/JPROC.2015.2425807

Dähne, S., Meinecke, F. C., Haufe, S., Höhne, J., Tangermann, M., Müller, K.-R., et al. (2014a). SPoC: a novel framework for relating the amplitude of neuronal oscillations to behaviorally relevant parameters. *Neuroimage* 86, 111–122. doi: 10.1016/j.neuroimage.2013.07.079

Dähne, S., Nikulin, V. V., Ramírez, D., Schreier, P. J., Müller, K.-R., and Haufe, S. (2014b). Finding brain oscillations with power dependencies in neuroimaging data. *Neuroimage* 96, 334–348. doi: 10.1016/j.neuroimage.2014.03.075

Dalmaijer, E. (2014). *Is the Low-cost Eyetribe Eye Tracker Any Good for Research?* Technical report, PeerJ PrePrints. Available online at: https://peerj.com/preprints/585/

De Jong, R., Coles, M. G., Logan, G. D., and Gratton, G. (1990). In search of the point of no return: the control of response processes. *J. Exp. Psychol. Hum. Percept. Perform.* 16, 164–182. doi: 10.1037/0096-1523.16.1.164

De Vos, M., Gandras, K., and Debener, S. (2014). Towards a truly mobile auditory brain–computer interface: exploring the P300 to take away. *Int. J. Psychophysiol.* 91, 46–53. doi: 10.1016/j.ijpsycho.2013.08.010

Debener, S., Emkes, R., De Vos, M., and Bleichner, M. (2015). Unobtrusive ambulatory EEG using a smartphone and flexible printed electrodes around the ear. *Sci. Rep.* 5:16743. doi: 10.1038/srep16743

Di Flumeri, G., Borghini, G., Aricò, P., Colosimo, A., Pozzi, S., Bonelli, S., et al. (2015). "On the use of cognitive neurometric indexes in aeronautic and air traffic management environments," in *Symbiotic Interaction, Vol. 9359, Lecture Notes in Computer Science*, eds B. Blankertz, G. Jacucci, L. Gamberini, A. Spagnolli, and J. Freeman (Berlin: Springer), 45–56. doi: 10.1007/978-3-319-24917-9_5

Dijksterhuis, C., de Waard, D., Brookhuis, K., Mulder, B., and de Jong, R. (2013). Classifying visuomotor workload in a driving simulator using subject specific spatial brain patterns. *Front. Neurosci.* 7:149. doi:10.3389/fnins.2013.00149

Ding, N., and Simon, J. Z. (2012). Emergence of neural encoding of auditory objects while listening to competing speakers. *Proc. Natl. Acad. Sci. U.S.A.* 109, 11854–11859. doi: 10.1073/pnas.1205381109

Dmochowski, J. P., Bezdek, M. A., Abelson, B. P., Johnson, J. S., Schumacher, E. H., and Parra, L. C. (2014). Audience preferences are predicted by temporal reliability of neural processing. *Nat. Commun.* 5:4567. doi: 10.1038/ncomms5567

Dmochowski, J. P., Sajda, P., Dias, J., and Parra, L. C. (2012). Correlated components of ongoing EEG point to emotionally laden attention–a possible marker of engagement? *Front. Hum. Neurosci.* 6:112. doi: 10.3389/fnhum.2012.00112

Dornhege, G., del R. Millán, J., Hinterberger, T., McFarland, D., and Müller, K.-R. (eds.) (2007). *Toward Brain-Computer Interfacing*. Cambridge, MA: MIT Press.

Elbert, T., Rockstroh, B., Lutzenberger, W., and Birbaumer, N. (1980). Biofeedback of slow cortical potentials. I. *Electroencephalogr. Clin. Neurophysiol.* 48, 293–301. doi: 10.1016/0013-4694(80)90265-5

Eugster, M. J., Ruotsalo, T., Spapé, M. M., Kosunen, I., Barral, O., Ravaja, N., et al. (2014). "Predicting term-relevance from brain signals," in *Proceedings of the 37th International ACM SIGIR Conference on Research & Development in Information Retrieval, SIGIR '14* (New York, NY: ACM), 425–434. doi: 10.1145/2600428.2609594

Faller, J., Scherer, R., Costa, U., Opisso, E., Medina, J., and Müller-Putz, G. R. (2014). A co-adaptive brain-computer interface for end users with severe motor impairment. *PLoS ONE* 9:e101168. doi: 10.1371/journal.pone.0101168

Fazli, S., Dähne, S., Samek, W., Bießmann, F., and Müller, K.-R. (2015). Learning from more than one data source: data fusion techniques for sensorimotor rhythm-based Brain-Computer Interfaces. *Proc. IEEE* 103, 891–906. doi: 10.1109/JPROC.2015.2413993

Fukunaga, K. (1990). *Introduction to Statistical Pattern Recognition, 2nd Edn.* Boston, MA: Academic Press.

Gaebler, M., Bießmann, F., Lamke, J. P., Müller, K. R., Walter, H., and Hetzer, S. (2014). Stereoscopic depth increases intersubject correlations of brain networks. *Neuroimage* 100, 427–434. doi: 10.1016/j.neuroimage.2014.06.008

Galin, D., Johnstone, J., and Herron, J. (1978). Effects of task difficulty on EEG measures of cerebral engagement. *Neuropsychologia* 16, 461–472. doi: 10.1016/0028-3932(78)90069-6

Gallegos-Ayala, G., Furdea, A., Takano, K., Ruf, C. A., Flor, H., and Birbaumer, N. (2014). Brain communication in a completely locked-in patient using bedside near-infrared spectroscopy. *Neurology* 82, 1930–1932. doi: 10.1212/WNL.0000000000000449

Gerson, A., Parra, L., and Sajda, P. (2006). Cortically-coupled computer vision for rapid image search. *IEEE Trans. Neural Syst. Rehabil. Eng.* 2, 174–179. doi: 10.1109/TNSRE.2006.875550

Gevins, A., Leong, H., Du, R., Smith, M. E., Le, J., DuRousseau, D., et al. (1995). Towards measurement of brain function in operational environments. *Biol. Psychol.* 40, 169–186. doi: 10.1016/0301-0511(95)05105-8

Gevins, A., and Smith, M. E. (2003). Neurophysiological measures of cognitive workload during human-computer interaction. *Theor. Issues Ergon. Sci.* 4, 113–131. doi: 10.1080/14639220210159717

Gevins, A., Smith, M. E., Leong, H., McEvoy, L., Whitfield, S., Du, R., et al. (1998). Monitoring working memory load during computer-based tasks with EEG pattern recognition methods. *Hum. Factors* 40, 79–91. doi: 10.1518/001872098779480578

Golenia, J.-E., Wenzel, M., and Blankertz, B. (2015). "Live demonstrator of EEG and eye-tracking input for disambiguation of image search results," in *Symbiotic Interaction, Vol. 9359, Lecture Notes in Computer Science*, eds B. Blankertz, G. Jacucci, L. Gamberini, A. Spagnolli, and J. Freeman (Berlin: Springer International Publishing), 81–86. doi: 10.1007/978-3-319-24917-9_8

Goverdovsky, V., Looney, D., Kidmose, P., and Mandic, D. P. (2016). In-ear EEG from viscoelastic generic earpieces: robust and unobtrusive 24/7 monitoring. *IEEE Sensors J.* 16, 271–277. doi: 10.1109/JSEN.2015.2471183

Graziano, M., Parra, L. C., and Sigman, M. (2015). Neural correlates of perceived confidence in a partial report paradigm. *J. Cogn. Neurosci.* 27, 1090–1103. doi: 10.1162/jocn_a_00759

Guger, C., Krausz, G., Allison, B. Z., and Edlinger, G. (2012). Comparison of dry and gel based electrodes for P300 brain-computer interfaces. *Front. Neurosci.* 6:60. doi: 10.3389/fnins.2012.00060

Gugler, M., Sannelli, C., Haufe, S., Schubert, R., Schrauf, M., Kincses, W. E., et al. (2010). "Intramodal attentional processing during a monotonous car driving simulation: an EEG study," in *Annual Meeting of the Cognitive Neuroscience Society* (Montreal, QC), 17:20.

Gwizdka, J., and Cole, M. J. (2011). "Inferring cognitive states from multimodal measures in information science," in *ICMI 2011 Workshop on Inferring Cognitive and Emotional States from Multimodal Measure* (Alicante), 1–4.

Haggard, P., and Eimer, M. (1999). On the relation between brain potentials and the awareness of voluntary movements. *Exp. Brain Res.* 126, 128–133. doi: 10.1007/s002210050722

Haji Mirza, S. N. H., Proulx, M., and Izquierdo, E. (2011). "Gaze movement inference for user adapted image annotation and retrieval," in *Proceedings of the 2011 ACM Workshop on Social and Behavioural Networked Media Access , SBNMA '11* (New York, NY: ACM), 27–32. doi: 10.1145/2072627.2072636

Hajimirza, S., Proulx, M., and Izquierdo, E. (2012). Reading users' minds from their eyes: a method for implicit image annotation. *IEEE Trans. Multimedia* 14, 805–815. doi: 10.1109/TMM.2012.2186792

Hardoon, D. R., and Pasupa, K. (2010). "Image ranking with implicit feedback from eye movements," in *Proceedings of the 2010 Symposium on Eye-Tracking Research & Applications , ETRA '10* (New York, NY: ACM), 291–298. doi: 10.1145/1743666.1743734

Hasson, U. (2004). Intersubject synchronization of cortical activity during natural vision. *Science* 303, 1634–1640. doi: 10.1126/science.1089506

Hasson, U., and Honey, C. J. (2012). Future trends in neuroimaging: neural processes as expressed within real-life contexts. *NeuroImage* 62, 1272–1278. doi: 10.1016/j.neuroimage.2012.02.004

Hasson, U., Malach, R., and Heeger, D. J. (2010). Reliability of cortical activity during natural stimulation. *Trends Cogn. Sci.* 14, 40–48. doi: 10.1016/j.tics.2009.10.011

Haufe, S., Kim, J.-W., Kim, I.-H., Sonnleitner, A., Schrauf, M., Curio, G., et al. (2014a). Electrophysiology-based detection of emergency braking intention in real-world driving. *J. Neural Eng.* 11:056011. doi: 10.1088/1741-2560/11/5/056011

Haufe, S., Meinecke, F., Görgen, K., Dähne, S., Haynes, J.-D., Blankertz, B., et al. (2014b). On the interpretation of weight vectors of linear models in multivariate neuroimaging. *NeuroImage* 87, 96–110. Neuroimage single best paper of 2014 Award. doi: 10.1016/j.neuroimage.2013.10.067

Haufe, S., Treder, M. S., Gugler, M. F., Sagebaum, M., Curio, G., and Blankertz, B. (2011). EEG potentials predict upcoming emergency brakings during simulated driving. *J. Neural Eng.* 8:056001. doi: 10.1088/1741-2560/8/5/056001

Hayashi, H., Shirai, H., Kameda, M., Kunifuji, S., and Miyahara, M. (2000). "Assessment of extra high quality images using both eeg and assessment words on high order sensations," in *2000 IEEE International Conference on Systems, Man, and Cybernetics*, Vol. 2 (Nashville, TN: IEEE), 1289–1294. doi: 10.1109/icsmc.2000.886031

Haynes, J. D. (2011). Decoding and predicting intentions. *Ann. N. Y. Acad. Sci.* 1224, 9–21. doi: 10.1111/j.1749-6632.2011.05994.x

Hill, N. J., Ricci, E., Haider, S., McCane, L. M., Heckman, S., Wolpaw, J. R., et al. (2014). A practical, intuitive brain–computer interface for communicating 'yes' or 'no' by listening. *J. Neural Eng.* 11:035003. doi: 10.1088/1741-2560/11/3/035003

Holm, A., Lukander, K., Korpela, J., Sallinen, M., and Muller, K. M. (2009). Estimating brain load from the EEG. *ScientificWorldJournal* 9, 639–651. doi: 10.1100/tsw.2009.83

ITU (2002). "Methodology for the subjective assessment of the quality of television pictures," in *Rec. ITU-R BT 500-11*. Available online at: https://www.itu.int/rec/R-REC-BT.500

ITU (2008). "Subjective video quality assessmentmethods formultimedia applications," in *Rec. ITU-T P.910*. Available online at: https://www.itu.int/rec/T-REC-P.910/en

Jäncke, L., Kühnis, J., Rogenmoser, L., and Elmer, S. (2015). Time course of EEG oscillations during repeated listening of a well-known aria. *Front. Hum. Neurosci.* 9:401. doi: 10.3389/fnhum.2015.00401

Jangraw, D. C., Wang, J., Lance, B. J., and Chang, S.-F. (2014). Neurally and ocularly informed graph-based models for searching 3d environments. *J. Neural Eng.* 11:046003. doi: 10.1088/1741-2560/11/4/046003

Kamienkowski, J. E., Ison, M. J., Quiroga, R. Q., and Sigman, M. (2012). Fixation-related potentials in visual search: a combined EEG and eye tracking study. *J. Vis.* 12:4. doi: 10.1167/12.7.4

Kamiya, J. (1969). "Operant control of the EEG alpha rhythm and some of its reported effects," in *Altered States of Consciousness: A Book of Readings*, ed C. Tart (New York, NY: Wiley), 489–501.

Kaunitz, L., Kamienkowski, J., Varatharajah, A., Sigman, M., Quiroga, R., and Ison, M. (2014). Looking for a face in the crowd: fixation-related potentials in an eye-movement visual search task. *Neuroimage* 89, 297–305. doi: 10.1016/j.neuroimage.2013.12.006

Kecklund, G., and Åkerstedt, T. (1993). Sleepiness in long distance truck driving: an ambulatory EEG study of night driving. *Ergonomics* 36, 1007–1017. doi: 10.1080/00140139308967973

Khaliliardali, Z., Chavarriaga, R., Gheorghe, L. A., and del R Millán, J. (2015). Action prediction based on anticipatory brain potentials during simulated driving. *J. Neural Eng.* 12:066006. doi: 10.1088/1741-2560/12/6/066006

Kim, I.-H., Kim, J.-W., Haufe, S., and Lee, S.-W. (2014). Detection of braking intention in diverse situations during simulated driving based on EEG feature combination. *J. Neural Eng.* 12:016001. doi. 10.1088/1741-2560/12/1/016001

Klimesch, W., Doppelmayr, M., Schwaiger, J., Auinger, P., and Winkler, T. (1999). Paradoxical'alpha synchronization in a memory task. *Cogn. Brain Res.* 7, 493–501. doi: 10.1016/S0926-6410(98)00056-1

Kohlmorgen, J., Dornhege, G., Braun, M., Blankertz, B., Müller, K.-R., Curio, G., et al. (2007). "Improving human performance in a real operating environment through real-time mental workload detection," in *Toward Brain-Computer Interfacing*, eds G. Dornhege, J. del R. Millán, T. Hinterberger, D. McFarland and K.-R. Müller (Cambridge, MA: MIT Press), 409–422.

Koles, Z. J. (1991). The quantitative extraction and topographic mapping of the abnormal components in the clinical EEG. *Electroencephalogr. Clin. Neurophysiol.* 79, 440–447. doi: 10.1016/0013-4694(91)90163-X

Kornhuber, H. H., and Deecke, L. (1965). Hirnpotentialänderungen bei willkürbewegungen und passiven bewegungen des menschen: bereitschaftspotential und reafferente potentiale. *Pflugers Arch.* 284, 1–17. doi: 10.1007/BF00412364

Kovacevic, N., Ritter, P., Tays, W., Moreno, S., and McIntosh, A. R. (2015). 'virtual dream': collective neurofeedback in an immersive art environment. *PLoS ONE* 10:e0130129. doi: 10.1371/journal.pone.0130129

Kroupi, E., Hanhart, P., Lee, J.-S., Rerabek, M., and Ebrahimi, T. (2014). "EEG correlates during video quality perception," in *European Sign Process Conference* (Lisbon).

Kübler, A., Nijboer, F., Mellinger, J., Vaughan, T. M., Pawelzik, H., Schalk, G., et al. (2005). Patients with ALS can use sensorimotor rhythms to operate a brain-computer interface. *Neurology* 64, 1775–1777. doi: 10.1212/01.WNL.0000158616.43002.6D

Legewie, H., Simonova, O., and Creutzfeldt, O. (1969). EEG changes during performance of various tasks under open-and closed-eyed conditions. *Electroencephalogr. Clin. Neurophysiol.* 27, 470–479. doi: 10.1016/0013-4694(69)90187-4

Libet, B. (1985). Unconscious cerebral initiative and the role of conscious will in voluntary action. *Behav. Brain Sci.* 8, 529–539. doi: 10.1017/S0140525X00044903

Libet, B., Gleason, C. A., Wright, E. W., and Pearl, D. K. (1983). Time of conscious intention to act in relation to onset of cerebral activity (readiness-potential). *Brain* 106, 623–642. doi: 10.1093/brain/106.3.623

Lindemann, L., Wenger, S., and Magnor, M. (2011). "Evaluation of video artifact perception using event-related potentials," in *Proc ACM SIGGRAPH Symp Appl Percept in Graph and Visualiz* (Toulouse), 53–58.

Looney, D., Kidmose, P., and Mandic, D. P. (2014). "Ear-EEG: user-centered and wearable BCI," in *Brain-Computer Interface Research*, eds C. Guger, B. Allison, and E. C. Leuthardt (Berlin: Springer), 41–50.

Lucier, A. (1965). *Music for Solo Performer for Enormously Amplified Brain Waves and Percussion, Score.* in *Chambers: Scores by Alvin Lucier. Interviews with the composer by Douglas Simon* (Middletown, CT: Wesleyan University Press), 67. The piece was premiered on 5 May 1965 at the Rose Art Museum of Brandeis University in Waltham, MA.

Markand, O. N. (1990). Alpha rhythms. *J. Clin. Neurophysiol.* 7, 163–190. doi: 10.1097/00004691-199004000-00003

McCall, J., and Trivedi, M. (2007). Driver behavior and situation aware brake assistance for intelligent vehicles. *Proc. IEEE* 95, 374–387. doi: 10.1109/JPROC.2006.888388

Mehta, R. K., and Parasuraman, R. (2013). Neuroergonomics: a review of applications to physical and cognitive work. *Front. Hum. Neurosci.* 7:889. doi: 10.3389/fnhum.2013.00889

Miklody, D., Uitterhoeve, W., v. Heel, D., Klinkenberg, K., and Blankertz, B. (2016). "Maritime cognitive workload assessment," in *Symbiotic Interaction, Vol. 9961, Lecture Notes in Computer Science*, eds L. Gamberini, A. Spagnolli, G. Jacucci, B. Blankertz, and J. Freeman (Springer International Publishing).

Mirkovic, B., Debener, S., Jaeger, M., and De Vos, M. (2015). Decoding the attended speech stream with multi-channel EEG: implications for online, daily-life applications. *J. Neural Eng.* 12:046007. doi: 10.1088/1741-2560/12/4/046007

Moldovan, A.-N., Ghergulescu, I., Weibelzahl, S., and Muntean, C. (2013). "User-centered eeg-based multimedia quality assessment," in *2013 IEEE International Symposium on Broadband Multimedia System and Broadcasting (BMSB)*, 1–8. doi: 10.1109/BMSB.2013.6621743

Morone, G., Pisotta, I., Pichiorri, F., Kleih, S., Paolucci, S., Molinari, M., et al. (2015). Proof of principle of a brain-computer interface approach to support poststroke arm rehabilitation in hospitalized patients: design, acceptability, and usability. *Arch. Phys. Med. Rehabil.* 96, S71–S78. doi: 10.1016/j.apmr.2014.05.026

Mullen, T. R., Kothe, C. A., Chi, Y. M., Ojeda, A., Kerth, T., Makeig, S., et al. (2015). Real-time neuroimaging and cognitive monitoring using wearable dry EEG. *IEEE Trans. Biomed. Eng.* 62, 2553–2567. doi: 10.1109/TBME.2015.2481482

Müller, K.-R., Tangermann, M., Dornhege, G., Krauledat, M., Curio, G., and Blankertz, B. (2008). Machine learning for real-time single-trial EEG-analysis: from brain-computer interfacing to mental state monitoring. *J. Neurosci. Methods* 167, 82–90. doi: 10.1016/j.jneumeth.2007.09.022

Mustafa, M., Guthe, S., and Magnor, M. (2012). Single-trial EEG classification of artifacts in videos. *ACM Trans. Appl. Percept.* 9:12. doi: 10.1145/2325722.2325725

Naumann, L., Schultze-Kraft, M., Dähne, S., and Blankertz, B. (2016). "Prediction of difficulty levels in video games from ongoing EEG," in *Symbiotic Interaction, Vol. 9961, Lecture Notes in Computer Science*, eds L. Gamberini, A. Spagnolli, G. Jacucci, B. Blankertz, and J. Freeman (Springer International Publishing).

Nicolae, I., Acqualagna, L., and Blankertz, B. (2015a). "Neural indicators of the depth of cognitive processing for user-adaptive neurotechnological applications," in *Engineering in Medicine and Biology Society (EMBC), 2015 37th Annual International Conference of the IEEE* (Milano: IEEE), 1484–1487.

Nicolae, I.-E., Acqualagna, L., and Blankertz, B. (2015b). "Tapping neural correlates of the depth of cognitive processing for improving human computer interaction," in *Symbiotic Interaction, Vol. 9359, Lecture Notes in Computer Science*, eds B. Blankertz, G. Jacucci, L. Gamberini, A. Spagnolli, and J. Freeman (Springer International Publishing), 126–131. doi: 10.1007/978-3-319-24917-9_13

Nikulin, V. V., Kegeles, J., and Curio, G. (2010). Miniaturized electroencephalographic scalp electrode for optimal wearing comfort. *Clin. Neurophysiol.* 121, 1007–1014. doi: 10.1016/j.clinph.2010.02.008

Noh, E., Herzmann, G., Curran, T., and de Sa, V. R. (2014). Using single-trial EEG to predict and analyze subsequent memory. *Neuroimage* 84, 712–723. doi: 10.1016/j.neuroimage.2013.09.028

Norcia, A., Ales, J., Cooper, E., and Wiegand, T. (2014). Measuring perceptual differences between compressed and uncompressed video sequences using the swept-parameter visual evoked potential. *J. Vis.* 14, 649–649. doi: 10.1167/14.10.649

Norton, J. J., Lee, D. S., Lee, J. W., Lee, W., Kwon, O., Won, P., et al. (2015). Soft, curved electrode systems capable of integration on the auricle as a persistent brain–computer interface. *Proc. Natl. Acad. Sci. U.S.A.* 112, 3920–3925. doi: 10.1073/pnas.1424875112

Oliveira, F. T., Aula, A., and Russell, D. M. (2009). "Discriminating the relevance of web search results with measures of pupil size," in *Proceedings of the SIGCHI Conference on Human Factors in Computing Systems, CHI '09* (New York, NY: ACM), 2209–2212. doi: 10.1145/1518701.1519038

O'Sullivan, J. A., Power, A. J., Mesgarani, N., Rajaram, S., Foxe, J. J., Shinn-Cunningham, B. G., et al. (2015). Attentional selection in a cocktail party environment can be decoded from single-trial EEG. *Cereb. Cortex* 25, 1697–1706. doi: 10.1093/cercor/bht355

Papadelis, C., Chen, Z., Kourtidou-Papadeli, C., Bamidis, P. D., Chouvarda, I., Bekiaris, E., et al. (2007). Monitoring sleepiness with on-board electrophysiological recordings for preventing sleep-deprived traffic accidents. *Clin. Neurophysiol.* 118, 1906–1922. doi: 10.1016/j.clinph.2007.04.031

Parasuraman, R., and Wilson, G. (2008). Putting the brain to work: Neuroergonomics past, present, and future. *Hum. Factors* 50:468. doi: 10.1518/001872008X288349

Pfurtscheller, G., and Aranibar, A. (1979). Evaluation of event-related desynchronization preceding and following voluntary self-paced movement. *Electroencephalogr. Clin. Neurophysiol.* 46, 138–146. doi: 10.1016/0013-4694(79)90063-4

Piper, S. K., Krueger, A., Koch, S. P., Mehnert, J., Habermehl, C., Steinbrink, J., et al. (2014). A wearable multi-channel fNIRS system for brain imaging in freely moving subjects. *Neuroimage* 85, 64–71. doi: 10.1016/j.neuroimage.2013.06.062

Pope, A. T., Bogart, E. H., and Bartolome, D. S. (1995). Biocybernetic system evaluates indices of operator engagement in automated task. *Biol. Psychol.* 40, 187–195. doi: 10.1016/0301-0511(95)05116-3

Porbadnigk, A. K., Antons, J.-N., Blankertz, B., Treder, M. S., Schleicher, R., Möller, S., et al. (2010). "Using ERPs for assessing the (sub)conscious perception of noise," in *Conference of Proceedings IEEE Engineering in Medicine and Biology Society* (Buenos Aires), 2690–2693.

Porbadnigk, A. K., Scholler, S., Blankertz, B., Ritz, A., Born, M., Scholl, R., et al. (2011). "Revealing the neural response to imperceptible peripheral flicker with machine learning," in *Conference of Proceedings IEEE Engineering in Medicine and Biology Society* (Boston, MA), 3692–3695.

Porbadnigk, A. K., Treder, M. S., Blankertz, B., Antons, J.-N., Schleicher, R., Möller, S., et al. (2013). Single-trial analysis of the neural correlates of speech quality perception. *J. Neural Eng.* 10:056003. doi: 10.1088/1741-2560/10/5/056003

Prinzel, L. J., Freeman, F. G., Scerbo, M. W., Mikulka, P. J., and Pope, A. T. (2003). Effects of a psychophysiological system for adaptive automation on performance, workload, and the event-related potential P300 component. *Hum. Factors* 45, 601–613. doi: 10.1518/hfes.45.4.601.27092

Purcell, D. W., John, S. M., Schneider, B. A., and Picton, T. W. (2004). Human temporal auditory acuity as assessed by envelope following responses. *J. Acoust. Soc. Am.* 116, 3581–3593. doi: 10.1121/1.1798354

Rämä, P., and Baccino, T. (2010). Eye-Fixation Related Potentials (efrps) during object identification. *Vis. Neurosci.* 27, 187–192. doi: 10.1017/S0952523810000283

Salvaris, M., and Haggard, P. (2014). Decoding intention at sensorimotor timescales. *PLoS ONE* 9:e85100. doi: 10.1371/journal.pone.0085100

Schaefer, R. S., Farquhar, J., Blokland, Y., Sadakata, M., and Desain, P. (2011). Name that tune: decoding music from the listening brain. *Neuroimage* 56, 843–849. doi: 10.1016/j.neuroimage.2010.05.084

Schmidt, E. A., Kincses, W. E., Schrauf, M., Haufe, S., Schubert, R., and Curio, G. (2007). "Assessing drivers' vigilance state during monotonous driving," in *Proceedings of the Fourth International Symposium on Human Factors in Driving Assessment, Training, and Vehicle Design* (Washington, DC), 138–145.

Schmidt, E. A., Schrauf, M., Simon, M., Fritzsche, M., Buchner, A., and Kincses, W. E. (2009). Drivers' misjudgement of vigilance state during prolonged monotonous daytime driving. *Accid. Anal. Prev.* 41, 1087–1093. doi: 10.1016/j.aap.2009.06.007

Scholler, S., Bosse, S., Treder, M. S., Blankertz, B., Curio, G., Müller, K.-R., et al. (2012). Towards a direct measure of video quality perception using EEG. *IEEE Trans. Image Process.* 21, 2619–2629. doi: 10.1109/TIP.2012.2187672

Schultze-Kraft, M., Birman, D., Rusconi, M., Allefeld, C., Görgen, K., Dähne, S., et al. (2016a). The point of no return in vetoing self-initiated movements. *Proc. Natl. Acad. Sci. U.S.A.* 113, 1080–1085. doi: 10.1073/pnas.1513569112

Schultze-Kraft, M., Dähne, S., Gugler, M., Curio, G., and Blankertz, B. (2016b). Unsupervised classification of operator workload from brain signals. *J. Neural Eng.* 13:036008. doi:10.1088/1741-2560/13/3/036008

Shih, J. J., Krusienski, D. J., and Wolpaw, J. R. (2012). Brain-computer interfaces in medicine. *Mayo Clin. Proc.* 87, 268–279. doi: 10.1016/j.mayocp.2011.12.008

Simon, M., Schmidt, E. A., Kincses, W. E., Fritzsche, M., Bruns, A., Aufmuth, C., et al. (2011). EEG alpha spindle measures as indicators of driver fatigue under real traffic conditions. *Clin. Neurophysiol.* 122, 1168–1178. doi: 10.1016/j.clinph.2010.10.044

Smith, M. E., Gevins, A., Brown, H., Karnik, A., Du, R., and Gevins, A. S. (2001). Monitoring task loading with multivariate EEG measures during complex forms of human-computer interaction. *Hum. Factors* 43, 366–380. doi: 10.1518/001872001775898287

Soekadar, S. R., Birbaumer, N., Slutzky, M. W., and Cohen, L. G. (2015). Brain-machine interfaces in neurorehabilitation of stroke. *Neurobiol. Dis.* 83, 172–179. doi: 10.1016/j.nbd.2014.11.025

Sonnleitner, A., Simon, M., Kincses, W. E., Buchner, A., and Schrauf, M. (2012). Alpha spindles as neurophysiological correlates indicating attentional shift in a simulated driving task. *Int. J. Psychophysiol.* 83, 110–118. doi: 10.1016/j.ijpsycho.2011.10.013

Sterman, M., and Friar, L. (1972). Suppression of seizures in an epileptic following sensorimotor {EEG} feedback training. *Electroencephalogr. Clin. Neurophysiol.* 33, 89–95. doi: 10.1016/0013-4694(72)90028-4

Stopczynski, A., Stahlhut, C., Larsen, J. E., Petersen, M. K., and Hansen, L. K. (2014). The smartphone brain scanner: a portable real-time neuroimaging system. *PLoS ONE* 9:e86733. doi: 10.1016/0013-4694(72)90028-4

Straebel, V., and Thoben, W. (2014). Alvin Lucier's music for solo performer: experimental music beyond sonification. *Organ. Sound* 19:17. doi: 10.1017/S135577181300037X

Sturm, I. (2016). *Analyzing the perception of natural music with EEG and ECoG.* Ph.D. thesis, Berlin Institute of Technology.

Sturm, I., Blankertz, B., Potes, C., Schalk, G., and Curio, G. (2014). ECoG high gamma activity reveals distinct cortical representations of lyrics passages, harmonic and timbre-related changes in a rock song. *Front. Hum. Neurosci.* 8:798. doi: 10.3389/fnhum.2014.00798

Sturm, I., Dähne, S., Blankertz, B., and Curio, G. (2015a). Multi-variate EEG analysis as a novel tool to examine brain responses to naturalistic music stimuli. *PLoS ONE* 10:e0141281. doi: 10.1371/journal.pone.0141281

Sturm, I., Treder, M., Miklody, D., Purwins, H., Dähne, S., Blankertz, B., et al. (2015b). Extracting the neural representation of tone onsets for separate voices of ensemble music using multivariate EEG analysis. *Psychomusicol. Music Mind Brain* 25, 366–379. doi: 10.1037/pmu0000104

Thompson, J. (2013). *Neural Decoding of Subjective Music Listening Experiences.* Ph.D. thesis, Dartmouth College Hanover, New Hampshire, Hanover.

Treder, M. S., Purwins, H., Miklody, D., Sturm, I., and Blankertz, B. (2014). Decoding auditory attention to instruments in polyphonic music using single-trial EEG classification. *J. Neural Eng.* 11:026009. doi: 10.1088/1741-2560/11/2/026009

Treder, M. S., Schmidt, N. M., and Blankertz, B. (2011). Gaze-independent brain-computer interfaces based on covert attention and feature attention. *J. Neural Eng.* 8:066003. doi: 10.1088/1741-2560/8/6/066003

Trivedi, M. M., and Cheng, S. Y. (2007). Holistic sensing and active displays for intelligent driver support systems. *Computer* 40, 60–68. doi: 10.1109/MC.2007.170

Ušćumlić, M., and Blankertz, B. (2016). Active visual search in non-stationary scenes: coping with temporal variability and uncertainty. *J. Neural Eng.* 13:016015. doi: 10.1088/1741-2560/13/1/016015

Ušćumlić, M., Hägele, M., and Blankertz, B. (2015). "EEG correlates of visual recognition while overtly tracking a moving object," in *Symbiotic Interaction, Vol. 9359, Lecture Notes in Computer Science*, eds B. Blankertz, G. Jacucci, L. Gamberini, A. Spagnolli, and J. Freeman (Berlin: Springer International Publishing), 166–171. doi: 10.1007/978-3-319-24917-9_18

van Erp, J., Lotte, F., and Tangermann, M. (2012). Brain-computer interfaces: beyond medical applications. *Computer* 45, 26–34. doi: 10.1109/MC.2012.107

Vidal, J. J. (1973). Toward direct brain-computer communication. *Annu. Rev. Biophys.* 2, 157–180. doi: 10.1146/annurev.bb.02.060173.001105

Von Lühmann, A., Herff, C., Heger, D., and Schultz, T. (2015). Towards a wireless open source instrument: functional near-infrared spectroscopy in mobile neuroergonomics and BCI applications. *Front. Hum. Neurosci.* 9:617. doi: 10.3389/fnhum.2015.00617

Walter, W., and Shipton, H. (1951). A toposcopic display system applied to neurophysiology. *J. Br. Inst. Radio Eng.* 11, 260–273. doi: 10.1049/jbire.1951.0040

Wenzel, M., Moreira, C., Lungu, I.-A., Bogojeski, M., and Blankertz, B. (2015). "Neural responses to abstract and linguistic stimuli with variable recognition latency," in *Symbiotic Interaction, Vol. 9359, Lecture Notes in Computer Science*, eds B. Blankertz, G. Jacucci, L. Gamberini, A. Spagnolli, and J. Freeman (Springer International Publishing), 172–178. doi: 10.1007/978-3-319-24917-9_19

Wenzel, M. A., Golenia, J.-E., and Blankertz, B. (2016). Classification of eye fixation related potentials for variable stimulus saliency. *Front. Neurosci.* 10:23. doi: 10.3389/fnins.2016.00023

Wolpaw, J. R., and Wolpaw, E. W., (eds.). (2012). *Brain-Computer Interfaces: Principles and Practice.* New York, NY: Oxford University Press.

Zander, T. O., and Kothe, C. (2011). Towards passive brain-computer interfaces: applying brain-computer interface technology to human-machine systems in general. *J. Neural Eng.* 8:025005. doi: 10.3389/fnins.2011.00053

Zander, T. O., Lehne, M., Ihme, K., Jatzev, S., Correia, J., Kothe, C., et al. (2011). A dry EEG-system for scientific research and brain–computer interfaces. *Front. Neurosci.* 5:53. doi: 10.3389/fnins.2011.00053

Zhang, H., Chavarriaga, R., Gheorghe, L. A., and Millán, J. d. R. (2015a). "Brain correlates of lane changing reaction time in simulated driving," in *2015 IEEE International Conference on Systems, Man, and Cybernetics (SMC2015)* (Hong Kong).

Zhang, H., Chavarriaga, R., Khaliliardali, Z., Gheorghe, L., Iturrate, I., and d R Millan, J. (2015b). EEG-based decoding of error-related brain activity in a real-world driving task. *J. Neural Eng.* 12:066028. doi: 10.1088/1741-2560/12/6/066028

17

Modulating pathological oscillations by rhythmic non-invasive brain stimulation—a therapeutic concept?

Lutz A. Krawinkel[1], *Andreas K. Engel*[2] *and Friedhelm C. Hummel*[1,3]*

[1] BrainImaging and NeuroStimulation (BINS) Laboratory, Department of Neurology, University Medical Center Hamburg-Eppendorf, Hamburg, Germany, [2] Department of Neurophysiology and Pathophysiology, University Medical Center Hamburg-Eppendorf, Hamburg, Germany, [3] Department of Neurology, Favoloro University, Medical School, Buenos Aires, Argentina

Edited by:
Manuel Fernando Casanova, University of Louisville, USA

Reviewed by:
Yu Liu, The University of Tennessee Health Science Center, USA
Estate M. Sokhadze, University of Louisville, USA

***Correspondence:**
Friedhelm C. Hummel, BrainImaging and NeuroStimulation (BINS) Laboratory, Department of Neurology, University Medical Center Hamburg-Eppendorf, Building O10, Martinistraße 52, 20246 Hamburg, Germany
f.hummel@uke.de

A large amount of studies of the last decades revealed an association between human behavior and oscillatory activity in the human brain. Alike, abnormalities of oscillatory activity were related with pathological behavior in many neuropsychiatric disorders, such as in Parkinson's disease (PD) or in schizophrenia (SCZ). As a therapeutic tool, non-invasive brain stimulation (NIBS) has demonstrated the potential to improve behavioral performance in patients suffering from neuropsychiatric disorders. Since evidence accumulates that NIBS might be able to modulate oscillatory activity and related behavior in a scientific setting, this review focuses on discussing potential interventional strategies to target abnormalities in oscillatory activity in neuropsychiatric disorders. In particular, we will review oscillatory changes described in patients after stroke, with PD or suffering from SCZ. Potential ways of targeting interventionally the underlying pathological oscillations to improve related pathological behavior will be further discussed.

Keywords: non-invasive brain stimulation, oscillatory activity, stroke, Parkinson's disease, schizophrenia

Importance of Oscillations for Information Processing in the Healthy Brain

Since Berger first described oscillatory activity of the brain in the 1920s, oscillations have been investigated extensively and research revealed clear relevance of human brain oscillations for information processing and behavior (Singer and Gray, 1995; Engel et al., 2001; Brown, 2003; Buzsáki and Draguhn, 2004; Pfurtscheller et al., 2005; Schoffelen et al., 2005; Fries, 2009; Jensen and Mazaheri, 2010).

Generally, an oscillation is a periodic fluctuation caused by changes in excitability of a group of neurons, measured on the scalp as differences in voltage with techniques like electroencephalography (EEG) or magnetencephalography (MEG). Oscillations are suggested to be able to temporally coordinate and control neuronal firing and are proposed to be one basic principle of information processing in the human brain (Engel et al., 2001; Varela et al., 2001; Buzsáki and Draguhn, 2004). Based on phenomenological observations, a division in frequency bands has been established. Usually, oscillation frequencies are categorized as delta-band (1.5–4 Hz), theta-band (4–7 Hz), alpha-band (8–12 Hz), beta-band (12–30 Hz) and gamma-band (30–80 Hz). Since this review will focus on specific aspects of pathological oscillatory activity, the next paragraph will briefly introduce selected relevant findings for each frequency band in the healthy brain.

Slow delta-band resting-state oscillations are prominent in sleep and are, like theta-band oscillations, associated with memory consolidation (Marshall et al., 2006; Rasch and Born, 2013). Alpha-band oscillations are prominent oscillations in the resting brain and alpha-band activity is associated with a wide range of brain functions like visual perception (Busch et al., 2009), working memory and short-term-memory retention (Palva and Palva, 2007). Alpha-band responses to eyes closing and opening respectively have been described since the first EEG-recordings and have been interpreted as desynchronization of affected neurons by information processing. This task-related suppression of alpha-band activity has been extensively investigated for other areas like motor cortex, and is called event-related desynchronization (Pfurtscheller, 1992; Klimesch et al., 2007). Besides event-related desynchronisation, there is event-related synchronization, which has been proposed to reflect cortical idling (Pfurtscheller et al., 1996). Furthermore, alpha-band activity was induced during inhibitory control processes (Hummel et al., 2002; Haegens et al., 2010; Jensen and Mazaheri, 2010; Sauseng et al., 2013). Beta-band oscillations are, like alpha-band oscillations, involved in perceptual processes (Engel and Fries, 2010). Another functional relevance of beta-band oscillations is sensorimotor control, their activity has been described during motor tasks and maintenance of contractions (Pfurtscheller and Lopes da Silva, 1999; Kilner et al., 2000; Engel and Fries, 2010). Since beta oscillations are described to be associated with a steady state of the motor system, it has been hypothesized that they signal the "status quo" (Gilbertson et al., 2005; Engel and Fries, 2010). Having been extensively investigated, task-related or evoked gamma-band oscillations respectively are thought to be involved into a broad range of behavioral components like visual perception and attention, and are associated with several memory functions (Singer and Gray, 1995; Tallon-Baudry et al., 1998; Herrmann et al., 2004; Jensen et al., 2007).

Moreover, besides local phenomena, mechanisms of oscillatory communication have been identified. For example synchronization of phases is suggested to be one basic principle for long range communication and is a component of connectivity measurements like coherence (Varela et al., 2001; Hummel and Gerloff, 2005; Schoffelen et al., 2005). Furthermore high frequency activity has been described as being depended on low frequency phase (Osipova et al., 2008; Jensen and Mazaheri, 2010; Buzsáki and Wang, 2012).

Underlining a potential causal relationship, both oscillatory activity and behavior were modulated by non-invasive brain stimulation (NIBS) in several studies. Before focussing on abnormal oscillations and pathological behavior, the influence of NIBS on oscillations of the healthy brain will be discussed in the next section.

Modulation of Oscillations by Rhythmic NIBS in the Healthy Brain

Several recent studies combining NIBS and EEG revealed that NIBS is able to modulate oscillations in the healthy brain (Plewnia et al., 2008; Pogosyan et al., 2009; Zaehle et al., 2010; Thut et al., 2011; Vernet et al., 2013). Generally, one basic technique of NIBS is Transcranial Magnetic Stimulation (TMS). By depolarization of neurons, a TMS single pulse applied over the hand knob area typically leads to a motor evoked potential in the contralateral hand (Hummel and Cohen, 2005; Hallett, 2007). Combining TMS with EEG, an increase of the intrinsic frequency of the TMS-affected area and their thalamic loops respectively has been observed (Rosanova et al., 2009). Another basic method of NIBS is Transcranial Electric Stimulation (TES). In contrast to TMS, TES is suggested to tune oscillators by modulating the membrane potential of neurons and their spontaneous firing rates (Nitsche and Paulus, 2000).

Regarding rhythmic applications of TMS, there is e.g., the theta burst stimulation (TBS) protocol, in which a triple pulse with an interpulse frequency of 50 Hz is applied in a theta rhythm. Applied continuously, TBS has an inhibitory effect, applied in an intermittent mode TBS has an excitatory effect (Huang et al., 2005; Hallett, 2007). Furthermore, repetitive TMS (rTMS) applied in a frequency below or at 1 Hz has an inhibitory effect, application of frequencies at faster rates (>5 Hz) leads to excitation (Pascual-Leone et al., 1994; Hummel and Cohen, 2005). Regarding patterned applications of TES, there is transcranial alternating current stimulation (tACS), a sinusoidal stimulation with spatially alternating anodal and cathodal components. Furthermore, there are transcranial random noise stimulation (tRNS) and direct current stimulation with a sinusoidal component, called oscillatory tDCS (Siebner and Ziemann, 2010).

Depending on their effect on oscillations, a division of rhythmic applications of NIBS into two concepts has been proposed (Siebner and Ziemann, 2010). On the one hand rhythmic NIBS can be applied in an oscillatory mode in the frequency of the targeted oscillation or its oscillator, respectively (Pogosyan et al., 2009; Zaehle et al., 2010; Thut et al., 2011). In the following, this mode will be called "direct", because there is a direct interference of stimulation frequency and the frequency of the oscillator. On the other hand, one can apply rhythmic NIBS in a non oscillatory mode, not reflecting the targeted oscillations or the frequency of the targeted oscillator. In this case NIBS is suggested to modulate underlying oscillatory mechanisms (Nitsche and Paulus, 2000; Lapenta et al., 2013; Vernet et al., 2013). This non oscillatory mode will be called "indirect" in the following.

In a study on "direct" modulation of ongoing oscillations, five pulses of TMS with an adjusted individual alpha frequency were able to entrain a parietal alpha oscillator specifically in its natural frequency (Thut et al., 2011). tACS entrained individual parietal-central alpha oscillations if applied in the endogenous frequency at the occipital pole (Zaehle et al., 2010). Furthermore, 10 Hz repetitive bifocal TMS over left primary motor cortex and over visual cortex led to an increase of alpha-band and lower beta coherence between the stimulated sites (Plewnia et al., 2008), supporting the exciting concept to not only influence local oscillatory activity but also long-range oscillatory interactions by NIBS.

Combining NIBS with EEG, "direct" applications of NIBS also modulated both oscillatory activity and behavioral components, thereby providing evidence for a causal role of oscillations and its modulation. In a visuomotor task tACS applied at 20 Hz reduced peak velocity on the one hand and increased coherence between scalp-recorded activity and EMG activity at 20 Hz on the other hand (Pogosyan et al., 2009). Recently it has been shown by concurrent EEG-tACS that 10 Hz stimulation can entrain parieto-occipital alpha activity and modulate target detection performance in an oddball task in a phase-dependent manner (Helfrich et al., 2014). In an auditory experiment perception thresholds were dependent on the phase of the entrained oscillation using 10 Hz oscillatory tDCS (Neuling et al., 2012). Furthermore slow wave oscillatory tDCS in a frequency of 0.75 Hz applied during non-rapid-eye-movement sleep induced an increase of slow wave oscillations and enhanced the retention of declarative memories (Marshall et al., 2006). However, this study was critically evaluated by the same group showing that the total amount of current and not the oscillatory component of the oscillatory tDCS might have been the main effective variable (Groppa et al., 2010).

As an "indirect" rhythmic application of NIBS, continuous theta burst stimulation (cTBS) increased theta-band power and decreased beta-band power in an eyes-closed resting experiment (Vernet et al., 2013). As an underlying mechanism the authors suggest that cTBS modulates synchronization of relevant oscillators. In a non resting setup cTBS increased event-related lower beta power applied over primary motor cortex for at least 30 min (Noh et al., 2012) and 40 trains of ten excitatory TMS pulses at 20 Hz increased alpha and beta-band event-related synchronization at the stimulation site (Veniero et al., 2011).

Like "direct" applications, also "indirect" applications were able to modulate both oscillations and behavior. Inhibitory 1 Hz rTMS on right prefrontal cortex reduced both response times for congruent cued targets and ipsilateral alpha amplitude (Sauseng et al., 2011). In another study 5 Hz tDCS (theta tDCS) decreased both slow wave activity, frontal slow EEG spindle power and consolidation of declarative memory (Marshall et al., 2011).

Taken together evidence is increasing that oscillations, being one basic principle of information processing in the human brain, can be modulated by NIBS. In many cases, this suggests a possible mechanism for how NIBS may exert its effects on cognitive processes or behavior.

In the following paragraph, alteration of oscillatory activity will be discussed as a pathophysiological mechanism in neuropsychiatric disorders. As examples, we will consider oscillatory changes in the alpha-band after stroke, beta-band changes in patients with Parkinson's disease (PD) and altered gamma-band activity in patients suffering from schizophrenia (SCZ). Next, we will discuss potential applications of rhythmic NIBS like rTMS and tACS in order to modulate pathological oscillations and potentially improve the clinical outcome in patients.

Role of Oscillatory Activity in the Pathophysiology of Neuropsychiatric Disorders

Stroke is one of the leading causes for acquired long-term disability in industrialized countries (Kolominsky-Rabas et al., 2001) and, therefore, studies on neurophysiological changes accompanying and following stroke have received considerable interest.

Several studies have observed changes in alpha-band activity recorded over the affected hemisphere (AH) after stroke in the resting brain (Tecchio et al., 2005, 2006; Dubovik et al., 2012; Westlake et al., 2012; Laaksonen et al., 2013). Thirty-two patients with stroke of the middle cerebral artery within the first 10 days (Tecchio et al., 2005) and 56 stroke patients in a chronic stage (Tecchio et al., 2006) showed a reduction of the individual alpha frequency in the AH. In 16 patients with affected upper limp function, amplitude of alpha-band oscillations increased in the AH compared to the unaffected hemisphere (UH) and to control subjects 1 month and 3 months after stroke (Laaksonen et al., 2013). In the latter study, alpha oscillations had a burst-like pattern and were found both in rolandic and in parietal regions. However, these changes in alpha-band activity did not correlate with the clinical outcome in patients (Tecchio et al., 2005, 2006; Laaksonen et al., 2013).

In contrast, two studies addressing interregional resting-state functional connectivity (FC, based on imaginary coherence, IC) were able to correlate changes of alpha-band activity with performance (Dubovik et al., 2012) and motor recovery (Westlake et al., 2012) after stroke. Twenty patients showed a decrease of alpha-band FC of central electrodes over the lesions to all other electrodes 3 months after stroke of middle or/and anterior cerebral artery (Dubovik et al., 2012). Moreover, motor functions correlated with IC values of the precentral gyrus and all other investigated brain regions. Since FC changes were not restricted to the boundaries of the lesions but restricted to a specific frequency, the authors emphasize that oscillatory changes are probably not due to tissue loss but to changes in affected tissue. Furthermore the study showed that changes in FC are probably due to changes in alpha phase synchrony rather than to changes in alpha amplitude (Stam et al., 2007; Dubovik et al., 2012). Another study found changes in alpha-band activity in the acute phase of stroke (Westlake et al., 2012). Greater initial functional alpha-band connectivity of ipsilesional primary sensory cortex and prefrontal cortex in the acute phase correlated with better clinical improvement 8–12 weeks after stroke in fourteen patients with motor impairment of the upper limb.

Next to changes in alpha-band activity, also changes of slow wave oscillations were found after brain injuries like head trauma and stroke (Lewine et al., 1999; Butz et al., 2004). In line with these results a shift from fast to slow rhythms could be observed after stroke (Dubovik et al., 2012) and slow delta wave oscillations of the UH have been shown to be correlated with clinical outcome after stroke (Tecchio et al., 2007). Patients with persisting abnormal slow wave oscillations (abnormal low frequency magnetic activity) had a significantly worse clinical outcome compared to patients without persisting slow wave oscillatory components (Laaksonen et al., 2013).

Besides clinical observations, slow wave activity has also been investigated in an animal stroke model, in which slow wave oscillations were associated with axonal sprouting after thermal-ischemic lesioning (Carmichael and Chesselet, 2002). In this model, a treatment with tetrodotoxin reduced both slow oscillations and axonal sprouting. In another study neuronal bursts were able to reduce inhibitory factors that surround axons (Ming et al., 2001). In a recent publication it could be shown that new patterns of axonal sprouting mediated recovery after stroke in an animal model (Overman et al., 2012). Taken together, these data provided first evidence that there might be an association of slow neuronal firing, axonal sprouting and behavioral recovery.

PD has a high prevalence in aging populations (von Campenhausen et al., 2005). Evidence is increasing that clinical symptoms of PD are related to abnormalities in beta-band activity (Levy et al., 2002; Kühn et al., 2008, 2009; Crowell et al., 2012; Heinrichs-Graham et al., 2014; Herz et al., 2014). Prominent beta-band activity has been recorded in the basal ganglia in animal models of PD and in PD patients with deep brain stimulation (DBS; Levy et al., 2000, 2002; Kühn et al., 2008; Bergmann et al., 2012; Heinrichs-Graham et al., 2014; Herz et al., 2014). Both dopamine treatment and DBS have been shown to reduce beta-band activity (Brown et al., 2001; Levy et al., 2002; Kühn et al., 2008). The modulation of beta-band activity by dopaminergic treatment (Kühn et al., 2009) and by DBS (Ray et al., 2008) was associated with a reduction of bradykinesia and rigidity. A recent study in PD also revealed that treatment with levodopa reinforced beta-band coupling between primary motor cortex and lateral premotor cortex (Herz et al., 2014). Another study demonstrated a lack of physiological event-related beta desynchronization which could be modulated by levodopa in PD (Heinrichs-Graham et al., 2014). Taken together, in PD abnormal beta oscillations are a consistent finding with a strong relation to abnormal behavior. Hence, beta-band oscillations could be a promising target for interventional strategies based on rhythmic NIBS.

SCZ has a life-time prevalence of 0.4% and belongs to the thirty most disabling disorders worldwide (Murray and Lopez, 1997; McGrath et al., 2008). Besides psychotic symptoms patients with SCZ show abnormalities in cognitive performance, e.g., in working memory, cognitive control and sensory gating. These cognitive deficits are, on the one hand, associated with clinical and functional outcome (Green et al., 2000; Gold, 2004; McGrath et al., 2008). On the other hand they are related with abnormalities in gamma-band oscillations (Johannesen et al., 2005; Uhlhaas et al., 2008; Barr et al., 2010; Sun et al., 2011). Compared to healthy controls, patients with SCZ showed excessive gamma-band oscillations in conditions with high memory load (Barr et al., 2010). Altered gamma-band activity was also found in the resting brain of SCZ patients (Andreou et al., 2014). Furthermore, evoked gamma power and phase synchronization were reduced after auditory stimulation in patients with SCZ (Light et al., 2006). In line with these results, after a 40 Hz binaural stimulation a reduced phase locking between primary auditory cortices was observed in patients with SCZ, which correlated with auditory hallucination scores (Mulert et al., 2011).

Moreover, combination of TMS and EEG has been used in SCZ research by using a TMS double pulse paradigm (Farzan et al., 2009) called long intracortical inhibition (LICI). LICI is an established, probably $GABA_B$ mediated measurement for cortical inhibition in motor cortex using motor-evoked potentials as a readout (McDonnell et al., 2006). Both $GABA_A$ and $GABA_B$ suggested to be involved in the generation of gamma-band oscillations (Wang and Buzsáki, 1996; Brown et al., 2007). Recently, EEG parameters were established as another readout for double pulse TMS paradigms in non motor areas like DLPFC (Daskalakis et al., 2008). A study in healthy subjects demonstrated that applying a TMS LICI protocol over DLPFC led to a decrease of gamma oscillations whereas gamma oscillations over motor cortex did not change after LICI application (Farzan et al., 2009). In contrast, patients with SCZ showed an impaired LICI-mediated inhibition of gamma oscillations in DLPFC compared to healthy participants and patients with bipolar disorder (Farzan et al., 2010a).

In summary, gamma-band oscillations have been related with cognitive performance in the healthy brain (Tallon-Baudry et al., 1998; Herrmann et al., 2004). In SCZ abnormal gamma-band activity was associated with behavioral impairment (Johannesen et al., 2005; Uhlhaas et al., 2008; Barr et al., 2010; Sun et al., 2011; Andreou et al., 2014). In line with these results, gamma-band activity could be one potential target of NIBS in SCZ.

Targeting Pathological Oscillations by Non-Invasive Brain Stimulation

This section will address the question of how rhythmic NIBS could be used to modulate pathological oscillations and thereby modulate behavior and clinical symptoms in stroke, PD and SCZ.

Several studies have demonstrated that NIBS can improve functional outcome of stroke patients (Hummel and Cohen, 2005; Hummel et al., 2005, 2006; Kim et al., 2006; Cazzoli et al., 2012; for review Schulz et al., 2013). To our knowledge, however, there is to date limited data on the effect of NIBS on oscillations in stroke. In six patients with severe hemiparesis, tDCS modulated alpha-band oscillations of sensorimotor areas during imaginary movements of the affected hand (Kasashima et al., 2012). Since detection of stable brain rhythms can be difficult in damaged brain areas after stroke, the aim of the latter study was to enhance oscillatory activity in the lesioned hemisphere by tDCS in order to be able to achieve a stable and well distinguishable brain signal for use in a brain-computer-interface (BCI). Event related alpha-band desynchronisation, a correlate of local activation, was significantly enhanced after tDCS stimulation compared to sham stimulation, making the signal more suitable for a BCI.

Although several studies have applied NIBS in stroke patients, only one case report has used rhythmic NIBS to modulate oscillations. In a patient with aphasia 10 Hz rTMS modulated both oscillatory activity and clinical outcome (Dammekens et al., 2014). In the treated patient the stroke lesion affected the left inferior frontal gyrus (IFG), which is part of the language network (Crosson et al., 2007). Generally, according to the concept of an interhemispheric rivalry in stroke (Murase et al., 2004; Duque et al., 2005), inhibitory rTMS protocols of 1 Hz stimulation frequency are applied to the healthy hemisphere in order to prevent interhemispheric maladaptive processes in contralesional networks. Another approach is to excite the damaged hemisphere with rTMS protocols with a frequency above 5 Hz (Lefaucheur, 2006). In the latter study, excitatory rTMS was applied over the damaged left IFG in daily sessions over 3 weeks leading to an increase of FC between left and right IFG in the theta- and high beta-band. Behaviorally, the patient improved on repetition tasks for naming and comprehension. In addition to being a case report, this study does certainly not establish a causal relation between modulation of oscillations and changes in behavior. Nevertheless, this study provides first hints that rhythmic NIBS might be effective in modulating both oscillatory activity and clinical outcome.

Based on the emerging understanding about the relationship between NIBS and the modulation or induction of oscillatory activity in the last decad, hypotheses on how to enhance brain functioning and ameliorate impaired behavior after focal brain lesions can be defined. These hypotheses would be amenable to evaluation in controlled clinical trials in stroke patients. Combining the evidence that (1) changes in alpha-band activity are correlated with recovery and performance after stroke (Dubovik et al., 2012; Westlake et al., 2012) and that (2) NIBS is able modulate alpha-band activity (Plewnia et al., 2008; Thut et al., 2011) one could consider applying rhythmic alpha-NIBS after stroke. As illustrated schematically in **Figure 1A**, bifocal TMS at alpha frequency could entrain alpha-band activity between lesioned areas and relevant neighboring regions. In this context, bifocal application should potentially be performed with a certain phase lag between the targeted areas. An application of less focal alpha tACS in a montage covering both targeted areas would be another option. In both cases rhythmic NIBS would potentially lead to a synchronization in the alpha-band of lesioned sites and relevant connected areas like ipsilateral and contralateral premotor cortices respectively (Johansen-Berg et al., 2002; Ward et al., 2003; Gerloff et al., 2006; Rehme et al., 2011; Dubovik et al., 2012; Westlake et al., 2012).

Another option to entrain alpha-band activity could be to add noise, as shown in **Figure 1B**. tRNS is a technique which has been used to modulate cortical excitability and BOLD activity (Terney et al., 2008; Saiote et al., 2013). It has been suggested that, by adding noise, tRNS is able to augment cortical oscillations of different frequencies (Antal and Paulus, 2013). In stroke patients, tRNS could elevate reduced alpha-band activity in affected parts of the brain back to suprathreshold levels (Moss et al., 2004) and thereby restore important connective functions. Analogue to the potential effects on the aging brain, rhythmic or patterned NIBS like tRNS, tACS and rTMS could be used to entrain recruitment of other brain areas to support both affected networks and functional outcome (Gutchess, 2014).

Regarding the results of reduced alpha peak frequency and increased alpha amplitude in the AH after stroke (Tecchio et al., 2005) one could argue that behavioral changes might be

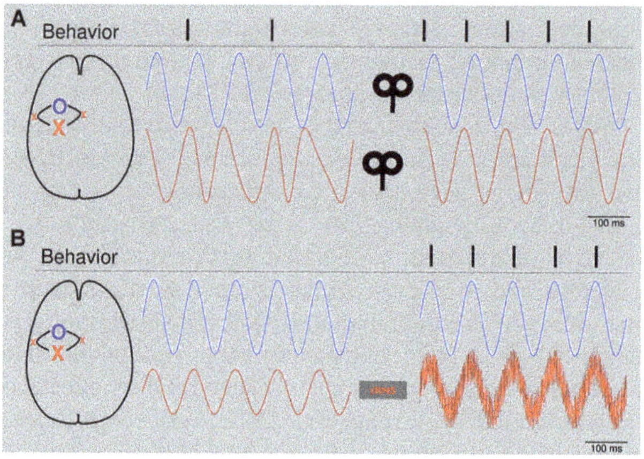

FIGURE 1 | (A) Schematic: Bifocal repetitive TMS (rTMS) restores alpha-band activity. After stroke, alpha oscillators (red line, left) of the affected area (red X, primary motor cortex) show unsteady phase properties. Since physiological behavior depends on a constant phase relation of alpha oscillations between the affected area and connected networks (blue O, blue line, left, premotor areas), the patient is impaired (behavior, left, e.g., muscle contractions). After application of bifocal, rTMS at alpha frequency over both areas with a lag reflecting physiological offset of oscillators, oscillatory activity is synchronized (blue and red line, right) in terms of a constant phase lag. Behavior improves (right). Please note that conditions are highly simplified. First, next to phase, also amplitude is important for signal processing. Second, in the presented physiological condition (right) phases are completely locked, which is artificial. Naturally, phases would fluctuate. **(B)** Schematic: tRNS augments alpha oscillators. After stroke alpha activity (red line, left) of the affected area (red X) is reduced. Threshold for establishing information processing with a related network (blue line, left) is not reached and dependent normal behavior is reduced. tRNS applied over the affected oscillator augments alpha activity by adding noise (red line, right). Information processing is re-established and behavior improves. Please note that conditions are very much simplified. In both cases, phase is totally locked without any phase lag. Biological signals would fluctuate.

related to alpha induced inhibition (Jensen and Mazaheri, 2010). In contrast to changes in FC (Dubovik et al., 2012; Westlake et al., 2012), these changes were not correlated with behavioral changes, however, and gaining clinical benefit by modulating these features of local oscillatory activity remains an untested possibility.

In addition to the modulation of electrophysiological dynamics, NIBS might also influence molecular environment of neurons. By modulating slow wave activity occurring after stroke (Tecchio et al., 2005; Dubovik et al., 2012; Laaksonen et al., 2013) related neural repair might be modulated. Since there is first evidence in an animal model that there might be an association of slow neuronal firing, axonal recovery and recovery of function (Ming et al., 2001; Carmichael and Chesselet, 2002; Overman et al., 2012), one should consider a slow frequency stimulation as performed before in different contexts (Marshall et al., 2011) to gain axonal sprouting and improve clinical outcome after brain injury like stroke.

As discussed in the preceding section, pathological beta oscillations are a consistent finding in basal ganglia correlated with behavioral changes in PD patients (Levy et al., 2002; Kühn et al., 2008, 2009; Crowell et al., 2012; Heinrichs-Graham et al., 2014; Herz et al., 2014). It is known that these abnormal beta-band oscillations can be modulated by established DBS protocols. In addition, a number of studies investigated the effects of NIBS on motor function in patients with PD. Applying 5 Hz rTMS over primary motor cortex led to a short term increase of motor function in six PD patients (Siebner et al., 2000). A 5 Hz rTMS protocol consisting of 2000 pulses per day over ten days led to significant reduction of motor impairment (Khedr et al., 2003). Moreover, rTMS over inferior frontal cortex modulated event-related potentials in the subthalamic nucleus (STN) in patients with implanted DBS electrodes (Rektor et al., 2010). Though different stimulation locations were used for both techniques, resting-state functional-connectivity MRI analysis revealed, that targets of stimulation might be nodes in the same network (Fox et al., 2014).

In our view, the clinical effectiveness of these two stimulation techniques and their probably network-associated ability to modulate cortex-basal ganglia dynamics point to the great potential of NIBS applications in PD. As discussed above, pathological beta oscillations could be a promising target for rhythmic NIBS. A recent study has demonstrated the possibility to enhance the "akinetic" effect of beta oscillations. In a task where subjects got a cue to stop a planned grip-movement, tACS stimulation with 20 Hz significantly reduced grip force in that condition (Joundi et al., 2012). One the one hand these results underline the potential impact of enhanced beta oscillations in "akinetic" disorders like PD. On the other hand, the results point out the ability of cortical NIBS to affect loops involving the basal ganglia.

To our knowledge, however, it has not been possible to reduce pathological beta oscillations in PD by NIBS. Potentially, reducing beta activity could be achieved by phase cancellation. Phase cancellation by application of tACS has already been used for tremor reduction in PD. Targeting tremor-associated oscillations in such an approach in patients with tremor-dominant PD led to an almost 50% suppression of resting tremor (Brittain et al., 2013). As a first step in the study, the individual tremor frequency of each patient was measured. In a second step, tremor-frequency adjusted tACS was applied over the primary motor cortex at different phase angles. Certain phase angles led to tremor reduction whereas stimulation at different angles led to an increase of tremor. This study underlines the great potential of individualized application of rhythmic NIBS and suggests the potential efficacy of phase cancellation. Based on monkey data, phase cancellation has also been suggested as a physiological mechanism for controlling tremor in spinal cord networks (Williams et al., 2010). As illustrated schematically in **Figure 2A**, phase cancellation might be applied to pathological beta oscillations in PD potentially targeting bradykinesia and rigidity (Ray et al., 2008; Kühn et al., 2009).

Since tremor shifted to a different frequency in some of the patients in the study by Brittain et al. (2013), tACS application should be adjusted to ongoing tremor activity to provide an effective modulation, as shown schematically in **Figure 2B**. To this end, online read-out techniques that allow stimulation in dependence on ongoing oscillatory activity (Berényi et al., 2012; Bergmann et al., 2012) will be highly advantageous in order to adjust NIBS to changing pathologic frequency and provide effective phase cancellation and reduction of symptoms. In a clinical setting such an "online", closed-loop approach has already been tested successfully: in PD DBS has been triggered based on recorded local field potentials (Little et al., 2013). These interventional strategies are interesting and potentially promising for amelioration of symptoms not well responsive to DBS.

In SCZ, combining single or double pulse TMS with EEG revealed abnormalities of cortical inhibition of gamma oscillations (Farzan et al., 2009, 2010b). Both studies point towards a scientific benefit of combining these methods and suggest that measurements on TMS-evoked oscillatory activity could be useful as a "biomarker" for neuropsychiatric disorders. Applying a similar approach, TMS evoked EEG activity has been proposed to add information to diagnostic procedures for chronic disorders of consciousness (Ragazzoni et al., 2013).

Abnormal gamma-band oscillations of patients with SCZ have been modulated by rTMS (Barr et al., 2011). In an N-back working memory task, subjects were asked to compare stimuli with those from previous trials. 20 Hz TMS applied bilaterally to DLPFC in reduced gamma activity in the SCZ patients (Barr et al., 2011). This approach, which is schematically presented in **Figure 2C**, could be considered as an "indirect" application, in which underlying gamma oscillators were modulated by an excitatory 20 Hz rTMS protocol not directly targeted at gamma frequencies. Since rTMS of a single session in the latter study did not change working memory behavior, the same group performed a pilot study with 20 Hz rTMS over DLPFC bilateraly for twenty sessions in a randomized double-blinded sham-controlled manner. This application led to a significant improvement of accuracy in working memory underlining that rTMS might potentially improve cognitive impairments in SCZ patients (Barr et al., 2013). Moreover, these results point towards the need for repetitive sessions of NIBS to gain long term effects. However, changes in gamma oscillations were not addressed in this follow-up study (Barr et al., 2013).

Taken together, application of rTMS seem to be promising for the treatment of negative symptoms of SCZ, although so far only demonstrated in proof-of-principle studies. Gamma oscillations show a high diversity in SCZ (Sun et al., 2011) and, hence, a direct link between the modulation of gamma oscillations and an improved cognitive performance in SCZ remains speculative. Nevertheless, further applications for the treatment of negative symptoms based on safe and low cost NIBS techniques addressing specifically gamma oscillations should be further developed and evaluated in detail in future studies.

Summary and Further Perspectives of NIBS

Evidence is increasing that NIBS may provide a novel and promising strategy to modulate both oscillatory activity and related behavior in the healthy brain. To date only a limited number of studies have employed NIBS to modulate oscillatory

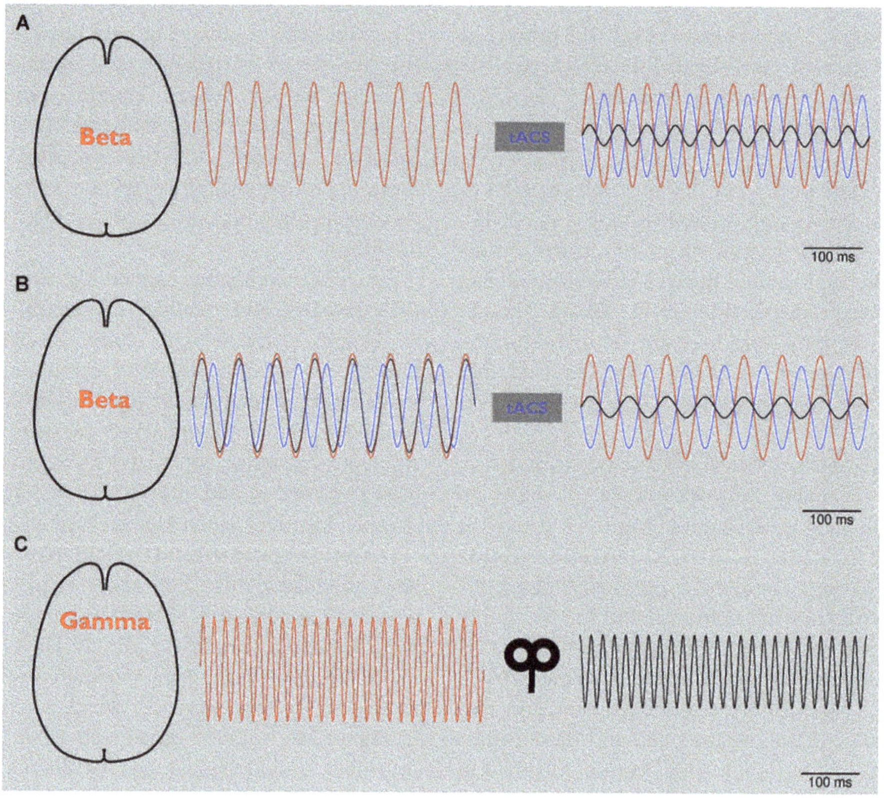

FIGURE 2 | (A) Schematic: tACS in Parkinson's disease (PD). Abnormal beta oscillations (red line, left and right) are related to rigidity and bradykinesia. Application of tACS with a phase lag of 180° (blue line, right) leads to a reduction of these pathological oscillations (black line, right) by phase cancellation (right). As a result, rigidity and bradykinesia are reduced. Please note that to date phase cancellation has been thought to be able to reduce tremor in PD by affecting tremor related cortical frequencies. To our knowledge, beta frequency has not yet been targeted by NIBS using the phase cancellation concept. **(B)** Schematic: tACS in PD using online readout techniques. Since it has been reported that during tACS application tremor frequency changed in patients with PD, more online readout techniques should be developed to adjust NIBS applications. After application of 20 Hz tACS (see panel **A**), pathological beta rhythm changes its frequency to 15 Hz (red line, left). tACS of 20 Hz with 180° phase lag (blue line, left) looses its effect (black line, left). After online adjustment, tACS shifts to 15 Hz (blue line, right). Pathological beta (red line, right) is again reduced (black line, right). **(C)** Schematic: rTMS in schizophrenia (SCZ). By modulating oscillators of abnormal gamma-band activity (red line, left), amplitude is reduced (black line, right) and related behavioral impairments are reduced.

abnormalities in neuropsychiatric disorders as a treatment strategy. As discussed above, this concept is supported by studies suggesting, for example, that tACS can reduce tremor in PD (Brittain et al., 2013) or that rhythmic TMS can improve both working memory (Barr et al., 2013) and impaired gamma activity in patients with SCZ (Barr et al., 2011). In stroke, NIBS might modulate both oscillatory activity and clinical performance (Dammekens et al., 2014). Taken together, the application of rhythmic NIBS in order to modulate underlying, disease related oscillations is a very promising approach.

Next steps will be the development and evaluation of safe and low-cost applications of patterned NIBS in order to target pathological oscillatory activity to achieve improvement of clinical symptoms of neuropsychiatric patients impacting on their daily life. Demonstrating the expected effects of NIBS in patients might have an incremental impact on treatment of neuropsychiatric disorders and subsequently the health system, as novel devices has been developed for home-based, self-application of NIBS. As soon as such approaches will be proven save in the home-based environment, they may offer a cost-effective strategy to significantly enhance treatment intensity.

Still one can argue critically that oscillatory changes after NIBS application are not a cause but a by-product merely associated with behavioral changes. However, combining NIBS with electrophysiological recordings bears great potential to establish the specificity and reliability of oscillations as biomarkers.

Acknowledgments

This work has been supported by the German Research Foundation (DFG, SFB936/A2/A3/C4) and by the European Union (ERC-2010-AdG-269716 "MULTISENSE").

References

Andreou, C., Nolte, G., Leicht, G., Polomac, N., Hanganu-Opatz, I. L., Lambert, M., et al. (2014). Increased resting-state gamma-band connectivity in first-episode schizophrenia. *Schizophr. Bull.* doi: 10.1093/schbul/sbu121. [Epub ahead of print].

Antal, A., and Paulus, W. (2013). Transcranial alternating current stimulation (tACS). *Front. Hum. Neurosci.* 7:317. doi: 10.3389/fnhum.2013.00317

Barr, M. S., Farzan, F., Arenovich, T., Chen, R., Fitzgerald, P. B., and Daskalakis, Z. J. (2011). The effect of repetitive transcranial magnetic stimulation on gamma oscillatory activity in schizophrenia. *PLoS One* 6:e22627. doi: 10.1371/journal.pone.0022627

Barr, M. S., Farzan, F., Rajji, T. K., Voineskos, A. N., Blumberger, D. M., Arenovich, T., et al. (2013). Can repetitive magnetic stimulation improve cognition in schizophrenia? Pilot data from a randomized controlled trial. *Biol. Psychiatry* 73, 510–517. doi: 10.1016/j.biopsych.2012.08.020

Barr, M. S., Farzan, F., Tran, L. C., Chen, R., Fitzgerald, P. B., and Daskalakis, Z. J. (2010). Evidence for excessive frontal evoked gamma oscillatory activity in schizophrenia during working memory. *Schizophr. Res.* 121, 146–152. doi: 10.1016/j.schres.2010.05.023

Berényi, A., Belluscio, M., Mao, D., and Buzsáki, G. (2012). Closed-loop control of epilepsy by transcranial electrical stimulation. *Science* 337, 735–737. doi: 10.1126/science.1223154

Bergmann, T. O., Mölle, M., Schmidt, M. A., Lindner, C., Marshall, L., Born, J., et al. (2012). EEG-guided transcranial magnetic stimulation reveals rapid shifts in motor cortical excitability during the human sleep slow oscillation. *J. Neurosci.* 32, 243–253. doi: 10.1523/JNEUROSCI.4792-11.2012

Brittain, J. S., Probert-Smith, P., Aziz, T. Z., and Brown, P. (2013). Tremor suppression by rhythmic transcranial current stimulation. *Curr. Biol.* 23, 436–440. doi: 10.1016/j.cub.2013.01.068

Brown, P. (2003). Oscillatory nature of human basal ganglia activity: relationship to the pathophysiology of Parkinson's disease. *Mov. Disord.* 18, 357–363. doi: 10.1002/mds.10358

Brown, J. T., Davies, C. H., and Randall, A. D. (2007). Synaptic activation of GABA(B) receptors regulates neuronal network activity and entrainment. *Eur. J. Neurosci.* 25, 2982–2990. doi: 10.1111/j.1460-9568.2007.05544.x

Brown, P., Oliviero, A., Mazzone, P., Insola, A., Tonali, P., and Di Lazzaro, V. (2001). Dopamine dependency of oscillations between subthalamic nucleus and pallidum in Parkinson's disease. *J. Neurosci.* 21, 1033–1038.

Busch, N. A., Dubois, J., and VanRullen, R. (2009). The phase of ongoing EEG oscillations predicts visual perception. *J. Neurosci.* 29, 7869–7876. doi: 10.1523/JNEUROSCI.0113-09.2009

Butz, M., Gross, J., Timmermann, L., Moll, M., Freund, H.-J., Witte, O. W., et al. (2004). Perilesional pathological oscillatory activity in the magnetoencephalogram of patients with cortical brain lesions. *Neurosci. Lett.* 355, 93–96. doi: 10.1016/j.neulet.2003.10.065

Buzsáki, G., and Draguhn, A. (2004). Neuronal oscillations in cortical networks. *Science* 304, 1926–1929. doi: 10.1126/science.1099745

Buzsáki, G., and Wang, X.-J. (2012). Mechanisms of gamma oscillations. *Annu. Rev. Neurosci.* 35, 203–225. doi: 10.1146/annurev-neuro-062111-150444

Carmichael, S. T., and Chesselet, M.-F. (2002). Synchronous neuronal activity is a signal for axonal sprouting after cortical lesions in the adult. *J. Neurosci.* 22, 6062–6070.

Cazzoli, D., Müri, R. M., Schumacher, R., von Arx, S., Chaves, S., Gutbrod, K., et al. (2012). Theta burst stimulation reduces disability during the activities of daily living in spatial neglect. *Brain* 135(Pt. 11), 3426–3439. doi: 10.1093/brain/aws182

Crosson, B., McGregor, K., Gopinath, K. S., Conway, T. W., Benjamin, M., Chang, Y., et al. (2007). Functional MRI of language in aphasia: a review of the literature and the methodological challenges. *Neuropsychol. Rev.* 17, 157–177. doi: 10.1007/s11065-007-9024-z

Crowell, A. L., Ryapolova-Webb, E. S., Ostrem, J. L., Galifianakis, N. B., Shimamoto, S., Lim, D. A., et al. (2012). Oscillations in sensorimotor cortex in movement disorders: an electrocorticography study. *Brain* 135(Pt. 2), 615–630. doi: 10.1093/brain/awr332

Dammekens, E., Vanneste, S., Ost, J., and De Ridder, D. (2014). Neural correlates of high frequency repetitive transcranial magnetic stimulation improvement in post-stroke non-fluent aphasia: a case study. *Neurocase* 20, 1–9. doi: 10.1080/13554794.2012.713493

Daskalakis, Z. J., Farzan, F., Barr, M. S., Maller, J. J., Chen, R., and Fitzgerald, P. B. (2008). Long-interval cortical inhibition from the dorsolateral prefrontal cortex: a TMS-EEG study. *Neuropsychopharmacology* 33, 2860–2869. doi: 10.1038/npp.2008.22

Dubovik, S., Pignat, J.-M., Ptak, R., Aboulafia, T., Allet, L., Gillabert, N., et al. (2012). The behavioral significance of coherent resting-state oscillations after stroke. *Neuroimage* 61, 249–257. doi: 10.1016/j.neuroimage.2012.03.024

Duque, J., Hummel, F., Celnik, P., Murase, N., Mazzocchio, R., and Cohen, L. G. (2005). Transcallosal inhibition in chronic subcortical stroke. *Neuroimage* 28, 940–946. doi: 10.1016/j.neuroimage.2005.06.033

Engel, A. K., and Fries, P. (2010). Beta-band oscillations–signalling the status quo? *Curr. Opin. Neurobiol.* 20, 156–165. doi: 10.1016/j.conb.2010.02.015

Engel, A. K., Fries, P., and Singer, W. (2001). Dynamic predictions: oscillations and synchrony in top-down processing. *Nat. Rev. Neurosci.* 2, 704–716. doi: 10.1038/35094565

Farzan, F., Barr, M. S., Levinson, A. J., Chen, R., Wong, W., Fitzgerald, P. B., et al. (2010a). Evidence for gamma inhibition deficits in the dorsolateral prefrontal cortex of patients with schizophrenia. *Brain* 133(Pt. 5), 1505–1514. doi: 10.1093/brain/awq046

Farzan, F., Barr, M. S., Levinson, A. J., Chen, R., Wong, W., Fitzgerald, P. B., et al. (2010b). Reliability of long-interval cortical inhibition in healthy human subjects: a TMS-EEG study. *J. Neurophysiol.* 104, 1339–1346. doi: 10.1152/jn.00279.2010

Farzan, F., Barr, M. S., Wong, W., Chen, R., Fitzgerald, P. B., and Daskalakis, Z. J. (2009). Suppression of gamma-oscillations in the dorsolateral prefrontal cortex following long interval cortical inhibition: a TMS-EEG study. *Neuropsychopharmacology* 34, 1543–1551. doi: 10.1038/npp.2008.211

Fox, M. D., Buckner, R. L., Liu, H., Chakravarty, M. M., Lozano, A. M., and Pascual-Leone, A. (2014). Resting-state networks link invasive and noninvasive brain stimulation across diverse psychiatric and neurological diseases. *Proc. Natl. Acad. Sci. U S A* 111, E4367–E4375. doi: 10.1073/pnas.1405003111

Fries, P. (2009). Neuronal gamma-band synchronization as a fundamental process in cortical computation. *Annu. Rev. Neurosci.* 32, 209–224. doi: 10.1146/annurev.neuro.051508.135603

Gerloff, C., Bushara, K., Sailer, A., Wassermann, E. M., Chen, R., Matsuoka, T., et al. (2006). Multimodal imaging of brain reorganization in motor areas of the contralesional hemisphere of well recovered patients after capsular stroke. *Brain* 129(Pt. 3), 791–808. doi: 10.1093/brain/awh713

Gilbertson, T., Lalo, E., Doyle, L., Di Lazzaro, V., Cioni, B., and Brown, P. (2005). Existing motor state is favored at the expense of new movement during 13–35 Hz oscillatory synchrony in the human corticospinal system. *J. Neurosci.* 25, 7771–7779. doi: 10.1523/jneurosci.1762-05.2005

Gold, J. M. (2004). Cognitive deficits as treatment targets in schizophrenia. *Schizophr. Res.* 72, 21–28. doi: 10.1016/j.schres.2004.09.008

Green, M. F., Kern, R. S., Braff, D. L., and Mintz, J. (2000). Neurocognitive deficits and functional outcome in schizophrenia: are we measuring the "right stuff"? *Schizophr. Bull.* 26, 119–136. doi: 10.1093/oxfordjournals.schbul.a033430

Groppa, S., Bergmann, T. O., Siems, C., Mölle, M., Marshall, L., and Siebner, H. R. (2010). Slow-oscillatory transcranial direct current stimulation can induce bidirectional shifts in motor cortical excitability in awake humans. *Neuroscience* 166, 1219–1225. doi: 10.1016/j.neuroscience.2010.01.019

Gutchess, A. (2014). Plasticity of the aging brain: new directions in cognitive neuroscience. *Science* 346, 579–582. doi: 10.1126/science.1254604

Haegens, S., Osipova, D., Oostenveld, R., and Jensen, O. (2010). Somatosensory working memory performance in humans depends on both engagement and disengagement of regions in a distributed network. *Hum. Brain Mapp.* 31, 26–35. doi: 10.1002/hbm.20842

Hallett, M. (2007). Transcranial magnetic stimulation: a primer. *Neuron* 55, 187–199. doi: 10.1016/j.neuron.2007.06.026

Heinrichs-Graham, E., Wilson, T. W., Santamaria, P. M., Heithoff, S. K., Torres-Russotto, D., Hutter-Saunders, J. A. L., et al. (2014). Neuromagnetic evidence of abnormal movement-related beta desynchronization in Parkinson's disease. *Cereb. Cortex* 24, 2669–2678. doi: 10.1093/cercor/bht121

Helfrich, R. F., Schneider, T. R., Rach, S., Trautmann-Lengsfeld, S. A., Engel, A. K., and Herrmann, C. S. (2014). Entrainment of brain oscillations by transcranial alternating current stimulation. *Curr. Biol.* 24, 333–339. doi: 10.1016/j.cub.2013.12.041

Herrmann, C. S., Munk, M. H. J., and Engel, A. K. (2004). Cognitive functions of gamma-band activity: memory match and utilization. *Trends Cogn. Sci.* 8, 347–355. doi: 10.1016/j.tics.2004.06.006

Herz, D. M., Florin, E., Christensen, M. S., Reck, C., Barbe, M. T., Tscheuschler, M. K., et al. (2014). Dopamine replacement modulates oscillatory coupling between premotor and motor cortical areas in Parkinson's disease. *Cereb. Cortex* 24, 2873–2883. doi: 10.1093/cercor/bht140

Huang, Y.-Z., Edwards, M. J., Rounis, E., Bhatia, K. P., and Rothwell, J. C. (2005). Theta burst stimulation of the human motor cortex. *Neuron* 45, 201–206. doi: 10.1016/j.neuron.2004.12.033

Hummel, F., Andres, F., Altenmüeller, E., Dichgans, J., and Gerloff, C. (2002). Inhibitory control of acquired motor programmes in the human brain. *Brain* 125(Pt. 2), 404–420. doi: 10.1093/brain/awf030

Hummel, F., Celnik, P., Giraux, P., Floel, A., Wu, W.-H., Gerloff, C., et al. (2005). Effects of non-invasive cortical stimulation on skilled motor function in chronic stroke. *Brain* 128(Pt. 3), 490–499. doi: 10.1093/brain/awh369

Hummel, F. C., and Cohen, L. G. (2005). Drivers of brain plasticity. *Curr. Opin. Neurol.* 18, 667–674. doi: 10.1097/01.wco.0000189876.37475.42

Hummel, F., and Gerloff, C. (2005). Larger interregional synchrony is associated with greater behavioral success in a complex sensory integration task in humans. *Cereb. Cortex* 15, 670–678. doi: 10.1093/cercor/bhh170

Hummel, F. C., Voller, B., Celnik, P., Floel, A., Giraux, P., Gerloff, C., et al. (2006). Effects of brain polarization on reaction times and pinch force in chronic stroke. *BMC. Neurosci.* 7:73. doi: 10.1186/1471-2202-7-73

Jensen, O., Kaiser, J., and Lachaux, J.-P. (2007). Human gamma-frequency oscillations associated with attention and memory. *Trends Neurosci.* 30, 317–324. doi: 10.1016/j.tins.2007.05.001

Jensen, O., and Mazaheri, A. (2010). Shaping functional architecture by oscillatory alpha activity: gating by inhibition. *Front. Hum. Neurosci.* 4:186. doi: 10.3410/f.6253958.6325058

Johannesen, J. K., Kieffaber, P. D., O'Donnell, B. F., Shekhar, A., Evans, J. D., and Hetrick, W. P. (2005). Contributions of subtype and spectral frequency analyses to the study of P50 ERP amplitude and suppression in schizophrenia. *Schizophr. Res.* 78, 269–284. doi: 10.1016/j.schres.2005.05.022

Johansen-Berg, H., Rushworth, M. F. S., Bogdanovic, M. D., Kischka, U., Wimalaratna, S., and Matthews, P. M. (2002). The role of ipsilateral premotor cortex in hand movement after stroke. *Proc. Natl. Acad. Sci. U S A* 99, 14518–14523. doi: 10.1073/pnas.222536799

Joundi, R. A., Jenkinson, N., Brittain, J.-S., Aziz, T. Z., and Brown, P. (2012). Driving oscillatory activity in the human cortex enhances motor performance. *Curr. Biol.* 22, 403–407. doi: 10.1016/j.cub.2012.01.024

Kasashima, Y., Fujiwara, T., Matsushika, Y., Tsuji, T., Hase, K., Ushiyama, J., et al. (2012). Modulation of event-related desynchronization during motor imagery with transcranial direct current stimulation (tDCS) in patients with chronic hemiparetic stroke. *Exp. Brain Res.* 221, 263–268. doi: 10.1007/s00221-012-3166-9

Khedr, E. M., Farweez, H. M., and Islam, H. (2003). Therapeutic effect of repetitive transcranial magnetic stimulation on motor function in Parkinson's disease patients. *Eur. J. Neurol.* 10, 567–572. doi: 10.1046/j.1468-1331.2003.00649.x

Kilner, J. M., Baker, S. N., Salenius, S., Hari, R., and Lemon, R. N. (2000). Human cortical muscle coherence is directly related to specific motor parameters. *J. Neurosci.* 20, 8838–8845.

Kim, Y.-H., You, S. H., Ko, M.-H., Park, J.-W., Lee, K. H., Jang, S. H., et al. (2006). Repetitive transcranial magnetic stimulation-induced corticomotor excitability and associated motor skill acquisition in chronic stroke. *Stroke* 37, 1471–1476. doi: 10.1161/01.str.0000221233.55497.51

Klimesch, W., Sauseng, P., and Hanslmayr, S. (2007). EEG alpha oscillations: the inhibition–timing hypothesis. *Brain Res. Rev.* 53, 63–88. doi: 10.1016/j.brainresrev.2006.06.003

Kolominsky-Rabas, P. L., Weber, M., Gefeller, O., Neundoerfer, B., and Heuschmann, P. U. (2001). Epidemiology of ischemic stroke subtypes according to TOAST criteria: incidence, recurrence and long-term survival in ischemic stroke subtypes: a population-based study. *Stroke* 32, 2735–2740. doi: 10.1161/hs1201.100209

Kühn, A. A., Kempf, F., Brücke, C., Gaynor Doyle, L., Martinez-Torres, I., Pogosyan, A., et al. (2008). High-frequency stimulation of the subthalamic nucleus suppresses oscillatory beta activity in patients with Parkinson's disease in parallel with improvement in motor performance. *J. Neurosci.* 28, 6165–6173. doi: 10.1523/JNEUROSCI.0282-08.2008

Kühn, A. A., Tsui, A., Aziz, T., Ray, N., Brücke, C., Kupsch, A., et al. (2009). Pathological synchronisation in the subthalamic nucleus of patients with Parkinson's disease relates to both bradykinesia and rigidity. *Exp. Neurol.* 215, 380–387. doi: 10.1016/j.expneurol.2008.11.008

Laaksonen, K., Helle, L., Parkkonen, L., Kirveskari, E., Mäkelä, J. P., Mustanoja, S., et al. (2013). Alterations in spontaneous brain oscillations during stroke recovery. *PLoS One* 8:e61146. doi: 10.1371/journal.pone.0061146

Lapenta, O. M., Minati, L., Fregni, F., and Boggio, P. S. (2013). Je pense donc je fais: transcranial direct current stimulation modulates brain oscillations associated with motor imagery and movement observation. *Front. Hum. Neurosci.* 7:256. doi: 10.3389/fnhum.2013.00256

Lefaucheur, J.-P. (2006). Stroke recovery can be enhanced by using repetitive transcranial magnetic stimulation (rTMS). *Neurophysiol. Clin.* 36, 105–115. doi: 10.1016/j.neucli.2006.08.011

Levy, R., Ashby, P., Hutchison, W. D., Lang, A. E., Lozano, A. M., and Dostrovsky, J. O. (2002). Dependence of subthalamic nucleus oscillations on movement and dopamine in Parkinson's disease. *Brain* 125(Pt. 6), 1196–1209. doi: 10.1093/brain/awf128

Levy, R., Hutchison, W. D., Lozano, A. M., and Dostrovsky, J. O. (2000). High-frequency synchronization of neuronal activity in the subthalamic nucleus of parkinsonian patients with limb tremor. *J. Neurosci.* 20, 7766–7775.

Lewine, J. D., Davis, J. T., Sloan, J. H., Kodituwakku, P. W., and Orrison, W. W. (1999). Neuromagnetic assessment of pathophysiologic brain activity induced by minor head trauma. *AJNR Am. J. Neuroradiol.* 20, 857–866.

Light, G. A., Hsu, J. L., Hsieh, M. H., Meyer-Gomes, K., Sprock, J., Swerdlow, N. R., et al. (2006). Gamma band oscillations reveal neural network cortical coherence dysfunction in schizophrenia patients. *Biol. Psychiatry* 60, 1231–1240. doi: 10.1016/j.biopsych.2006.03.055

Little, S., Pogosyan, A., Neal, S., Zavala, B., Zrinzo, L., Hariz, M., et al. (2013). Adaptive deep brain stimulation in advanced Parkinson's disease. *Ann. Neurol.* 74, 449–457. doi: 10.1002/ana.23951

Marshall, L., Helgadóttir, H., Mölle, M., and Born, J. (2006). Boosting slow oscillations during sleep potentiates memory. *Nature* 444, 610–613. doi: 10.1038/nature05278

Marshall, L., Kirov, R., Brade, J., Mölle, M., and Born, J. (2011). Transcranial electrical currents to probe EEG brain rhythms and memory consolidation during sleep in humans. *PLoS One* 6:e16905. doi: 10.1371/journal.pone.0016905

McDonnell, M. N., Orekhov, Y., and Ziemann, U. (2006). The role of GABA(B) receptors in intracortical inhibition in the human motor cortex. *Exp. Brain Res.* 173, 86–93. doi: 10.1007/s00221-006-0365-2

McGrath, J., Saha, S., Chant, D., and Welham, J. (2008). Schizophrenia: a concise overview of incidence, prevalence and mortality. *Epidemiol. Rev.* 30, 67–76. doi: 10.1093/epirev/mxn001

Ming, G., Henley, J., Tessier-Lavigne, M., Song, H., and Poo, M. (2001). Electrical activity modulates growth cone guidance by diffusible factors. *Neuron* 29, 441–452. doi: 10.1016/s0896-6273(01)00217-3

Moss, F., Ward, L. M., and Sannita, W. G. (2004). Stochastic resonance and sensory information processing: a tutorial and review of application. *Clin. Neurophysiol.* 115, 267–281. doi: 10.1016/j.clinph.2003.09.014

Mulert, C., Kirsch, V., Pascual-Marqui, R., McCarley, R. W., and Spencer, K. M. (2011). Long-range synchrony of γ oscillations and auditory hallucination symptoms in schizophrenia. *Int. J. Psychophysiol.* 79, 55–63. doi: 10.1016/j.ijpsycho.2010.08.004

Murase, N., Duque, J., Mazzocchio, R., and Cohen, L. G. (2004). Influence of interhemispheric interactions on motor function in chronic stroke. *Ann. Neurol.* 55, 400–409. doi: 10.1002/ana.10848

Murray, C. J., and Lopez, A. D. (1997). Global mortality, disability and the contribution of risk factors: global burden of disease study. *Lancet* 349, 1436–1442. doi: 10.1016/s0140-6736(96)07495-8

Neuling, T., Rach, S., Wagner, S., Wolters, C. H., and Herrmann, C. S. (2012). Good vibrations: oscillatory phase shapes perception. *Neuroimage* 63, 771–778. doi: 10.1016/j.neuroimage.2012.07.024

Nitsche, M. A., and Paulus, W. (2000). Excitability changes induced in the human motor cortex by weak transcranial direct current stimulation. *J. Physiol.* 527(Pt. 3), 633–639. doi: 10.1111/j.1469-7793.2000.t01-1-00633.x

Noh, N. A., Fuggetta, G., Manganotti, P., and Fiaschi, A. (2012). Long lasting modulation of cortical oscillations after continuous theta burst transcranial magnetic stimulation. *PLoS One* 7:e35080. doi: 10.1371/journal.pone.0035080

Osipova, D., Hermes, D., and Jensen, O. (2008). Gamma power is phase-locked to posterior alpha activity. *PLoS One* 3:e3990. doi: 10.1371/journal.pone.0003990

Overman, J. J., Clarkson, A. N., Wanner, I. B., Overman, W. T., Eckstein, I., and Maguire, J. L. (2012). A role for ephrin-A5 in axonal sprouting , recovery and activity-dependent plasticity after stroke. *Proc. Natl. Acad. Sci. U S A* 109, E2230–E2239. doi: 10.1073/pnas.1204386109

Palva, S., and Palva, J. M. (2007). New vistas for alpha-frequency band oscillations. *Trends Neurosci.* 30, 150–158. doi: 10.1016/j.tins.2007.02.001

Pascual-Leone, A., Valls-Solé, J., Wassermann, E. M., and Hallett, M. (1994). Responses to rapid-rate transcranial magnetic stimulation of the human motor cortex. *Brain* 117(Pt. 4), 847–858. doi: 10.1093/brain/117.4.847

Pfurtscheller, G. (1992). Event-related synchronization (ERS): an electrophysiological correlate of cortical areas at rest. *Electroencephalogr. Clin. Neurophysiol.* 83, 62–69. doi: 10.1016/0013-4694(92)90133-3

Pfurtscheller, G., and Lopes da Silva, F. H. (1999). Event-related EEG/MEG synchronization and desynchronization: basic principles. *Clin. Neurophysiol.* 110, 1842–1857. doi: 10.1016/s1388-2457(99)00141-8

Pfurtscheller, G., Neuper, C., Brunner, C., and da Silva, F. L. (2005). Beta rebound after different types of motor imagery in man. *Neurosci. Lett.* 378, 156–159. doi: 10.1016/j.neulet.2004.12.034

Pfurtscheller, G., Stancák, A. Jr., and Neuper, C. (1996). Event-related synchronization (ERS) in the alpha band-an electrophysiological correlate of cortical idling: a review. *Int. J. Psychophysiol.* 24, 39–46. doi: 10.1016/s0167-8760(96)00066-9

Plewnia, C., Rilk, A. J., Soekadar, S. R., Arfeller, C., Huber, H. S., Sauseng, P., et al. (2008). Enhancement of long-range EEG coherence by synchronous bifocal transcranial magnetic stimulation. *Eur. J. Neurosci.* 27, 1577–1583. doi: 10.1111/j.1460-9568.2008.06124.x

Pogosyan, A., Gaynor, L. D., Eusebio, A., and Brown, P. (2009). Boosting cortical activity at beta-band frequencies slows movement in humans. *Curr. Biol.* 19, 1637–1641. doi: 10.1016/j.cub.2009.07.074

Ragazzoni, A., Pirulli, C., Veniero, D., Feurra, M., Cincotta, M., Giovannelli, F., et al. (2013). Vegetative versus minimally conscious states: a study using TMS-EEG, sensory and event-related potentials. *PLoS One* 8:e57069. doi: 10.1371/journal.pone.0057069

Rasch, B., and Born, J. (2013). About sleep's role in memory. *Physiol. Rev.* 93, 681–766. doi: 10.1152/physrev.00032.2012

Ray, N. J., Jenkinson, N., Wang, S., Holland, P., Brittain, J. S., Joint, C., et al. (2008). Local field potential beta activity in the subthalamic nucleus of patients with Parkinson's disease is associated with improvements in bradykinesia after dopamine and deep brain stimulation. *Exp. Neurol.* 213, 108–113. doi: 10.1016/j.expneurol.2008.05.008

Rehme, A. K., Eickhoff, S. B., Wang, L. E., Fink, G. R., and Grefkes, C. (2011). Dynamic causal modeling of cortical activity from the acute to the chronic stage after stroke. *Neuroimage* 55, 1147–1158. doi: 10.1016/j.neuroimage.2011.01.014

Rektor, I., Baláz, M., and Bocková, M. (2010). Cognitive event-related potentials and oscillations in the subthalamic nucleus. *Neurodegener. Dis.* 7, 160–162. doi: 10.1159/000289228

Rosanova, M., Casali, A., Bellina, V., Resta, F., Mariotti, M., and Massimini, M. (2009). Natural frequencies of human corticothalamic circuits. *J. Neurosci.* 29, 7679–7685. doi: 10.1523/JNEUROSCI.0445-09.2009

Saiote, C., Polanía, R., Rosenberger, K., Paulus, W., and Antal, A. (2013). High-frequency TRNS reduces BOLD activity during visuomotor learning. *PLoS One* 8:e59669. doi: 10.1371/journal.pone.0059669

Sauseng, P., Feldheim, J. F., Freunberger, R., and Hummel, F. C. (2011). Right prefrontal TMS disrupts interregional anticipatory EEG alpha activity during shifting of visuospatial attention. *Front. Psychol.* 2:241. doi: 10.3389/fpsyg.2011.00241

Sauseng, P., Gerloff, C., and Hummel, F. C. (2013). Two brakes are better than one: the neural bases of inhibitory control of motor memory traces. *Neuroimage* 65, 52–58. doi: 10.1016/j.neuroimage.2012.09.048

Schoffelen, J.-M., Oostenveld, R., and Fries, P. (2005). Neuronal coherence as a mechanism of effective corticospinal interaction. *Science* 308, 111–113. doi: 10.1126/science.1107027

Schulz, R., Gerloff, C., and Hummel, F. C. (2013). Non-invasive brain stimulation in neurological diseases. *Neuropharmacology* 64, 579–587. doi: 10.1016/j.neuropharm.2012.05.016

Siebner, H. R., Rossmeier, C., Mentschel, C., Peinemann, A., and Conrad, B. (2000). Short-term motor improvement after sub-threshold 5-Hz repetitive transcranial magnetic stimulation of the primary motor hand area in Parkinson's disease. *J. Neurol. Sci.* 178, 91–94. doi: 10.1016/s0022-510x(00)00370-1

Siebner, H. R., and Ziemann, U. (2010). Rippling the cortex with high-frequency (>100 Hz) alternating current stimulation. *J. Physiol.* 588(Pt. 24), 4851–4852. doi: 10.1113/jphysiol.2010.200857

Singer, W., and Gray, C. M. (1995). Visual feature integration and the temporal correlation hypothesis. *Annu. Rev. Neurosci.* 18, 555–586. doi: 10.1146/annurev.neuro.18.1.555

Stam, C. J., Nolte, G., and Daffertshofer, A. (2007). Phase lag index: assessment of functional connectivity from multi channel EEG and MEG with diminished bias from common sources. *Hum. Brain Mapp.* 28, 1178–1193. doi: 10.1002/hbm.20346

Sun, Y., Farzan, F., Barr, M. S., Kirihara, K., Fitzgerald, P. B., Light, G. A., et al. (2011). γ Oscillations in schizophrenia: mechanisms and clinical significance. *Brain Res.* 1413, 98–114. doi: 10.1016/j.brainres.2011.06.065

Tallon-Baudry, C., Bertrand, O., Peronnet, F., and Pernier, J. (1998). Induced gamma-band activity during the delay of a visual short-term memory task in humans. *J. Neurosci.* 18, 4244–4254.

Tecchio, F., Pasqualetti, P., Zappasodi, F., Tombini, M., Lupoi, D., Vernieri, F., et al. (2007). Outcome prediction in acute monohemispheric stroke via magnetoencephalography. *J. Neurol.* 254, 296–305. doi: 10.1007/s00415-006-0355-0

Tecchio, F., Zappasodi, F., Pasqualetti, P., Tombini, M., Caulo, M., Ercolani, M., et al. (2006). Long-term effects of stroke on neuronal rest activity in rolandic cortical areas. *J. Neurosci. Res.* 83, 1077–1087. doi: 10.1002/jnr.20796

Tecchio, F., Zappasodi, F., Pasqualetti, P., Tombini, M., Salustri, C., Oliviero, A., et al. (2005). Rhythmic brain activity at rest from rolandic areas in acute mono-hemispheric stroke: a magnetoencephalographic study. *Neuroimage* 28, 72–83. doi: 10.1016/j.neuroimage.2005.05.051

Terney, D., Chaieb, L., Moliadze, V., Antal, A., and Paulus, W. (2008). Increasing human brain excitability by transcranial high-frequency random noise stimulation. *J. Neurosci.* 28, 14147–14155. doi: 10.1523/JNEUROSCI.4248-08.2008

Thut, G., Veniero, D., Romei, V., Miniussi, C., Schyns, P., and Gross, J. (2011). Rhythmic TMS causes local entrainment of natural oscillatory signatures. *Curr. Biol.* 21, 1176–1185. doi: 10.1016/j.cub.2011.05.049

Uhlhaas, P. J., Haenschel, C., Nikolić, D., and Singer, W. (2008). The role of oscillations and synchrony in cortical networks and their putative relevance for the pathophysiology of schizophrenia. *Schizophr. Bull.* 34, 927–943. doi: 10.1093/schbul/sbn062

Varela, F., Lachaux, J. P., Rodriguez, E., and Martinerie, J. (2001). The brainweb: phase synchronization and large-scale integration. *Nat. Rev. Neurosci.* 2, 229–239. doi: 10.1038/35067550

Veniero, D., Brignani, D., Thut, G., and Miniussi, C. (2011). Alpha-generation as basic response-signature to transcranial magnetic stimulation (TMS) targeting the human resting motor cortex: a TMS/EEG co-registration study. *Psychophysiology* 48, 1381–1389. doi: 10.1111/j.1469-8986.2011.01218.x

Vernet, M., Bashir, S., Yoo, W.-K., Perez, J. M., Najib, U., and Pascual-Leone, A. (2013). Insights on the neural basis of motor plasticity induced by theta burst stimulation from TMS-EEG. *Eur. J. Neurosci.* 37, 598–606. doi: 10.1111/ejn.12069

von Campenhausen, S., Bornschein, B., Wick, R., Bötzel, K., Sampaio, C., Poewe, W., et al. (2005). Prevalence and incidence of Parkinson's disease in Europe. *Eur. Neuropsychopharmacol.* 15, 473–490. doi: 10.1016/j.euroneuro.2005.04.007

Wang, X. J., and Buzsáki, G. (1996). Gamma oscillation by synaptic inhibition in a hippocampal interneuronal network model. *J. Neurosci.* 16, 6402–6413.

Ward, N. S., Brown, M. M., Thompson, A. J., and Frackowiak, R. S. J. (2003). Neural correlates of motor recovery after stroke: a longitudinal fMRI study. *Brain* 126(Pt. 11), 2476–2496. doi: 10.1093/brain/awg245

Westlake, K. P., Hinkley, L. B., Bucci, M., Guggisberg, A. G., Byl, N., Findlay, A. M., et al. (2012). Resting state α-band functional connectivity and recovery after stroke. *Exp. Neurol.* 237, 160–169. doi: 10.1016/j.expneurol.2012.06.020

Williams, E. R., Soteropoulos, D. S., and Baker, S. N. (2010). Spinal interneuron circuits reduce approximately 10-Hz movement discontinuities by phase cancellation. *Proc. Natl. Acad. Sci. U S A* 107, 11098–11103. doi: 10.1073/pnas.0913373107

Zaehle, T., Rach, S., and Herrmann, C. S. (2010). Transcranial alternating current stimulation enhances individual alpha activity in human EEG. *PLoS One* 5:e13766. doi: 10.1371/journal.pone.0013766

18

Self-regulation of blood oxygenation level dependent response: primary effect or epiphenomenon?

Andrea Caria [1,2]*

[1] *Department of Psychology and Cognitive Science, University of Trento, Rovereto, Italy,* [2] *Institute of Medical Psychology and Behavioral Neurobiology, Eberhard-Karls-University of Tübingen, Tübingen, Germany*

Keywords: real-time fMRI, BOLD signal, neurofeedback, self-regulation

Edited by:
Manuel Fernando Casanova, University of Louisville, USA

Reviewed by:
Hari S. Sharma, Uppsala University, Sweden
Victor Manuel Pulgar, Wake Forest School of Medicine, USA

Correspondence:
Andrea Caria
andrea.caria@unitn.it

In the last decade, several studies indicated that neuronal activity can be volitionally modulated using real-time fMRI (rtfMRI) based neurofeedback. Human participants through rtfMRI paradigms can learn to regulate the blood oxygenation level dependent (BOLD) response in several localized cortical and subcortical regions (for extended reviews see Caria et al., 2012; Weiskopf, 2012; Sulzer et al., 2013). Increasing evidence also indicated that strengthening or weakening specific BOLD activity using rtfMRI training leads to significant changes in cognitive, emotional and motor behavior (Caria et al., 2012; Weiskopf, 2012; Sulzer et al., 2013). These findings suggested that rtfMRI might represent an important novel approach in cognitive neuroscience by potentially providing indications of cause-and-effect relationships between brain and behavior, and also in clinical applications (Subramanian et al., 2011; Linden et al., 2012; Ruiz et al., 2013; Sitaram et al., 2014).

Although rtfMRI studies extend and enrich a large body of literature demonstrating operant learning of neuronal oscillations, skepticism still exists on the validity and reliability of studies showing learned control of the BOLD response. In particular, it is still debated whether this phenomenon is a primary effect of learning or it just an epiphenomenon resulting, for instance, from repeated execution of some mental processes.

Here, I will discuss specific psychophysiological and neurophysiological mechanisms presumably underlying learned regulation of the BOLD response to attempt to clarify its nature.

OPERANT LEARNING OF THE BOLD RESPONSE

Direct manipulation of brain activity grounds on the principles of operant conditioning that describe the relationship between changes in behavior (in this case the neurophysiological response) as consequence of contingent environmental events. Reinforcement is the mechanism that allows participants to increase the frequency of specific brain activity and to shape the desired pattern of neuronal activations. During operant learning of the BOLD response participants are reinforced proportionally to how much the ongoing metabolic signal approach or resemble the target level of activation in single or multiple regions of interest. The information of the ongoing signal fluctuations, provided as explicit visual feedback to the participants, represents the intrinsic reward.

Operant learning is an important approach for manipulating brain functions (Birbaumer and Kimmel, 1979) acting on intrinsic physiological properties of neuronal activity, which have been extensively shown to undergo classical and operant conditioning (Kandel and Schwartz, 1982).

The application of operant control principles to metabolic signals builds on several previous experiments demonstrating operant control of neuroeletric activity in non-human and human animals (Birbaumer and Kimmel, 1979; Fetz, 2007). Studies on volitional control of neural activity dates back to the late sixties and seventies when operant conditioning of central nervous system activity was demonstrated (Olds, 1965; Fetz, 1969; Shinkman et al., 1974). CNS unit conditioning was shown by operantly rewarding rats to increase the activity of midbrain neurons using intracranial stimulation (Olds, 1965). In 1969, Fetz demonstrated conditioning of the activity of single neurons in precentral cortex in anesthetized monkeys by reinforcing high rates of neuronal discharge with food reward and auditory or visual feedback of unit firing rates (Fetz, 1969). More recently, Brain-Computer Interface and Brain-Machine interface studies reported volitional control of cortical cell activity, in particular in the motor cortex, in both animals and humans (Serruya et al., 2002; Taylor et al., 2002; Carmena et al., 2003; Moritz et al., 2008), with food reward and visual feedback of neuronal ensembles' activity. Altogether these findings robustly proved that neuronal activity from localized brain areas can be manipulated through operant conditioning.

On the other hand, there are unclear aspects of operant conditioning of the BOLD response in humans that make rtfMRI neurofeedback paradigms not fully established. Among these is the role of mental and cognitive processes for learning. Some rtfMRI studies indicated that successful BOLD regulation relies on the use of mental imagery (Chiew et al., 2012; Banca et al., 2015; Blefari et al., 2015). In particular, these studies suggested that strategies based on mental imagery are important for learning BOLD control considering the partial common substrates for internal representations and overt behavior, which holds in particular for the primary motor (Jeannerod, 1995; Roth et al., 1996; Jeannerod and Frak, 1999; Niyazov et al., 2005) and visual areas (Kosslyn and Thompson, 2003; Klein et al., 2004; Slotnick et al., 2005). On the contrary, other studies indicated that a combination of cognitive strategies (mental imagery) and feedback information is critical for participants to learn BOLD regulation, and that cognitive and imagery alone is not sufficient (decharms et al., 2005; Bray et al., 2007; Caria et al., 2010; Scharnowski et al., 2012). In particular, mere repetition of mental strategies leads to an initial increase of BOLD signal but to a rapid decrease in the following consecutive runs (Caria et al., 2010). In fact, fMRI adaptation paradigms (Kourtzi and Kanwisher, 2001) show that task repetition leads to a decrease of the BOLD signal.

In addition, while it is true that imagery and cognitive processing certainly affect learning and physiological regulation, studies on operant control of brain oscillations suggest that feedback is more important than instructions for successful slow cortical potentials regulation (Roberts et al., 1989; Birbaumer et al., 1990). There are indications from EEG based neurofeedback studies that mental imagery is efficacious initially but it would be then dropped when participants become more confident with self-regulation (Leuthardt et al., 2004). Ultimately, control of neuroelectric activity turns to a highly implicit process over training, and the contribution of higher order cognitive processes becomes negligible. Indeed, control of neurophysiological signals can even be attained when participants have little or no direct experience of it (Rockstroh et al., 1984). However, until now there exist no clear demonstrations that these mechanisms, although plausible, hold also for learned metabolic signals.

In most rtfMRI studies participants were aware of the responses leading to reward. Only one study reported to have employed implicit visual task and feedback to learn BOLD control in V1/V2 areas, however participants still reported to have used explicit mental strategies (Shibata et al., 2011).

In short, the fact that operant control of brain activity, even single cell responses is possible also in animals speaks against a fundamental influence of cognitive factors on the effect of operant brain regulation. On the other hand, it is conceivable that in human participants the combination of specific conscious processes and operant strategies might support retention of learned BOLD control out of the laboratory setting, and might facilitate the (re-)activation of impaired or dormant mechanisms, in particular in patients.

WHAT NEUROPHYSIOLOGICAL MECHANISMS MEDIATE LEARNED BOLD CONTROL?

A further issue of rtfMRI experiments is the unclear neurophysiology of the BOLD signal, which prevents us to univocally interpret the behavioral changes induced by operant learning of the metabolic signal. We know from previous investigations on instrumental learning of neuroelectric signals that the brain has intrinsic neurophysiological processes allowing regulation of neural activity even in the absence of external stimuli (Wolpaw et al., 2002; Birbaumer and Cohen, 2007; Fetz, 2007). While no specific receptors directly support regulation of brain oscillations, it exists a complex neurovascular system that regulates and controls the BOLD signal.

At least three main blood flow regulatory mechanisms have been described: cerebral autoregulation—the brain ability to maintain a constant flow through changes of cerebral perfusion pressure—neurogenic regulation—the cerebral blood flow modulation through extensive arborization of perivascular nerves—and flow-metabolism coupling, or functional hyperemia—the brain capacity to vary blood flow to match metabolic activity (Peterson et al., 2011). Endothelial cells and astrocytes play a central role in all these regulatory mechanisms (Iadecola and Nedergaard, 2007): the former by providing several vasoactive factors for the regulation of cerebral blood flow and the latter because of their anatomical position that physically links the cerebral microvasculature with synapses.

Learned increase and decrease of BOLD activity might indeed be associated with variations in the flow-metabolism coupling. Local changes in neural activity have been shown to influence BOLD signal (Buxton et al., 2004; Logothetis and Wandell, 2004; Lee et al., 2010) through variations in cerebral blood flow (CBF), cerebral blood volume (CBV) and cerebral metabolic rate of oxygen consumption (CMRO2). It has been also demonstrated that changes in the coupling ratio of CBF and CMRO2 in response to neural activity strongly affect the BOLD response (Kim and Ogawa, 2012; Buxton et al., 2014). Considering such complexity of the neurovascular system, it is thus conceivable that learned control of the BOLD response might be based on these sophisticated regulatory mechanisms.

An intriguing perspective for rtfMRI neurofeedback arises from the hypothesis proposing that modulation of brain activity is directly and causally affected by changes of metabolic signals (Moore and Cao, 2008). Specifically, it has been conjectured that the brain vascular system, being a complex and interconnected network under tight regulatory control that occurs in close communication with neurons and glia, might directly contribute to information processing (Moore and Cao, 2008). Accordingly, the hemodynamic processes would not only support metabolic demand but also directly shape brain functions; self-regulation of metabolic signals might thus induce changes of neuronal activations. In line with this perspective non-invasive direct electrical stimulation (e.g., using transcranial direct electric stimulation, tDCS) targeting cerebral microvessels has been proposed to enhance brain functions trough changes of cerebrovascular function (Dutta, 2015; Pulgar, 2015).

So far, despite the increasing number of hypotheses and studies aiming to clarify the nature of the BOLD response, the neurometabolic coupling of this signal remains unclear. It has been shown that the BOLD fMRI response correlates with local field potentials (Logothetis et al., 2001; Viswanathan and Freeman, 2007), with spiking activity (Heeger and Ress, 2002), and with both LFP and spiking activity (Mukamel et al., 2005). In addition, BOLD signal can reflect different brain processing such as excitatory and inhibitory activity, neuromodulation, and bottom-up and top-down signals (Viswanathan and Freeman, 2007; Logothetis, 2008; Lee et al., 2010).

On the basis of this evidence it is difficult to infer whether the net effect of self-regulation of BOLD signal is excitatory, inhibitory or a combination or both. On the other hand, rtfMRI studies, although sometimes controversial, often reported an improvement of subjects' performance associated with increased amplitude of the BOLD response (decharms et al., 2005; Bray et al., 2007; Rota et al., 2009; Caria et al., 2010; Scharnowski et al., 2012, 2015; Zhang et al., 2013; Blefari et al., 2015). For instance, studies showed a decrease in reaction times for task execution associated with increase activity of the primary motor cortex (M1), and for task initiation after up-regulation of the SMA (Scharnowski et al., 2015). M1 activity was also positively correlated with accuracy improvement of performance during an isometric pinching task (Blefari et al., 2015) In the visual domain, increased visual perception was induced by increased BOLD response in the visual cortex (Scharnowski et al., 2012). Moreover, enhanced emotional response was associated with increased percentage BOLD signal change in the left anterior insula (Caria et al., 2010). Importantly, these studies reported poorer performance either during initial regulation runs or after down-regulation. Altogether these findings suggest that learned increase of the BOLD response might be associated with increased excitatory activity. This assumption would be also supported by studies showing improved memory performance associated with decreased BOLD activity in the parahippocampal cortex (Yoo et al., 2012; Scharnowski et al., 2015), which was then interpreted as result of increased brain resources for memory encoding because of decreased cortical processing (Yoo et al., 2012). Indeed, increased BOLD signal might occur from increased net excitation associated with glutamatergic activity (Logothetis, 2008). However, this represents only one possible interpretation, as larger BOLD signal can also be induced by concurrent increase of both glutamatergic and GABAergic activity, with changes in hemodynamic responses reflecting balanced local recurrent activity (Logothetis, 2008). In line with this alternative mechanism, it has been shown that enhanced perceptual sensitivity induced by fMRI feedback training results from a mixture of positive and negative activated voxels in the targeted regions of interest rather than from uniform positive or negative activity (Shibata et al., 2011).

Therefore, fMRI neurofeedback might also rely on, and possibly alter, the capacity of the cerebral cortex to generate persistent activity in the absence of sensory stimulation (Haider et al., 2006), which would in turn influence neuronal responsiveness to a wide range of inputs (Shu et al., 2003a). In addition, as the ongoing network activity can be turned on and off by synaptic inputs via electrical stimulation (Shu et al., 2003b), it can also be postulated its self-regulation via operant conditioning.

CONCLUSIONS

In short, the observed behavioral changes induced by rtfMRI training might be related to several plausible neurophysiological processes, and it is still not possible to conclusively ascertain the actual mechanism on the basis of the current results. Multimodal measurements such as simultaneous EEG-rtfMRI acquisition, as well as alternative real-time functional imaging methods such as MR perfusion and MR spectroscopy, might help to clarify the neurophysiological mechanisms underlying learned control of the BOLD response. Nevertheless, there exist clear indications that self-regulation of BOLD signal is not an epiphenomenon but a primary effect of operant learning, which can rely on precise neurovascular regulatory mechanisms.

AUTHOR CONTRIBUTIONS

The author confirms being the sole contributor of this work and approved it for publication.

ACKNOWLEDGMENTS

This work is part of the BRAINTRAIN European research network (Collaborative Project) supported by the European Commission under the Health Cooperation Work Programme of the 7th Framework Programme (Grant agreement n° 602186).

REFERENCES

Banca, P., Sousa, T., Catarina Duarte, I., and Castelo-Branco, M. (2015). Visual motion imagery neurofeedback based on the hMT+/V5 complex: evidence for a feedback-specific neural circuit involving neocortical and cerebellar regions. *J. Neural Eng.* 12:066003. doi: 10.1088/1741-2560/12/6/066003

Birbaumer, N., and Cohen, L. G. (2007). Brain-computer interfaces: communication and restoration of movement in paralysis. *J. Physiol.* 579, 621–636. doi: 10.1113/jphysiol.2006.125633

Birbaumer, N., Elbert, T., Canavan, A. G., and Rockstroh, B. (1990). Slow potentials of the cerebral cortex and behavior. *Physiol. Rev.* 70, 1–41.

Birbaumer, N., and Kimmel, H. (1979). *Biofeedback and Self-Regulation.* Hillsdale, NJ: Erlbaum.

Blefari, M. L., Sulzer, J., Hepp-Reymond, M. C., Kollias, S., and Gassert, R. (2015). Improvement in precision grip force control with self-modulation of primary motor cortex during motor imagery. *Front. Behav. Neurosci.* 9:18. doi: 10.3389/fnbeh.2015.00018

Bray, S., Shimojo, S., and O'doherty, J. P. (2007). Direct instrumental conditioning of neural activity using functional magnetic resonance imaging-derived reward feedback. *J. Neurosci.* 27, 7498–7507. doi: 10.1523/JNEUROSCI.2118-07.2007

Buxton, R. B., Griffeth, V. E., Simon, A. B., Moradi, F., and Shmuel, A. (2014). Variability of the coupling of blood flow and oxygen metabolism responses in the brain: a problem for interpreting BOLD studies but potentially a new window on the underlying neural activity. *Front. Neurosci.* 8:139. doi: 10.3389/fnins.2014.00139

Buxton, R. B., Uludag, K., Dubowitz, D. J., and Liu, T. T. (2004). Modeling the hemodynamic response to brain activation. *Neuroimage* 23(Suppl. 1), S220–S233. doi: 10.1016/j.neuroimage.2004.07.013

Caria, A., Sitaram, R., and Birbaumer, N. (2012). Real-time fMRI: a tool for local brain regulation. *Neuroscientist* 18, 487–501. doi: 10.1177/1073858411407205

Caria, A., Sitaram, R., Veit, R., Begliomini, C., and Birbaumer, N. (2010). Volitional control of anterior insula activity modulates the response to aversive stimuli. A real-time functional magnetic resonance imaging study. *Biol. Psychiatry* 68, 425–432. doi: 10.1016/j.biopsych.2010.04.020

Carmena, J. M., Lebedev, M. A., Crist, R. E., O'doherty, J. E., Santucci, D. M., Dimitrov, D. F., et al. (2003). Learning to control a brain-machine interface for reaching and grasping by primates. *PLoS Biol.* 1:E42. doi: 10.1371/journal.pbio.0000042

Chiew, M., Laconte, S. M., and Graham, S. J. (2012). Investigation of fMRI neurofeedback of differential primary motor cortex activity using kinesthetic motor imagery. *Neuroimage* 61, 21–31. doi: 10.1016/j.neuroimage.2012.02.053

decharms, R. C., Maeda, F., Glover, G. H., Ludlow, D., Pauly, J. M., Soneji, D., et al. (2005). Control over brain activation and pain learned by using real-time functional MRI. *Proc. Natl. Acad. Sci. U.S.A.* 102, 18626–18631. doi: 10.1073/pnas.0505210102

Dutta, A. (2015). Bidirectional interactions between neuronal and hemodynamic responses to transcranial direct current stimulation (tDCS): challenges for brain-state dependent tDCS. *Front. Syst. Neurosci.* 9:107. doi: 10.3389/fnsys.2015.00107

Fetz, E. E. (1969). Operant conditioning of cortical unit activity. *Science* 163, 955–958. doi: 10.1126/science.163.3870.955

Fetz, E. E. (2007). Volitional control of neural activity: implications for brain-computer interfaces. *J. Physiol.* 579, 571–579. doi: 10.1113/jphysiol.2006.127142

Haider, B., Duque, A., Hasenstaub, A. R., and Mccormick, D. A. (2006). Neocortical network activity *in vivo* is generated through a dynamic balance of excitation and inhibition. *J. Neurosci.* 26, 4535–4545. doi: 10.1523/JNEUROSCI.5297-05.2006

Heeger, D. J., and Ress, D. (2002). What does fMRI tell us about neuronal activity? *Nat. Rev. Neurosci.* 3, 142–151. doi: 10.1038/nrn730

Iadecola, C., and Nedergaard, M. (2007). Glial regulation of the cerebral microvasculature. *Nat. Neurosci.* 10, 1369–1376. doi: 10.1038/nn2003

Jeannerod, M. (1995). Mental imagery in the motor context. *Neuropsychologia* 33, 1419–1432. doi: 10.1016/0028-3932(95)00073-C

Jeannerod, M., and Frak, V. (1999). Mental imaging of motor activity in humans. *Curr. Opin. Neurobiol.* 9, 735–739. doi: 10.1016/S0959-4388(99)00038-0

Kandel, E. R., and Schwartz, J. H. (1982). Molecular biology of learning: modulation of transmitter release. *Science* 218, 433–443. doi: 10.1126/science.6289442

Kim, S. G., and Ogawa, S. (2012). Biophysical and physiological origins of blood oxygenation level-dependent fMRI signals. *J. Cereb. Blood Flow Metab.* 32, 1188–1206. doi: 10.1038/jcbfm.2012.23

Klein, I., Dubois, J., Mangin, J. F., Kherif, F., Flandin, G., Poline, J. B., et al. (2004). Retinotopic organization of visual mental images as revealed by functional magnetic resonance imaging. *Brain Res. Cogn. Brain Res.* 22, 26–31. doi: 10.1016/j.cogbrainres.2004.07.006

Kosslyn, S. M., and Thompson, W. L. (2003). When is early visual cortex activated during visual mental imagery? *Psychol. Bull.* 129, 723–746. doi: 10.1037/0033-2909.129.5.723

Kourtzi, Z., and Kanwisher, N. (2001). Representation of perceived object shape by the human lateral occipital complex. *Science* 293, 1506–1509. doi: 10.1126/science.1061133

Lee, J. H., Durand, R., Gradinaru, V., Zhang, F., Goshen, I., Kim, D. S., et al. (2010). Global and local fMRI signals driven by neurons defined optogenetically by type and wiring. *Nature* 465, 788–792. doi: 10.1038/nature09108

Leuthardt, E. C., Schalk, G., Wolpaw, J. R., Ojemann, J. G., and Moran, D. W. (2004). A brain-computer interface using electrocorticographic signals in humans. *J. Neural Eng.* 1, 63–71. doi: 10.1088/1741-2560/1/2/001

Linden, D. E., Habes, I., Johnston, S. J., Linden, S., Tatineni, R., Subramanian, L., et al. (2012). Real-time self-regulation of emotion networks in patients with depression. *PLoS ONE* 7:e38115. doi: 10.1371/journal.pone.0038115

Logothetis, N. K. (2008). What we can do and what we cannot do with fMRI. *Nature* 453, 869–878. doi: 10.1038/nature06976

Logothetis, N. K., Pauls, J., Augath, M., Trinath, T., and Oeltermann, A. (2001). Neurophysiological investigation of the basis of the fMRI signal. *Nature* 412, 150–157. doi: 10.1038/35084005

Logothetis, N. K., and Wandell, B. A. (2004). Interpreting the BOLD signal. *Annu. Rev. Physiol.* 66, 735–769. doi: 10.1146/annurev.physiol.66.082602.092845

Moore, C. I., and Cao, R. (2008). The hemo-neural hypothesis: on the role of blood flow in information processing. *J. Neurophysiol.* 99, 2035–2047. doi: 10.1152/jn.01366.2006

Moritz, C. T., Perlmutter, S. I., and Fetz, E. E. (2008). Direct control of paralysed muscles by cortical neurons. *Nature* 456, 639–642. doi: 10.1038/nature07418

Mukamel, R., Gelbard, H., Arieli, A., Hasson, U., Fried, I., and Malach, R. (2005). Coupling between neuronal firing, field potentials, and FMRI in human auditory cortex. *Science* 309, 951–954. doi: 10.1126/science.1110913

Niyazov, D. M., Butler, A. J., Kadah, Y. M., Epstein, C. M., and Hu, X. P. (2005). Functional magnetic resonance imaging and transcranial magnetic stimulation: effects of motor imagery, movement and coil orientation. *Clin. Neurophysiol.* 116, 1601–1610. doi: 10.1016/j.clinph.2005.02.028

Olds, J. (1965). Operant conditioning of single unit responses. *Excerpta Med. Int. Cong. Series* 87, 372–380.

Peterson, E. C., Wang, Z., and Britz, G. (2011). Regulation of cerebral blood flow. *Int. J. Vasc. Med.* 2011:823525. doi: 10.1155/2011/823525

Pulgar, V. M. (2015). Direct electric stimulation to increase cerebrovascular function. *Front. Syst. Neurosci.* 9:54. doi: 10.3389/fnsys.2015.00054

Roberts, L. E., Birbaumer, N., Rockstroh, B., Lutzenberger, W., and Elbert, T. (1989). Self-report during feedback regulation of slow cortical potentials. *Psychophysiology* 26, 392–403. doi: 10.1111/j.1469-8986.1989.tb01941.x

Rockstroh, B., Birbaumer, N., Elbert, T., and Lutzenberger, W. (1984). Operant control of EEG and event-related and slow brain potentials. *Biofeedback Self Regul.* 9, 139–160. doi: 10.1007/BF00998830

Rota, G., Sitaram, R., Veit, R., Erb, M., Weiskopf, N., Dogil, G., et al. (2009). Self-regulation of regional cortical activity using real-time fMRI: the right inferior frontal gyrus and linguistic processing. *Hum. Brain Mapp.* 30, 1605–1614. doi: 10.1002/hbm.20621

Roth, M., Decety, J., Raybaudi, M., Massarelli, R., Delon-Martin, C., Segebarth, C., et al. (1996). Possible involvement of primary motor cortex in mentally simulated movement: a functional magnetic resonance imaging study. *Neuroreport* 7, 1280–1284. doi: 10.1097/00001756-199605170-00012

Ruiz, S., Lee, S., Soekadar, S. R., Caria, A., Veit, R., Kircher, T., et al. (2013). Acquired self-control of insula cortex modulates emotion recognition and brain network connectivity in schizophrenia. *Hum. Brain Mapp.* 34, 200–212. doi: 10.1002/hbm.21427

Scharnowski, F., Hutton, C., Josephs, O., Weiskopf, N., and Rees, G. (2012). Improving visual perception through neurofeedback. *J. Neurosci.* 32, 17830–17841. doi: 10.1523/JNEUROSCI.6334-11.2012

Scharnowski, F., Veit, R., Zopf, R., Studer, P., Bock, S., Diedrichsen, J., et al. (2015). Manipulating motor performance and memory through real-time fMRI neurofeedback. *Biol. Psychol.* 108, 85–97. doi: 10.1016/j.biopsycho.2015.03.009

Serruya, M. D., Hatsopoulos, N. G., Paninski, L., Fellows, M. R., and Donoghue, J. P. (2002). Instant neural control of a movement signal. *Nature* 416, 141–142. doi: 10.1038/416141a

Shibata, K., Watanabe, T., Sasaki, Y., and Kawato, M. (2011). Perceptual learning incepted by decoded fMRI neurofeedback without stimulus presentation. *Science* 334, 1413–1415. doi: 10.1126/science.1212003

Shinkman, P. G., Bruce, C. J., and Pfingst, B. E. (1974). Operant conditioning of single-unit response patterns in visual cortex. *Science* 184, 1194–1196. doi: 10.1126/science.184.4142.1194

Shu, Y., Hasenstaub, A., Badoual, M., Bal, T., and Mccormick, D. A. (2003a). Barrages of synaptic activity control the gain and sensitivity of cortical neurons. *J. Neurosci.* 23, 10388–10401.

Shu, Y., Hasenstaub, A., and Mccormick, D. A. (2003b). Turning on and off recurrent balanced cortical activity. *Nature* 423, 288–293. doi: 10.1038/nature01616

Sitaram, R., Caria, A., Veit, R., Gaber, T., Ruiz, S., and Birbaumer, N. (2014). Volitional control of the anterior insula in criminal psychopaths using real-time fMRI neurofeedback: a pilot study. *Front. Behav. Neurosci.* 8:344. doi: 10.3389/fnbeh.2014.00344

Slotnick, S. D., Thompson, W. L., and Kosslyn, S. M. (2005). Visual mental imagery induces retinotopically organized activation of early visual areas. *Cereb. Cortex* 15, 1570–1583. doi: 10.1093/cercor/bhi035

Subramanian, L., Hindle, J. V., Johnston, S., Roberts, M. V., Husain, M., Goebel, R., et al. (2011). Real-time functional magnetic resonance imaging neurofeedback for treatment of Parkinson's disease. *J. Neurosci.* 31, 16309–16317. doi: 10.1523/JNEUROSCI.3498-11.2011

Sulzer, J., Haller, S., Scharnowski, F., Weiskopf, N., Birbaumer, N., Blefari, M. L., et al. (2013). Real-time fMRI neurofeedback: progress and challenges. *Neuroimage* 76, 386–399. doi: 10.1016/j.neuroimage.2013.03.033

Taylor, D. M., Tillery, S. I., and Schwartz, A. B. (2002). Direct cortical control of 3D neuroprosthetic devices. *Science* 296, 1829–1832. doi: 10.1126/science.1070291

Viswanathan, A., and Freeman, R. D. (2007). Neurometabolic coupling in cerebral cortex reflects synaptic more than spiking activity. *Nat. Neurosci.* 10, 1308–1312. doi: 10.1038/nn1977

Weiskopf, N. (2012). Real-time fMRI and its application to neurofeedback. *Neuroimage* 62, 682–692. doi: 10.1016/j.neuroimage.2011.10.009

Wolpaw, J. R., Birbaumer, N., Mcfarland, D. J., Pfurtscheller, G., and Vaughan, T. M. (2002). Brain-computer interfaces for communication and control. *Clin. Neurophysiol.* 113, 767–791. doi: 10.1016/S1388-2457(02)00057-3

Yoo, J. J., Hinds, O., Ofen, N., Thompson, T. W., Whitfield-Gabrieli, S., Triantafyllou, C., et al. (2012). When the brain is prepared to learn: enhancing human learning using real-time fMRI. *Neuroimage* 59, 846–852. doi: 10.1016/j.neuroimage.2011.07.063

Zhang, G., Yao, L., Zhang, H., Long, Z., and Zhao, X. (2013). Improved working memory performance through self-regulation of dorsal lateral prefrontal cortex activation using real-time fMRI. *PLoS ONE* 8:e73735. doi: 10.1371/journal.pone.0073735

19

Prefrontal tDCS decreases pain in patients with multiple sclerosis

Samar S. Ayache[1,2,3†], Ulrich Palm[1,4†], Moussa A. Chalah[1,2], Tarik Al-Ani[1], Arnaud Brignol[5], Mohamed Abdellaoui[6], Dalia Dimitri[6], Marc Sorel[1], Alain Créange[1,6] and Jean-Pascal Lefaucheur[1,2]*

[1] EA 4391, Excitabilité Nerveuse et Thérapeutique, Université Paris-Est-Créteil, Créteil, France, [2] Service de Physiologie – Explorations Fonctionnelles, Hôpital Henri Mondor, Assistance Publique – Hôpitaux de Paris, Créteil, France, [3] Neurology Division, Lebanese American University Medical Center - Rizk Hospital, Beirut, Lebanon, [4] Department of Psychiatry and Psychotherapy, Ludwig-Maximilian-University, Munich, Germany, [5] Département d'Informatique et de Recherche Opérationnelle, Université de Montréal, Montréal, QC, Canada, [6] Service de Neurologie, Hôpital Henri Mondor, Assistance Publique – Hôpitaux de Paris, Créteil, France

Edited by:
*Mikhail Lebedev,
Duke University, USA*

Reviewed by:
*Matteo Feurra,
National Research University, Higher School of Economics, Russia
Koen Cuypers,
Hasselt University - KU Leuven, Belgium*

***Correspondence:**
*Samar S. Ayache
samarayache@gmail.com*

†These authors have contributed equally to this work.

Background: In the last few years, transcranial direct current stimulation (tDCS) has emerged as an appealing therapeutic option to improve brain functions. Promising data support the role of prefrontal tDCS in augmenting cognitive performance and ameliorating several neuropsychiatric symptoms, namely pain, fatigue, mood disturbances, and attentional impairment. Such symptoms are commonly encountered in patients with multiple sclerosis (MS).

Objective: The main objective of the current work was to evaluate the tDCS effects over the left dorsolateral prefrontal cortex (DLPFC) on pain in MS patients.Our secondary outcomes were to study its influence on attention, fatigue, and mood.

Materials and Methods: Sixteen MS patients with chronic neuropathic pain were enrolled in a randomized, sham-controlled, and cross-over study.Patients randomly received two anodal tDCS blocks (active or sham), each consisting of three consecutive daily tDCS sessions, and held apart by 3 weeks. Evaluations took place before and after each block. To evaluate pain, we used the Brief Pain Inventory (BPI) and the Visual Analog Scale (VAS). Attention was assessed using neurophysiological parameters and the Attention Network Test (ANT). Changes in mood and fatigue were measured using various scales.

Results: Compared to sham, active tDCS yielded significant analgesic effects according to VAS and BPI global scales.There were no effects of any block on mood, fatigue, or attention.

Conclusion: Based on our results, anodal tDCS over the left DLPFC appears to act in a selective manner and would ameliorate specific symptoms, particularly neuropathic pain. Analgesia might have occurred through the modulation of the emotional pain network. Attention, mood, and fatigue were not improved in this work. This could be partly attributed to the short protocol duration, the small sample size, and the heterogeneity of our MS cohort. Future large-scale studies can benefit from comparing the tDCS effects over different cortical sites, changing the stimulation montage, prolonging the duration of protocol, and coupling tDCS with neuroimaging techniques for a better understanding of its possible mechanism of action.

Keywords: pain, attention, multiple sclerosis, transcranial direct current stimulation, dorsolateral prefrontal cortex

INTRODUCTION

Multiple sclerosis (MS) is a chronic progressive inflammatory disease of the central nervous system, and represents the major cause of non-traumatic disability in young adults (Noseworthy et al., 2000; Compston and Coles, 2008). During the course of the disease, the patients may develop sensorimotor, cognitive, emotional, and behavioral symptoms. For instance, although MS was previously considered a painless disease, chronic pain has been recently reported as a debilitating symptom (Ehde et al., 2005), with a prevalence varying between 29 and 86% (O'Connor et al., 2008). The lower limbs dysesthesias remain the most common and difficult to treat painful symptoms, attributed to demyelination and axonal degeneration processes involving the central sensory pathways (O'Connor et al., 2008). Psychiatric comorbidities are also common (Marrie et al., 2015). In particular, anxiety and depression were found to occur in about 21.9 and 23.7% of MS patients, respectively (Marrie et al., 2015). Moreover, up to 75% of MS patients can face fatigue at some point during the disease course; such a symptom was found to have a drastic impact on their quality of life (Chalah et al., 2015). Furthermore, abnormalities in the attentional capacities have been described in MS patients (Urbanek et al., 2010; Crivelli et al., 2012; Omisade et al., 2012; Vázquez-Marrufo et al., 2014; Ayache et al., 2015).

The interaction between pain and attention has gained an increasing interest in the last decade. Although pain serves as a warning signal for responding to potential hazards, its relationship with the intensity of a stimulus is not linear. It is rather modulated by several factors, among which attention appears to play a major role (Van Damme et al., 2010). On the one hand, distraction was documented to decrease the perceived intensity of provoked pain (Legrain et al., 2002). On the other hand, pain can capture the attentional processes, in a way that prohibits good performance on cognitive tasks, even with a voluntary neglect of the nociceptive stimuli (Eccleston and Crombez, 1999; Legrain et al., 2009a,b; Van Damme et al., 2010). In this perspective, the neurocognitive model of attention to pain explains the aforementioned interaction by two modes of selection: the top-down attention, which prioritizes relevant information and prevents irrelevant stimuli such as pain from capturing attention, and the bottom-up attention by which unintentional stimulus captures the attention (Legrain et al., 2009a).

The current advances in neuroimaging and neurophysiological modalities have unveiled the key role of the dorsolateral prefrontal cortex (DLPFC) in the circuits of pain (Lorenz et al., 2003), fatigue (Chalah et al., 2015), depression (Gobbi et al., 2014), and attention (Petersen and Posner, 2012), including the attentional circuit dedicated to noxious stimuli (Legrain et al., 2009a). Among the available literature regarding experimental pain, one study has revealed negative correlations between the activation patterns within the DLPFC bilaterally and each of pain intensity and unpleasantness (Lorenz et al., 2003). Here, the DLPFC was thought to modulate pain perception through corticosubcortical and corticocortical pathways. In addition, DLPFC seems to be a major component of the so-called cortico-striato-thalamo-cortical fatigue loop in MS (Chalah et al., 2015). Moreover, the middle frontal gyrus, which embeds the DLPFC, was found to be selectively related to depression in MS (Gobbi et al., 2014). Furthermore, DLPFC constitutes a main component of the attentional circuits, particularly the fronto-parietal executive control network (Petersen and Posner, 2012). This was based on lesions studies in human where the DLPFC appears to be involved in switching from one set of tasks to the other (Petersen and Posner, 2012). Nevertheless, experimental research investigating the interaction between bottom-up and top-down attention has highlighted the role of DLPFC in processing the painful stimuli (Legrain et al., 2009a). By maintaining the attentional load, this cortical area prioritizes goal-relevant information in order to prevent the attentional capture by pain (Legrain et al., 2009a). Therefore, one can assume that acting on DLPFC might have an impact on pain perception, attentional resources, mood, and fatigue.

Noninvasive brain stimulation (NIBS) is currently being investigated for the management of neuropsychiatric symptoms when pharmacological interventions fail. Among those techniques, transcranial direct current stimulation (tDCS) has gained a particular interest in recent years, and appears to be a promising tool for the treatment of several neurological disorders. It acts by changing the cortical excitability (Nitsche and Paulus, 2000, 2001; Nitsche and Fregni, 2007; Nitsche et al., 2008), notably by depolarizing (activating) and hyperpolarizing (inhibiting) the cortical circuits, in the case of anodal and cathodal stimulation, respectively.

In the present work, we applied anodal tDCS over the left DLPFC. Our primary endpoint was to evaluate its effects on neuropathic pain in MS patients. Our secondary outcomes were to assess its impact on attention, mood, and fatigue.

MATERIALS AND METHODS

Ethics Statement

This is a prospective, randomized, cross-over, sham-controlled study, conducted according to the declaration of Helsinki, and approved by the local ethical committee (CPP-Ile de France VI, registered as N° 2012-A00721-42). The trial is registered at the Deutsches Register Klinischer Studien (drks-neu.uniklinik-freiburg.de) and has the following registration number: DRKS00005296. All participants were well instructed about the protocol and voluntarily gave their written informed consent prior to inclusion.

Study Participants

Patients were enrolled by M.A., M.S., D.D., and A.C. from the Neurology department of Henri Mondor Hospital, Créteil, France, between November 2012 and November 2014 according to the following criteria: (i) a definite MS diagnosis according to the 2010 revised McDonald criteria (Polman et al., 2011); (ii) age between 18 and 70 years; (iii) right handedness based on the Edinburgh inventory (Oldfield, 1971); and (iv) a history of neuropathic pain since more than 3 months as per the Neuropathic Pain Symptom Inventory (NPSI; Bouhassira et al., 2004), with an intensity >40 on the visual analog scale from 0 to 100 (VAS_{0-100}), obtained as the average of daily scores over a representative week.

Exclusion criteria consisted of the following: (i) MS relapses within the last 2 months; (ii) changes in pharmacological and physical therapies during the last month; (iii) the presence of comorbid neurodegenerative or psychiatric disorders; (iv) history of substance abuse; (v) absence of measurable pain related evoked potentials (PREPs) at the right hand; (vi) severe deficit in the visual acuity or fields as documented by an ophthalmic exam; and (vii) severe right upper limb impairment as per the Medical Research Council scale for muscle power (MRC) (Medical Research Council, 1981). For the latter, we applied the MRC score to the four muscle groups involved in pinching, wrist extension, forearm flexion, and arm abduction, so that the sum of their scores could vary between 0 (null strength) and 20 (full strength); an MRC score <12 excluded the individual from participation.

A standard neurological examination was performed in all patients including a documentation of the disability level based on the expanded disability status scale (EDSS; Kurtzke, 1983), and a thorough pain evaluation.

tDCS

A battery driven multi-channel direct current stimulator (Starstim, Neuroelectrics, Barcelona, Spain) delivered the direct current over the scalp through sponge electrodes (surface area $= 25\,cm^2$), soaked in a saline solution to minimize the risk of skin irritation (Palm et al., 2014). The stimulation electrodes were directly positioned on an adult sized cap worn by the patients, and labeled according to the 10–20 EEG system of electrode positioning (Starstim, Neuroelectrics, Barcelona, Spain). To stimulate the left DLPFC, the anode was placed over F3, and its corresponding cathode over the right supraorbital region (**Figure 1**). The used current intensity was 2 mA (total current density over the stimulated area: $0.06\,mA/cm^2$) which is below the threshold for tissue damage (Poreisz et al., 2007; Nitsche et al., 2008). For the active stimulation, the current was ramped up during the first 15 s to a maximum of 2 mA that was maintained throughout the 20-min stimulation session. As for the sham stimulation, the current was ramped down immediately after ramping up in order to achieve an effective blinding (Gandiga et al., 2006; Ambrus et al., 2012).

Sham or active anodal tDCS blocks were tested in a random order and were held apart by at least 3 weeks. Each block consisted of three consecutive daily tDCS sessions. The stimulations were performed by well-trained physicians. The sessions took place in a quiet and illuminated room. The patients were at rest in an armchair and were not performing any cognitive task. Only the performing physician (S.S.A) was aware of the stimulation mode (real or sham tDCS). The evaluators (U.P and M.A.C) and the patients were blind to it.

Primary Outcomes: Pain Scales

For pain evaluation, we relied on the self-reported VAS_{0-100} and the short version of the Brief Pain Inventory (BPI). The latter is a validated and reliable tool to measure pain intensity and its interference with patient's life (Cleeland and Ryan, 1994).

Secondary Outcomes

Cognitive Task

Attention was evaluated using a computerized test: The Attention Network Test (ANT; Fan et al., 2002). Briefly, this test evaluates the three main attentional networks: the alerting network that consists of controlling vigilance and task performance, the orienting network responsible for the orientation to external stimuli, and the executive function network in charge of conflict resolution (Fan et al., 2002; Petersen and Posner, 2012). The test was performed in a quiet room, with the participants sitting in front of a monitor aligned to their midsagittal plane. The stimulus consists of a row of five horizontal black arrows, against a white background: a "central" arrow surrounded on each side by two others called "flankers" which can be pointing left- or right-ward. Several possible conditions arise: a "congruent" condition takes place when the flankers and the central arrow are in same direction; an "incongruent" condition occurs when the flankers and the central arrow are in opposite direction; and a "neutral" condition occurs when the flankers are replaced instead by four strokes. The participants indicated the direction of the central arrow by clicking on the left or right mouse buttons, with either the right index or the right middle finger, when the central arrowhead pointed to the left or right, respectively. During the total duration of the test, the subjects are asked to fix a central cross, and are informed about a warning "cue," which consists of a star-shaped signal that may precede the stimulus in question, and thus might either help or not in localizing the latter. Here, four possibilities exist: "no cue" condition when there is no preceding signal, "center cue" condition when it appears at the center of the screen, "double cue" condition when signals are simultaneously provided above and below the central cross, and a "spatial" cue condition when the signal is presented either up or down the cross. We used the 1.3.0 version of ANT, which includes one practice sequence (24 trials), and three identical sequences of 96 trials each, separated by an optional resting period. The participants should answer correctly as fast as possible, and the test provides the mean accuracy (MA) and the mean reaction time (MRT), which reflect the errors rate and the time required by the participant to answer, respectively. Moreover, all conditions are analyzed to assess the integrity of the attentional networks. For instance, the alerting network is evaluated when the participant fixes the central cross; the orienting network is put into play when the warning signal is presented prior to the stimulus; and the executive function network is recruited when the subject is trying to solve the conflict and takes a decision in order to answer.

Neuropsychological Assessment

Mood and fatigue were evaluated using the 14-item Hospital Anxiety and Depression Scale (HADS; Snaith and Zigmond, 1986) and the 21-item Modified Fatigue Impact Scale (MFIS), respectively (Fatigue guidelines development panel of the multiple sclerosis council for clinical practice guidelines, 1998; Téllez et al., 2005). MFIS accounts for the physical (9 items), cognitive (10 items), and psychosocial (2 items) components of fatigue.

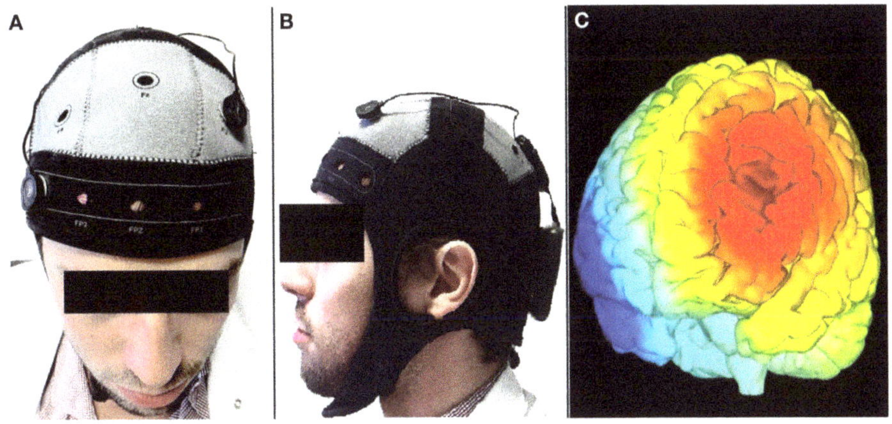

FIGURE 1 | An illustration of the tDCS montage in this study (Starstim, Neuroelectrics, Barcelona, Spain); with a cathode over AF8 (A), an anode over F3 (A,B) according to the international 10–20 EEG system. A simulation of the electric field generated between F3 (in red) and AF8 (in blue) is shown in **(C)**.

Neurophysiological Testing

Pain related evoked potentials (PREPs)

PREPs can be generated at the cortical level by a variety of noxious stimuli (Kakigi et al., 2005; Arendt-Nielsen and Andersen, 2006), namely the lasers (Arendt-Nielsen and Chen, 2003). Their amplitudes serve as physiological correlates for the amount of attention paid toward noxious stimuli, and reflect the functionality of the involved neural networks (Garcia-Larrea et al., 2002; Lorenz and Garcia-Larrea, 2003). A concentric planar electrode—which was previously found to be an alternative to laser in inducing PREPs—has served the purpose in this work (Kaube et al., 2000; Lefaucheur et al., 2012).

The first step consisted of defining the pain perception threshold (PPT). The PPT was determined by the method of limits, which consists of raising the stimulus intensity from zero to the point where the stimulus is perceived as painful sensation at intensity of 60–70 on VAS_{0-100}. The threshold was determined three times. The average of the three trials was defined as the PPT.

Stimulation was carried out using a concentric electrode designed to excite the superficial skin layers, hence the nociceptive axons (Lefaucheur et al., 2012). Stimuli were applied at the first dorsal interosseous space of the right hand, the cutaneous area located on the dorsal and lateral aspect of the hand between the extensor pollicis longus tendon and the extensor indicis tendon. A single stimulus was a train of three pulses that lasts 0.5 ms, with an inter-pulse interval (IS) of 5 ms.

After determining the PPT, two sets of twenty stimuli were performed at irregular intervals, at VAS_{60-70}.The PREPs were recorded via 10 mm Genuine Grass Gold Cup Electrodes (Grass Products, Astro-Med, Inc., Natus Neurology, Warwick, RI 02886 U.S.A.), fixed to the scalp surface using a special paste (Grass Products, Astro-Med, Inc., Natus Neurology, Warwick, RI 02886 U.S.A.). The electrodes were positioned as the following: the recording one at Cz (international 10–20 EEG system of electrode positioning), the reference one at the left earlobe, and the ground one with a Velcro strap around the right forearm (Ref NT-S07ALPINE ground electrode with Velcro Strap, Alpine Biomed, Skovlunde, Denmark). In addition, electro-oculogram was obtained via pre-gelled adhesive surface electrodes (Ref 9013S0242, Alpine Biomed, Skovlunde, Denmark) placed at the right infraorbital lateral margin.

The recorded signal was bandpass filtered at 0.5–30 Hz and stored for analysis using a Keypoint machine (Dantec Dynamics, Bristol, United Kingdom). The final step consisted of averaging the signals offline, and excluding the contaminated recordings (saccadic eye movements or blinks, and raw signals above 70 V). We then analyzed the collected N2-P2 responses and measured their baseline-to-peak amplitudes, peak-to-peak amplitudes, and latencies.

Frontal midline theta activity

The frontal midline theta (FmΘ) is an oscillatory activity in the theta band (4–7 Hz) that appears in the medial frontal region at any time during the performance of a cognitive task, reaching 6–7 Hz in frequency and 30–60 mV in amplitude (Ishihara and Yoshi, 1972; Mizuki et al., 1980). We looked for this activity by recording EEG during the second ANT sequence. The recording electrodes were located on the patients' cap at Fpz and Fz (according to the international 10–20 EEG system of electrode positioning), and connected to the recording device (Starstim, Neuroelectrics, Barcelona, Spain). The raw EEG signals were stored for offline processing and analysis. These signals were then pass-band-filtered in the frequency range [0.5–30 Hz] to keep only the rhythms of interest delta, theta, alpha and beta.

An important step before doing any analysis would be to reject ocular and blink artifacts that are highly abundant in raw data. For this, prior to any analysis, we applied on all data an algorithm that detects, localizes, and rejects artifacts in a single-channel biosignal. An example of the artifact rejection is shown in **Figure 2**.

EEG analysis

EEG analysis was performed by T.A. and A.B. To obtain a good estimate of the percentage held by the dominant

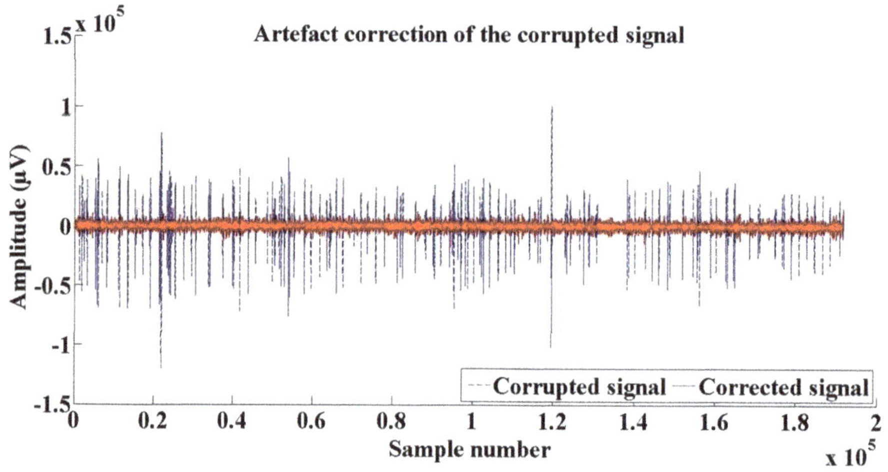

FIGURE 2 | An example of artifact rejection in a single EEG record.

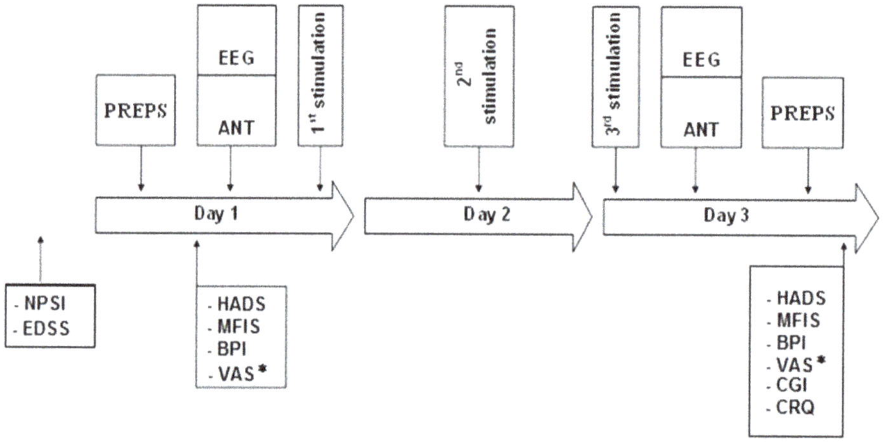

FIGURE 3 | Schematic diagram of the experimental protocol. Two tDCS blocks, each consisting of 3 consecutive daily stimulations of either sham tDCS or active tDCS (randomized order); held apart by a 3-week interval.ANT, Attention Network Test; BPI, Brief Pain Inventory; CGI, Clinical Global Impression; CRQ, Comfort Rating Questionnaire; EEG, recording at Fpz and Pz during ANT; EDSS, Expanded Disability Status Scale; HADS, Hospital Anxiety and Depression Scale; MFIS, Modified Fatigue Impact Scale; NPSI, Neuropathic Pain Symptoms Inventory; PREPs, Pain Related Evoked Potentials; VAS*, Visual Analog Scale for pain assessed 7 days prior to the first stimulation session (D1) and 7 days after the last stimulation session (D3) of each block.

rhythms (delta, theta, alpha, and beta) in a given raw EEG signals we determined the frequencies that dominate each signal.

First, the signals were band-pass filtered in the frequency bands [0.5–3.5 Hz], [4–7 Hz], [8–12 Hz], and [13–30 Hz] corresponding to the rhythms delta, theta, alpha, and beta respectively. To take into account the difference in the amplitudes of these rhythms, we determined the gradient of their amplitudes, looked for their envelopes, and calculated the modulus of the Hilbert transform of the gradients in question (Marple, 1999). At each sample of the given EEG signal, we selected the maximum modulus. Finally, the percentage of each frequency band in the given EEG signal of each patient was determined.

Experimental Protocol

After the inclusion session, patients were randomized to receive either sham or active tDCS block (**Figure 3**). The randomization schedule was generated by U.P. prior to the beginning of the study using a dedicated software ("true" random number generation without any restriction, stored in a computer until the patient was assigned to the intervention).

Keeping in mind the fluctuating nature of neuropathic pain, and the effects of circadian rhythm on attentional capacities, the patients underwent the experimental protocol at the same time of the day (Knight and Mather, 2013). They were also asked to restrict stimulants consumption, like caffeine or nicotine, at least 3 h prior to their appointment. No blocks were performed during summer time to avoid any influence of temperature on fatigue (Chalah et al., 2015).

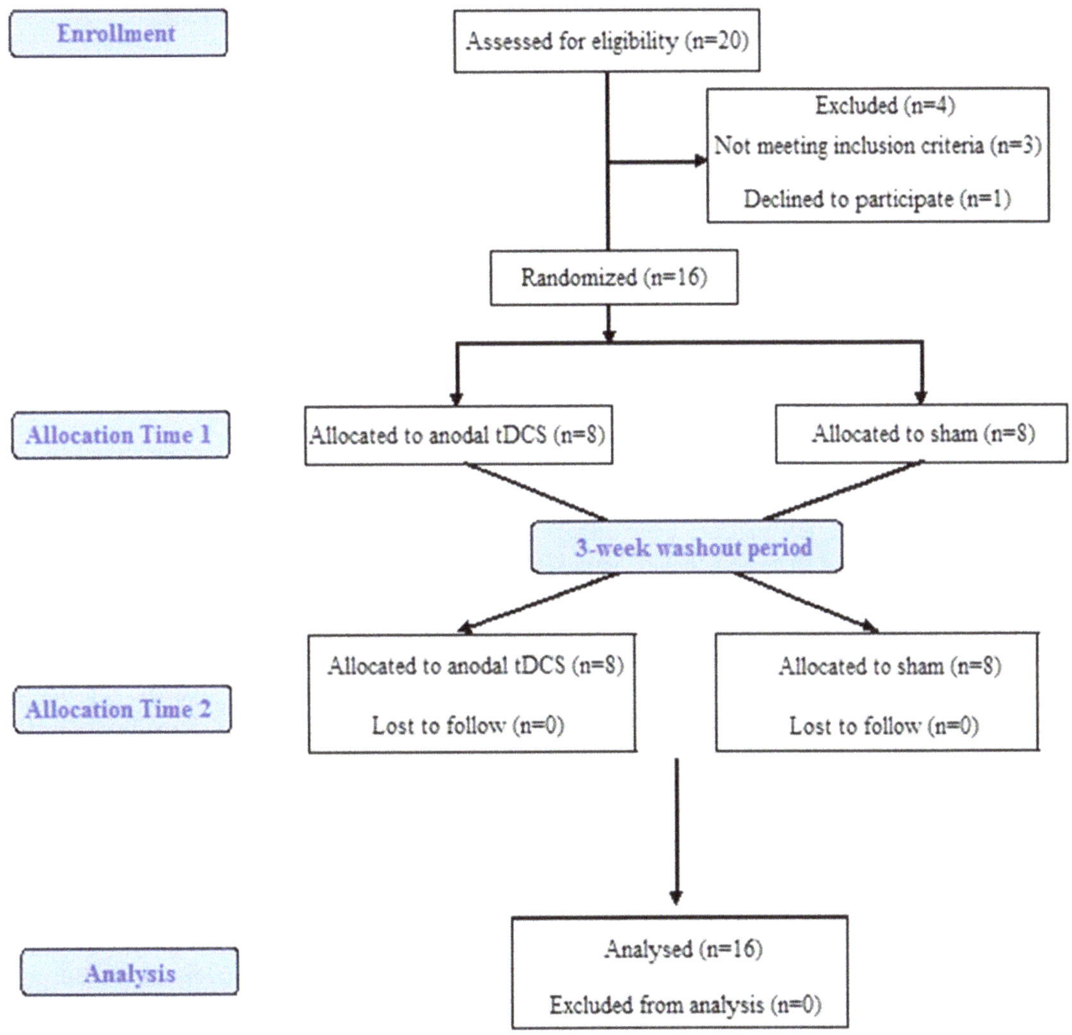

FIGURE 4 | Schematic flow chart of patients through the study.

The patients daily recorded the average of their pain intensity 1 week before and 1 week after each block using VAS_{0-100}. At the first day of each block (D1), they were asked to fill questionnaires for pain (BPI), fatigue (MFIS), anxiety and depression (HADS). This was followed by PREPs recording, the performance of ANT test, and finally the tDCS session. The latter was repeated at the second (D2) and third (D3) day of each block. At D3, the above-mentioned evaluations were repeated following the stimulation session, and the patients' degree of satisfaction regarding the protocol was assessed using the Comfort Rating Questionnaire (CRQ) and the Global Clinical Impression (GCI). At the end of each block, the patients were asked to guess the mode of stimulation (active/sham). A schematic diagram is shown in **Figure 3**.

Data Analysis

For the ANT parameters, we excluded from the analysis the reaction times of trials with either error or with a reaction time value above or below the mean ± 2 standard deviations (SD). Statistical analyses were performed using the StatView and InStat software. Our Data followed normal distributions according to the method of Kolmogorov and Smirnov. Data collected before and after each block were analyzed with paired *t*-tests, and those with a $p < 0.05$ were considered significant. This included PREPs (amplitudes and latencies), ANT parameters (MA and RT), frontal theta activity percentages, and self-rating questionnaires scores for pain (VAS_{0-100}, BPI), fatigue (MFIS), anxiety and depression (HADS).

RESULTS

Demographic and Clinical Data

Twenty MS patients were enrolled, and four were excluded (one declined to participate, and three were not eligible). Sixteen patients (13 women, 3 men, mean age 48.9 ± 10.0 years, age range 38–67 years) completed the study (**Figure 4** illustrates the flowchart of all participants). All had neuropathic pain; their mean NPSI was 5.12 ± 2.4

at enrollment. Their mean EDSS was 4.25 ± 1.4. Eleven patients had relapsing remitting MS (RRMS), four were in the secondary progressive phase (SPMS) and one had a primary progressive type (PPMS). The mean disease duration was 11.8 ± 9.4 years and the progressive phase duration was 6 ± 3.2 years.

All patients had concomitant medication intake, consisting of antiepileptic drugs (nine patients; one of them with two drugs), antidepressants (nine patients, one of them with two drugs), opioids (five patients, one of them with two drugs) and immunomodulating agents (13 patients). Pharmacological treatment was continued and kept stable throughout the experimental protocol.

Adverse Effects, Comfort Rating, and Blinding Integrity

After both active and sham stimulation, six patients reported insomnia. Nausea was reported by five patients after active stimulation and by four patients after sham stimulation. Severe headache occurred in three patients after active stimulation and in one patient after sham stimulation. Phosphenes were reported by one patient after sham stimulation.

No significant difference was found between both conditions regarding the CRQ sum scores during (p = 0.96) and after stimulation (p = 0.43). No significant differences were observed between both stimulation conditions on the overall discomfort (p = 0.79) or the mean GCI (p = 0.82; Friedman test). Details are provided in **Table 1**.

TABLE 1 | Confort rating questionnaire (CRQ) and global clinical impression (GCI) for sham and active tDCS.

	Sham	tDCS	paired t-test
CRQ sum scores during stimulation	18.3 ± 12.3	19.1 ± 11.5	$P = 0.96$
CRQ sum scores after stimulation	20.7 ± 13.8	17.5 ± 9.6	$P = 0.43$
Overall discomfort after stimulation	2.4 ± 2.0	2.6 ± 2.3	$P = 0.79$
Mean GCI after stimulation	4.6 ± 0.8	4.6 ± 0.9	$P = 0.82$

Pain Perception

The mean VAS_{0-100} pain ratings 7 days before and 7 days after stimulation showed significant decrease after active tDCS (p = 0.024), but no change after sham tDCS (p = 0.66). Analogously, the mean VAS_{0-100} pain ratings for days 1–3 before and after stimulation showed significant decrease after active tDCS (p = 0.021), and no improvement after sham tDCS (p = 0.56).

Active stimulation resulted in a significant improvement of BPI global score (p = 0.02), and its interference subscale (p = 0.01), but had no significant effects on the severity subscale. Sham did not have any significant effects on BPI scores or its subscales. Pain scores are found in **Table 2**.

Cognitive Results

There were no significant changes in any of the ANT parameters after both sham and active stimulation (**Table 3**).

Neuropsychological Scores

The baseline mean global MFIS score, HADS anxiety and depression subscales were 52.6 ± 12.2, 9.2 ± 4.0, and 6.6 ± 3.2, respectively.

No significant differences were observed following both stimulation conditions for the MFIS total scores, HADS total scores and subscales. The neuropsychological scores are detailed in **Table 4**.

Neurophysiological Testing

PREPs

PREPs results did not significantly differ between active and sham stimulation (**Table 5**).

EEG Results

A trendwise or significant increase in the theta band was observed following sham and active stimulation, respectively. Theta Fpz showed a trendwise increase after sham stimulation (p = 0.09), and theta Fz showed significant increase after sham stimulation (p = 0.04). After active stimulation, theta Fpz and Fz increased by trend (p = 0.09 and p = 0.09, respectively; **Table 5**).

DISCUSSION

This study aimed to explore the impact of prefrontal tDCS on pain in 16 MS patients. Active anodal but not sham tDCS showed significant analgesic effects on VAS_{0-100} pain ratings in the first 3 days and over 1 week after stimulation. These effects were further reflected by a significant decrease in the BPI total score and its interference subscale following only active stimulation. No relevant changes in BPI severity subscale were found after either stimulation conditions. Similarly, neither intervention had any effects on PREPs (amplitudes and latencies), ANT parameters, fatigue and mood scales. Lastly, a trendwise or a significant increase in the frontal theta activity was observed following active or sham stimulation, respectively.

Effects on Pain

The most prominent effect of tDCS treatment was analgesia. Such findings are of high interest and in line with previous studies. In fact, the DLPFC is known to have a crucial role in modulating pain (Lorenz et al., 2003). Interestingly, changes in pain perception following tDCS have been documented in several experimental protocols where anodal tDCS over the DLPFC increased the pain thresholds induced by electrical and heat stimuli in healthy volunteers (Boggio et al., 2008; Mylius et al., 2012).

As for the BPI scale, the fact that anodal tDCS over the prefrontal cortex ameliorated the interference but not the severity subscale might be accounted by the pathophysiologic mechanisms of pain. Actually, a pain matrix was conceptualized and includes three interacting networks (Garcia-Larrea and Peyron, 2013). A first order nociceptive network comprises

TABLE 2 | VAS and BPI scores (Mean ± SD) before and after sham and active tDCS.

	Before sham	After sham	Paired *t*-test	Before tDCS	After tDCS	Paired *t*-test
VAS mean/7days	52.1 ± 19.6	50.3 ± 19.7	*P* = 0.66	51.2 ± 19.2	43.1 ± 26.2	*P* = 0.02
VAS mean/Day 1–3	48.8 ± 22.0	51.3 ± 18.8	*P* = 0.56	53.1 ± 20.2	43.1 ± 26.2	*P* = 0.02
BPI global score	9.9 ± 3.5	9.2 ± 3.4	*P* = 0.19	9.2 ± 3.4	8.2 ± 3.5	*P* = 0.02
BPI severity subscale	4.8 ± 2.4	4.6 ± 2.1	*P* = 0.40	4.8 ± 2.4	4.3 ± 2.1	*P* = 0.15
BPI interference subscale	5.0 ± 1.5	4.6 ± 1.6	*P* = 0.18	4.5 ± 1.6	3.9 ± 1.6	*P* = 0.01

TABLE 3 | ANT results (Mean ± SD) before and after sham and active tDCS.

	Before sham	After sham	Paired *t*-test	Before tDCS	After tDCS	Paired *t*-test
ANT alertness	61.7 ± 60.5	58.8 ± 66.0	*P* = 0.78	36.5 ± 42.0	52.1 ± 36.0	*P* = 0.08
ANT orientation	53.7 ± 33.2	53.4 ± 27.5	*P* = 0.98	41.0 ± 30.5	50.2 ± 27.4	*P* = 0.33
ANT conflict	143.0 ± 67.9	141.8 ± 53.2	*P* = 0.95	143.1 ± 75.8	153.9 ± 69.0	*P* = 0.43
ANT mean reaction time	768.3 ± 95.0	766.1 ± 130.3	*P* = 0.94	725.4 ± 93.8	742.3 ± 99.7	*P* = 0.38
ANT accuracy	86.1 ± 21.7	90.2 ± 14.6	*P* = 0.43	92.4 ± 9.2	88.4 ± 15.0	*P* = 0.17

TABLE 4 | Neuropsychological results (Mean ± SD) before and after sham and active tDCS.

	Before sham	After sham	*t*-test	Before tDCS	After tDCS	*t*-test
Mean HADS total score	14.4 ± 5.9	14.5 ± 6.5	*P* = 0.80	14.1 ± 6.3	13.6 ± 5.8	*P* = 0.52
Mean HADS anxiety	8.1 ± 3.4	8.3 ± 3.9	*P* = 0.70	7.7 ± 3.0	7.6 ± 3.6	*P* = 0.90
Mean HADS depression	6.3 ± 3.0	6.2 ± 3.3	*P* = 0.81	6.4 ± 3.9	6.0 ± 3.3	*P* = 0.35
MFIS global score	48.2 ± 15.5	47.4 ± 17.7	*P* = 0.76	49.5 ± 14.4	49.0 ± 15.2	*P* = 0.42

the posterior operculoinsular area receiving spinothalamic projections. A second order network consists of the posterior parietal, prefrontal and anterior insular areas, and is responsible of the transition from cortical nociception to conscious perception. A third network is composed of the orbitofrontal, perigenual and limbic areas, by which the pain perception can be modified in function of expectations, emotions and beliefs. Therefore, our results suggest that tDCS could have acted on the second and third order networks of the pain matrix where the prefrontal cortex majorly contributes (Garcia-Larrea and Peyron, 2013).

Effects on Attention

Concerning attention, ANT variables did not significantly change after any of the tDCS interventions. In fact, we hypothesized that tDCS over the DLPFC could improve attentional capacities by modifying the sensitivity of stimulus-specific neural responses, in a way that enhances the top-down selection type or inhibits the bottom-up one; notably, by amplifying or inhibiting the activity of neurons which respond, respectively, to relevant or irrelevant stimuli (Desimone and Duncan, 1995). In accordance with our speculation, anodal tDCS over the left DLPFC have found to improve the attentional bias acquisition in one study (Clarke et al., 2014), and sustained attention in another one (Nelson et al., 2014). However, the lack of significant improvement of ANT parameters in our study can be explained by many facts. First, ANT is known to represent a complex task which measures three different attentional networks and hence involves several cortico-cortical and cortico-subcortical connections. Second, in contrast to previous tDCS studies in healthy subjects, MS patients are known to have a dysfunction in the attentional networks, notably in the alerting and/or the orienting ones (Urbanek et al., 2010; Crivelli et al., 2012; Omisade et al., 2012; Vázquez-Marrufo et al., 2014; Ayache et al., 2015) which might have prevented tDCS from causing any improvement. Third, our tDCS design might not have been optimal to ameliorate ANT variables. It is noteworthy that a lateralization in the attentional performance exists between left and right hemispheric structures (Corbetta and Shulman, 2002; Raz and Buhle, 2006; Lückmann et al., 2014). In fact, the left and right hemispheres are thought to be involved in phasic and tonic alertness, respectively (Raz and Buhle, 2006). In this model, the right DLPFC has an executory capacity which enables it to monitor the attentional performance and hence regulates it accordingly, while the right inferior parietal region seems to have a role in endogenous and exogenous alerting. In line with this topography, one study found that anodal tDCS over the right frontal cortex (F10 of the 10–10 EEG system of electrodes positioning) could improve the alerting network of attention (Coffman et al., 2012). Another study compared the effects of anodal tDCS over different cortical targets in terms of attentional improvement and showed significant effects following the stimulation of the right posterior parietal cortex (PPC) but not the left DLPFC (Roy et al., 2015). This suggests that unlike our design, which targeted the left hemisphere, stimulation of

TABLE 5 | Neurophysiological (EEG and PREPS) results (Mean ± SD) before and after sham and active tDCS.

	Before sham	After sham	Paired *t*-test	Before tDCS	After tDCS	Paired *t*-test
Theta Fpz	51.1 ± 14.6	58.9 ± 10.2	$P = 0.09$	53.8 ± 13.9	62.1 ± 11.1	$P = 0.09$
Theta Fz	53.9 ± 9.8	59.3 ± 7.9	$P = 0.04$	54.9 ± 15.1	62.6 ± 10.5	$P = 0.09$
Mean N2 latency	118.9 ± 34.8	131.7 ± 25.6	$P = 0.16$	138.1 ± 44.6	141.8 ± 33.2	$P = 0.66$
Mean P2 latency	178.0 ± 48.8	187.0 ± 36.0	$P = 0.41$	202.2 ± 58.5	199.6 ± 45.9	$P = 0.80$
Mean N2 amplitude	11.3 ± 7.6	14.1 ± 6.5	$P = 0.16$	12.6 ± 9.9	12.0 ± 7.4	$P = 0.77$
Mean P2 amplitude	10.5 ± 4.3	10.4 ± 7.6	$P = 0.96$	15.1 ± 10.7	13.2 ± 9.4	$P = 0.57$
Mean N2-P2 amplitude	21.4 ± 8.9	22.4 ± 9.2	$P = 0.64$	25.2 ± 9.0	23.6 ± 13.0	$P = 0.50$

the right fronto-parietal structures might have better effects on attention. Fourth, our protocol consisted of performing ANT before the first stimulation session (D1) and after the last one (D3) of each block, but did not contain a "within-day control" of attention. This was based on the hypothesis that a tDCS-induced cumulative effect might result from the repetition of the stimulation sessions. However, three consecutive daily sessions might not be enough to induce such an effect, and therefore a within-day control for attention would have revealed better outcomes. Fifth, concerning the tDCS montage adopted in this study, the anode was placed at the left DLPFC while its reference electrode was the right supraorbital region. We should note that the chosen reference is not neutral. In fact the orbitofrontal cortex has an important role inemotional and cognitive processing, including the attentional processes to emotional stimuli. Therefore, applying a cathodal stimulation on that region might have impacted our results.

These data altogether suggest that future studies might benefit from comparing the effects of tDCS over different cortical areas (e.g., left/right DLPFC and left/right PPC), prolonging the duration of the stimulation period, adding a within-day control for attention, and adopting a different reference site, before drawing any conclusion.

Effects on Mood and Fatigue

As for mood changes, although there are evidence regarding the antidepressant effects of anodal tDCS over the DLPFC (Kalu et al., 2012; Loo et al., 2012; Berlim et al., 2013; Brunoni et al., 2013), the lack of mood changes in our patients cohort can be attributed to the short stimulation period adapted in this study. In this perspective, depression studies have shown dose-dependent effects of tDCS in mood improvement that could extend over several weeks. Our results are supported by another study where no improvement in mood scores has occurred following five tDCS sessions over the left DLPFC (Saiote et al., 2014).

Concerning fatigue, we found no effects of tDCS on the MFIS scores. A lack of improvement in fatigue following tDCS has already been reported by two studies (Ferrucci et al., 2014; Saiote et al., 2014).

Effects on Neurophysiological Parameters

PREPs

PREPs amplitudes were not changed following both active and sham tDCS. Although PREPs can correlate with the subjective pain sensation, it is commonly accepted that PREPs amplitude reflects the integrity of the spino-thalamo-cortical tract (Casey et al., 1996; Wu et al., 1999; Garcia-Larrea et al., 2002). In this view, most of the neuroimaging studies have demonstrated that MS patients with neuropathic pain had several demyelinating lesions within the spinal cord, brainstem, and thalamus (Seixas et al., 2014). Furthermore, PREPs amplitude is known to depend on the attentional level toward the stimulated limb (Garcia-Larrea et al., 2002), in this context, attentional dysfunction has been frequently reported in MS patients. Taken together, these disturbances might have prohibited tDCS from having any effect on PREPs parameters in our cohort.

EEG

As for the frontal midline theta activity, their increase following both stimulation blocks can be explained by different approaches. In fact, anxiety improvement has previously been correlated with the appearance of such waves following anxiolytic treatment (Mizuki et al., 1983, 1989). In addition, an emotionally positive state was found to be associated with theta power in frontal midline leads (Aftanas and Golocheikine, 2001). In this perspective, it might be possible that medical care itself, regardless of stimulation block type, had accounted for a subtle decrease in patients' anxiety, despite the absence of any significant changes in HADS scores.

Limitations

It is important to note that, in our patients' cohort, the observed tDCS effects could have been influenced by antiepileptic treatments. The latter are known to inhibit long-term-potentiation induced neuroplasticity changes by blockade of voltage-gated ion channels (Nitsche et al., 2012). However, in most of the studies dealing with chronic neuropathic pain, patients commonly suffer from a severe pain which is resistant to multiple drugs. Particularly, the available tDCS studies for central neuropathic pain have included patients taking antiepileptics, antidepressants, and opioid analgesics (Fregni et al., 2006; Soler et al., 2010; Wrigley et al., 2013). Similar to our work, the authors asked their patients to keep their routine medications throughout the study period. Another limitation would be the lack of functional or structural neuroimaging data in our work. Future studies can benefit from combining imaging with tDCS application, in order to understand the mechanisms of action of tDCS on the studied brain networks, and to correlate the clinical response to gray matter and white matter pathologies (Chalah et al., 2015). In addition, the small sample size and heterogeneity of our MS cohort could have prohibited the emergence of any positive effect in terms of attention, mood and fatigue. Finally, MS-related symptoms can fluctuate during the course of the disease; such a fluctuation should be taken into account prior to the interpretation of any intervention results. In this context, our study could have benefited from testing the difference between baseline scores prior to tDCS and sham conditions. However, we believe that our inclusion criteria (e.g., the presence of a neuropathic pain since more than 3 months with an intensity greater than 40 on VAS; the absence of MS relapses since at last 2 months, a stable therapy since 1 month) might have restricted such an influence. We also controlled for the impact of some variables on attention, pain, and fatigue; namely by restricting the consumption of psychostimulants, and performing the stimulation block at the same time during the day, with no blocks occurring in summer.

AUTHOR CONTRIBUTIONS

MA, MS, DD, and AC: enrolled patients from the neurology department of Henri Mondor Hospital. SA, UP, and MC: performed the stimulation sessions and collected the data. SA and JL: designed the study, developed the methodology, interpreted the data and wrote the final draft. MC and UP: wrote the first draft. TA and AB: analyzed the EEG data.

REFERENCES

Aftanas, L. I., and Golocheikine, S. A. (2001). Human anterior and frontal midline theta and lower alpha reflect emotionally positive state and internalized attention: high-resolution EEG investigation of meditation. *Neurosci. Lett.* 310, 57–60. doi: 10.1016/S0304-3940(01)02094-8

Ambrus, G. G., Al-Moyed, H., Chaieb, L., Sarp, L., Antal, A., and Paulus, W. (2012). The fade-in-short stimulation–fade out approach to sham tDCS–reliable at 1 mA for naïve and experienced subjects, but not investigators. *Brain Stimul.* 5, 499–504. doi: 10.1016/j.brs.2011.12.001

Arendt-Nielsen, L., and Andersen, O. K. (2006). Electrophysiological assessment of pain. *Suppl. Clin. Neurophysiol.* 59, 241–249. doi: 10.1016/S1567-424X(09)70037-6

Arendt-Nielsen, L., and Chen, A. C. (2003). Lasers and other thermal stimulators for activation of skin nociceptors in humans. *Neurophysiol. Clin.* 33, 259–268. doi: 10.1016/j.neucli.2003.10.005

Ayache, S. S., Palm, U., Chalah, M. A., Nguyen, R., Farhat, W. H., Créange, A., et al. (2015). Orienting network dysfunction in progressive multiple sclerosis. *J. Neurol. Sci.* 351, 206–207. doi: 10.1016/j.jns.2015.02.044

Berlim, M. T., Van den Eynde, F., and Daskalakis, Z. J. (2013). Clinical utility of transcranial direct current stimulation (tDCS) for treating major depression a systematic review and meta-analysis of randomized, double-blind and sham-controlled trials. *J. Psychiatr. Res.* 47, 1–7. doi: 10.1016/j.jpsychires.2012.09.025

Boggio, P. S., Zaghi, S., Lopes, M., and Fregni, F. (2008). Modulatory effects of anodal transcranial direct current stimulation on perception and pain thresholds in healthy volunteers. *Eur. J. Neurol.* 15, 1124–1130. doi: 10.1111/j.1468-1331.2008.02270.x

Bouhassira, D., Attal, N., Fermanian, J., Alchaar, H., Gautron, M., Masquelier, E., et al. (2004). Development and validation of the neuropathic pain symptom inventory. *Pain* 108, 248–257. doi: 10.1016/j.pain.2003.12.024

Brunoni, A. R., Valiengo, L., Baccaro, A., Zanão, T. A., de Oliveira, J. F., Goulart, A., et al. (2013). The sertraline vs. electrical current therapy for treating depression clinical study results from a factrial randomized, controlled trial. *JAMA Psychiatry* 70, 383–391. doi: 10.1001/2013.jamapsychiatry.32

Casey, K. L., Beydoun, A., Boivie, J., Sjolund, B., Holmgren, H., Leijon, G., et al. (1996). Laser-evoked cerebral potentials and sensory function in patients with central pain. *Pain* 64, 485–491. doi: 10.1016/0304-3959(95)00143-3

Chalah, M. A., Riachi, N., Ahdab, R., Créange, A., Lefaucheur, J. P., and Ayache, S. S. (2015). Fatigue in multiple sclerosis: neural correlates and the role of non-invasive brain stimulation. *Front. Cell. Neurosci.* 9:460. doi: 10.3389/fncel.2015.00460

Clarke, P. J., Browning, M., Hammond, G., Notebaert, L., and MacLeod, C. (2014). The causal role of the dorsolateral prefrontal cortex in the modification of attentional bias: evidence from transcranial direct current stimulation. *Biol. Psychiatry* 76, 946–952. doi: 10.1016/j.biopsych.2014.03.003

Cleeland, C. S., and Ryan, K. M. (1994). Pain assessment: global use of the Brief Pain Inventory. *Ann. Acad. Med. Singapore* 23, 129–138.

Coffman, B. A., Trumbo, M. C., and Clark, V. P. (2012). Enhancement of object detection with transcranial direct current stimulation is associated with increased attention. *BMC Neurosci.* 13:108. doi: 10.1186/1471-2202-13-108

Compston, A., and Coles, A. (2008). Multiple sclerosis. *Lancet* 372, 1502–1517. doi: 10.1016/S0140-6736(08)61620-7

Corbetta, M., and Shulman, G. L. (2002). Control of goal-directed and stimulus-driven attention in the brain. *Nat. Rev. Neurosci.* 3, 201–215. doi: 10.1038/nrn755

Crivelli, L., Farez, M. F., González, C. D., Fiol, M., Amengual, A., Leiguarda, R., et al. (2012). Alerting network dysfunction in early multiple sclerosis. *J. Int. Neuropsychol. Soc.* 18, 757–763. doi: 10.1017/S1355617712000410

Desimone, R., and Duncan, J. (1995). Neural mechanisms of selective visual attention. *Annu. Rev. Neurosci.* 18, 193–222. doi: 10.1146/annurev.ne.18.030195.001205

Eccleston, C., and Crombez, G. (1999). Pain demands attention: a cognitive-affective model of the interruptive function of pain. *Psychol. Bull.* 125, 356–366. doi: 10.1037/0033-2909.125.3.356

Ehde, D. M., Osborne, T. L., and Jensen, M. P. (2005). Chronic pain in persons with multiple sclerosis. *Phys. Med. Rehabil. Clin. N. Am.* 16, 503–512. doi: 10.1016/j.pmr.2005.01.001

Fan, J., McCandliss, B. D., Sommer, T., Raz, A., and Posner, M. I. (2002). Testing the efficiency and independence of attentional networks. *J. Cogn. Neurosci.* 14, 340–347. doi: 10.1162/089892902317361886

Fatigue guidelines development panel of the multiple sclerosis council for clinical practice guidelines (1998). *Fatigue and Multiple Sclerosis. Evidence-Based Management Strategies for Fatigue in Multiple Sclerosis.* Washington, DC: Paralyzed Veterans of America.

Ferrucci, R., Vergari, M., Cogiamanian, F., Bocci, T., Ciocca, M., Tomasini, E., et al. (2014). Transcranial direct current stimulation (tDCS) for fatigue in multiple sclerosis. *NeuroRehabilitation* 34, 121–127. doi: 10.3233/NRE-131019

Fregni, F., Boggio, P. S., Lima, M. C., Ferreira, M. J., Wagner, T., Rigonatti, S. P., et al. (2006). A sham-controlled, phase II trial of transcranial direct current stimulation for the treatment of central pain in traumatic spinal cord injury. *Pain* 122, 197–209. doi: 10.1016/j.pain.2006.02.023

Gandiga, P. C., Hummel, F. C., and Cohen, L. G. (2006). Transcranial DC stimulation (tDCS): a tool for double-blind sham-controlled clinical studies in brain stimulation. *Clin. Neurophysiol.* 117, 845–850. doi: 10.1016/j.clinph.2005.12.003

Garcia-Larrea, L., Convers, P., Magnin, M., André-Obadia, N., Peyron, R., Laurent, B., et al. (2002). Laser-evoked potential abnormalities in central pain patients: the influence of spontaneous and provoked pain. *Brain* 125, 2766–2781. doi: 10.1093/brain/awf275

Garcia-Larrea, L., and Peyron, R. (2013). Pain matrices and neuropathic pain matrices: a review. *Pain* 154(Suppl. 1), S29–S43. doi: 10.1016/j.pain.2013.09.001

Gobbi, C., Rocca, M. A., Riccitelli, G., Pagani, E., Messina, R., Preziosa, P., et al. (2014). Influence of the topography of brain damage on depression and fatigue in patients with multiple sclerosis. *Mult. Scler.* 20, 192–201. doi: 10.1177/1352458513493684

Ishihara, T., and Yoshi, N. (1972). Multivariate analytic study of EEG and mental activity in juvenile delinquents. *Electroencephalogr. Clin. Neurophysiol.* 33, 71–80. doi: 10.1016/0013-4694(72)90026-0

Kakigi, R., Inui, K., and Tamura, Y. (2005). Electrophysiological studies on human pain perception. *Clin. Neurophysiol.* 116, 743–763. doi: 10.1016/j.clinph.2004.11.016

Kalu, U. G., Sexton, C. E., Loo, C. K., and Ebmeier, K. P. (2012). Transcranial direct current stimulation in the treatment of major depression: a meta-analysis. *Psychol. Med.* 42, 1791–1800. doi: 10.1017/S0033291711003059

Kaube, H., Katsarava, Z., Käufer, T., Diener, H., and Ellrich, J. (2000). A new method to increase nociception specificity of the human blink reflex. *Clin. Neurophysiol.* 111, 413–416. doi: 10.1016/S1388-2457(99)00295-3

Knight, M., and Mather, M. (2013). Look out-it's your off-peak time of day! Time of day matters more for alerting than for orienting or executive attention. *Exp. Aging Res.* 39, 305–321. doi: 10.1080/0361073X.2013.779197

Kurtzke, J. F. (1983). Rating neurologic impairment in multiple sclerosis: an expanded disability status scale (EDSS). *Neurology* 33, 1444–1452. doi: 10.1212/WNL.33.11.1444

Lefaucheur, J. P., Ahdab, R., Ayache, S. S., Lefaucheur-Ménard, I., Rouie, D., Tebbal, D., et al. (2012). Pain-related evoked potentials: a comparative study between electrical stimulation using a concentric planar electrode and laser stimulation using a CO2 laser. *Neurophysiol. Clin.* 42, 1999–1206. doi: 10.1016/j.neucli.2011.12.003

Legrain, V., Damme, S. V., Eccleston, C., Davis, K. D., Seminowicz, D. A., and Crombez, G. A. (2009a). A neurocognitive model of attention to pain: behavioral and neuroimaging evidence. *Pain* 144, 230–232. doi: 10.1016/j.pain.2009.03.020

Legrain, V., Guérit, J. M., Bruyer, R., and Plaghki, L. (2002). Attentional modulation of the nociceptive processing into the human brain: selective spatial attention, probability of stimulus occurrence, and target detection effects on laser evoked potentials. *Pain* 99, 21–39. doi: 10.1016/S0304-3959(02)00051-9

Legrain, V., Perchet, C., and García-Larrea, L. (2009b). Involuntary orienting of attention to nociceptive events: neural and behavioral signatures. *J. Neurophysiol.* 102, 2423–2434. doi: 10.1152/jn.00372.2009

Loo, C. K., Alonzo, A., Martin, D., Mitchell, P. B., Galvez, V., and Sachdev, P. (2012). Transcranial direct current stimulation for depression 3-week, randomised, sham-controlled trial. *Br. J. Psychiatry* 200, 52–59. doi: 10.1192/bjp.bp.111.097634

Lorenz, J., and Garcia-Larrea, L. (2003). Contribution of attentional and cognitive factors to laser evoked brain potentials. *Neurophysiol. Clin.* 33, 293–301. doi: 10.1016/j.neucli.2003.10.004

Lorenz, J., Minoshima, S., and Casey, K. L. (2003). Keeping pain out of mind: the role of the dorsolateral prefrontal cortex in pain modulation. *Brain* 126, 1079–1091. doi: 10.1093/brain/awg102

Lückmann, H. C., Jacobs, H. I., and Sack, A. T. (2014). The cross-functional role of frontoparietal regions in cognition: internal attention as the overarching mechanism. *Prog. Neurobiol.* 116, 66–86. doi: 10.1016/j.pneurobio.2014.02.002

Marple, S. L. (1999). Computing the discrete-time analytic signal via FFT. *IEEE Trans. Signal Process.* 47, 2600–2603. doi: 10.1109/78.782222

Marrie, R. A., Reingold, S., Cohen, J., Stuve, O., Trojano, M., Sorensen, P. S., et al. (2015). The incidence and prevalence of psychiatric disorders in multiple sclerosis: a systematic review. *Mult. Scler.* 21, 305–317. doi: 10.1177/1352458514564487

Medical Research Council (1981). *Aids to the Examination of the Peripheral Nervous System, Memorandum no. 45.* London: Her Majesty's Stationery Office.

Mizuki, Y., Hashimoto, M., Tanaka, T., Inanaga, K., and Tanaka, M. A. (1983). New physiological tool for assessing anxiolytic effects in humans: frontal midline theta activity. *Psychopharmacology (Berl.)* 80, 311–314. doi: 10.1007/BF00432111

Mizuki, Y., Suetsugi, M., Imai, T., Kai, S., Kajimura, N., and Yamada, M. (1989). A physiological marker for assessing anxiety level in humans: frontal midline theta activity. *J. Psychiatry Neurol.* 43, 619. doi: 10.1111/j.1440-1819.1989.tb03096.x

Mizuki, Y., Tanaka, M., Isozaki, H., Nishijima, H., and Inanaga, K. (1980). Periodic appearance of theta rhythm in the frontal midline area during performance of a mental task. *Electroencephalogr. Clin. Neurophysiol.* 49, 345–351. doi: 10.1016/0013-4694(80)90229-1

Mylius, V., Jung, M., Menzler, K., Haag, A., Khader, P. H., Oertel, W. H., et al. (2012). Effects of transcranial direct current stimulation on pain perception and working memory. *Eur. J. Pain* 16, 974–982. doi: 10.1002/j.1532-2149.2011.00105.x

Nelson, J. T., McKinley, R. A., Golob, E. J., Warm, J. S., and Parasuraman, R. (2014). Enhancing vigilance in operators with prefrontal cortex transcranial direct current stimulation (tDCS). *Neuroimage* 85 (Pt 3), 909–917. doi: 10.1016/j.neuroimage.2012.11.061

Nitsche, M. A., Cohen, L. G., Wassermann, E. M., Priori, A., Lang, N., Antal, A., et al. (2008). Transcranial direct current stimulation: state of the art 2008. *Brain Stimul.* 1, 206–223. doi: 10.1016/j.brs.2008.06.004

Nitsche, M. A., and Fregni, F. (2007). Transcranial direct current stimulation- an adjuvant tool for the treatment of neuropsychiatric disease. *Curr. Psychiatry Rev.* 3, 222–232. doi: 10.2174/157340007781369649

Nitsche, M. A., Muller-Dahlhaus, F., Paulus, W., and Ziemann, U. (2012). The pharmacology of neuroplasticity induced by noninvasive brain stimulation: building models for the clinical use of CNS active drugs. *J. Physiol.* 590, 4641–4662. doi: 10.1113/jphysiol.2012.232975

Nitsche, M. A., and Paulus, W. (2000). Excitability changes induced in the human motor cortex by weak transcranial direct current stimulation. *J. Physiol.* 527, 633–639. doi: 10.1111/j.1469-7793.2000.t01-1-00633.x

Nitsche, M. A., and Paulus, W. (2001). Sustained excitability elevations induced by transcranial DC motor cortex stimulation in humans. *Neurology* 57, 1899–1901. doi: 10.1212/WNL.57.10.1899

Noseworthy, J. H., Lucchinetti, C., Rodriguez, M., and Weinshenker, B. G. (2000). Multiple sclerosis. *N. Engl. J. Med.* 343, 938–952. doi: 10.1056/NEJM200009283431307

O'Connor, A. B., Schwid, S. R., Herrmann, D. N., Markman, J. D., and Dworkin, R. H. (2008). Pain associated with multiple sclerosis: systematic review and proposed classification. *Pain* 137, 96–111. doi: 10.1016/j.pain.2007.08.024

Oldfield, R. C. (1971). The assessment and analysis of handedness: the Edinburgh inventory. *Neuropsychologia* 9, 97–113. doi: 10.1016/0028-3932(71)90067-4

Omisade, A., Fisk, J. D., Klein, R. M., Schmidt, M., Darvesh, S., and Bhan, V. (2012). Information processing and magnetic resonance imaging indices of brain pathology in multiple sclerosis. *Int. J. MS Care* 14, 84–89. doi: 10.7224/1537-2073-14.2.84

Palm, U., Feichtner, K. B., Hasan, A., Gauglitz, G., Langguth, B., Nitsche, M. A., et al. (2014). The role of contact media at the skin-electrode interface during transcranial direct current stimulation (tDCS). *Brain Stimul.* 7, 762–764. doi: 10.1016/j.brs.2014.06.006

Petersen, S. E., and Posner, M. I. (2012). The attention system of the human brain: 20 years after. *Annu. Rev. Neurosci.* 35, 73–89. doi: 10.1146/annurev-neuro-062111-150525

Polman, C. H., Reingold, S. C., Banwell, B., Clanet, M., Cohen, J. A., Filippi, M., et al. (2011). Diagnostic criteria for multiple sclerosis: 2010 revisions to the McDonald criteria. *Ann. Neurol.* 69, 292–302. doi: 10.1002/ana.22366

Poreisz, C., Boros, K., Antal, A., and Paulus, W. (2007). Safety aspects of transcranial direct current stimulation concerning healthy subjects and patients. *Brain Res. Bull.* 72, 208–214. doi: 10.1016/j.brainresbull.2007.01.004

Raz, A., and Buhle, J. (2006). Typologies of attentional networks. *Nat. Rev. Neurosci.* 7, 367-379. doi: 10.1038/nrn1903

Roy, L. B., Sparing, R., Fink, G. R., and Hesse, M. D. (2015). Modulation of attention functions by anodal tDCS on right PPC. *Neuropsychologia* 74, 96–107. doi: 10.1016/j.neuropsychologia.2015.02.028

Saiote, C., Goldschmidt, T., Timäus, C., Steenwijk, M. D., Opitz, A., Antal, A., et al. (2014). Impact of transcranial direct current stimulation on fatigue in multiple sclerosis. *Restor. Neurol. Neurosci.* 32, 423–436. doi: 10.3233/RNN-130372

Seixas, D., Foley, P., Palace, J., Lima, D., Ramos, I., and Tracey, I. (2014). Pain in multiple sclerosis: a systematic review of neuroimaging studies. *Neuroimage Clin.* 5, 322–331. doi: 10.1016/j.nicl.2014.06.014

Snaith, R. P., and Zigmond, A. S. (1986). The hospital anxiety and depression scale. *Br. Med. J. (Clin. Res. Ed.)* 292, 344. doi: 10.1136/bmj.292.6516.344

Soler, M. D., Kumru, H., Pelayo, R., Vidal, J., Tormos, J. M., Fregni, F., et al. (2010). Effectiveness of transcranial direct current stimulation and visual illusion on neuropathic pain in spinal cord injury. *Brain* 133, 2565–2577. doi: 10.1093/brain/awq184

Téllez, N., Río, J., Tintoré, M., Nos, C., Galán, I., and Montalban, X. (2005). Does the Modified Fatigue Impact Scale offer a more comprehensive assessment of fatigue in MS? *Mult. Scler.* 11, 198–202. doi: 10.1191/1352458505ms1148oa

Urbanek, C., Weinges-Evers, N., Bellmann-Strobl, J., Bock, M., Dörr, J., Hahn, E., et al. (2010). Attention Network Test reveals alerting network dysfunction in multiple sclerosis. *Mult. Scler.* 16, 93–99. doi: 10.1177/1352458509350308

Van Damme, S., Legrain, V., Vogt, J., and Crombez, G. (2010). Keeping pain in mind: a motivational account of attention to pain. *Neurosci. Biobehav. Rev.* 34, 204–213. doi: 10.1016/j.neubiorev.2009.01.005

Vázquez-Marrufo, M., Galvao-Carmona, A., González-Rosa, J. J., Hidalgo-Muñoz, A. R., Borges, M., Ruiz-Peña, J. L., et al. (2014). Neural correlates of alerting and orienting impairment in multiple sclerosis patients. *PLoS ONE* 12:e97226. doi: 10.1371/journal.pone.0097226

Wrigley, P. J., Gustin, S. M., McIndoe, L. N., Chakiath, R. J., Henderson, L. A., and Siddall, P. J. (2013). Longstanding neuropathic pain after spinal cord injury is refractory to transcranial direct current stimulation: a randomized controlled trial. *Pain* 154, 2178–2184. doi: 10.1016/j.pain.2013.06.045

Wu, Q., García-Larrea, L., Mertens, P., Beschet, A., Sindou, M., and Mauguière, F. (1999). Hyperalgesia with reduced laser evoked potentials in neuropathic pain. *Pain* 80, 209–214. doi: 10.1016/S0304-3959(98)00206-1

EEG negativity in fixations used for gaze-based control: toward converting intentions into actions with an eye-brain-computer interface

Sergei L. Shishkin [1]*, *Yuri O. Nuzhdin* [1], *Evgeny P. Svirin* [1], *Alexander G. Trofimov* [2], *Anastasia A. Fedorova* [1], *Bogdan L. Kozyrskiy* [1,3] *and Boris M. Velichkovsky* [1,4,5]

[1] Department of Neurocognitive Technologies, Kurchatov Complex of NBICS Technologies, National Research Centre "Kurchatov Institute," Moscow, Russia, [2] Department of Cybernetics, National Research Nuclear University MEPhI, Moscow, Russia, [3] Department of Computer Systems and Technologies, National Research Nuclear University MEPhI, Moscow, Russia, [4] Centre for Cognitive Programs and Technologies, Russian State University for Humanities, Moscow, Russia, [5] Department of Psychology, Technische Universität Dresden, Dresden, Germany

Edited by:
Mikhail Lebedev,
Duke University, USA

Reviewed by:
George C. McConnell,
Stevens Institute of Technology, USA
Witali Dunin-Barkowski,
Scientific Research Institute of System Analysis (RAS), Russia

***Correspondence:**
Sergei L. Shishkin
sergshishkin@mail.ru

We usually look at an object when we are going to manipulate it. Thus, eye tracking can be used to communicate intended actions. An effective human-machine interface, however, should be able to differentiate intentional and spontaneous eye movements. We report an electroencephalogram (EEG) marker that differentiates gaze fixations used for control from spontaneous fixations involved in visual exploration. Eight healthy participants played a game with their eye movements only. Their gaze-synchronized EEG data (fixation-related potentials, FRPs) were collected during game's control-on and control-off conditions. A slow negative wave with a maximum in the parietooccipital region was present in each participant's averaged FRPs in the control-on conditions and was absent or had much lower amplitude in the control-off condition. This wave was similar but not identical to stimulus-preceding negativity, a slow negative wave that can be observed during feedback expectation. Classification of intentional vs. spontaneous fixations was based on amplitude features from 13 EEG channels using 300 ms length segments free from electrooculogram contamination (200–500 ms relative to the fixation onset). For the first fixations in the fixation triplets required to make moves in the game, classified against control-off data, a committee of greedy classifiers provided 0.90 ± 0.07 specificity and 0.38 ± 0.14 sensitivity. Similar (slightly lower) results were obtained for the shrinkage Linear Discriminate Analysis (LDA) classifier. The second and third fixations in the triplets were classified at lower rate. We expect that, with improved feature sets and classifiers, a hybrid dwell-based Eye-Brain-Computer Interface (EBCI) can be built using the FRP difference between the intended and spontaneous fixations. If this direction of BCI development will be successful, such a multimodal interface may improve the fluency of interaction and can possibly become the basis for a new input device for paralyzed and healthy users, the EBCI "Wish Mouse."

Keywords: brain-computer interfaces, human-computer interfaces, gaze interaction, assistive technology, eye tracking, detection of intention, slow cortical potentials, stimulus-preceding negativity

INTRODUCTION

A brain-computer interface (BCI) is a tool of control and communication without using muscles or peripheral nerves, through the use of brain signals only (Wolpaw et al., 2002). The lay public often expects that such tools should directly and effortlessly converts internal intents into actions in the outside physical world. In reality, however, BCIs provide much slower interaction comparing to traditional human-machine interfaces, such as mouse and keyboard computer input. Most of mental operations and states cannot be detected from the electroencephalogram (EEG) or other non-invasive brain signals on single-trial basis within seconds. A typical BCI does not recognize the user's whishes or action plans directly; to send a command, a user needs to execute one of a limited range of motor imagery, cognitive or perceptual tasks that can evoke recognizable brain signals. Such tasks are typically unrelated to the current activity and their use imposes additional mental load and decreases the fluency of BCI use. Invasive BCIs are promising, but high risks and costs associated with brain surgery require further efforts to make this technology acceptable even for severely paralyzed patients (Lahr et al., 2015; Bowsher et al., 2016; Waldert, 2016).

Can a machine recognize our intentions more directly at least in certain situations? Consider, for example, using a computer Graphical User Interface (GUI) by a healthy person. When he or she decides to click a screen button or a link, they need to take a mouse with their hand, move the cursor to the screen button or link and then click the mouse button (**Figure 1, upper panel**). Imagine that the computer analyzes his or her brain signals and can detect signal patterns related to the intention to make an action, so that the mouse is no longer needed. It is likely that, under these settings, the user could better focus on their main activity, because they would not need to switch to any motor task (**Figure 1, bottom panel**).

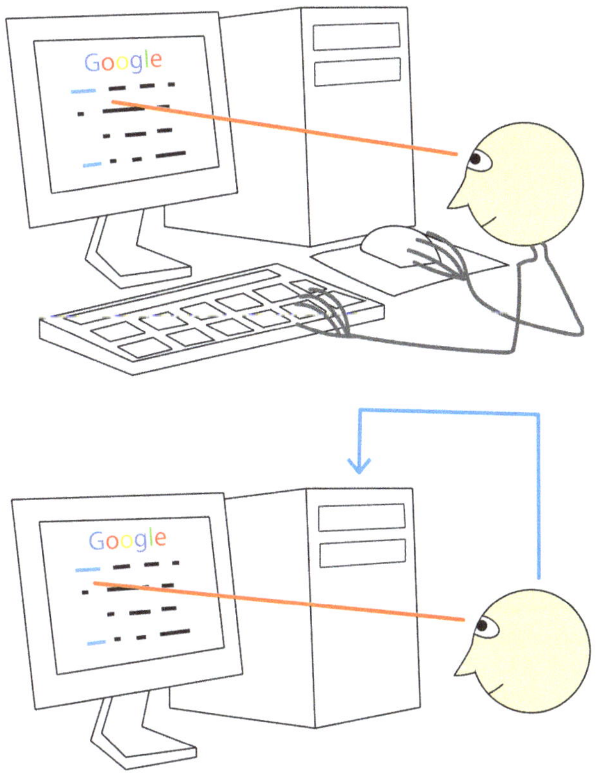

FIGURE 1 | A direct way to convey your desire to a computer: just look! When using a monitor, we normally look at a screen button or a link before clicking on them (upper panel). Between looking and clicking, we take the mouse (if we are not holding it all time), locate the cursor, move the cursor to the button or link, check if it reached the target. Gaze fixation at a given monitor location, however, can be promptly recognized with an eye tracker. If our intention to click would be recognized with some technology based on brain signal analysis (**lower panel, blue line**), computer control could be obtained without the above listed range of motor and sensory activities. (Generally, detection of gaze fixations alone is not enough due to the Midas touch problem, see text for details).

In this case, gaze positioning would play important role, and eye muscles need to be used intensively. However, the same is true for the operation of any non-invasive BCI when high information transfer rate is demonstrated: it is always a gaze-dependent operation, in a partial contradiction to Wolpaw et al. (2002) strict definition of a BCI. The user of such BCIs (the Steady State Visual Evoked Potential based BCI, SSVEP BCI; the codebook Visual Evoked Potential based BCI, cVEP BCI; the P300 wave based BCI, P300 BCI, when it is used by healthy people and some of the EEG electrodes are placed over the visual areas) selects one of a number of spatially distinct stimuli with his or her gaze, and the BCI task is actually to find where the user is looking by analyzing the brain's fully automatic response to stimulation.

In other words, these BCIs play the role of an eye tracker, and the brain's response to stimuli is used in such BCIs somewhat similarly to the use of the corneal reflection in a video based eye tracker. Moreover, a BCI that uses spatially distinct visual stimuli is an eye tracker with limited capabilities: unlike the usual eye trackers, it cannot determine coordinates of an arbitrary gaze position, but only indicate at which one of the stimuli the user is looking. Although attention is involved, and attempts were made to use overt and covert attention as separate BCI control channels, its direct (not gaze-mediated) effect is low comparing to gaze dependent effects. This is one of the main reasons why performance of the same BCI systems is, unfortunately, much lower in severely paralyzed users who do not control their gaze well (e.g., Sellers et al., 2010). In addition, as these BCIs depend on repetitive presentation of visual stimuli, GUIs should be significantly modified to become compatible with them.

The technology that enables direct interaction with computers using eye gaze also exists and is already used to assist paralyzed people in such tasks as typing and web browsing, with better performance than typical BCIs offer (Bolt, 1982; Jacob, 1990, 1991; Velichkovsky et al., 1997; Majaranta and Bulling, 2014). In a frequent variant of this technology, a video based eye tracker captures gaze direction. Intentionally prolonged gaze fixations (dwells) on elements of GUI, such as screen buttons, are detected and converted into equivalents of mouse clicks. It was, however, recognized early in the development of gaze-based interaction that the eye movements and fixations used for sending commands in such interfaces are similar to eye movements and fixations that are a part of normal eye behavior unrelated to interaction, such as viewing (Jacob, 1990, 1991). The interaction systems that are based on gaze direction, therefore, cannot distinguish between attempts to issue a command and the visual gaze fixations, and this leads to the Midas touch problem (Jacob, 1990, 1991): wherever the user looks, a command is activated, even if he or she has no intention to produce any command.

It was also stated at that early stage of developing gaze-base interaction with computers that the main issue in this field is "appropriate interaction techniques that incorporate eye movements into the user-computer dialogue in a convenient and natural way" (Jacob, 1990, p. 11). Such techniques have not been developed so far, despite many attempts to solve the Midas touch problem. For example, if only fixations on screen buttons exceeding a long (1000 ms or longer) threshold produce "clicks," erroneous command activations will be rare, but the need to use such long fixation will slow down the control and make it tiresome. Impressive speed of interaction was recently achieved with dwell-free typing approach (Kristensson and Vertanen, 2012; Sarcar et al., 2013; Pedrosa et al., 2015), however, it seems to impose high attentional demands. Another recently developed approach to increase the speed is to use, as a marker of control, a saccade to a new position of interest that naturally occurs immediately after the feedback at the position where the user currently looks for control (Publicover et al., 2016). In this case, short fixation duration thresholds can be used because unintended selection are typically not confirmed by such well-timed saccades. This system, by definition, cannot work when the user does not respond to feedback quickly enough. Thus, attentional demands imposed by this system can also be high. Other attempts to provide markers for command-related gaze fixations or eye movements (see, e.g., Velichkovsky et al., 1997; Majaranta and Bulling, 2014, for reviews) possessed the same or other drawbacks.

One may expect that brain state and/or course of brain activity differs strongly during gaze fixations related to attempts to send a command and gaze fixations related to other activities, such as free viewing or mind wandering. A "click" on a fixated GUI element could be made on the basis of fast detection of brain activity patterns that correlate with the intention to activate a command (**Figure 1, bottom panel**). The joint use of the information from "eyes and brains" for GUI control ("point with your eye and click with your mind!") was proposed as early as in 1996 (Velichkovsky and Hansen, 1996).

Several attempts to enhance gaze based control with a "mental click" recognized by BCI has been made. However, the use of additional mental tasks, such as motor imagery (e.g., in Zander et al., 2010) or mental concentration (Kim et al., 2015) does not seem to be effective, because BCIs cannot reliably recognize such activity within a fixation unless it is very long. Moreover, the use of additional mental task may itself interfere with the main mental activity. It is, therefore, not surprising that in a recent extensive review of hybrid BCIs only 3 of 55 reviewed journal papers addressed the Midas touch problem (Banville and Falk, 2016; see also other reviews on hybrid BCIs by Pfurtscheller et al., 2010; Müller-Putz et al., 2015). It seems that mechanistically combining gaze based technologies with existing BCIs cannot lead to the development of an efficient input system.

Zander and colleagues (Ihme and Zander, 2011; Protzak et al., 2013) proposed to make use of the EEG patterns that naturally accompany gaze based control. Their works were based on the "passive BCI" approach, i.e., the detection of brain signal patterns that naturally accompany the brain activities of interest, without the need from the user to do anything voluntarily to evoke these patterns (Zander and Kothe, 2011). The passive BCI approach seems to be exactly what is needed for detecting intentions in the most unobtrusive way, while gaze dwells effectively reveal the time intervals where the markers of intentions can be searched for in the brain signals. The EEG was collected during fixations intentionally used for control and during non-controlling fixations and successfully classified off-line (Ihme and Zander, 2011; Protzak et al., 2013). However, gaze dwell time thresholds were again quite long, 2000 ms in Ihme and Zander (2011) and 1000 ms in Protzak et al. (2013). Moreover, the participant task in both studies involved visual search, and the classification could rely mainly on fixation-related potential (FRP) components related to finding a target, rather than to intention to act.

When a target is searched for among a range of distractors, one may use the EEG potentials that accompany target detection, such as the P300 wave. Recent studies of the FRPs in the visual search tasks demonstrated that finding an object, area or position of interest can be detected using a combination of eye tracking and EEG (Healy and Smeaton, 2011; Kamienkowski et al., 2012; Brouwer et al., 2013; Kaunitz et al., 2014; Devillez et al., 2015; Finke et al., 2016; Ušćumlić and Blankertz, 2016; Wenzel et al., 2016). In particular, Finke et al. (2016) reported high performance, with area under ROC curve (AUC) of about 0.9, for classification of short target vs. non-target fixations. Similar phenomena could be a basis of classification in studies by Ihme and Zander (2011) and Protzak et al. (2013). This approach, however, is limited, because a click on a screen button or link is not always required immediately after they are found. In many applications, the user should be at least given an option to execute control in less automatic way. The P300 wave, which plays important role in this approach, can decrease and even vanish under many conditions, for example, when the target is always found at the same position. Classification of FRPs can be also related to the effects from planning a saccade to a new location of interest (Graupner et al., 2011; Nikolaev et al., 2013), but its possible use in BCI is limited for similar reasons. An effective general-purpose interface may include algorithms for supporting fast responses to just-found targets, but has to be primarily focused on more direct procedures of intention detection.

The current study followed the proposals of Zander and colleagues (Ihme and Zander, 2011; Protzak et al., 2013), i.e., it relied on finding EEG (FRP) markers for gaze dwells intentionally used for control. However, we aimed on investigating the possibility to find the FRP markers of controlling fixations when relatively short (500 ms) dwell time threshold is used. Fixations of this length are frequently observed in normal viewing, and do not require significant effort when they should be produced voluntarily. Special attention was paid to equalizing irrelevant factors that could confound the difference between the fixations used for control and spontaneous fixations. We took a straightforward approach of collecting the synchronized gaze and EEG data from the participants in a realistic scenario, when they played a game with their gaze only. The gaze controlled variant of a known, sufficiently engaging computer game was designed for this study, to make possible obtaining a large number of fixations of required duration, both intentionally used for control and spontaneous ones.

Results from a pilot study of the FRP markers of controlling fixations and summaries of the current work were presented at a few conferences (Shishkin et al., 2015, 2016b,c). This publication provides the detailed description of the approach, methodology and results.

METHODS

Participants

The study was conducted in 8 healthy participants (age 21–48, mean 29, one female) in accordance with the Declaration of Helsinki and the local institutional regulations. All participants gave written informed consent. They had normal or corrected to normal vision. Two of them (participants 6 and 7) had no previous experience with gaze based control. The others already participated in a few pilot experiments with the same gaze controlled game as in this study.

Apparatus and Software Used in Online Experiments

Electroencephalogram (EEG) was recorded at 500 Hz and 24 bit voltage resolution with an *actiCHamp* amplifier and *actiCAP* active electrodes (Brain Products, Germany) from 19 positions (Fz, F3, F4, Cz, C3, C4, Pz, P1, P2, P3, P4, POz, PO3, PO4, PO7, PO8, Oz, O1, and O2). More electrodes were placed in the posterior area than in the anterior one, because our pilot studies indicated that the marker for controlling fixations was likely to be found in the occipitoparietal region. Reference EEG electrodes were located at earlobes. Electrooculogram (EOG) was captured with the same amplifier and active electrode set. For horizontal EOG, electrodes were placed about 1 cm from the outer canthi. Vertical EOG was recorded with an electrode about 2 cm below the right eye and another one at Fp2 position (this location was preferred to more standard lower locations to avoid interference with the forehead rest). Ground electrode was located at AFz. Electrode impedances were kept below 20 KOhm. Gaze coordinates were recorded monocularly at 500 Hz sampling rate with the *EyeLink 1000 Plus* video based eye tracker (SR Research, Canada).

Recording of EEG and EOG, their synchronization with the eye gaze data, online processing of the eye gaze data and running the gaze controlled game were made with custom programs under *Resonance*, a framework for prototyping multimodal (hybrid) BCIs being developed by one of the authors of this study (Y.O.N.). For offline synchronization of the data, markers were sent from the eye tracker computer's parallel port to the EEG amplifier's TTL port in the beginning of each game. To control the stability of synchronization, this procedure was repeated in the end of the games (the time difference was typically no larger than two samples).

Dwells were detected online using a spatial (dispersion-based) criterion: gaze position range on each of X and Y coordinates should not exceed 2° for the specified dwell time (500 or 1000 ms, depending on condition). This criterion was chosen for two practical reasons: first, it could be easily implemented in the online software; secondly, it provided subjective experience of reliable control, according to our observations in the pilot experiments with the gaze controlled game used in this study. Several additional criteria had also to be met: no dwell detected in a 3 × 3° squared region centered around the previous click's position for previous 3000 ms, and no dwell detected in any position for 500 ms or 1000 ms (depending on condition). Each time all these criteria were met, a "click" was produced in the game (an event with the same effect as of a computer mouse click), and this time minus 500 or 1000 ms (for 500 or 1000 ms conditions, relatively) was designated as the beginning of the dwell event. The location of each "click" was computed as medians of X and Y coordinates of the gaze within the dwell time interval (excluding subintervals corresponding to the blinks reported by the eye tracker).

For simplicity, we call in this paper all the detected intentional and spontaneous dwell events "fixations." Although the criteria for their detection were rather loose and, theoretically, small amplitude saccades and re-fixations could happen within the dwell interval, it seemed unlikely that they could bias our analysis results.

The Gaze Controlled Game

To collect the EEG during diverse, intensive and realistic gaze-mediated interaction with a computer, we designed a gaze controlled game *EyeLines*. It was based on a computer game *Lines* (or *Color Lines*) ("Color Lines," in Wikipedia. Retrieved June 27, 2016, from http://en.wikipedia.org/wiki/ColorLines). Like the original game, the *EyeLines* is a simple computer puzzle game, with the goal to construct as many "lines" from colored balls as possible. The player is presented with a square board on which three colored balls appear in the beginning of the game. On each turn, the player has to move one ball to a free cell on the board. When the required or higher number of balls with the same color form a "full" line, either horizontal, vertical or diagonal, these balls disappear. If no such line is formed, three new balls randomly selected out of seven different colors are put on random cells. The game is over when the board is full.

In *Lines*, a move is typically made with a mouse click first on a ball and then on a free cell where it should be moved. In *EyeLines* (**Figure 2**), gaze dwells are used as an equivalent to mouse clicks, following the approach most often used in gaze controlled software. To avoid unwanted actions resulting from spontaneous long fixations and also to make possible collecting sufficient number of such fixations, gaze based control in the game board was off by default. After deciding which ball to move and to which free cell, a participant had to switch control on by gaze dwell on the only location where control was permanently on. This location was an additional cell (the *button*) positioned outside the game board either left, as in **Figure 2**, or right to it.

The participants were instructed to make the moves in the game by three subsequent *controlling fixations*: on the *button*, on a *ball* and on a *free cell* where the ball should be moved. A 500 or 1000 ms dwell time threshold was used (same in all games that constituted one experiment block) for all these actions. When fixation duration exceeded the threshold, a visual feedback was given. It was specific to each action: dwell on the button led to appearing, in this separate cell, a ball of color different from the board balls (the participants were told that this indicates switching the board control on); dwell on a ball within the board led to ball selection indicated by a gray square frame that appeared around the ball; dwell on a free cell led to moving the selected ball into this cell.

When control was off, fixations on the balls made no effect. They were considered as presumably spontaneous fixations (used for viewing or related to mind wandering) and constituted a separate type of *non-controlling fixations*.

To ensure more reliable gaze based control and to reduce complexity of the gameplay (so that even novices could make sufficient number of moves per game without long practice), we made some features of *EyeLines* simpler comparing to typical implementations of *Lines*. In particular, the board size was made 7 × 7 instead of 9 × 9 in "classical" *Lines*, and the minimal number of balls required to form a full line was decreased from five to four. To support more detectable gaze fixations, a dot was put in the center of each ball and each free cell, the balls were drawn as plane circles (not as "3d like" spheres, to avoid asymmetrical features that could significantly shift the gaze from the center), and cells were designed as small squares with substantial spaces between them (**Figure 2**).

The game was presented on a 27″ LCD monitor positioned at the distance of 60 cm from participant's eyes. The game board subtended 18 × 18° on the monitor screen.

Procedure

Participants were seated in a chair in front of the monitor. Chin and forehead rest was used to ensure stable head positioning. Participants were asked to relax and make no bodily movements during calibration and playing the game. They were instructed to make moves in the game by still looking sequentially at the button, the ball and the free cell, each time until they saw the feedback. After a move was completed, they could freely look at the board and fixate any ball or free cell for any time without evoking any action, until they dwelled at the button again for a time exceeding the threshold.

Participants were told to refrain from hurrying up with each move and to find "better" moves whenever possible, but not to think for too long time. In the preliminary experiments, however, we found that the *EyeLines* players often tend to makes moves as fast as possible even when they were urged not to do so. Due to this, sufficient number of non-controlling fixations could be not always collected. Therefore, an additional feature was introduced to *EyeLines*: after each 4–8 moves the cell outside the board that indicated the button's position disappeared from the screen for 10 s and the dwell on its former position had no effect, so that the participant could not make moves during this time. The participants were told that they had to use this time for planning the further moves. In addition to encouraging higher number of long fixations within this time, this trick presumably could help to prevent the participants from playing the game at too fast pace.

To those participants who had no prior experience with *EyeLines* or *Lines*, rules of the game were explained prior to EEG electrode mounting. They played two games with short duration (2 min) for practice.

In the main part of the experiment, all the participants played, in total, eight games with maximum duration of 5 min. The session was divided into two blocks of equal size, differed by the dwell time threshold, which was set at either 500 or 1000 ms. The order of the blocks was randomly assigned to the participants (three of the eight started with the 500 ms threshold block). The switch-on button position (left or right to the board) was alternated every game throughout the session. Its position in the first game was also chosen randomly (counterbalanced over the group). A 5 to 10 min rest was offered between the blocks, and shorter (typically up to minute) rest intervals were inserted between the games. Prior to each game, a nine-point calibration of the eye tracker was run.

Offline Data Analysis

In this study, all EEG analysis, including classification, was made offline using the EEG data collected during the online gaze-based control. However, to make single-trial FRP classification performance evaluation realistic, the procedures for signal processing, feature extraction and application of the classifier to the new data were designed so that they could be used online without introducing any significant delay.

Signal preprocessing and segmentation were made mainly with *R*, while *MATLAB* (*MathWorks*) was used for visualization and classification. EEGLAB (Delorme and Makeig, 2004) routines *eegplot* and *topoplot* were used, relatively, for manual checking the quality of EEG/EOG epochs and for plotting scalp topographies. MANOVA was performed using *STATISTICA 7* (*StatSoft*).

Electroencephalogram (EEG) was re-referenced offline to linked earlobes, and bipolar EOG was calculated as the difference of amplitude in right/left and upper/lower channels, respectively. Line noise in EEG and EOG was reduced with 50 Hz notch filter (2nd order Butterworth). For creating the ERP time plots (but not for the other types of analysis), low-pass 7 Hz filter (2nd order Butterworth) was also applied.

For EEG and EOG analysis, [−500 +1500] ms epochs were extracted related to the start of four types of fixations exceeding the dwell time threshold: three types of controlling fixations (button, ball and free cell) and one type of non-controlling fixations. As non-controlling fixations, only fixations on balls made without fixating the button prior to them were considered; fixations of this kind on free cells were very rare and could not be used in the analysis. Data were analyzed separately for 500 and 1000 ms dwell threshold conditions. In some cases, they were also divided into subconditions related to left and right position of the button.

Fixation-related potentials (FRPs), by definition, are synchronized with the eye movements and, therefore, can be systematically contaminated by EOG artifacts. To deal with

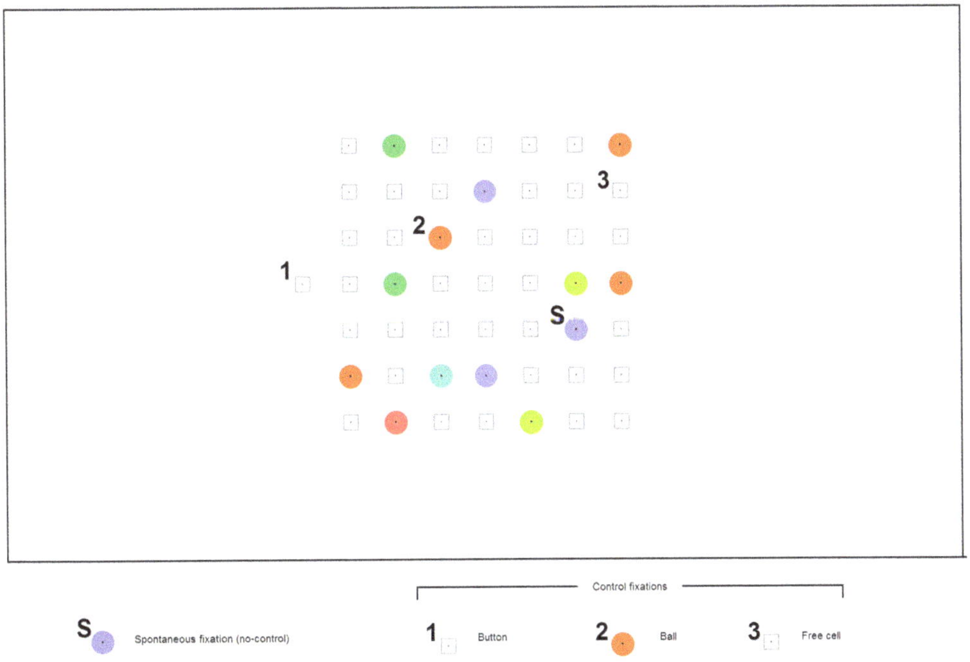

FIGURE 2 | An example screenshot of the *EyeLines* display. The participants moved the color balls in order to construct lines from balls of the same color. Each move was made with gaze fixations only. A participant could make any number of spontaneous fixations (S) without any visible effect; however, their time was recorded. A dwell on the button (1) lead to appearing a ball in the button position, indicating that "control is on." After this, a dwell on any ball in the game board (2) led to its "selection" (a frame appeared around it), and then the ball could be placed to a new position by a dwell on a free cell (3). (The digits 1, 2, 3, and the letter "S" were not a part of the actual display and were added to the screenshot for illustrative purposes).

this problem, we set the baseline interval and borders of the EEG time intervals used for analysis and classification within the fixation. Our pilot studies suggested that the difference between the EEG amplitude in controlling and non-controlling fixations in the *EyeLines* game was most pronounced in the late part of fixation. In contrast, the amplitude of the lambda wave, the component of the fixation-related potentials with the latency of about 100 ms from fixation start, did not exhibit pronounced dependence on gaze-based control. To make the baseline less sensitive to the lambda wave and other visual components that could be irrelevant for control detection, we decided to use as the baseline 200–300 ms interval relative to the fixation start. No high-pass filter was used (the EEG amplifier used in this study allowed for DC recording), so the amplitude shifts related to eye movements could not influence the fixation interval through the transient response of the filter. Because our study was focused on the EEG features that could be used in fast online classification of the controlling and non-controlling fixations, the upper border of the analyzed interval was set at 500 ms both in 500 ms and 1000 ms dwell threshold conditions.

After baseline subtraction, we checked the number of epochs with amplitude higher than 70 μV in 200–500 ms interval in any channel, per fixation type, condition and participant. The highest incidence of such epochs was only five, while in most cases no such epochs were observed at all. Therefore, no artifact rejection procedure was applied to the data.

Feature Extraction and Classification

Electroencephalogram (EEG) features were extracted from only 13 posterior channels (P1, P2, P3, P4, Pz, PO3, PO4, PO7, PO8, POz, O1, O2, and Oz). Due to low number of non-controlling fixations exceeding 1000 ms threshold, the classifier was trained using only the data from the condition where this threshold was used. Therefore, the right border of the interval for feature selection was set as the lowest dwell threshold in our experiment, i.e., 500 ms. (In online mode, not implemented in this study but supposed to be the main application of its results, a fixation exceeding this threshold should be classified as soon as possible, thus features could be taken only before the threshold.) The left border was set at 200 ms after the fixation start, to exclude the EOG artifacts. As in the EEG analysis described above, mean amplitude of the 200–300 ms baseline interval was subtracted from the EEG amplitudes channelwise, and no filter was used (except for the 50 Hz notch filter during EEG recording).

To capture the development of the negative wave, we used overlapping windows of 50 ms length and time step 20 ms (200–250, 220–270, and 440–490 ms, total $n = 13$ windows). The feature vector (169 features) for each fixation k was composed of the mean values of EEG amplitude $m_k(i, c)$ computed for each of these windows ($i = 1$–8) in each channel ($c = 1$–13).

One class of the data was the non-controlling fixations. The other class was formed either from the button fixations only (Trainset 1) or from all controlling fixations (Trainset 2). Trainset

1 was used because button FRPs differed most strongly from the non-controlling fixations, so their classification could provide an upper estimate of the performance. It is also possible that only the first fixation in a controlling sequence of fixations should be detected in the EBCI. Trainset 2 was used to explore how well the classifier could be used with different type of controlling fixations without additional tuning to each of them.

Two classification approaches were applied to the data separately. The first one was the Linear Discriminate Analysis (LDA) with shrinkage regularization (Blankertz et al., 2011) implemented in Fieldtrip toolbox for EEG/MEG-analysis (Oostenveld et al., 2011, http://www.ru.nl/neuroimaging/fieldtrip), further referred to as Shrinkage LDA. The second approach, the Committee of Greedy Classifiers, further referred to as Committee, was to create a pool of weak threshold classifiers performing in one-dimensional feature spaces (one classifier per feature), to select classifiers with a greedy algorithm and to use them in a classifier committee. More specifically, each weak classifier was trained independently on one of the 169 features, and a greedy algorithm was used to select 15 features and corresponding classifiers from the pool (at the first iteration, the classifier which had the minimal classification error was chosen to become a committee member; at each of further iterations, the classifier which minimized the error of committee was added to it). The Committee classified fixations by simple voting of the selected weak classifiers (Trofimov et al., 2015).

Thresholds for the classifiers were adjusted using validation subsets to obtain at least 0.90 specificity. The reason to aim on relatively high specificity in expense of sensitivity was that in EBCIs, i.e., interfaces based on combining gaze based control and the BCI technology, low sensitivity of an EEG classifier can be partly compensated by additional gaze based control routines. In particular, if users found that the interface does not respond to their intention as fast as they expect, they can simply dwell longer, so that the interface may recognize the intention without the EEG, just with an additional, longer dwell time threshold. In contrast, the specificity of the interface should be kept high in most cases, because too frequent false alarms can be annoying and even dangerous (e.g., in robotic applications).

For each classifier, performance was estimated separately for training and testing using either Trainset 1 or Trainset 2, and for testing on data from either 500 ms or 1000 ms dwell threshold conditions, to estimate if the same classifier could be used effectively for different types of data.

Five-fold cross-validation was used for estimation of the classifiers' performance, except for the cases when training and testing was done on different subtypes of fixations. Details on how the data were divided into training, validating and testing subsets are given in notes under relevant tables (**Tables 2–5**) in the *Results* section.

RESULTS

Behavioral Data

Each participant was able to play *EyeLines* with gaze control only, i.e., without any manual input. The control was very stable: participants reported that they encountered from 1 to 4 errors per session, including ball selections or free cell selection incorrectly recognized by the software, as well as their own errors. Offline analysis of gaze data showed that there were also rare cases when the participants dwelled on two or more balls in a row when control was on, or attempted to make a move that violated the rules and therefore was not actually executed; these cases were excluded from the analysis, except for some of the rarest cases which were difficult to separate due to technical reasons (the latter lead to slightly higher number of ball selections comparing to button activation events). On average, a participant made about 150 moves in the condition with 500 ms dwell threshold and about 120 moves in the condition with 1000 ms dwell threshold.

The number of controlling and non-controlling threshold-exceeding fixations collected in the experiment is given in **Table 1**. About 160 spontaneous fixations of 500 ms or longer duration were collected with 500 ms threshold, while the number of 1000 ms or longer spontaneous fixations was about 15 times lower. Except for these long spontaneous fixations, the number of collected fixations was sufficient for analysis, varying from 74 for free cell selection with 1000 ms threshold (in participant 2), to 208 for non-controlling fixation with 500 ms threshold (in the same participant). The number of controlling fixations was higher in every participant in the 500 ms compared to 1000 ms threshold conditions (see **Table 1**), possibly due to the restriction of the total game duration that was same in both conditions. However, the size of this difference was small in all participants (varying from 20 to 34%), therefore, no correction of the EEG analysis procedure was needed.

Overview of the Fixation-Related Potentials (FRPs)

Our main interest was to characterize the EEG features that can be used for online detection of the dwell-based gaze control and, therefore, should appear earlier than the dwell time threshold. In the current study, for the sake of simplicity, we focused only on amplitude (not spectral and not synchrony based) features, on current fixation (not the preceding one) and only on the features that could not be affected by eye movement artifacts.

Before starting to analyze the FRPs, we had to check if the EEG at the output of our preprocessing algorithm was sufficiently free from the EOG contamination. The highest contamination could be expected in the case of button fixations, when the gaze fixated an extreme position and the horizontal EOG could be added to the EEG signal especially strongly and systematically. **Figure 3** shows FRPs (as a "butterfly plot") and EOG for the button events averaged separately for left and right button positions. While the EOG contamination was evident in the FRP waveforms before the start of the fixation (0 on the time scale) and after approximately 250 ms following the dwell threshold at 500 ms (right vertical line), the horizontal EOG had very low amplitude in the 200–500 ms range. This interval was used for the analysis of EEG amplitude in both 500 and 1000 ms dwell time threshold conditions.

Figure 3 reveals a nearly linear negative trend in most of the EEG channels used in the study, possibly related to the

TABLE 1 | Number of controlling and non-controlling (spontaneous) fixations exceeding the dwell time threshold in the 500 ms and 1000 ms threshold conditions (collapsed over left-button and right-button conditions).

Sbj.	500 ms fixation threshold					1000 ms fixation threshold				
	Non-controlling fixations	Controlling fixations				Non-controlling fixations	Controlling fixations			
		All	Button	Ball	Free cell		All	Button	Ball	Free cell
1	114	444	150	148	146	9	369	124	123	122
2	208	364	120	128	116	15	271	101	96	74
3	144	408	138	139	131	13	325	109	108	108
4	200	549	184	184	181	24	446	150	148	148
5	162	435	147	148	140	4	338	113	113	112
6	124	527	176	180	171	5	428	145	142	141
7	123	442	151	153	138	7	358	122	121	115
8	194	517	171	175	171	9	378	125	127	126
Mean	158.6	460.8	154.6	156.9	149.3	10.8	364.1	123.6	122.3	118.3
Std.	38.0	64.1	21.2	20.4	22.7	6.5	56.0	16.9	17.1	22.6

expectation of the visual feedback (note that the experiment was organized in such a way that the gaze dwells intentionally used for control led to an equivalent of mouse click on the fixated position of the screen). Since we already used an interval near the start of this trend (200–300 ms) as the baseline, an average over an interval near the threshold can be used as a robust estimate of the trend. To view the topography of this negativity, we averaged EEG amplitude over 400–500 ms interval and plotted the results. **Figure 4** shows grand average maps (individual maps had a similar pattern). According to this figure, the negativity was prominent in the parietooccipital area in all conditions. The maps also demonstrate a left-right asymmetry in Button condition that depended on button position: it was slightly stronger in the hemisphere contralateral to the gaze controlled switch-on button position where gaze dwelled in these fixations. Specifically, the difference between PO4 and PO3 amplitude in Button fixations with 500 ms dwell threshold was -0.4 ± 1.7 μV (M ± SD) in left button condition and $+2.2 \pm 1.3$ μV in right button condition. The difference was significant, according to paired Student's *t*-test [$t_{(7)} = -3.2, p = 0.02$]. In Ball fixations, no difference between the two positions of the button was observed [the corresponding values were $+ 0.5 \pm 0.9$ μV and $+ 0.3 \pm 0.8$ μV, $t_{(7)} = 0.5, p = 0.6$].

Note that Button fixations were the most extreme fixations required for playing the game (the switch-on button was positioned left or right to the game board), while Ball fixations were all within the game board. The presence of the laterality effect in the Button but not in the Ball fixations means that it was not related to the direction of the previous saccade but is not sufficient to decide whether it was related to the current fixation or to the direction of the saccade to the next position that could be planned within this fixation. Nevertheless, the laterality effect is interesting because it was not reported so far for the Stimulus-Preceding Negativity (SPR) that could be the closest "relative" of the observed negative variation in the psychophysiological literature (see Discussion for more details).

In the rest of the amplitude analysis, POz electrode was used, because it the negativity that marked control-on fixations was typically highest at this location.

Factors Influencing the FRPs

Generally, FRPs may depend on many factors that may vary significantly during gaze interaction. These effects may negatively affect the stability of EBCI classifiers built using the FRPs or can be used for increasing the amplitude of the FRPs markers and, thus, for improving the EBCI performance. Detailed analysis of such effects could not be performed within the current study. However, we were interested to estimate if the negativity in the intentional fixation can be influenced by several factors which were well controlled in our experiment: left or right position of the switch-on "button" (which was already shown to produce a laterality effect), dwell time threshold (low effect of this factor would suggest that varying time of the feedback can be applied in online operation of EBCI likely without strong reduction of performance) and fixation type (it was most important to confirm the difference between spontaneous (non-controlling) and controlling fixations, but the difference between different types of controlling fixations should also be taken into account in EBCI development).

For this analysis, each participant's POz amplitudes averaged over 400–500 ms interval (with 200–300 ms baseline) for each fixation type and dwell time threshold were submitted to a 3-way MANOVA, with the following repeated measures factors:

- Button Position, with 2 levels: Left and Right,
- Dwell Threshold, with 2 levels: 500 ms and 1000 ms dwell time,
- Fixation Type, with 4 levels: Button, Ball, Free Cell, No-Control.

Significant effect was found for Fixation Type [Wilk's $\lambda = 0.06$, $F_{(3, 5)} = 24.6$, $p = 0.002$], whereas the Button Position effect [Wilk's $\lambda = 0.96$, $F_{(1, 7)} = 0.32$, $p = 0.6$], Dwell Threshold effect [Wilk's $\lambda = 0.99$, $F_{(1, 7)} = 0.02$, $p = 0.9$] and all interactions

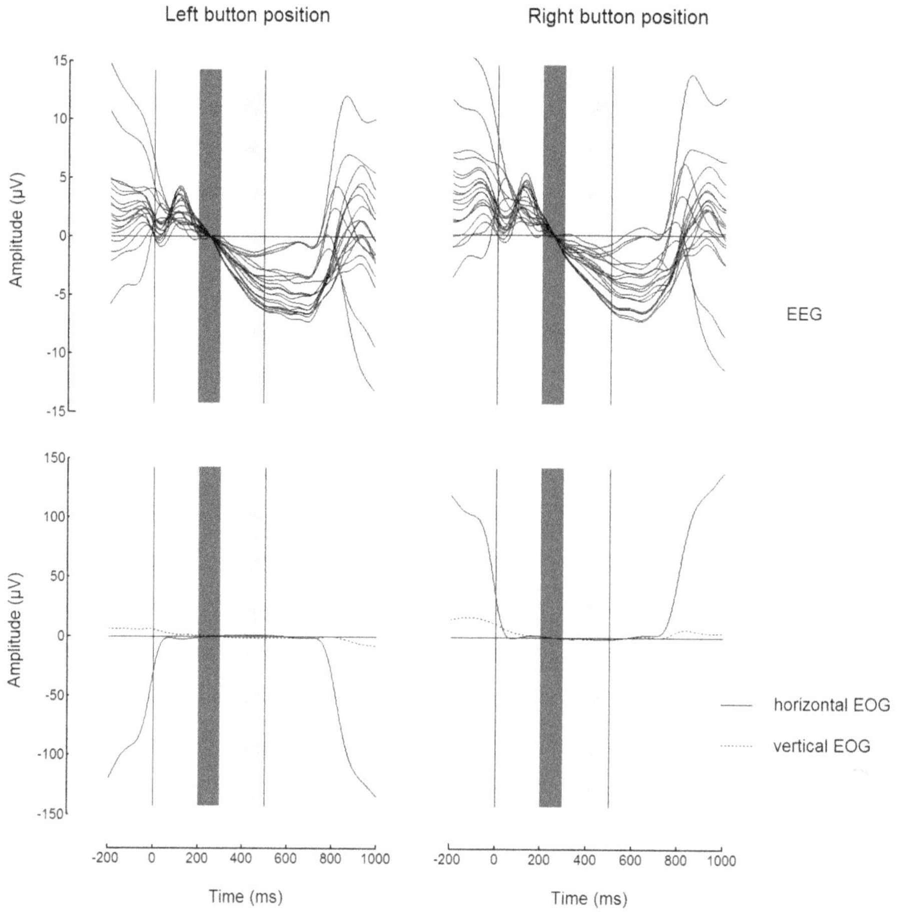

FIGURE 3 | Butterfly plots showing grand average ($n = 8$) superimposed channels with fixation-related potentials (FRPs, upper panels) and corresponding electrooculogram (EOG, lower panels) for fixations on button. The signals were low-pass filtered at 7 Hz and baseline corrected (high-pass filtering was not used). Note the similarity between the waveforms for left and right button positions (in the left and in the right, respectively) within most of the fixation interval. Zero millisecond corresponds to the beginning of fixation. The baseline interval (200–300 ms) is shown by dark gray bars. The light gray bars show 400–500 ms interval from which the EEG amplitudes were averaged to obtain estimates of the trend over the fixation used in the subsequent analysis (**Figures 4**, **5**). Dwell time threshold was 500 ms (marked with the vertical lines in the right edges of the light gray bars).

between factors were not significant. According to *post-hoc* Tukey HSD test, amplitude at POz in 400–500 ms interval was significantly more negative in Button comparing to No-Control fixations ($p = 0.0002$), in Ball comparing to No-Control fixations ($p = 0.01$) and in Button comparing to Free Cell fixations ($p = 0.0007$). In Ball fixations, POz was nearly significantly more negative than in Free Cell fixations ($p = 0.064$), while the difference between No-Control and Free Cell fixation as well as between Button and Ball fixations was not significant ($p = 0.18$ and $p = 0.8$, respectively).

Mean amplitudes and confidence intervals are shown in **Figure 5**. Individual data generally followed the same pattern, with largest POz amplitude in Button fixations. With 500 ms dwell threshold, POz amplitude ranged −3.6 to −10.3 μV in the Left button condition (−5.5 ± 2.1 μV) and −3.4 to −7.4 μV (5.1 ± 1.4 μV) in the Right button condition (the values in the parenthesis are M ± SD). POz amplitude in No-Control fixations, however, tended to be also negative (Left button: −0.4 to −4.0 μV, −2.0 ± 1.3 μV; Right button: +0.6 to −3.2 μV, −1.1 ± 1.2 μV).

Individual and averaged over the groups FRPs at POz for Button fixations and both 500 ms and 1000 ms thresholds are shown, separately for the left and right button conditions, in **Figure 6**. Note that in the 200–500 ms interval the signal pattern was similar for all the compared conditions, and the amplitudes and time courses were, in general, very similar in different dwell threshold and button position conditions (**Figure 6**). Importantly, during Button and Ball fixations the negativity at POz was developed over the first 500 ms in all participants (this was not the case only in the Free cell fixations for several participants).

FRPs time courses for all fixation types averaged over the left and right button positions are presented in **Figure 7** (only for the 500 ms dwell threshold condition). This figure confirms the difference between fixation types: subsequent fixations were progressively weaker within the triplets used to make moves.

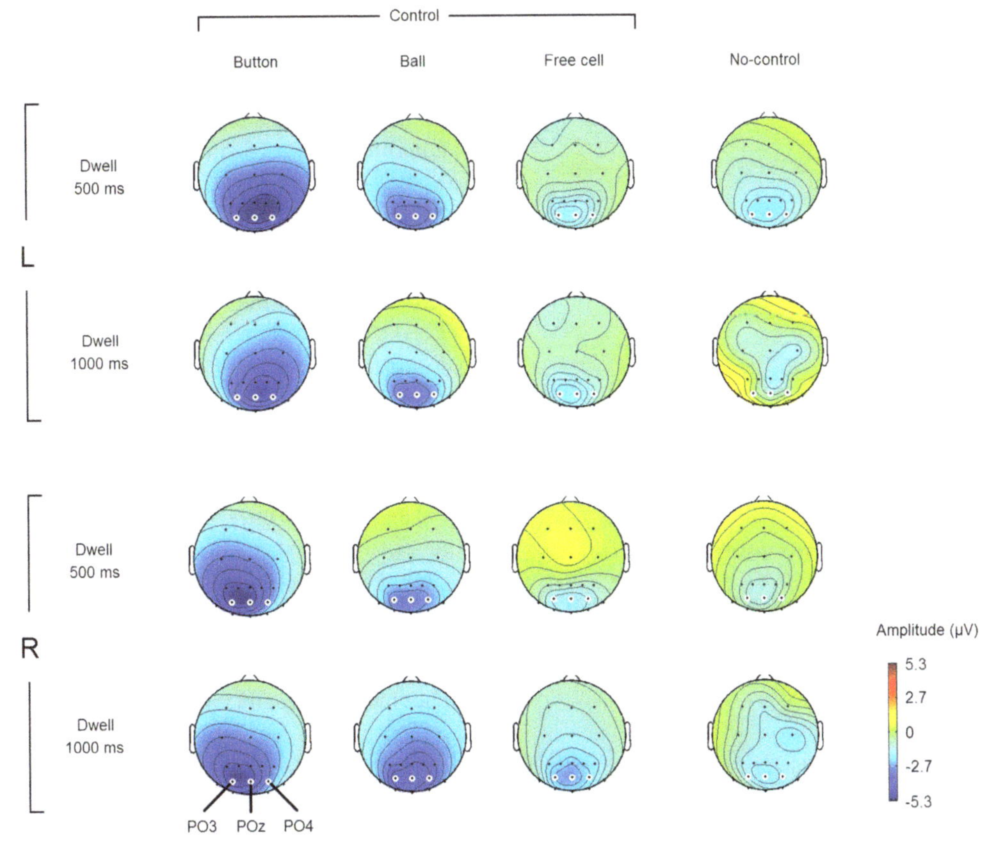

FIGURE 4 | Grand average (*n* = 8) amplitude topography of the negative potential developed within different types of fixations and different dwell time thresholds. L, left button position; R, right button position (note that the switch-on button was "clicked" not manually but by gaze fixations only). Amplitude estimates were obtained by averaging over 400–500 ms interval relative to fixation start (baseline 200–300 ms). Small white circles highlight the electrodes which were used in statistical analysis (POz, PO3, and PO4). Note that non-controlling fixations were rare in Dwell 1000 ms condition (see **Table 1**), thus the corresponding maps can be considered only as a rough estimate.

More detailed analysis is needed to estimate possible impact of the negativity from previous fixation(s) on the baseline, that could, theoretically, cause this progressive decrease. Also, additional experiments and analysis are needed to rule out the possibility that it was an extreme eye position that enabled high effect in Button fixations and to rule out possible effects that the preceding high-amplitude saccade could have on it or (through its effect on the lambda wave) even on the beginning of the baseline (cf. Nikolaev et al., 2016).

Figure 7 shows that, although No-Control fixations were accompanied by the negativity at POz in some participants, its growth tended to terminate in these fixations earlier than in the controlling fixations. It was possible that the participants sometimes forgot to switch control on before fixating a ball and quickly recognized their fault but could made a saccade before the dwell time threshold, so such fixations were erroneously considered as non-controlling ones in our analysis.

Classification

Finally, we estimated the possibilities to use the EEG marker of the gaze dwells used for intentional control by training statistical classifiers on the collected data and testing their performance offline under different settings that could be generally reproduced in online operation of the hybrid gaze interaction/BCI system (EBCI). Only 300 ms long EEG segments corresponding to fixations (200–500 ms relative to fixation onset) were used for single-trial classification.

The classifiers were trained using non-controlling fixations as the non-target class. The target class was represented either by Button fixations only (Trainset 1), or by all controlling fixations (Trainset 2). For the LDA classifier with the shrinkage regularization, performance results are provided in **Table 2** (Trainset 1) and **Table 3** (Trainset 2). For the committee of weak classifiers selected by the greedy algorithm, performance results are presented in **Table 4** (Trainset 1) and **Table 5** (Trainset 2).

As follows from **Tables 2–5**, the procedure for setting the classifier threshold using the validation subset provided a good approximation to the target specificity value of 0.90. Insufficient number of the non-controlling fixations in the 1000 ms dwell threshold condition (see **Table 1**) made calculation of specificity for this condition impossible. For the 500 ms dwell threshold data and LDA classifier, specificity was almost the same for

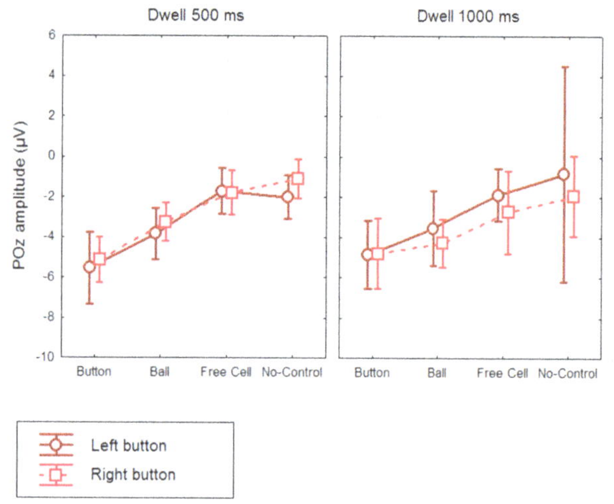

FIGURE 5 | Grand mean ($n = 8$) values and 95% confidence intervals of the negative potential at POz developed within different types of fixations, using different dwell time thresholds and button positions. Amplitude estimates were obtained by averaging over 400.500 ms interval relative to fixation start (baseline 200. 300 ms). Note that No-Control fixations were rare in Dwell 1000 ms condition (see **Table 1**), thus the average for these data can be considered only as a rough estimate.

Trainset 1 and Trainset 2: M ± SD was 0.87 ± 0.11 and 0.86 ± 0.15, respectively. A similar pattern was observed in the case of the committee of classifiers, but the mean values were slightly higher comparing to LDA: 0.90 ± 0.07 and 0.91 ± 0.07, respectively, for Trainset 1 and Trainset 2. Since the average number of non-controlling fixations in 4 games with the 500 ms dwell threshold was about 160 (**Table 1**) and one game lasted 5 min or (rarely) slightly less, the rate of 500 ms or longer non-controlling fixations was about $160/(4 \times 5) = 8\ \text{min}^{-1}$, and the specificity of 0.9 corresponded to $8\times(1-0.9) = 0.8$ false alarms per minute.

It was not possible to compare the two classifiers using ROC AUC values (the index which integrates performance estimates for different thresholds), because they could be computed not in all cases. However, given that the specificity values did not strongly differ between the classifiers and the training sets, we decided to compare the sensitivity values directly between different settings (**Figure 8**). We run a single 4-way MANOVA analysis on all sensitivity data, with the following repeated measures factors:

- Classifier, with 2 levels: Shrinkage LDA, Committee of Greedy Classifiers,
- Training Set, with 2 levels: Trainset 1 (only fixations on button as controlling fixations), Trainset 2 (all controlling fixations),
- Threshold, with 2 levels: 500 ms dwell time, 1000 ms dwell time,
- Fixation Type, with 3 levels: Button, Ball, Free Cell.

MANOVA results are presented in **Table 6**. They generally followed the effects observed in the analysis of EEG amplitudes reported above, such as significant main effect for Fixation Type factor (sensitivity was significantly higher for Button fixations, according to *post-hoc* analysis). Main effect and almost all interactions were not significant for Classifier, except for Classifier × Training Set × Dwell Threshold interaction ($p = 0.04$). There was a tendency of better sensitivity provided by the committee of classifiers comparing to the LDA in the case of training on all types of fixations and applying the classifier to 1000 ms data ($p = 0.08$, *post-hoc* Tukey test).

Although main effect was not significant for Training Set ($p = 0.32$), its interaction with Fixation Type was significant ($p = 0.012$). *Post-hoc* analysis revealed that the classifiers that were trained using all controlling fixations (Trainset 2) overperformed the classifiers trained on Button fixations only (Trainset 1) in the case of Ball and Free Cell fixations ($p = 0.005$ for both of them). With Trainset 1, sensitivity for the fixations not used for training (Button and Free Cell) was close to random level, especially with LDA classifier (**Table 2**), while improvement for Button fixations in the case of Trainset 1 did not reached statistical significance ($p = 0.09$, *post-hoc* Tukey test).

As one could expect, the classifier was more sensitive when the train and test data were recorded with the same dwell time threshold ($p = 0.0002$ for main effect of the factor Threshold). However, as follows from **Tables 2, 3**, the average difference was relatively small (on average, not higher than 0.03 for Trainset 1 and not higher than 0.06 for Trainset 2).

DISCUSSION

This study, for the first time, demonstrated that gaze fixations used for the interaction with a computer can be differentiated from spontaneous fixations using EEG markers from short time intervals (here, 200–500 ms relative to fixation start). This result opens the perspective of developing a hybrid "eye-brain computer interface," the EBCI, as an unobtrusive communication and control tool both for paralyzed patients with preserved gaze control and for healthy users.

In addition, with special measures taken to obtain the fixation-related EEG potentials (FRPs) free from contamination with EOG artifacts, we revealed and quantitatively characterized a pattern differentiating the controlling and no-controlling (spontaneous) fixations in each of the eight participants.

The analysis of FRPs is challenging due to the systematic contamination of the EEG from electrical potential shifts accompanying the eyeball movements. Such contamination cause problems either when the EOG artifacts appear in the time intervals that are the main focus of analysis or when they are present during intervals used for baseline correction (Finke et al., 2016; Nikolaev et al., 2016). In addition, EEG components within the first 200 ms after fixation onset depend on the size of saccade preceding the fixation (Nikolaev et al., 2016). In our study, only the 200–500 ms interval relative to fixation start was used for FRP analysis and classification of fixations to avoid any interference. Moreover, we did not filter out low frequencies, to avoid contamination that can extend into this interval due to strong transient response after saccade-related shift of the EOG potential, and set the baseline intervals borders within the analyzed interval, i.e., at 200–300 ms relative

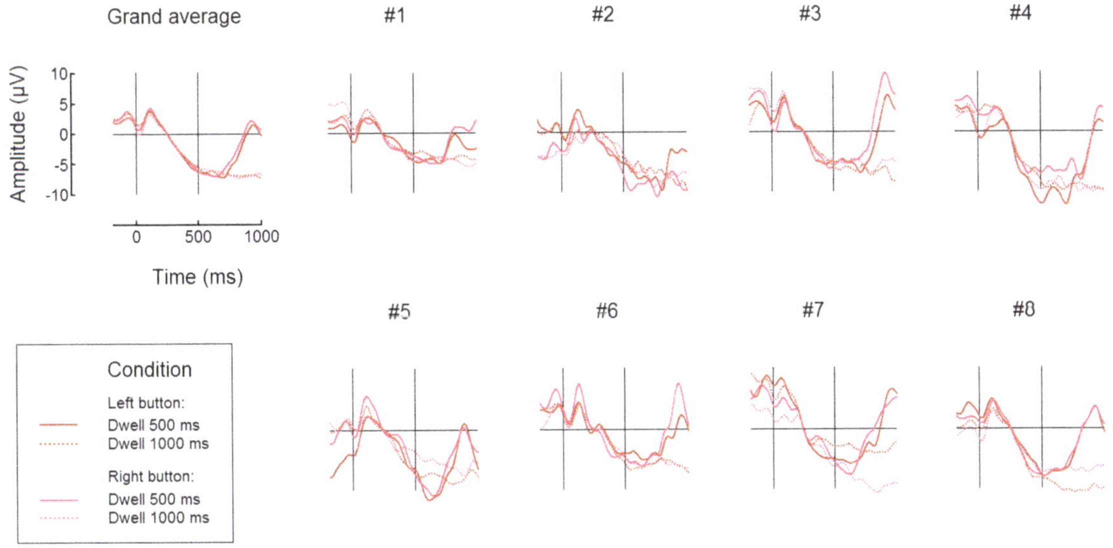

FIGURE 6 | Comparing different dwell time thresholds and button positions: grand average ($n = 8$) and individual FRP waveforms observed at POz in Button fixations. Fixation start and the 500 ms dwell time threshold are denoted by vertical lines. Filtering and baseline as in **Figure 3**.

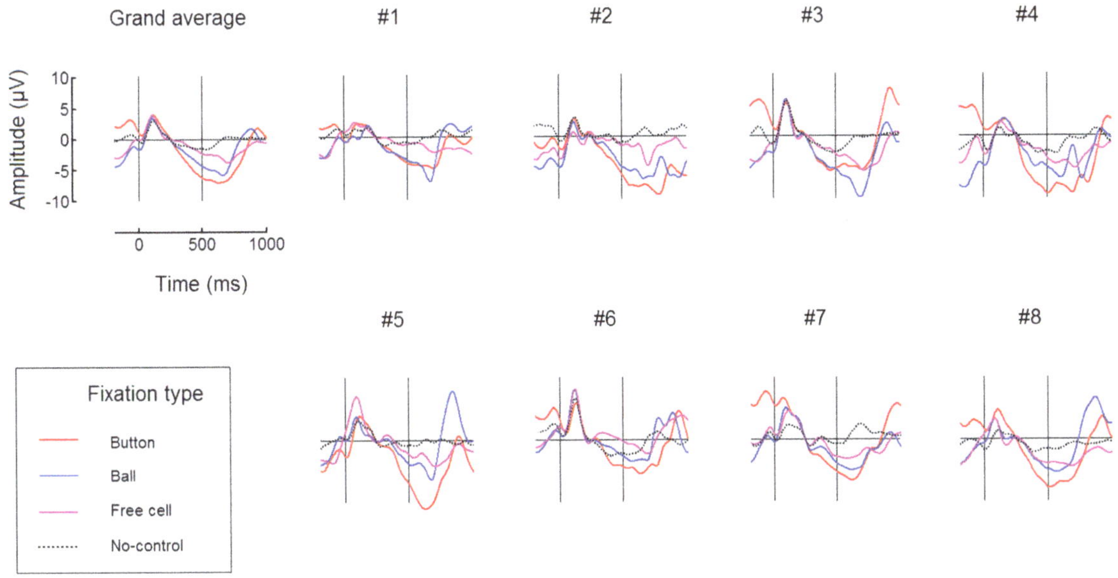

FIGURE 7 | Comparing different types of fixations: grand average ($n = 8$) and individual FRP waveforms observed at POz with 500 ms dwell time threshold. Here, left and right button data were averaged. Fixation start and the dwell time threshold are denoted by vertical lines. Filtering and baseline as in **Figure 3**.

to fixation onset. Positioning of the baseline in this interval means that results should be interpreted with care taking into account possible dampening of the activity of interest due to its presence in the subtracted signal. However, for demonstrating the possibility of developing an EBCI it was more important to prove that we obtained an EEG marker that was free from EOG contamination. As **Figure 3** shows, the EOG contamination indeed was absent in the 200–500 ms interval of the analyzed data that could be affected by it most strongly, i.e., in Button fixations.

The Negative EEG Wave

The topography of the EEG amplitudes in the 400–500 ms interval relative to fixation onset revealed a negativity focused at POz (**Figure 4**). Surprisingly, it was already developed in this interval even when the dwell threshold was 1000 ms. In the first and second of the three dwells used to make a move in the game (Button and Ball fixations), the EEG negativity at POz was strong in the 400–500 ms interval in all participants and significantly differed from the values in long non-controlling (spontaneous) fixations.

TABLE 2 | Performance of the LDA classifier with shrinkage regularization trained using only fixations on button as target fixations (Trainset 1).

Sbj.	Test on fixations with 500 ms threshold					Test on fixations with 1000 ms threshold		
	Specificity	Sensitivity			AUC	Sensitivity		
		Button	Ball	Free cell	Button	Button	Ball	Free cell
1	0.87 ± 0.13	0.23 ± 0.17	0.05	0.12	0.64 ± 0.06	0.16	0.07	0.09
2	0.85 ± 0.10	0.29 ± 0.22	0.15	0.09	0.67 ± 0.09	0.28	0.08	0.05
3	0.84 ± 0.09	0.51 ± 0.24	0.26	0.29	0.76 ± 0.07	0.41	0.20	0.30
4	0.92 ± 0.12	0.29 ± 0.21	0.08	0.08	0.70 ± 0.08	0.30	0.05	0.11
5	0.83 ± 0.14	0.38 ± 0.11	0.20	0.29	0.77 ± 0.03	0.45	0.30	0.28
6	0.87 ± 0.09	0.23 ± 0.06	0.09	0.11	0.64 ± 0.07	0.19	0.12	0.13
7	0.93 ± 0.05	0.15 ± 0.09	0.03	0.02	0.57 ± 0.03	0.07	0.04	0.04
8	0.86 ± 0.11	0.43 ± 0.18	0.05	0.15	0.76 ± 0.04	0.34	0.13	0.10
Mean	0.87	0.31	0.11	0.14	0.69	0.28	0.12	0.14
Std.	0.11	0.20	0.08	0.10	0.09	0.13	0.09	0.10

For training, recordings with 500 ms dwell threshold were used. On these recordings, 5-fold cross-validation was used to estimate, as M ± SD over folds, sensitivity and Area Under [ROC] Curve (AUC) for Button fixations, as well as specificity, in the 500 ms dwell threshold data. For each fold, the classifier was trained on 80% of the set, its threshold was adjusted on 8% aiming to obtain 90% specificity, and testing was done on 12%. In the case of testing on Ball and Free cell fixations, as well as for all 1000 ms dwell threshold data, the train and test sets were not overlapped and, therefore, the classifier was applied to all test data. Sensitivity is the same as True Positive Rate (TPR), here, the rate of correct classification of the intentional dwells. Specificity is equal to one minus the False Positive Rate (FPR); FPR is the same as the rate of false alarms, and in this work it corresponds to incorrectly classifying a spontaneous fixation as the controlling one (i.e., an intentional dwell).

The EEG negativity that was characteristic for the fixations used for control in our study was growing along the course of fixations, while Ihme and Zander (2011) and Protzak et al. (2013) reported EEG markers (also in the form of negativity) early within the controlling fixations. This difference could be caused by the differences in study design and processing approaches. In particular, the FRP in the study by Ihme and Zander (2011) could be influenced by EOG (although it unlikely influenced the classification results, according to the classifier weight scalp maps), while Protzak et al. (2013) focused on a time interval that immediately followed finding the target by the participants and could contain related activity. However, the FRPs presented in the latter work also showed, in the later part of the fixation intervals (mostly not used for classification), a deflection in negative direction, that could resemble the negative wave observed in our study if the authors would choose the baseline in the same time interval as we did it.

When a fixation is intentionally used for sending a command to computer, a user is expecting a feedback signal. In such situations, Stimulus Preceding Negativity (SPN) is observed. This EEG phenomenon can have a form of sustained negativity in anterior areas (unlikely to be detected with our baseline) and a sharp growth of negativity in parietal areas (Brunia, 1988; Brunia and Van Boxtel, 2001; Van Boxtel and Böcker, 2004; Brunia et al., 2011; Kotani et al., 2015). However, in our study the negativity was shifted to the hemisphere contralateral to the fixated location in the condition where the gaze was strongly shifted to the left or to the right (dwell on the switch-on button), an effect not known for SPN. Saccade preparation (possibly accompanying Button and Ball fixations, and, in some cases, even Free cell fixations) is characterized by a similar negative wave in the parietal area and is stronger in the hemisphere contralateral to saccade direction (Klostermann et al., 1994; Berchicci et al., 2012; Krebs et al., 2012). However, in our experiment the saccades following dwell on the button should be made in the direction opposite to the fixation location, i.e., the negativity had higher amplitude in the hemisphere ipsilateral to the direction of the saccade that followed the dwell; one may hypothesize that the mechanism enabling an intentional fixation at some location may have something in common with planning a saccade to this location, but we failed to find an evidence for this in the literature. Other slow negative EEG components related to preparation for action, Contingent Negative Variation (CNV) and Readiness Potential (RP), have more anterior localization.

Thus, we could not reliably identify the nature of the negative wave that marked the intentionally used gaze fixations, and additional studies are needed to clarify this question. In particular, it will be of practical importance to understand if the amplitude decreases within the controlling triplets (Button–Ball–Free cell) was just the order effect (the feedback for the second and especially third fixations in the sequence could be less informative, or affected by a refractory effect, etc.), or it resulted from factors specific to gaze position and object properties. Note, however, that when the classifier was trained on all types of data its performance was nonrandom even for Free cell fixations. If the EEG markers of intention to act will turn to be sensitive to various factors (properties of fixations, fixated objects, visual context, previous fixations, previous or planned saccades, variations in difficulty of maintaining a fixation intentionally, etc.; see, e.g., Nikolaev et al., 2016), different classifiers could be used for each specific case.

TABLE 3 | Performance of the LDA classifier with shrinkage regularization trained using all controlling fixations as target fixations (Trainset 2).

Sbj.	Test on fixations with 500 ms threshold									Test on fixations with 1000 ms threshold		
	Specificity	Sensitivity				AUC				Sensitivity		
		All	Button	Ball	Free cell	All	Button	Ball	Free cell	But-ton	Ball	Free cell
1	0.90 ± 0.16	0.18 ± 0.19	0.21 ± 0.21	0.17 ± 0.18	0.18 ± 0.18	0.63 ± 0.06	0.64 ± 0.10	0.61 ± 0.05	0.64 ± 0.06	0.13	0.09	0.08
2	0.85 ± 0.07	0.28 ± 0.10	0.34 ± 0.17	0.30 ± 0.08	0.20 ± 0.13	0.63 ± 0.02	0.66 ± 0.06	0.64 ± 0.02	0.58 ± 0.05	0.30	0.24	0.16
3	0.96 ± 0.05	0.19 ± 0.12	0.24 ± 0.21	0.15 ± 0.10	0.15 ± 0.11	0.63 ± 0.04	0.70 ± 0.10	0.60 ± 0.06	0.59 ± 0.08	0.20	0.10	0.09
4	0.83 ± 0.17	0.32 ± 0.18	0.41 ± 0.19	0.26 ± 0.21	0.27 ± 0.17	0.64 ± 0.02	0.69 ± 0.07	0.62 ± 0.03	0.60 ± 0.03	0.34	0.24	0.32
5	0.83 ± 0.09	0.21 ± 0.08	0.25 ± 0.14	0.19 ± 0.08	0.21 ± 0.11	0.64 ± 0.03	0.67 ± 0.03	0.61 ± 0.03	0.66 ± 0.05	0.19	0.16	0.14
6	0.70 ± 0.25	0.32 ± 0.23	0.36 ± 0.27	0.30 ± 0.23	0.37 ± 0.28	0.59 ± 0.06	0.59 ± 0.06	0.56 ± 0.05	0.63 ± 0.07	0.31	0.21	0.27
7	0.90 ± 0.09	0.12 ± 0.09	0.19 ± 0.11	0.12 ± 0.06	0.13 ± 0.11	0.56 ± 0.01	0.60 ± 0.02	0.55 ± 0.03	0.56 ± 0.05	0.07	0.07	0.09
8	0.92 ± 0.05	0.26 ± 0.16	0.24 ± 0.15	0.28 ± 0.15	0.30 ± 0.19	0.71 ± 0.06	0.68 ± 0.07	0.72 ± 0.05	0.74 ± 0.06	0.26	0.27	0.21
Mean	0.86	0.24	0.28	0.22	0.23	0.63	0.65	0.61	0.63	0.23	0.17	0.17
Std.	0.15	0.17	0.08	0.07	0.19	0.04	0.04	0.05	0.06	0.09	0.08	0.09

For training, recordings with 500 ms dwell threshold were used. On these recordings, 5-fold cross-validation was used to estimate, as M ± SD over folds, all the performance indices. For each fold, the classifier was trained on 80% of the set, its threshold was adjusted on 8% aiming to obtain 90% specificity, and testing was done on 12%. In the case of testing on 1000 ms dwell threshold data, the train and test sets were not overlapped and, therefore, the classifier was applied to all test data.

EBCI Performance

To enable fluent interaction, an EBCI should use short EEG segments. Our results demonstrated, for the first time, that EEG segments as short as 300 ms were sufficient to detect gaze fixations intentionally used for control.

In this study, the classifier threshold was adjusted for achieving specificity of about 0.9, that corresponded to false alarm rate of about 0.8 per minute. This rate is far from perfect, but can be acceptable in certain situations provided that the errors can be easily corrected. For example, in a game like *EyeLines*, if it was controlled on-line with an EBCI always switched on (with no need for the switch-on button), the player could simply attempt to choose another ball if a wrong one was selected, so the wrong selection would go harmless. (To complete the move, a free cell should be selected after the selection of a ball, but spontaneous dwells on free cells are not frequent even if the player do not make any effort to refrain from them, and can be easily avoided intentionally in the case of erroneous ball selection).

The best group average value of sensitivity, among all conditions and processing schemas, was only 0.38 ± 0.14 (in one participant, it was 20, and in others, ranged 0.31 to 0.47). This value was obtained for Button fixations using Trainset 1 (only Button fixations as the target class, non-controlling fixations as the non-target class) and the committee of greedy classifiers. Such sensitivity, of course, is not sufficient if the command always should be issued using the classifier.

However, as Protzak et al. (2013) suggested, an additional gaze dwell threshold can be used to ensure issuing a command even if it was not recognized by the BCI component of the system. We observed the high similarity of the FRPs before the 500 ms from the fixation onset under the 500 ms and 1000 ms dwell threshold conditions (**Figures 4**, **6**) and the relatively small decrease of the 500 ms trained classifier sensitivity when it was applied to the data from the 1000 ms condition (**Figure 8**). These results are in accordance with the recommendation by Protzak et al. (2013), demonstrating that the use of two thresholds will not likely lead to substantial drop in the classifier performance.

Classifier sensitivity followed the pattern observed for the amplitude of the negative wave that served as the marker of the controlling fixations, tending to decrease within the triplets of gaze dwells (Button–Ball–Free cell). The factors that are responsible for this decrease are yet to be determined, but it is likely that the key role was played by the order of dwells that closely followed each other. There are serious alternatives for the dwell-based EBCI in fast serial operation, such as dwell-free (Kristensson and Vertanen, 2012; Sarcar et al., 2013; Pedrosa et al., 2015) or response-based control (Publicover et al., 2016). The EBCI, thus, can be more suitable for single "clicks" or for starting a sequence, so that the rest of it will be entered using one of these alternative approaches.

Although the LDA classifier with shrinkage regularization is one of the methods of choice for ERP based BCIs (see, e.g., Blankertz et al., 2011), a simple classification approach based on the committee of greedy classifiers demonstrated at least comparable performance with our FRP data. In future studies, other classification approaches should be tested for the

TABLE 4 | Performance of the committee of 15 greedy classifiers trained using only fixations on button as target fixations (Trainset 1).

Sbj.	Test on fixations with 500 ms threshold				Test on fixations with 1000 ms threshold		
	Specificity	Sensitivity			Sensitivity		
		Button	Ball	Free cell	Button	Ball	Free cell
1	0.92 ± 0.04	0.31 ± 0.08	0.16	0.14	0.23	0.24	0.13
2	0.92 ± 0.03	0.40 ± 0.16	0.17	0.12	0.17	0.17	0.16
3	1.00 ± 0.00	0.20 ± 0.06	0.06	0.02	0.07	0.05	0.06
4	0.83 ± 0.04	0.44 ± 0.08	0.28	0.18	0.36	0.27	0.17
5	0.85 ± 0.06	0.45 ± 0.10	0.20	0.17	0.31	0.19	0.17
6	0.90 ± 0.06	0.39 ± 0.12	0.14	0.14	0.20	0.13	0.11
7	0.86 ± 0.06	0.47 ± 0.16	0.33	0.25	0.34	0.31	0.27
8	0.95 ± 0.04	0.41 ± 0.06	0.17	0.17	0.35	0.13	0.07
Mean	0.90	0.38	0.19	0.15	0.25	0.19	0.14
Std.	0.07	0.14	0.08	0.07	0.10	0.08	0.07

For training, recordings with 500 ms dwell threshold were used. On these recordings, 5-fold cross-validation was used to estimate, as M ± SD over folds, sensitivity for Button fixations and specificity in the 500 ms dwell threshold data. For each fold, the classifier was trained on 80% and tested on 20% of the set. In the case of testing on Ball and Free cell fixations, as well as for all 1000 ms dwell threshold data, the train and test sets were not overlapped and, therefore, the classifier was applied to all test data.

TABLE 5 | Performance of the committee of 15 greedy classifiers trained using all controlling fixations as target fixations (Trainset 2).

Sbj.	Test on fixations with 500 ms threshold					Test on fixations with 1000 ms threshold		
	Specificity	Sensitivity				Sensitivity		
		All	Button	Ball	Free cell	Button	Ball	Free cell
1	0.92 ± 0.08	0.22 ± 0.02	0.28 ± 0.07	0.22 ± 0.05	0.15 ± 0.03	0.25	0.27	0.17
2	0.91 ± 0.05	0.24 ± 0.08	0.30 ± 0.06	0.23 ± 0.09	0.18 ± 0.12	0.21	0.17	0.14
3	0.96 ± 0.04	0.18 ± 0.03	0.18 ± 0.04	0.19 ± 0.05	0.18 ± 0.09	0.11	0.10	0.12
4	0.91 ± 0.04	0.20 ± 0.02	0.30 ± 0.06	0.19 ± 0.01	0.10 ± 0.05	0.21	0.20	0.09
5	0.93 ± 0.06	0.26 ± 0.06	0.23 ± 0.11	0.24 ± 0.06	0.30 ± 0.09	0.22	0.24	0.19
6	0.93 ± 0.03	0.33 ± 0.06	0.34 ± 0.12	0.29 ± 0.04	0.36 ± 0.09	0.24	0.19	0.32
7	0.92 ± 0.08	0.26 ± 0.04	0.31 ± 0.11	0.27 ± 0.02	0.19 ± 0.06	0.29	0.21	0.17
8	0.84 ± 0.06	0.45 ± 0.07	0.50 ± 0.10	0.42 ± 0.12	0.43 ± 0.09	0.46	0.39	0.37
Mean	0.91	0.27	0.31	0.26	0.24	0.25	0.22	0.20
Std.	0.07	0.10	0.09	0.07	0.13	0.10	0.08	0.10

For training, recordings with 500 ms dwell threshold were used. On these recordings, 5-fold cross-validation was used to estimate, as M ± SD over folds, all the performance indices. For each fold, the classifier was trained on 80% and tested on 20% of the set. In the case of testing on 1000 ms dwell threshold data, the train and test sets were not overlapped and, therefore, the classifier was applied to all test data.

EBCI, especially those that were successful with similar data patterns, such as Locality Preserving Projections algorithm that provided good results for movement-related potentials (Xu et al., 2014). A relatively low intersubject variability of the negativity that marked the controlling fixations suggests that the classifier training can provide higher results when trained on the same data with priors obtained from other participants.

A thorough search for better feature sets can result in even higher improvement in performance. For example, in a preliminary study adding wavelet features extracted from the same data to the amplitude features provided significant increase of AUC up to 0.75 ± 0.04 (M ± SD for the same group) for shrinkage LDA classifier (Shishkin et al., 2016a). Note that in the current study we avoided using any data from the EEG earlier than 200 ms after fixation onset for most reliable exclusion of any contamination by artifacts, although earlier EEG samples from the fixation interval and pre-saccadic activity may include additional useful information. Moreover, our baseline choice could prevent extraction of any activity that was stable within our interval (e.g., the anterior component of SPN). Non-EEG information, especially gaze data and data about the fixated objects, their environment, possible types of current activity of the user and so on can be used as additional features, or, in some cases, for selecting a classifier (e.g., specific classifiers can be trained for different steps in sequences of actions, as in action triplets in our game). If sufficiently large amounts of gaze-synchronized EEG data will be harvested during the use of EBCIs, it will become possible to apply deep learning algorithms (LeCun et al., 2015; see also Nurse et al., 2016, on deep learning implementation at TrueNorth chip for EEG/ECoG/LFP data) that are able to find hidden patterns in the data and strongly improve classification performance.

However, it is possible that the sensitivity will not be improved to values close to 100%. What can be the added value of the BCI component if its sensitivity would be, for example, about 0.7, and the long dwells (without a BCI!) should be yet used in the rest of trials? We expect that even in this case the hybrid EBCI can provide advantage over usual gaze-based interaction when the interaction should require as little effort as possible. Indeed, the user will not need to take care about his or her attention and gaze to prevent unwanted "clicks," to confirm the command, etc., except to be ready to fixate slightly longer in certain cases. Moreover, it is possible that many of the misses are caused by low attentional concentration. In such cases, it might be even useful to avoid too fast interface response.

It is also possible that practice will lead to more stable and higher EEG marker amplitude through the operant conditioning mechanism. Practice can improve intentional regulation of the slow cortical potentials when they are used for BCI-based communication (Neumann et al., 2004), and the same may appear to be also true for the EBCI based on SPN-like slow activity. To test this hypothesis, the FRP dynamics and EBCI performance can be studied during prolonged use of the online EBCI. The use of additional, longer dwell time threshold makes possible intensive practice even with low sensitivity of the classifier. It was thus important that the study demonstrated high similarity of the 200–500 ms interval of FRPs of controlling fixations with 500 ms and 1000 ms dwell time thresholds.

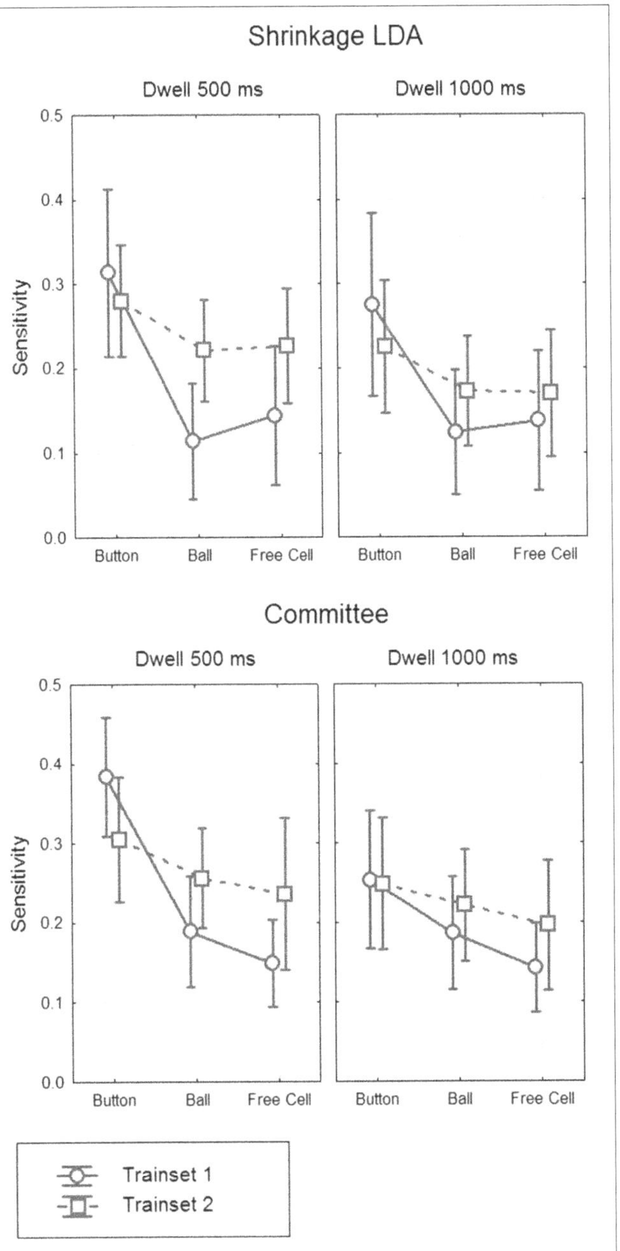

FIGURE 8 | Classifier sensitivity on the test data. Grand mean ($n = 8$) values and 95% confidence intervals for different classifiers, different types of fixations and different dwell time thresholds. The target (controlling) class in the train data was either button fixations (Trainset 1) only or all controlling fixations (Trainset 2).

Fast Fixation-Based EBCIs: An Emerging Class of Effective Hybrid BCIs

The gaze fixation and FRP data complement each other when used as an input to a hybrid interface: the fixation onset provides the temporal marker required for EEG segmentation and FRP extraction, the FRP provides features for a passive BCI classifier that automatically recognizes target finding (in the case of visual search) or issuing a command (in intentional dwell-based control), and the gaze position indicates the target (Protzak et al., 2013; Finke et al., 2016). This combination may enable fluent interaction both in visual search (Finke et al., 2016; see also Introduction) and in intentional dwell-based control (Protzak et al., 2013, and the current study).

These two types of interaction are rather different. In a visual search, the user typically makes the decision about what target he or she is looked for in advance, but the target location is not known and should be found during exploration of a scene. In intentional control, the scene and all objects in it can be well known to the user, who should be given an option not to evoke any interaction even when looking at them until the decision to interact will be made. Moreover, it is not unlikely that such an EBCI will be able to make "clicks" even at freely chosen places without any defined objects, for example, when used for drawing. While the P300 wave is important in the search tasks (Finke et al., 2016), in the intentional dwell-based interaction a negative SPN-like wave and no signs of P300 were observed (**Figures 6**, **7** in the current paper). Nevertheless, in both cases the BCI task is the same: to detect a target fixation among non-target fixations, in other words, just to provide "yes" or "no" answer for each fixation. Given the limitations of non-invasive brain signals and

TABLE 6 | Four-way MANOVA results for sensitivity.

Factor	*Wilks' λ*	*F*	*df*	*p*
Classifier	0.90	0.80	1, 7	0.40
Training Set	0.86	1.15	1, 7	0.32
Dwell Threshold	**0.12**	**52.06**	**1, 7**	**0.0002**
Fixation Type	**0.06**	**44.68**	**2, 6**	**0.0002**
Classifier × Training Set	1.00	0.01	1, 7	0.94
Classifier × Dwell Threshold	0.87	1.05	1, 7	0.34
Training Set × Dwell Threshold	**0.46**	**8.23**	**1, 7**	**0.024**
Classifier × Fixation Type	0.54	2.55	2, 6	0.16
Training Set × Fixation Type	**0.23**	**10.18**	**2, 6**	**0.012**
Dwell Threshold × Fixation Type	**0.06**	**44.71**	**2, 6**	**0.0002**
Classifier × Training Set × Dwell Threshold	**0.52**	**6.34**	**1, 7**	**0.040**
Classifier × Training Set × Fixation Type	0.47	3.45	2, 6	0.10
Classifier × Dwell Threshold × Fixation Type	0.53	2.68	2, 6	0.15
Training Set × Dwell Threshold × Fixation Type	**0.35**	**5.62**	**2, 6**	**0.042**
Classifier × Training Set × Dwell Threshold × Fixation Type	0.77	0.91	2, 6	0.45

Significant effects ($p < 0.05$) are shown in bold. Factors and their levels are described in the text.

the need to use single-trial data, it is important that the BCI task is made as simple as this. Gaze single-trial data provide much more reach information, but they lack the modalities that can be extracted from brain signals. Therefore, it is natural to combine the gaze and brain state data in a multimodal (hybrid) human-machine interface (Velichkovsky and Hansen, 1996).

It seems possible that some other psychophysiological paradigms of interaction with computer GUI elements (and, possibly, with other visual media, virtual and real objects, robot parts, etc.) can be also useful for evoking brain activity that can be quickly recognized and used to act at a fixated location. Due to similarity of the input data, all such tasks can be implemented in interfaces, for the use in different situations, with the same hardware and even software. A "second-order-hybrid" BCI built in this way may provide a highly fluent and natural means of interaction. Other functions of passive BCI (Zander and Kothe, 2011) and brain state monitoring (Van Erp et al., 2012), such as based on estimation of attention level for different objects or using error potential detection, also can benefit from fixation-based EEG segmentation and can be easily incorporated into the same system to support adaptation (immediate or based on long-term data analysis) of the interface and connected machines to the user's attentive states and interests.

Augmentation of Human-Computer Interaction with Passive Dwell-Based EBCIs

Although in most cases computers assist people in their mental, not physical activities, for every interaction with a computer the motor system should be used. Effects of physical workload on mental activity have not been much studied (DiDomenico and Nussbaum, 2011), and effects of light physical load on some specific kinds of mental activity, such as creative and/or highly focused, seems not been investigated at all. It is not unlikely that even a light physical load can interfere with mental work, at least in certain individuals, and that full freeing from physical activity can provide certain benefits, at least in certain cases of high focus on a mental task. In addition, certain forms of computer use, e.g., viewing artistic images, may benefit from enabling this activity in a highly relaxed state, without any use of skeletal muscles. To test the hypothesis that the non-motor interaction with computers can provide special benefits for the intellectual activities requires an interface enabling such interaction in unobtrusive way. Such an interface must have much better performance than the existing BCIs and without the burden of the Midas touch problem (or of existing solutions to it) associated with the gaze control technologies. EBCIs may become the first type of interface suitable for this.

With a tool for the separation of intentional and spontaneous fixations, potential benefits of the gaze based interaction could be high, due to the natural co-ordination between gaze and action. A user often fixates their gaze on a GUI button or a link earlier than approaches them with the mouse cursor (Huang et al., 2012; Liebling and Dumais, 2014) or before manually touching it on a touchscreen (Weill-Tessier et al., 2016). Fixating gaze at action location prior to reaching it or prior to the action is also observed when locations or objects in the physical world are reached and manipulated (Land et al., 1999; Neggers and Bekkering, 2000; Johansson et al., 2001). Gaze leadership should not be overemphasized: for known locations, the mouse typically leads the gaze, and the gaze often goes to a new location before the mouse click occurs (Liebling and Dumais, 2014), a behavior that is impossible with a dwell-based EBCI. In addition, it is not likely that it will not be possible to significantly reduce the dwell duration in dwell-based EBCIs comparing to our settings, where it was at least 500 ms plus the time of reaction to feedback. For serial operation and automatized actions, dwell-free approaches seem more relevant to optimize gaze based interaction. However, gaze dwells are a natural mean to convey intentions in social interactions, and it seems natural to use them in interaction with computers as well. What the dwell-based passive EBCI may offer is not speed but fluency of operation: it could become a tool to convert intentions into actions seamlessly and without any involvement of motor system. Ideally, such an EBCI will not require from the user anything more than just looking and willing to act.

The use of passive BCIs can be not the only way to enable such a fluent interaction. For example, for the interaction with anthropomorphic robots that could be considered as partners rather than tools, we proposed to use "joint attention" gaze patterns (gaze gesture sequences) that are developed in infancy and can be automatically used by adults. Most of our participants easily found the ways to interact with a simple model of an anthropomorphic robot which responded to such patterns, although no information was provided to them about these patterns (Fedorova et al., 2015). However, we believe that for a certain range of tasks the use of dwell-based EBCIs will be optimal.

From the Wish Switch to the Wish Mouse

Gray Walter, who discovered the CNV, created the first BCI, the "wish switch" (Regan, 1989, p. 218) as early as in 1964. It sent a command to a projector to present the next picture when the patient was just going to press the button to advance the projector. The BCI was directly connected to the patient's motor cortex and could detect "the wish" even before the actual button press (Graimann et al., 2010). Later, Gray Walter proposed separate use of the CNV components, the Expectancy Wave (for direct control) and earlier Intention Wave ("so that the subject has the desired experience before any action has been taken"—Walter, 1966), but it seems that such experiments were never made.

Later on, slow negative potentials that could be related to expectation and intention (but possibly to other mental activities as well) were used, together with positive deflections, by Birbaumer and his colleagues in their "Thought Translation Device" (e.g., Neumann et al., 2003, 2004), and the Lateralized Readiness Potential (LRP) was used in the Berlin BCI group's early works (Blankertz et al., 2002, 2003). Computer screen color control through a BCI, that presumably responded to individual's wishes (here, unconscious ones), was demonstrated by Kaplan et al. (2005) with the use of rhythmic EEG components instead of the negative deflections. The majority of BCI studies were focused on techniques that do not respond to wishes and intents directly, such as motor imagery and responses to stimuli. Recently, slow premotor potentials were employed for developing neurorehabilitation BCIs (Niazi et al., 2011; Ibáñez et al., 2014; Lew et al., 2014; Xu et al., 2014; Jiang et al., 2015; Shakeel et al., 2015). But probably only the works by Zander's group (Ihme and Zander, 2011; Protzak et al., 2013) addressed the direct conversion of intentions into actions in line with the elegant approach by Gray Walter, now also enhanced with gaze capabilities. In the current work, we demonstrated that this combination can be efficient in realistic settings, and described an EEG marker for the controlling gaze fixations. As we discussed above, this marker is similar to SPN, the phenomenon that is again a member of the family of slow negative cortical potentials related to anticipation (Van Boxtel and Böcker, 2004).

Gaze is an ideal complement to brain activity in an interface aiming on a direct conversion of intentions into actions: it is itself driven by interest and wishes, but is able to convey the information about location, not easily available even from invasive brain signal recordings. Thus, combining eye tracking with the detection of FRP correlates of the wish to make a click at the fixated location will lead to creation of a "wish mouse," a tool that will possibly provide unusually fluent interaction with computers both for people with motor disabilities and for healthy individuals.

CONCLUSION

This study demonstrated that intentional gaze fixations for 500 ms, used to control a computer interface through eye tracking technology, can be discriminated from spontaneous gaze fixations of the same duration using only 300 ms EEG segments. This was done by recording EEG from healthy participants who played a game with real-time control by 500 ms gaze fixations and by running an offline BCI simulation. We also described an EEG marker for the controlling gaze fixations, which was prominent in all our 8 participants. The marker was a negativity with occipitoparietal focus, similar to Stimulus-Preceding Negativity (SPN) but differed from it by its lateralization. In the subsequent work, we plan to test the online version of the Eye-Brain-Computer Interface (EBCI) using this EEG marker.

AUTHOR CONTRIBUTIONS

SS designed the study. SS, YN, AT, ES, and AF developed the methodology. AF, ES, and YN collected the data. SS, AT, ES, BK, YN, and AF analyzed the data. SS wrote the first draft. AF and SS drew the picture for **Figure 1**. SS and BV wrote the final draft. BV and SS supervised all aspects of the research.

FUNDING

This work was partly supported by the Russian Science Foundation, grant 14-28-00234 (all parts of the work except for the literature analysis and the development of the greedy classifier committee) and by the Russian Foundation for Basic Research, grant ofi-m 15-29-01344 (the development of the greedy classifier committee).

ACKNOWLEDGMENTS

The authors would like to thank Alex Ossadtchi and Andrey Nikolaev for useful comments and suggestions.

REFERENCES

Banville, H., and Falk, T. H. (2016). Recent advances and open challenges in hybrid brain-computer interfacing: a technological review of non-invasive human research. *Brain Comput. Interfaces* 3, 9–46. doi: 10.1080/2326263X.2015.1134958

Berchicci, M., Stella, A., Pitzalis, S., Spinelli, D., and Di Russo, F. (2012). Spatio-temporal mapping of motor preparation for self-paced saccades. *Biol. Psychol.* 90, 10–17. doi: 10.1016/j.biopsycho.2012.02.014

Blankertz, B., Curio, G., and Muller, K. R. (2002). Classifying single trial EEG: Towards brain computer interfacing. *Adv. Neural Inf. Process. Syst.* 14, 157–164.

Blankertz, B., Dornhege, G., Schäfer, C., Krepki, R., Kohlmorgen, J., Müller, K. R., et al. (2003). Boosting bit rates and error detection for the classification of fast-paced motor commands based on single-trial EEG analysis. *IEEE Trans. Neural Syst. Rehabil. Eng.* 11, 127–131. doi: 10.1109/TNSRE.2003.814456

Blankertz, B., Lemm, S., Treder, M., Haufe, S., and Müller, K. R. (2011). Single-trial analysis and classification of ERP components—a tutorial. *Neuroimage* 56, 814–825. doi: 10.1016/j.neuroimage.2010.06.048

Bolt, R. A. (1982). "Eyes at the interface," in *Proceedings of the 1982 Conference on Human Factors in Computing Systems (CHI '82)*, (New York, NY: ACM), 360–362. doi: 10.1145/800049.801811

Bowsher, K., Civillico, E. F., Coburn, J., Collinger, J., Contreras-Vidal, J. L., Denison, T., et al. (2016). Brain–computer interface devices for patients with paralysis and amputation: a meeting report. *J. Neural Eng.* 13:023001. doi: 10.1088/1741-2560/13/2/023001

Brouwer, A. M., Reuderink, B., Vincent, J., van Gerven, M. A., and van Erp, J. B. (2013). Distinguishing between target and nontarget fixations in a visual search task using fixation-related potentials. *J. Vis.* 13:17. doi: 10.1167/13.3.17

Brunia, C. H., Hackley, S. A., van Boxtel, G. J., Kotani, Y., and Ohgami, Y. (2011). Waiting to perceive: reward or punishment? *Clin. Neurophysiol.* 122, 858–868. doi: 10.1016/j.clinph.2010.12.039

Brunia, C. H. M. (1988). Movement and stimulus preceding negativity. *Biol. Psychol.* 26, 165–178. doi: 10.1016/0301-0511(88)90018-X

Brunia, C. H. M., and Van Boxtel, G. J. M. (2001). Wait and see. *Int. J. Psychophysiol.* 43, 59–75. doi: 10.1016/S0167-8760(01)00179-9

Delorme, A, and Makeig, S. (2004). EEGLAB: an open source toolbox for analysis of single-trial EEG dynamics including independent component analysis. *J. Neurosci. Methods* 134, 9–21. doi: 10.1016/j.jneumeth.2003.10.009

Devillez, H., Guyader, N., and Guérin-Dugué, A. (2015). An eye fixation–related potentials analysis of the P300 potential for fixations onto a target object when exploring natural scenes. *J. Vis.* 15:20. doi: 10.1167/15.13.20

DiDomenico, A., and Nussbaum, M. A. (2011). Effects of different physical workload parameters on mental workload and performance. *Int. J. Ind. Ergon.* 41, 255–260. doi: 10.1016/j.ergon.2011.01.008

Fedorova, A. A., Shishkin, S. L., Nuzhdin, Y. O., and Velichkovsky, B. M. (2015). "Gaze based robot control: the communicative approach," in *2015 7th International IEEE/EMBS Conference on Neural Engineering (NER)*, 751–754.

Finke, A., Essig, K., Marchioro, G., and Ritter, H. (2016). Toward FRP-based brain-machine interfaces–single-trial classification of fixation-related potentials. *PLoS ONE* 11:e0146848. doi: 10.1371/journal.pone.0146848

Graimann, B., Allison, B., and Pfurtscheller, G. (eds.). (2010). "Brain–Computer Interfaces: A Gentle Introduction," in *Brain–Computer Interfaces, The Frontiers Collection* (Berlin: Springer-Verlag), 1–27.

Graupner, S.-T., Pannasch, S., and Velichkovsky, B. M. (2011). Saccadic context indicates information processing within visual fixations: evidence from event-related potentials and eye-movements analysis of the distractor effect. *Int. J. Psychophysiol.* 80, 54–62. doi: 10.1016/j.ijpsycho.2011.01.013

Healy, G., and Smeaton, A. F. (2011). "Eye fixation related potentials in a target search task," in *33rd Annual International Conference of the IEEE Engineering in Medicine and Biology Society (EMBC'11)* (Boston, MA), 4203–4206.

Huang, J., White, R., and Buscher, G. (2012). "User see, user point: gaze and cursor alignment in web search," in *Proceedings of the SIGCHI Conference on Human Factors in Computing Systems (CHI '12)* (New York, NY: ACM), 1341–1350. doi: 10.1145/2207676.2208591

Ibáñez, J., Serrano, J. I., Del Castillo, M. D., Monge-Pereira, E., Molina-Rueda, F., Alguacil-Diego, I., et al. (2014). Detection of the onset of upper-limb movements based on the combined analysis of changes in the sensorimotor rhythms and slow cortical potentials. *J. Neural Eng.* 11:056009. doi: 10.1088/1741-2560/11/5/056009

Ihme, K., and Zander, T. O. (2011). "What you expect is what you get? Potential use of contingent negative variation for passive BCI systems in gaze-based HCI," in *International Conference on Affective Computing and Intelligent Interaction* (Berlin, Heidelberg: Springer), 447–456.

Jacob, R. J. (1990). "What you look at is what you get: eye movement-based interaction techniques," in *Proceedings of the SIGCHI Conference on Human Factors in Computing Systems (CHI '90)*, eds J. Carrasco Chew and J. Whiteside (New York, NY: ACM), 11–18. doi: 10.1145/97243.97246

Jacob, R. J. (1991). The use of eye movements in human-computer interaction techniques: what you look at is what you get. *ACM Trans. Inf. Syst.* 9, 152–169. doi: 10.1145/123078.128728

Jiang, N., Gizzi, L., Mrachacz-Kersting, N., Dremstrup, K., and Farina, D. (2015). A brain–computer interface for single-trial detection of gait initiation from movement related cortical potentials. *Clin. Neurophysiol.* 126, 154–159. doi: 10.1016/j.clinph.2014.05.003

Johansson, R. S., Westling, G., Bäckström, A., and Flanagan, J. R. (2001). Eye–hand coordination in object manipulation. *J. Neurosci.* 21, 6917–6932.

Kamienkowski, J. E., Ison, M. J., Quiroga, R. Q., and Sigman, M. (2012). Fixation-related potentials in visual search: a combined EEG and eye tracking study. *J. Vis.* 12:4. doi: 10.1167/12.7.4

Kaplan, A. Y., Lim, J. J., Jin, K. S., Park, B. W., Byeon, J. G., and Tarasova, S. U. (2005). Unconscious operant conditioning in the paradigm of brain-computer interface based on color perception. *Intern. J. Neuroscience.* 115, 781–802. doi: 10.1080/00207450590881975

Kaunitz, L. N., Kamienkowski, J. E., Varatharajah, A., Sigman, M., Quiroga, R. Q., and Ison, M. J. (2014). Looking for a face in the crowd: fixation-related potentials in an eye-movement visual search task. *Neuroimage* 89, 297–305. doi: 10.1016/j.neuroimage.2013.12.006

Kim, M., Kim, B. H., and Jo, S. (2015). Quantitative evaluation of a low-cost noninvasive hybrid interface based on EEG and eye movement. *IEEE Trans. Neural Syst. Rehabil. Eng.* 23, 159–168. doi: 10.1109/TNSRE.2014.2365834

Klostermann, W., Kömpf, D., Heide, W., Yerleger, R., Wauschkuhn, B., and Seyfert, T. (1994). The presaccadic cortical negativity prior to self-paced saccades with and without visual guidance. *Electroencephalogr. Clin. Neurophysiol.* 91, 219–228. doi: 10.1016/0013-4694(94)90072-8

Kotani, Y., Ohgami, Y., Ishiwata, T., Arai, J. I., Kiryu, S., and Inoue, Y. (2015). Source analysis of stimulus-preceding negativity constrained by functional magnetic resonance imaging. *Biol. Psychol.* 111, 53–64. doi: 10.1016/j.biopsycho.2015.08.005

Krebs, R. M., Boehler, C. N., Zhang, H. H., Schoenfeld, M. A., and Woldorff, M. G. (2012). Electrophysiological recordings in humans reveal reduced location-specific attentional-shift activity prior to recentering saccades. *J. Neurophysiol.* 107, 1393–1402. doi: 10.1152/jn.00912.2010

Kristensson, P. O., and Vertanen, K. (2012). "The potential of dwell-free eye-typing for fast assistive gaze communication," in *Proceedings of the Symposium on Eye Tracking Research and Applications (ETRA '12)*, eds S. N. Spencer (New York, NY: ACM), 241–244. doi: 10.1145/2168556.2168605

Lahr, J., Schwartz, C., Heimbach, B., Aertsen, A., Rickert, J., and Ball, T. (2015). Invasive brain–machine interfaces: a survey of paralyzed patients' attitudes, knowledge and methods of information retrieval. *J. Neural Eng.* 12:043001. doi: 10.1088/1741-2560/12/4/043001

Land, M., Mennie, N., and Rusted, J. (1999). The roles of vision and eye movements in the control of activities of daily living. *Perception* 28, 1311–1328. doi: 10.1068/p2935

LeCun, Y., Bengio, Y., and Hinton, G. (2015). Deep learning. *Nature* 521, 436–444. doi: 10.1038/nature14539

Lew, E.Y., Chavarriaga, R., Silvoni, S., and Millán, J. D. R. (2014). Single trial prediction of self-paced reaching directions from EEG signals. *Front. Neurosci.* 8:222. doi: 10.3389/fnins.2014.00222

Liebling, D. J., and Dumais, S. T. (2014). "Gaze and mouse coordination in everyday work," in *Proceedings of the 2014 ACM International Joint Conference on Pervasive and Ubiquitous Computing: Adjunct Publication (UbiComp '14 Adjunct)* (New York, NY: ACM), 1141–1150. doi: 10.1145/2638728.2641692

Majaranta, P., and Bulling, A. (2014). "Eye tracking and eye-based human-computer interaction," in *Advances in Physiological Computing: Human-Computer Interaction Series*, eds S. H. Fairclough and K. Gilleade (London: Springer-Verlag), 39–65.

Müller-Putz, G., Leeb, R., Tangermann, M., Höhne, J., Kübler, A., Cincotti, F., et al. (2015). Towards noninvasive hybrid brain-computer interfaces: framework, practice, clinical application, and beyond. *Proc. IEEE* 103, 926–943. doi: 10.1109/JPROC.2015.2411333

Neggers, S. F. W., and Bekkering, H. (2000). Ocular gaze is anchored to the target of an ongoing pointing movement. *J. Neurophysiol.* 83, 639–651.

Neumann, N., Hinterberger, T., Kaiser, J., Leins, U., Birbaumer, N., and Kübler, A. (2004). Automatic processing of self-regulation of slow cortical potentials: evidence from brain-computer communication in paralysed patients. *Clin. Neurophysiol.* 115, 628–635. doi: 10.1016/j.clinph.2003.10.030

Neumann, N., Kübler, A., Kaiser, J., Hinterberger, T., and Birbaumer, N. (2003). Conscious perception of brain states: mental strategies for brain–computer communication. *Neuropsychologia* 41, 1028–1036. doi: 10.1016/S0028-3932(02)00298-1

Niazi, I. K., Jiang, N., Tiberghien, O., Nielsen, J. F., Dremstrup, K., and Farina, D. (2011). Detection of movement intention from single-trial movement-related cortical potentials. *J. Neural Eng.* 8:066009. doi: 10.1088/1741-2560/8/6/066009

Nikolaev, A. R., Jurica, P., Nakatani, C., Plomp, G., and van Leeuwen, C. (2013). Visual encoding and fixation target selection in free viewing: presaccadic brain potentials. *Front. Syst. Neurosci.* 7:26. doi: 10.3389/fnsys.2013.00026

Nikolaev, A. R., Meghanathan, R. N., and van Leeuwen, C. (2016). Combining EEG and eye movement recording in free viewing: Pitfalls and possibilities. *Brain Cogn.* 107, 55–83. doi: 10.1016/j.bandc.2016.06.004

Nurse, E., Mashford, B. S., Yepes, A. J., Kiral-Kornek, I., Harrer, S., and Freestone, D. R. (2016). "Decoding EEG and LFP signals using deep learning: heading TrueNorth," in *Proceedings of the ACM International Conference on Computing Frontiers* (Boulder, CO). 259–266.

Oostenveld, R., Fries, P., Maris, E., and Schoffelen, JM (2011). FieldTrip: open source software for advanced analysis of MEG, EEG, and Invasive electrophysiological data. *Comput. Intell. Neurosci.* 2011:156869. doi: 10.1155/2011/156869

Pedrosa, D., Pimentel, M. D. G., Wright, A., and Truong, K. N. (2015). Filteryedping: design challenges and user performance of dwell-free eye typing. *ACM Trans. Accessible Comput.* 6:3. doi: 10.1145/2724728

Pfurtscheller, G., Allison, B. Z., Bauernfeind, G., Brunner, C., Solis-Escalante, T., Scherer, R., et al. (2010). The hybrid BCI. *Front. Neurosci.* 4:3. doi: 10.3389/fnpro.2010.00003

Protzak, J., Ihme, K., and Zander, T. O. (2013). "A passive brain-computer interface for supporting gaze-based human-machine interaction," in *International Conference on Universal Access in Human-Computer Interaction* (Heidelberg, Berlin: Springer), 662–671.

Publicover, N. G., Marggraff, L. J., and Drake, E. F. (2016). *Systems and Methods for Biomechanically-Based Eye Signals for Interacting with Real and Virtual Objects*. U.S. Patent Application No. 20160085302.

Regan, D. (1989). *Human Brain Electrophysiology: Evoked Potentials and Evoked Magnetic Fields in Science and Medicine*. Amsterdam: Elsevier.

Sarcar, S., Panwar, P., and Chakraborty, T. (2013). "EyeK: an efficient dwell-free eye gaze-based text entry system," in *Proceedings of the 11th Asia Pacific Conference on Computer Human Interaction (APCHI '13)* (New York, NY: ACM), 215–220. doi: 10.1145/2525194.2525288

Sellers, E. W., Vaughan, T. M., and Wolpaw, J. R. (2010). A brain-computer interface for long-term independent home use. *Amyotroph. Lateral Scler.* 11, 449–455. doi: 10.3109/17482961003777470

Shakeel, A., Navid, M. S., Anwar, M. N., Mazhar, S., Jochumsen, M., and Niazi, I. K. (2015). A review of techniques for detection of movement intention using movement related cortical potentials. *Comput. Math. Methods Med.* 2015:346217. doi: 10.1155/2015/346217

Shishkin, S. L., Kozyrskiy, B. L., Trofimov, A. G., Nuzhdin, Y. O., Fedorova, A. A., Svirin, E. P., et al. (2016a). Improving eye-brain-computer interface performance by using electroencephalogram frequency components. *Bull. RSMU* 2, 36–41.

Shishkin, S. L., Nuzhdin, Y. O., Svirin, E. P., Fedorova, A. A., Slobodskoy-Plusnin, Y. Y., Trofimov, A. G., et al. (2015). "Toward a fluent eye-brain-computer interface: EEG negativity marks visual fixations used to control a game," in *7th International IEEE EMBS Conference on Neural Engineering (IEEE/EMBS NER2015)* (Montpellier: Late Breaking Research Papers), 055–0463.

Shishkin, S. L., Nuzhdin, Y. O., Svirin, E. P., Trofimov, A. G., Fedorova, A. A., Dubynin, I. A., et al. (2016b). "Semi-direct mind-to-machine interface using gaze and intention markers," in *7th International Conference on Cognitive Science* (Svetlogorsk), 68-69.

Shishkin, S. L., Nuzhdin, Y. O., Trofimov, A. G., Svirin, E. P., Fedorova, A. A., Dubynin, I. A., et al. (2016c). Fixation-based eye-brain-computer interfaces: approaching a better human-computer symbiosis. *OperaMed. Physiol.* 2016(Suppl. S2), 83–84. Proceedings of Volga Neuroscience Meeting 2016. doi: 10.20388/OMP2016.00S2.005

Trofimov, A. G., Ivanitsky, I. I., and Velichkovsky, B. M. (2015). [*A greedy algorithm for constructing a committee of classifiers for the EEG signal.*] Vestnik Natsional'nogo Issledovatel'skogo Yadernogo Universiteta "MIFI" [Herald of the National Research Nuclear University MEPhI] 4, 537–544.

Uščumlić, M., and Blankertz, B. (2016). Active visual search in non-stationary scenes: coping with temporal variability and uncertainty. *J. Neural Eng.* 13:016015. doi: 10.1088/1741-2560/13/1/016015

Van Boxtel, G. J., and Böcker, K. B. (2004). Cortical measures of anticipation. *J. Psychophysiol.* 18, 61–76. doi: 10.1027/0269-8803.18.23.61

Van Erp, J. B., Lotte, F., and Tangermann, M. (2012). Brain-computer interfaces: beyond medical applications. *Computer* 45, 26–34. doi: 10.1109/MC.2012.107

Velichkovsky, B. M., and Hansen, J. P. (1996). "New technological windows into mind: there is more in eyes and brains for human-computer interaction," in *Proceedings of the SIGCHI Conference on Human Factors in Computing Systems (CHI '96)*, ed M. J. Tauber (New York, NY: ACM), 496–503. doi: 10.1145/238386.238619

Velichkovsky, B., Sprenger, A., and Unema, P. (1997). "Towards gaze-mediated interaction: collecting solutions of the "Midas touch problem," in *Proceedings of IFIP TC13 International Conference on Human-Computer Interaction (INTERACT'97)*, eds S. Howard, J. Hammond, and G. Lindgaard (London: Chapman and Hall), 509–516.

Waldert, S. (2016). Invasive vs. non-invasive neuronal signals for brain-machine interfaces: Will one prevail? *Front. Neurosci.* 10:295. doi: 10.3389/fnins.2016.00295

Walter, W. G. (1966). Expectancy waves and intention waves in the human brain and their application to the direct cerebral control of machines. *Electroenceph. Clin. Neurophysiol.* 21, 616.

Weill-Tessier, P., Turner, J., and Gellersen, H. (2016). "How do you look at what you touch? A study of touch interaction and gaze correlation on tablets," in *Proceedings of the Ninth Biennial ACM Symposium on Eye Tracking Research & Applications (ETRA '16)* (New York, NY: ACM), 329–330. doi: 10.1145/2857491.2888592

Wenzel, M. A., Golenia, J. E., and Blankertz, B. (2016). Classification of eye fixation related potentials for variable stimulus saliency. *Front. Neurosci.* 10:23. doi: 10.3389/fnins.2016.00023

Wolpaw, J. R., Birbaumer, N., McFarland, D. J., Pfurtscheller, G., and Vaughan, T. M. (2002). Brain–computer interfaces for communication and control. *Clin. Neurophysiol.* 113, 767–791. doi: 10.1016/S1388-2457(02)00057-3

Xu, R., Jiang, N., Lin, C., Mrachacz-Kersting, N., Dremstrup, K., and Farina, D. (2014). Enhanced low-latency detection of motor intention from EEG for closed-loop brain-computer interface applications. *IEEE Trans. Biomed. Eng.* 61, 288–296. doi: 10.1109/TBME.2013.2294203

Zander, T. O., Gaertner, M., Kothe, C., and Vilimek, R. (2010). Combining eye gaze input with a brain-computer interface for touchless human–computer interaction. *Int. J. Hum. Comput. Interact.* 27, 38–51. doi: 10.1080/10447318.2011.535752

Zander, T. O., and Kothe, C. (2011). Towards passive brain–computer interfaces: applying brain–computer interface technology to human–machine systems in general. *J. Neural Eng.* 8:025005. doi: 10.1088/1741-2560/8/2/025005

The overlooked potential for social factors to improve effectiveness of brain-computer interfaces

Cheryl Ann Sexton *

Department of Physiology and Pharmacology, Wake Forest University, School of Medicine, Winston-Salem, NC, USA

Keywords: brain-computer interface (BCI), neurorehabilitatation, social neuroscience, social behavior, augmenting cognition, neural prosthesis

Edited by:
Mikhail Lebedev, Duke University, USA

Reviewed by:
Femke Nijboer, Leiden University, Netherlands
Jérémie Mattout, Lyon Neuroscience Research Center, France
Paul Root Wolpe, Emory University, USA

Correspondence:
Cheryl Ann Sexton, csexton@wakehealth.edu

Introduction

The surge in development of brain-computer interface (BCI) devices is highly focused on the algorithms, mechanics, and neurophysics of their production (Lebedev and Nicolelis, 2006; Lebedev et al., 2011; Opris, 2013). Here I propose that capitalizing on research findings from the field of social neuroscience can enhance training and effectiveness of BCI devices. BCIs are not just about individual brains but also about brains in interaction with other brains. Learning in a social context is more effective than non-social instruction and countless neurophysiology studies have demonstrated that social interaction actually alters physiology, including changes in neuroplasticity and arousal. Importantly, social interaction also consists of emotional responses that have powerful rewarding qualities and incur reciprocal action. Interdisciplinary cooperation between social neuroscience and BCI innovation has been proposed to promote development of more effective BCIs that demonstrate adaptability during interaction (Mattout, 2012). The challenges of BCI illiteracy, or BCI inefficiency, suggests a vital need to consider all possible contributing factors to decrease the failure rate seen in up to a third of users (Vidaurre and Blankertz, 2010). Additionally, it has been suggested that BCI inefficiency can be reduced by addressing flaws in human training approaches, which have been largely neglected (Lotte et al., 2013). Therefore, the social cues and contexts a patient has when BCIs are integrated and employed should not be overlooked for their potential to improve effectiveness.

Social Intelligence

The human brain, like other primate brains, has evolved to be exquisitely tuned to social interactions (Ghazanfar and Santos, 2004). In fact, sociality might have been the primary force driving the evolution of primate intelligence (Jolly, 1966; Humphrey, 1976; Dunbar and Shultz, 2007). Thus, it is no leap to assume that cognitive abilities would be influenced by social interactions (Ybarra et al., 2008). Importantly, cognitive abilities do not exist as abstract mental activities independent of body and world (Barrett and Henzi, 2005). We are born into an environment that consists of others acting and interacting; successfully navigating this social milieu requires the development of many cognitive skills. These essential capacities include memory, learning, decision-making, and behavioral inhibition as well as more complex abilities such as communicating, problem-solving, teaching, mentalizing, and inferring others' mental states (Gariépy et al., 2014).

Social Cues and Contexts

Social contexts include observing and participating in exchanges between individuals, and responding to cues integral to social behavior. These cues include complex stimuli that require simultaneous processing of multiple sensory inputs, including olfactory, auditory, tactile, and visual cues. The emotional responses of self and others are also social cues. Whom we are interacting with matters, as well as the connection we feel with them along a continuum ranging from perceived social isolation to bonding and attachment (Cacioppo and Cacioppo, 2012). The mere presentation of cues specific to social interaction, such as language or images of the same species, is enough to cause neurophysiological changes in brain and behavior. In primates, many studies take advantage of the fact that pictures of objects, abstract images, or other species are not as rewarding as pictures of conspecifics (Wilson and Goldman-Rakic, 1994). Even the nature of the stimulus is relevant—we have a preference for biological movement over robotic movement for encoding behavior (Tai et al., 2004) and children learn new behaviors better from humans than from robots or androids (robots that look like humans) (Moriguchi et al., 2010a,b). The special effectiveness of social stimuli was recently shown when superimposing familiar face images onto the P300 Speller character matrix for ERP-based BCI performance increased accuracy and speed in healthy individuals (Kaufmann et al., 2011) and patients (Kaufmann et al., 2013).

Social Neurophysiology

Neurophysiological effects of social context and stimuli are distributed throughout the nervous system. Multiple areas of the brain respond to social conditions as assessed by a variety of methods, including transcranial magnetic stimulation, functional magnetic resonance imaging, electrophysiology, and molecular studies. To comprehensively describe all the neurological findings is not possible here so only a few are highlighted (see for reviews: Beer and Ochsner, 2006; Adolphs, 2009). The anterior cingular cortex (ACC) integrates complex stimuli, empathy, and decision making (Lavin et al., 2013). The striatum is a vital area for social interaction and reward (Báez-Mendoza and Schultz, 2013). In the inferior fronto-parietal areas, the mirror neuron system (discussed further below) is essential for social learning (reviewed in Rizzolatti and Sinigaglia, 2010). Differences in genetic expression are seen when zebra finches, a social songbird, sing to females directly rather than singing undirected song (Jarvis et al., 1998). Social behavior induces neurogenesis in the adult hippocampus in rodents (Gheusi et al., 2009; Lieberwirth and Wang, 2014; Peretto and Paredes, 2014). The early findings that social enrichment improves cognitive performance, neuronal growth, and overall brain mass (reviewed by Rosenzweig, 2007) followed by decades of confirmation, has led to the now standard practice that animals in research programs are provided appropriate social interactions (Guide for the Care and Use of Laboratory Animals, 2011). Conversely, decades of research have shown social stress during early development results in a number of behavioral and neurochemical deficits in multiple brain areas. For example, social isolation during rearing impairs neurogenesis in the dentate gyrus of the mouse hippocampus as revealed by deficits in spatial memory task (Ibi et al., 2008), and cell proliferation, cell survival, and neuronal differentiation are negatively affected by isolation during adulthood in female prairie voles (Lieberwirth and Wang, 2012).

Cognitive Function

Continuing development of BCIs that treat neurological and psychiatric disorders involving cognitive and emotional impairments suggests the need for the most comprehensive techniques to facilitate success. The research reviewed above clearly shows that cognition is changed by the qualities of social exchanges or social cues. For example, executive function can be increased (Ybarra et al., 2008) or reduced (Richeson et al., 2005) depending on the type of social interaction and even the identity of the actor. Where an individual falls along the continuum of social isolation (e.g., neglect, exclusion) to social connection has important consequences for cognitive abilities. In older adults, correlations between perceived isolation and poor cognitive responses have been shown (Tilvis et al., 2004; Wilson et al., 2007; Dickinson et al., 2011). In fact, brain and behavioral responses differ depending on the specific feeling of isolation/connection to the person with whom one is interacting (Cacioppo and Cacioppo, 2012).

Learning Socially

The social environment can arguably be said to be the richest environment for learning the most complex cognitive skills, pointing out the importance of training methods. A special quality about live social interaction is that it acutely primes the induction of novel responses (Gottlieb, 1991). For example, juvenile sparrows will learn the songs of another species when demonstrated by a live tutor that they do not learn from tape recordings (Baptista and Petrinovich, 1984). The use of social reinforcement has been noted to be particularly useful to improve BCI integration (reviewed in Lotte et al., 2013). Even if social feedback is provided by an android, behavioral change is better than when a computer display provides factual feedback (Ham and Midden, 2014). This suggests that when biofeedback systems are used (e.g., EEG, fMRI, MEG), engaging a person who communicates feedback in addition to computer displays could facilitate acceptance and speed of acquisition during training.

An essential learning substrate lies within the mirror neurons found in the cortical areas in humans; these neurons fire when observing or imitating another's behavior, evoking in the recipient the representational state of the observer's action or emotion (Rizzolatti and Craighero, 2004; Rizzolatti and Sinigaglia, 2010). This allows mere observation of an action to increase motor memory encoding (Stefan et al., 2005; Celnik et al., 2006). Methods in stroke rehabilitation based on the mirror neuron system—action observation, motor imagery, and imitation—take advantage of this opportunity to rebuild motor function (Garrison et al., 2010). Similarly, action observation has been proposed to interact with motor training in neurorehabilitation (Pomeroy et al., 2005), suggesting that cognitive training may also be possible by capitalizing on these mechanisms. For example, in a study with older adults, the combination of physical training and action observation together elicited encoding whereas conditions with only physical training or action observation failed. It is therefore suggested that employing a person who demonstrates the same action as the patient during BCI training would facilitate an increase in encoding more than just using imagery.

Brain-to-brain Coupling

Complex joint behaviors such as communication and social coordination depend on synchronous interactions. Interpersonal synchrony promotes a variety of positive outcomes, including affiliation, liking, rapport, and emotional support satisfaction. It is challenging to measure brain activity simultaneously from two people, but studies that examine inter-person variables such as synchrony have found revealing results using neuroimaging methods (summarized by Konvalinka and Roepstorff, 2012). Inter-personal entrainment of behavior between people occurs when engaged in rhythmic behavior, such as finger-tapping (Konvalinka et al., 2010) or chair-rocking (Richardson et al., 2007) resulting in unintentional coordination. Inducing synchronous activity induces brain-to-brain coupling, which might increase the efficiency of partnerships engaged with BCI use. Indeed, it has been suggested that our joint cognition with other minds increases their efficiency as a unit, particularly when in compromised situations (Wegner et al., 1991). Intriguing results with a multiuser BCI video game based on motor imagery showed improved utility, effectiveness, and engagement (Bonnet et al., 2013), suggesting methods using interacting brains would help reduce BCI illiteracy.

Brain-to-brain Transfer

Perhaps the most outstanding example of social interaction effect is the demonstration of brain-to-brain transfer of information via computer. In a recent study, the neural firing pattern code of a rat performing a memory task was transferred to a recipient rat, who then responded correctly more often than when stimulated with a random code or without stimulation (Deadwyler et al., 2013). Further, a study revealed that sensory information from a rat transmitted via computer included bidirectional reward contingency information that changed behavior of both donor and a naïve recipient rat in a location thousands of miles away (Pais-Vieira et al., 2013). Even human brain to rat brain transfer has been achieved (Yoo et al., 2013). These examples suggest that the day when neural signals can be transmitted between individuals is not out of the realm of possibility.

Recommendations

BCIs used for neurological rehabilitation require progressive practice with feedback and reward (Dobkin, 2007); here I suggest that capitalizing on social factors will result in better outcomes. The social environment provides a context particularly relevant for fostering the development and change of cognition. Given that the presence of social factors facilitates learning suggests that attention should be given to the conditions by which the BCI is integrated. For example, engage a loved one or a trusted facilitator who can supply emotionally rewarding feedback in training and treatment protocols. Use rewards of social stimuli, such as images of people or positive language, to enhance training, and deliver rewards with people instead of only computer displays. Pay attention to the emotional environment to ensure it is conducive for promoting change. Be aware that socially isolated patients will be more sensitive to negative cues and stimuli. Capitalize on the processes of imitation and action observation to stimulate responses of the mirror neuron system; in other words, have the patient and facilitator do the same task. Even if the patient is unable to perform the task, mere observation can stimulate motor neuron responses. Employ synchronization tasks between the facilitator and patient to increase trust and brain coupling. Finally, most revolutionary, use healthy individuals as donors to stimulate the patient via inter-brain coupling with brain-to-brain interfaces. In conclusion, just as it is essential that BCI development and use rely on the accurate use of technical principles, it is vital not to overlook the value of applying findings from social neuroscience in order to maximize the effectiveness of BCI implementation and integration.

References

Adolphs, R. (2009). The social brain: neural basis of social knowledge. *Annu. Rev. Psychol.* 60, 693–716. doi: 10.1146/annurev.psych.60.110707.163514

Báez-Mendoza, R., and Schultz, W. (2013). The role of the striatum in social behavior. *Front. Neurosci.* 7:233. doi: 10.3389/fnins.2013.00233

Baptista, L. F., and Petrinovich, L. (1984). Social interaction, sensitive phases and the song template hypothesis in the white-crowned sparrow. *Anim. Behav.* 32, 172–181. doi: 10.1016/S0003-3472(84)80335-8

Barrett, L., and Henzi, P. (2005). The social nature of primate cognition. *Proc. Biol. Sci.* 272, 1865–1875. doi: 10.1098/rspb.2005.3200

Beer, J. S., and Ochsner, K. N. (2006). Social cognition: a multi level analysis. *Brain Res.* 1079, 98–105. doi: 10.1016/j.brainres.2006.01.002

Bonnet, L., Lotte, F., and Lecuyer, A. (2013). Two brains, one game: design and evaluation of a multiuser BCI video game based on motor imagery. *IEEE Trans. Comput. Intell. AI Games* 5, 185–198. doi: 10.1109/TCIAIG.2012.2237173

Cacioppo, S., and Cacioppo, J. T. (2012). Decoding the invisible forces of social connections. *Front. Integr. Neurosci.* 6:51. doi: 10.3389/fnint.2012.00051

Celnik, P., Stefan, K., Hummel, F., Duque, J., Classen, J., and Cohen, L. G. (2006). Encoding a motor memory in the older adult by action observation. *Neuroimage* 29, 677–684. doi: 10.1016/j.neuroimage.2005.07.039

Deadwyler, S. A., Berger, T. W., Sweatt, A. J., Song, D., Chan, R. H. M., Opris, I., et al. (2013). Donor/recipient enhancement of memory in rat hippocampus. *Front. Syst. Neurosci.* 7:120. doi: 10.3389/fnsys.2013.00120

Dickinson, W. J., Potter, G. G., Hybels, C. F., McQuoid, D. R., and Steffens, D. C. (2011). Change in stress and social support as predictors of cognitive decline in older adults with and without depression. *Int. J. Geriatr. Psychiatry* 26, 1267–1274. doi: 10.1002/gps.2676

Dobkin, B. H. (2007). Brain-computer interface technology as a tool to augment plasticity and outcomes for neurological rehabilitation. *J. Physiol.* 579 (Pt 3), 637–642. doi: 10.1113/jphysiol.2006.123067

Dunbar, R. I. M., and Shultz, S. (2007). Evolution in the social brain. *Science* 317, 1344–1347. doi: 10.1126/science.1145463

Gariépy, J.-F., Watson, K. K., Du, E., Xie, D. L., Erb, J., Amasino, D., et al. (2014). Social learning in humans and other animals. *Front. Neurosci.* 8:58. doi: 10.3389/fnins.2014.00058

Garrison, K. A., Winstein, C. J., and Aziz-Zadeh, L. (2010). The mirror neuron system: a neural substrate for methods in stroke rehabilitation. *Neurorehabil. Neural Repair* 24, 404–412. doi: 10.1177/1545968309354536

Ghazanfar, A. A., and Santos, L. R. (2004). Primate brains in the wild: the sensory bases for social interactions. *Nat. Rev. Neurosci.* 5, 603–616. doi: 10.1038/nrn1473

Gheusi, G., Ortega-Perez, I., Murray, K., and Lledo, P.-M. (2009). A niche for adult neurogenesis in social behavior. *Behav. Brain Res.* 200, 315–322. doi: 10.1016/j.bbr.2009.02.006

Gottlieb, G. (1991). Social induction of malleability in ducklings. *Anim. Behav.* 41, 953–962.

Guide for the Care and Use of Laboratory Animals (2011). *Guide for the Care and Use of Laboratory Animals, 8th Edn.* The National Academies Press. Available online at: http://www.nap.edu/catalog/12910/guide-for-the-care-and-use-of-laboratory-animals-eighth (Accessed December 30, 2014).

Ham, J., and Midden, C. J. H. (2014). A persuasive robot to stimulate energy conservation: the influence of positive and negative social feedback and task similarity on energy-consumption behavior. *Int. J. Soc. Robot.* 6, 163–171. doi: 10.1007/s12369-013-0205-z

Humphrey, N. (1976). "The social function of intellect," in *Growing Points in Ethology*, eds P. P. G. Bateson and R. A. Hinde. Available online at: http://www.humphrey.org.uk/papers/1976SocialFunction.pdf.

Ibi, D., Takuma, K., Koike, H., Mizoguchi, H., Tsuritani, K., Kuwahara, Y., et al. (2008). Social isolation rearing-induced impairment of the hippocampal neurogenesis is associated with deficits in spatial memory and emotion-related behaviors in juvenile mice. *J. Neurochem.* 105, 921–932. doi: 10.1111/j.1471-4159.2007.05207.x

Jarvis, E., Scharff, C., Grossman, M., Ramos, J., and Nottebohm, F. (1998). For whom the bird sings: context-dependent gene expression. *Neuron* 21, 775–788.

Jolly, A. (1966). Lemur social behavior and primate intelligence. *Science* 153, 501–506.

Kaufmann, T., Schulz, S. M., Grunzinger, C., and Kubler, A. (2011). Flashing characters with famous faces improves ERP-based brain–computer interface performance. *J. Neural Eng.* 8, 1–10. doi: 10.1088/1741-2560/8/5/056016

Kaufmann, T., Schulz, S. M., Köblitz, A., Renner, G., Wessig, C., and Kübler, A. (2013). Face stimuli effectively prevent brain-computer interface inefficiency in patients with neurodegenerative disease. *Clin. Neurophysiol.* 124, 893–900. doi: 10.1016/j.clinph.2012.11.006

Konvalinka, I., and Roepstorff, A. (2012). The two-brain approach: how can mutually interacting brains teach us something about social interaction? *Front. Hum. Neurosci.* 6:215. doi: 10.3389/fnhum.2012.00215

Konvalinka, I., Vuust, P., Roepstorff, A., and Frith, C. D. (2010). Follow you, follow me: continuous mutual prediction and adaptation in joint tapping. *Q. J. Exp. Psychol.* 63, 2220–2230. doi: 10.1080/17470218.2010.497843

Lavin, C., Melis, C., Mikulan, E., Gelormini, C., Huepe, D., and Ibañez, A. (2013). The anterior cingulate cortex: an integrative hub for human socially-driven interactions. *Front. Neurosci.* 7:64. doi: 10.3389/fnins.2013.00064

Lebedev, M. A., and Nicolelis, M. A. L. (2006). Brain–machine interfaces: past, present and future. *Trends Neurosci.* 29, 536–546. doi: 10.1016/j.tins.2006.07.004

Lebedev, M. A., Tate, A. J., Hanson, T. L., Li, Z., O'Doherty, J. E., Winans, J. A., et al. (2011). Future developments in brain-machine interface research. *Clinics* 66 Suppl. 1, 25–32. doi: 10.1590/S1807-59322011001300004

Lieberwirth, C., and Wang, Z. (2012). The social environment and neurogenesis in the adult mammalian brain. *Front. Hum. Neurosci.* 6:118. doi: 10.3389/fnhum.2012.00118

Lieberwirth, C., and Wang, Z. (2014). Social bonding: regulation by neuropeptides. *Front. Neurosci.* 8:171. doi: 10.3389/fnins.2014.00171

Lotte, F., Larrue, F., and Mühl, C. (2013). Flaws in current human training protocols for spontaneous brain-computer interfaces: lessons learned from instructional design. *Front. Hum. Neurosci.* 7:568. doi: 10.3389/fnhum.2013.00568

Mattout, J. (2012). Brain-computer interfaces: a neuroscience paradigm of social interaction? A matter of perspective. *Front. Hum. Neurosci.* 6:114. doi: 10.3389/fnhum.2012.00114

Moriguchi, Y., Kanda, T., Ishiguro, H., and Itakura, S. (2010a). Children perseverate to a human's actions but not to a robot's actions. *Dev. Sci.* 13, 62–68. doi: 10.1111/j.1467-7687.2009.00860.x

Moriguchi, Y., Minato, T., Ishiguro, H., Shinohara, I., and Itakura, S. (2010b). Cues that trigger social transmission of disinhibition in young children. *J. Exp. Child Psychol.* 107, 181–187. doi: 10.1016/j.jecp.2010.04.018

Opris, I. (2013). Inter-laminar microcircuits across neocortex: repair and augmentation. *Front. Syst. Neurosci.* 7:80. doi: 10.3389/fnsys.2013.00080

Peretto, P., and Paredes, R. G. (2014). "Social cues, adult neurogenesis, and reproductive behavior," in *Neurobiology of Chemical Communication, Chapter 13*, ed C. Mucignat-Caretta (Boca Raton, FL: CRC Press). Available online at: http://www.ncbi.nlm.nih.gov/books/NBK200979/?report=reader

Pais-Vieira, M., Lebedev, M., Kunicki, C., Wang, J., and Nicolelis, M. A. L. (2013). A brain-to-brain interface for real-time sharing of sensorimotor information. *Sci. Rep.* 3:1319. doi: 10.1038/srep01319

Pomeroy, V. M., Clark, C. A., Miller, J. S. G., Baron, J.-C., Markus, H. S., and Tallis, R. C. (2005). The potential for utilizing the 'mirror neurone system' to enhance recovery of the severely affected upper limb early after stroke: a review and hypothesis. *Neurorehabil. Neural Repair* 19, 4–13. doi: 10.1177/1545968304274351

Richardson, M. J., Marsh, K. L., Isenhower, R. W., Goodman, J. R. L., and Schmidt, R. C. (2007). Rocking together: dynamics of intentional and unintentional interpersonal coordination. *Hum. Mov. Sci.* 26, 867–891. doi: 10.1016/j.humov.2007.07.002

Richeson, J. A., Trawalter, S., and Shelton, J. N. (2005). African Americans' implicit racial attitudes and the depletion of executive function after interracial interactions. *Soc. Cogn.* 23, 336–352. doi: 10.1521/soco.2005.23.4.336

Rizzolatti, G., and Craighero, L. (2004). The mirror-neuron system. *Annu. Rev. Neurosci.* 27, 169–192. doi: 10.1146/annurev.neuro.27.070203.144230

Rizzolatti, G., and Sinigaglia, C. (2010). The functional role of the parieto-frontal mirror circuit: interpretations and misinterpretations. *Nat. Rev. Neurosci.* 11, 264–274. doi: 10.1038/nrn2805

Rosenzweig, M. R. (2007). "Modification of brain circuits through experience," in *Neural Plasticity and Memory: From Genes To Brain Imaging*, ed F. Bermudez-Rattoni (Boca Raton, FL: CRC Press), 67–94. Available online at: http://www.mendeley.com/research/modification-brain-circuits-through-experience/?utm_source=desktop&utm_medium=1.12.4&utm_campaign=open_catalog&userDocumentId={719b8420-1b4f-49b3-85a7-f60344a6bbfe}.

Stefan, K., Cohen, L. G., Duque, J., Mazzocchio, R., Celnik, P., Sawaki, L., et al. (2005). Formation of a motor memory by action observation. *J. Neurosci.* 25, 9339–9346. doi: 10.1523/JNEUROSCI.2282-05.2005

Tai, Y. F., Scherfler, C., Brooks, D. J., Sawamoto, N., and Castiello, U. (2004). The human premotor cortex is 'mirror' only for biological actions. *Curr. Biol.* 14, 117–120. doi: 10.1016/j.cub.2004.01.005

Tilvis, R. S., Kahonen-Vare, M. H., Jolkkonen, J., Valvanne, J., Pitkala, K. H., and Strandberg, T. E. (2004). Predictors of cognitive decline and mortality of aged people over a 10-year period. *J. Gerontol. A Biol. Sci. Med. Sci.* 59, M268–M274. doi: 10.1093/gerona/59.3.M268

Vidaurre, C., and Blankertz, B. (2010). Towards a cure for BCI illiteracy. *Brain Topogr.* 23, 194–198. doi: 10.1007/s10548-009-0121-6

Wegner, D. M., Erber, R., and Raymond, P. (1991). Transactive memory in close relationships. *J. Pers. Soc. Psychol.* 61, 923–929.

Wilson, F. A. W., and Goldman-Rakic, P. S. (1994). Viewing preferences of rhesus monkeys related to memory for complex pictures, colours and faces. *Behav. Brain Res.* 60, 79–89.

Wilson, R. S., Krueger, K. R., Arnold, S. E., Schneider, J. A., Kelly, J. F., Barnes, L. L., et al. (2007). Loneliness and risk of alzheimer disease. *Arch. Gen. Psychiatry* 64, 234–240. doi: 10.1001/archpsyc.64.2.234

Ybarra, O., Burnstein, E., Winkielman, P., Keller, M. C., Manis, M., Chan, E., et al. (2008). Mental exercising through simple socializing: social interaction promotes general cognitive functioning. *Pers. Soc. Psychol. Bull.* 34, 248–259. doi: 10.1177/0146167207310454

22

A dynamical model improves reconstruction of handwriting from multichannel electromyographic recordings

Elizaveta Okorokova [1], *Mikhail Lebedev* [2], *Michael Linderman* [3] *and Alex Ossadtchi* [1, 4*]

[1] Centre for Cognition and Decision Making, National Research University Higher School of Economics, Moscow, Russia, [2] Department of Neurobiology, Duke University, Durham, NC, USA, [3] Department of Biomedical Engineering, Norconnect Inc., Ogdensburg, NY, USA, [4] Laboratory of Control of Complex Systems, Institute of Problems of Mechanical Engineering, Russian Academy of Sciences, St. Petersburg, Russia

Edited by:
Giovanni Mirabella,
Sapienza University of Rome, Italy

Reviewed by:
Giancarlo Ferrigno,
Politecnico di Milano, Italy
Giuseppe D'Avenio,
Istituto Superiore di Sanità, Italy

***Correspondence:**
Alex Ossadtchi
ossadtchi@gmail.com

In recent years, several assistive devices have been proposed to reconstruct arm and hand movements from electromyographic (EMG) activity. Although simple to implement and potentially useful to augment many functions, such myoelectric devices still need improvement before they become practical. Here we considered the problem of reconstruction of handwriting from multichannel EMG activity. Previously, linear regression methods (e.g., the Wiener filter) have been utilized for this purpose with some success. To improve reconstruction accuracy, we implemented the Kalman filter, which allows to fuse two information sources: the physical characteristics of handwriting and the activity of the leading hand muscles, registered by the EMG. Applying the Kalman filter, we were able to convert eight channels of EMG activity recorded from the forearm and the hand muscles into smooth reconstructions of handwritten traces. The filter operates in a causal manner and acts as a true predictor utilizing the EMGs from the past only, which makes the approach suitable for real-time operations. Our algorithm is appropriate for clinical neuroprosthetic applications and computer peripherals. Moreover, it is applicable to a broader class of tasks where predictive myoelectric control is needed.

Keywords: handwriting, electromyography, pattern recognition, dynamical modeling, the Kalman Filter, the Wiener Filter

1. INTRODUCTION

Handwriting is a unique development of human culture. A skill learned during the early childhood, it remains among the primary means of communication and self-expression throughout the course of life. From the physiological point of view, handwriting is a complex interplay between the nervous system and the numerous muscles of the upper extremity. Despite several attempts to study this intricate activity theoretically (Plamondon and Maarse, 1989; McKeague, 2005) and experimentally (Linderman et al., 2009; Huang et al., 2010; Li et al., 2013), it is still not well understood and can not be reliably replicated in prostheses.

The relationship between the muscle force and the pen trajectory is complicated by the motor redundancy phenomenon (Bernstein, 1967; Guigon et al., 2006). One and the same movement can be accomplished via basically infinite number of muscle activation patterns. Relatively fine spatial scale inherent to the handwriting process and the natural variations of the limb's kinematic variables further complicate the issue.

Additional obstacle in studying the physiology of handwriting is the difficulty of measuring the muscle force directly. Surface and intramuscular Electromyography (EMG) are the common methods to register neuromuscular activity during a motor task. Surface EMG is a non-invasive method which implies placing the electrodes on the skin above the muscles of interest. Being easy and safe to implement, this technique, however, does not yield sufficiently accurate biomechanical measurements, due to the complex relationship between the EMG and muscle force, complicated anatomy of muscles and the inability to record from all the muscles involved, especially from the deep muscles. Intramuscular EMG (iEMG) is invasive and uses needle electrodes inserted into the muscle tissue to yield more spatially specific measurements with less leakage and disturbance. The invasive nature of iEMG limits its utility.

Both EMG registration methods posit several substantial difficulties, primarily related to signal quality and associated issues of noise filtering and source extraction from the observed data. Nonetheless, it was shown that even the surface EMG carries valuable information about the neuromuscular interactions and can therefore be used effectively in modeling and interpreting movements (Reaz et al., 2006; Ahsan et al., 2009).

Despite the evident difficulties of measuring and interpreting neuromuscular activity with the currently available techniques, understanding such complex motor tasks as handwriting is important for both theoretical and practical reasons. Once we learn how to model the relationship between EMG patterns and pen movements during handwriting, we can introduce this knowledge to many rapidly expanding fields and practices, including biomedical engineering, robotics and biofeedback therapy. For instance, we can substantially improve the existing treatment and rehabilitation techniques for patients with a loss or an injury of an upper limb (Xiao and Menon, 2014), create rules for diagnostics of motor diseases based on handwriting (Van Gemmert et al., 1999; Stanford, 2004; Silveri et al., 2007), and even assist young children in learning how to write (Carter and Russell, 1985). Besides, an accurate model and methodolgies for building such models, establishing the correspondence between the handwriting and muscle activation patterns has a potential to become a foundation for creating intelligent neural prosthesis with a substantial number of degrees of freedom and fine spatial scale (Chan et al., 2000; Ohnishi et al., 2007; Shenoy et al., 2008; Bu et al., 2009; Castellini and van der Smagt, 2009).

However, such appealing advances and practices are still in their infancy. To date, the existing research on decoding of handwriting from electromyography is small and restricted to laboratory conditions. Several papers addressed the question of written character classification based on surface EMG, which involved implementation of machine-learning techniques to distinguish between muscle activation patterns for different written characters, such as digits, alphabet letters or simple geometric shapes. Linderman et al. (2009) classified symbols from 0 to 9, using eight bipolar surface electrodes placed on the hand and the forearm muscles. They implemented Fisher Linear Discriminant Analysis to obtain, on average, 90% accuracy of classification across subjects. Huang et al. (2010) used Dynamic Time Warping (DTW) to classify symbols based on 6-channel EMG recordings. Their average classification accuracy was 98.25% for digits, 97.89% for Chinese symbols and 84.29% for Latin capital letters. Li et al. (2013) improved the DTW algorithm by substituting Euclidean Distance with Mahalanobis Distance, to increase classification precision to almost 95%. In their experiment, subjects were instructed to write lower-case letters, while 4-channel EMG signals were recorded from their forearm.

The other studies considered a rather complex task of on-line decoding of the pen traces, based on the incoming EMG signals from the measurement electrodes. Among the most successful methods known to the authors, is the Wiener Filter (Linderman et al., 2009), which allows to attain accuracy of reconstruction of $47 \pm 2\%$ for X-coordinate and $63 \pm 15\%$ for Y-coordinate, measured by the coefficient of determination. However, the method used the data samples from the future, which would lead to extra delays in cases when used in the on-line mode.

In this paper, we consider the same multisubject data-set as in Linderman et al. (2009) and present our approach to EMG-based pen tracking that by taking into account the dynamic model of the pen coordinate process allows to outperform the previously reported techniques. The main idea behind our method is to fuse two information sources available about the process of handwriting. The first information source comes from the physical and the kinematic characteristics of handwriting. The second information source comes from the multichannel electromyography that indirectly measures the strength of the upper extremity muscles, activated to move the pen. To perform the fusion of the two sources optimally, we employ the Linear Kalman Filter (Kalman, 1960), which is a well-known recursive algorithm for dynamic statistical model-based inference.

2. MATERIALS AND METHODS

2.1. The Kalman Filter

2.1.1. Preliminary Remarks

In its classical formulation the Kalman Filter (KF) (Kalman, 1960) is an algorithm that fuses several (usually two) noisy sources of information to produce an estimate of the dynamical system's state vector, which is optimal in the "minimum squared error" sense. The method is over 50 years old, but it is still very popular, due to its intuitive structure, ease of implementation and computational efficiency.

In our application, the first information source is the dynamical model that captures the physical properties of the arm-wrist-pen device and is formalized as a multivariate autoregressive (MVAR) process, whose parameters are estimated from the data. The noisy vector of EMG measurements is the second source of information, whose relation to the pen coordinate is modeled via multivariate linear regression equation with coefficients determined from the training data-set.

For simplicity, the derivations provided in this section are based on the assumption of multivariate normality of the fused sources (Faragher, 2012), which is essential for the Kalman Filter to be the optimal estimator (the best among all other kinds). However, in the general Kalman Filter framework, this does not have to be the case (Arulampalam et al., 2002). When the assumption of normality does not hold, it is still possible to derive the KF equations based on the orthogonality principle (e.g., Jazwinski, 2007), which would guarantee the KF to be the best linear estimator, but not necessarily be optimal. In this case, it might be possible to increase accuracy by employing non-linear techniques that exploit higher order dependencies in the data, such as the Extended Kalman Filter (Julier and Uhlmann, 1997) or its "distribution-free" version, called Unscented Kalman Filter (Wan and Van Der Merwe, 2000). However, since the majority of trials in our multisubject dataset appear to test positively for the normality (see Appendix, Section Testing the Assumptions of the Model) the extent of improvement furnished by the use of the non-linear approaches is hard to predict theoretically. This leaves the question in the empirical realm to be addressed in the future studies.

As demonstrated by the statistical tests described in the Appendix (Section Testing the Assumptions of the Model), we could not reject the hypothesis of independence for the majority of trials. Based on this and, for the simplicity reasons, we base our developments in this paper on the assumption of independence of the two fused sources. In case the independence assumption is violated, the performance gained by taking into account the dynamics of the reconstructed process could have been more sizable should we use a slightly modified form of equations (Shimkin, 2009) to account for the non-trivial cross-covariance structure of the residuals. However, the extent to which modeling the cross-covariance structure of residuals would improve the performance is not entirely clear, due to the inherent non-stationarity and the associated estimation errors.

2.1.2. State Transition Model

As the first information source, we assume that, at each time moment t, the system evolves from the previous state at time $t-1$, according to the rule:

$$\boldsymbol{s}_t = \boldsymbol{A}\boldsymbol{s}_{t-1} + \boldsymbol{v}_t \tag{1}$$

where

- $\boldsymbol{s}_t = [x_t, y_t, \dot{x}_t, \dot{y}_t, \ddot{x}_t, \ddot{y}_t, ..., x_{t-K+1}, y_{t-K+1}, \dot{x}_{t-K+1}, \dot{y}_{t-K+1}, \ddot{x}_{t-K+1}, \ddot{y}_{t-K}]^T$ is a $6K \times 1$ state vector containing pen coordinates and their first and second rates of change for the window of K time moments starting from t;
- $\boldsymbol{A}$ is a $[6K \times 6K]$ state transition matrix, which performs the mapping between the state vectors at the two consecutive time moments;
- $\boldsymbol{v}_t$ is a $[6K \times 1]$ vector containing process noise, which is assumed to be drawn from a multivariate Gaussian distribution with zero mean and covariance matrix $\boldsymbol{Q}$.

Based on Equation (1), we can derive the following expressions connecting the mean and the covariance matrix of the state vector at the two consecutive time moments.

- $\boldsymbol{\mu}_{1t} = \boldsymbol{A}\boldsymbol{\mu}_{1(t-1)}$ is a 6K-dimensional mean state vector at time t;
- $\boldsymbol{\Sigma}_{1t} = \boldsymbol{A}\boldsymbol{\Sigma}_{1(t-1)}\boldsymbol{A}^T + \boldsymbol{Q}$ is a $6K \times 6K$ positive-definite covariance matrix of the state vector at time t.

Detailed derivations of the model parameters can be found in the Appendix (Section Testing the Assumptions of the Model).

2.1.3. Measurement Model

Usually, in the KF framework, the measurement equation appears in the $\boldsymbol{z} = F(\boldsymbol{s})$ form, describing the way the process to be estimated ($\boldsymbol{s}$) is related to the available vector of indirect measurements ($\boldsymbol{z}$). However, in our application, due to causal and physiological reasons, it is more natural to think that the EMG registered muscle activity gives rise to the pen movement. Therefore, we use the "inverse" form of what is usually called the observation equation in the KF framework and write

$$\boldsymbol{s}_t = \boldsymbol{H}\boldsymbol{z}_t + \boldsymbol{w}_t \tag{2}$$

where

- $\boldsymbol{z}_t$ is a $[8L \times 1]$ observation vector containing L groups of eight EMG measurements corresponding to the $[t-L+1, t]$ window of L most recent samples;
- $\boldsymbol{H}$ is a $[6K \times 8L]$ measurement transformation matrix, mapping the measurement domain to the state vector domain;
- $\boldsymbol{w}_t$ is a $[8L \times 1]$ vector of measurement noise with zero mean and covariance matrix $\boldsymbol{R}$. Additionally, the measurement noise $\boldsymbol{w}_t$ is assumed to be independent from the process noise $\boldsymbol{v}_t$.

The $6K$-dimensional state mean vector at time t is given by

$$\boldsymbol{\mu}_{2t} = E[\boldsymbol{s}_t] = \boldsymbol{H}\boldsymbol{z}_t. \tag{3}$$

Since we do not model $\boldsymbol{z}_t$ as a stochastic process, the covariance matrix of $\boldsymbol{s}_t$ reduces to covariance matrix of the measurement noise, so that $\boldsymbol{\Sigma}_{2t} = E[\boldsymbol{w}_t\boldsymbol{w}_t^T] = \boldsymbol{R}$. Note that this noise is assumed to be stationary.

2.1.4. Information Fusion

As outlined in the previous two subsections, we have two independent sources of information about the state vector. The first endogenous source bases its predictions on the dynamical characteristics of the pen coordinates during the handwriting and yields $f_1(\boldsymbol{s}_t|\boldsymbol{s}_{t-1})$ as the state vector distribution (red distribution in **Figure 1**). The second source is exogenous and uses externally registered EMG signals to suggest $f_2(\boldsymbol{s}_t|\boldsymbol{z}_t)$ as the state vector distribution (blue distribution in **Figure 1**). In order to reconstruct the state vector, optimally taking into account the predictions from both sources, we perform the statistical fusion of the estimates based on the dynamical and the measurement models. The schematic procedure of the source fusion is illustrated in **Figure 1**.

The joint conditional estimate of the state vector is distributed as $f_{fused}(\boldsymbol{s}_t|\boldsymbol{s}_{t-1}, \boldsymbol{z}_t)$ (green distribution in **Figure 1**). Assuming independence of the sources, the problem of finding $f(\boldsymbol{s}_t|\boldsymbol{s}_{t-1}, \boldsymbol{z}_t)$

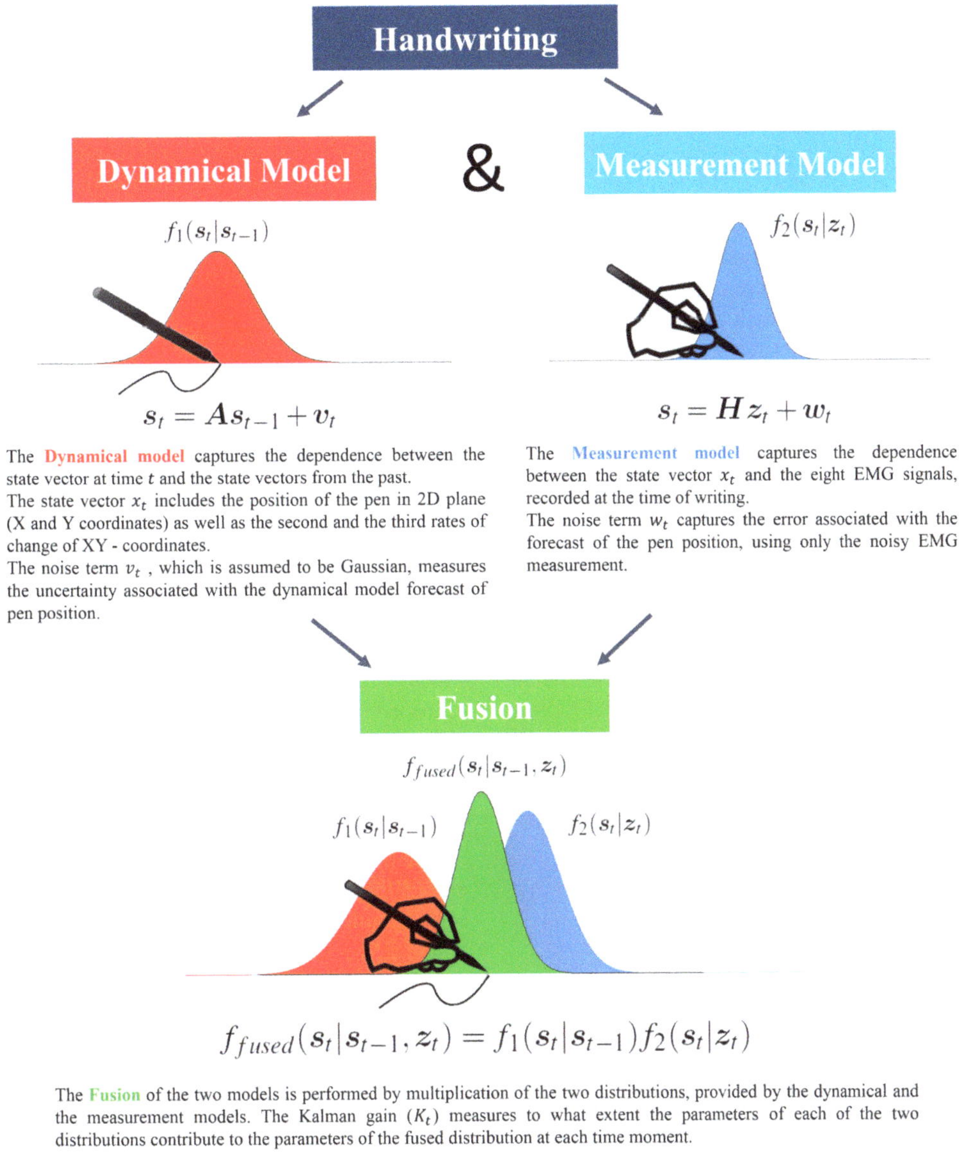

FIGURE 1 | Information Fusion by means of the Kalman Filter allows to improve reconstruction accuracy by adaptively balancing the contribution from the two information sources.

reduces to a simple multiplication of the two probability density functions, i.e.,

$$f_{fused}(s_t|s_{t-1}, z_t) = f_1(s_t|s_{t-1})f_2(s_t|z_t) \tag{4}$$

The product of two multivariate normal distributions is also a multivariate normal (Rencher, 2003). Its mean and covariance can be easily expressed in terms of the mean vectors and the covariance matrices of each of the two normal multipliers.

Specifically, $\mathbf{\Sigma}_{fused}$ is the covariance matrix of the fused distribution can be computed as

$$\mathbf{\Sigma}_{fused} = (\mathbf{\Sigma}_{1t}^{-1} + \mathbf{\Sigma}_{2t}^{-1})^{-1}, \tag{5}$$

and the $6K$-dimensional mean vector of the fused distribution is found to be the following weighted sum of the two mean vectors of the fused information sources:

$$\boldsymbol{\mu}_{fused} = \mathbf{\Sigma}_{fused}(\mathbf{\Sigma}_{1t}^{-1}\boldsymbol{\mu}_{1t} + \mathbf{\Sigma}_{2t}^{-1}\boldsymbol{\mu}_{2t}), \tag{6}$$

It is instructive to reformulate the expressions for the mean and the covariance matrix of the new distribution and to separate the influence of the two distributions being fused.

Using the matrix inversion lemma (Henderson and Searle, 1981), and setting

$$K_t = \mathbf{\Sigma}_{1t}(\mathbf{\Sigma}_{1t} + \mathbf{\Sigma}_{2t})^{-1} \tag{7}$$

we can rewrite Equations (5) and (6) as

$$\boldsymbol{\Sigma}_{fused} = \boldsymbol{\Sigma}_{1t} - \boldsymbol{K}_t\boldsymbol{\Sigma}_{1t}. \tag{8}$$

and

$$\boldsymbol{\mu}_{fused} = (\boldsymbol{I} - \boldsymbol{K}_t)\boldsymbol{\mu}_{1t} + \boldsymbol{K}_t\boldsymbol{\mu}_{2t}. \tag{9}$$

For detailed derivation of the parameters see the Appendix.

The term $\boldsymbol{K}_t$ in Equation (7), commonly known as the Kalman Gain, plays a crucial role of the dynamic scaling factor reflecting the distribution of trust in each of the two information sources. It depends on the relative amount of uncertainty present in the estimates by each of the information sources alone, and varies over time.

Since covariance matrices are positive definite, Equation (8) shows that by fusing the two distributions we reduce the variation associated with the state estimate, proportionally to the Kalman gain. At the same time, the fused mean (Equation 9) becomes the weighted average of the endogenously predicted and the measurements-based mean estimates.

2.1.5. The Algorithm

Based on the above equations we are now ready to formulate the algorithm for calculating the Kalman Filter estimate. At each time moment the computation can be split into three consecutive steps.

1. Endogenous state prediction and error covariance update:

$$\hat{\boldsymbol{s}}_{t|t-1} = \boldsymbol{\mu}_{1t} = \boldsymbol{A}\hat{\boldsymbol{s}}_{t-1|t-1} \tag{10}$$

$$\boldsymbol{P}_{t|t-1} = \boldsymbol{\Sigma}_{1t} = \boldsymbol{A}\boldsymbol{P}_{t-1|t-1}\boldsymbol{A}^T + \boldsymbol{Q} \tag{11}$$

2. Kalman Gain Calculation:

$$\boldsymbol{K}_t = \boldsymbol{\Sigma}_{1t}(\boldsymbol{\Sigma}_{1t} + \boldsymbol{\Sigma}_{2t})^{-1} = P_{t|t-1}(\boldsymbol{P}_{t|t-1} + \boldsymbol{R})^{-1} \tag{12}$$

3. Measurement Update:

$$\hat{\boldsymbol{s}}_{t|z} = \boldsymbol{\mu}_{2t} = \boldsymbol{H}\boldsymbol{z}_t \tag{13}$$

$$\hat{\boldsymbol{s}}_{t|t} = \hat{\boldsymbol{s}}_{t|t-1} + \boldsymbol{K}_t(\hat{\boldsymbol{s}}_{t|z} - \hat{\boldsymbol{s}}_{t|t-1}) \tag{14}$$

$$\boldsymbol{P}_{t|t} = \boldsymbol{P}_{t|t-1} - \boldsymbol{K}_t\boldsymbol{P}_{t|t-1} \tag{15}$$

In order to relate our approach to the classical KF paradigm in the equations above, we assigned the variables used in the previous subsection to the standard symbols, commonly employed in the KF literature. In the above algorithm, the first step is to use the State Transition Equation only and to calculate the so-called *a priori* estimate $\hat{\boldsymbol{s}}_{t|t-1}$, with associated variance $\boldsymbol{P}_{t|t-1}$ (Equations 10 and 11).

Then, we calculate the Kalman Gain based on the *a priori* covariance matrix and the covariance matrix of the Measurement Model (Equation 12).

Finally, the *a posteriori* estimate $\hat{\boldsymbol{s}}_{t|t}$ is computed by adjusting the endogenous *a priori* estimate with the EMG measurements. The amount of adjustment is governed by the time-varying Kalman Gain (Equation 14) and the innovations process $\hat{\boldsymbol{s}}_{t|z} - \hat{\boldsymbol{s}}_{t|t-1}$, informing the algorithm on the amount of mismatch between the endogenous and exogenous estimates. The *a posteriori* uncertainty, associated with the prediction, based on the two models, is given by $\boldsymbol{P}_{t|t}$ (Equation 15), which shows that, in the final estimate, the *a priori* uncertainty gets reduced proportionally to the Kalman Gain.

2.2. The Experiment

2.2.1. Data

Six healthy participants were instructed to write symbols from 0 to 9, repeating each symbol approximately 50 times. At the same time, muscle activity was recorded with eight bipolar-surface EMG electrodes, placed on each participants leading hand muscles: *opponens pollicis*, *abductor pollicis brevis*, *medial and lateral heads of first dorsal interrosseus*, and four forearm muscles: *flexor carpi radialis*, *extensor digitorum*, *extensor carpi ulnaris*, and *extensor carpi radialis*. The reference electrode was placed on each subject's forehead. Position of the pen was recorded using the special digitizing tablet, yielding a pair of coordinates in the two-dimensional space. For a detailed illustration of the experiment set-up, see Linderman et al. (2009).

2.2.2. Preprocessing

Before applying the algorithm, we preprocessed EMG signals to extract the envelope via the standard rectification procedure. For each channel separately, we first calculated the absolute value of the EMG signals and then low-pass filtered the result with a second-order Butterworth Filter with the cut-off frequency of F_c. We optimized the value of the cut-off frequency based on the training subset of the recorded data to obtain the best reconstruction performance. In the final results reported here $F_c = 2$ Hz. Additionally, we have applied square-root transformation to each signal's envelope, obtained via the described rectification procedure.

2.2.3. Training and Testing

Half of the trials of each symbol was randomly assigned to training the parameters of the model, while the remaining half was used for testing the performance (**Figure 2**). During training, the parameters of the dynamical model (Equation 1) and the measurement model (Equation 2) were estimated. We applied Ordinary Least Squares Method to estimate matrix $\boldsymbol{A}$ in the state transition equation and matrix $\boldsymbol{H}$ in the measurement equation. Covariance matrices $\boldsymbol{R}$ and $\boldsymbol{Q}$ were estimated based on the residuals of the two fitted models. Note that estimation of the covariance matrices of the error processes is particularly simple here, since, at the model identification step, we have the direct access to both state vector and the actual EMG measurements, thanks to the experimental setup described in Linderman et al. (2009). **Figure 2** shows the data flow diagram in the model identification and coordinate reconstruction modes.

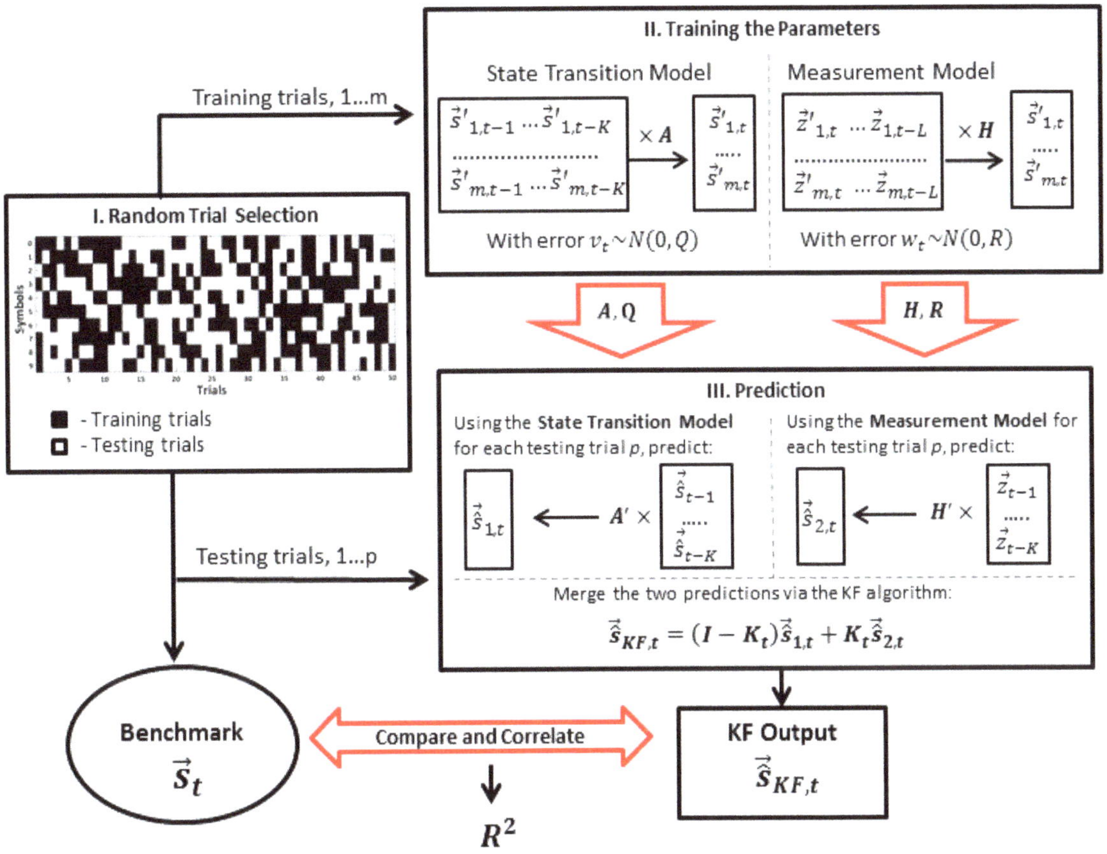

FIGURE 2 | Implementation of the Kalman Filter algorithm. For each participant of the experiment, the trials are randomly divided into training trials (black) and testing trials (white). Then, the training trials are used for learning of the parameters of the state transition model (matrices A and Q) and the measurement model (matrices H and R). The EMG data from the testing trials and the learned matrices are then used for the prediction of the state vector in both models. Finally, the predictions of the two models are merged via the Kalman filter algorithm and the result of the filter is compared to the actual state vector. The squared correlation coefficient (R^2) is used as a measure of efficiency of reconstruction.

We used two basic experimental designs to calibrate our pen tracking algorithm.

1. Within-Group Design
   A single set of parameters ($\boldsymbol{A}$, $\boldsymbol{H}$, $\boldsymbol{R}$, and $\boldsymbol{Q}$) was estimated using the training trials from all symbols at the same time and then tested on the remaining test trials.
2. Between-Group Design
   A separate set of parameters ($\boldsymbol{A}^n$, $\boldsymbol{H}^n$, $\boldsymbol{R}^n$ and $\boldsymbol{Q}^n$, $n \in 0, ..9$) was estimated for each symbol and then tested within the data from the trials of the same symbol.

Note that for Within-Group Design, only one set of matrices was estimated by pooling all the training samples together, while in Between-Group Design the four matrices were estimated separately for each of the ten symbols. Then, the out-of-training sample measurements were used to reconstruct handwriting via the recursive process outlined in Section 2.1.5.

The testing procedure was the same within each experimental design (see **Figure 2**). For each trial, the starting pen location point was set to zero vector. Then, the estimate of the pen position was computed recursively (Section 2.1.5). Reconstruction accuracy was measured by the squared correlation coefficient $\boldsymbol{R}^2$ between the actual coordinate and its fused estimate (**Figure 2**). This criterion corresponds to the percentage of energy in the actual pen traces (Total Sum of Squares - $\boldsymbol{SS}_t$) explained by the reconstructed ones (Explained Sum of Squares $\boldsymbol{SS}_e$), i.e.,

$$R^2 = \frac{SS_e}{SS_t} = \frac{\sum_{i=1}^{N} (\hat{s}_i - \bar{s})^2}{\sum_{i=1}^{N} (s_i - \bar{s})^2} \tag{16}$$

The accuracy was computed within each trial, and then averaged across trials for each symbol. Confidence intervals were computed to account for the standard errors associated with the variation across the participants.

2.2.4. Comparison with Other Models

We compared the accuracy of our model to the accuracy of the Wiener Filter (WF) estimate, which was originally tested on the same data-set by Linderman et al. (2009). The Wiener Filter approach is directly equivalent to predicting the pen coordinates, using only the measurement equation of the KF-framework alone (Equation 2). In other words, the Kalman filter is the Wiener filter, accompanied by information about the system's physical properties. Therefore, a comparison between the two models would not only show the possible improvement associated with the Kalman Filter, but also highlight the isolated benefit furnished by employing the dynamical properties of the system.

In the framework of handwriting recognition from electromyography reported in Linderman et al. (2009), the pen trace at time t was represented as a linear combination of EMG signals recorded in the non-causal interval of t: $[t - \delta_1, t + \delta_2]$. The unknown weights, mapping rectified EMG signals into the pen-tip coordinate vector, were estimated using the Ordinary Least Squares Method. It is important to stress that, in contrast to the approach reported in Linderman et al. (2009), our reconstruction procedures (both Kalman Filter and Wiener Filter based) operate causally and use only the samples from the immediate past. For each time moment t, only the samples from the $[t - \delta_1, t]$ interval were used. It is, therefore, interesting and instructive to test, whether or not the use of the dynamical model compensates for the reduced amount of information in the external measurements. In the situation when both methods use the same amount of exogenously registered data, the Kalman Filter is expected to outperform the Wiener Filter. To test the hypothesis, we performed the coordinate reconstruction with the two filters, fixing all other external parameters related to the data preprocessing step and compared their performance on the testing set of trials.

3. RESULTS

3.1. Finding Optimal Model Order

The dynamical model (Equation 1) and the measurement model (Equation 2) contain model order parameters K and L, corresponding to the number of past samples used. In order to find the optimal values of these parameters, we applied the cross-validation procedure. We used $\boldsymbol{R}^2$ as a metric of the goodness of reconstruction achieved (**Figure 3**).

To search for the combination of K and L that delivers the highest performance, we looked for the values of these parameters that maximize the $g = E(\boldsymbol{R}^2)/std(\boldsymbol{R}^2)$ ratio. The expected value $E(\boldsymbol{R}^2)$ and the standard deviation $std(\boldsymbol{R}^2)$ were computed over the trials in the data-set used for cross-validation. Therefore, high values of g correspond to the combination of high accuracy and stability of the reconstruction quality. **Figure 4** shows the average over all subjects value of g and $\boldsymbol{R}^2$.

Based on these maps, we set $K = 1$ and $L = 2$ to obtain the results reported in this paper. Note that the number of optimal measurement lags was reduced from 20 to 2, comparing to the original paper by Linderman et al. (2009), which significantly reduces computational complexity of the problem and reduces the response time of the system and potentially allows to track brisker movements.

3.2. Within-Group Design

We first trained one set of parameters for all symbols and used it to reconstruct pen traces from the EMG data in the testing set. **Figure 5** shows the result of reconstruction of several trials of each character for one of the participants. Despite being noisy

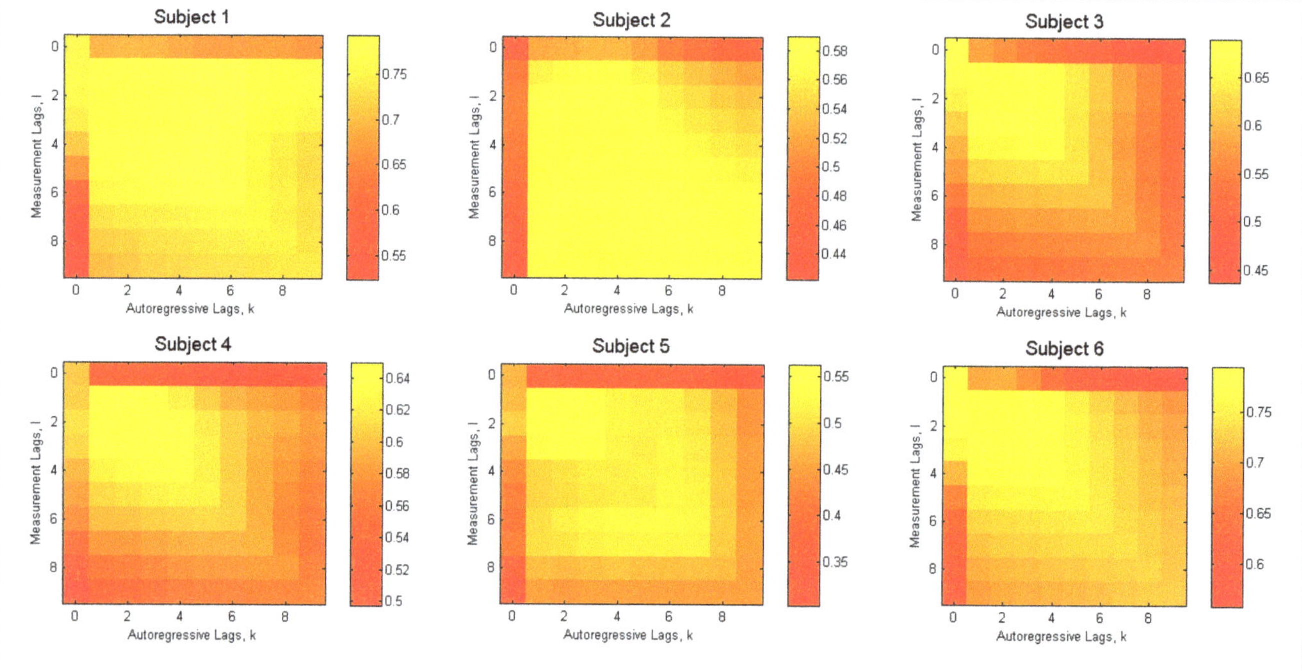

FIGURE 3 | Reconstruction accuracy as a function of model order parameters (*K* and *L*) for 6 subjects separately.

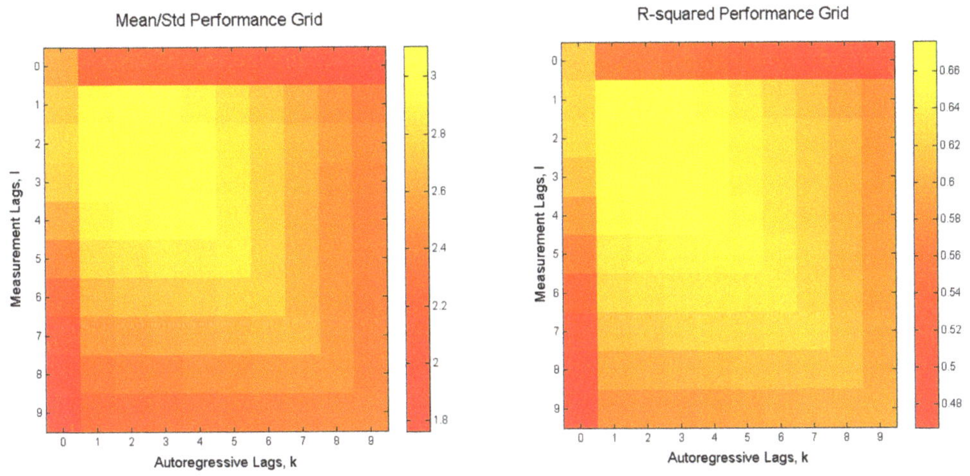

FIGURE 4 | Average reconstruction accuracy as a function of model order parameters (K and L). Left: average over all 6 subjects value of g. **Right:** Average over all 6 subjects value of R^2 for the mean reconstruction accuracy in the two coordinates $(X + Y)//2$.

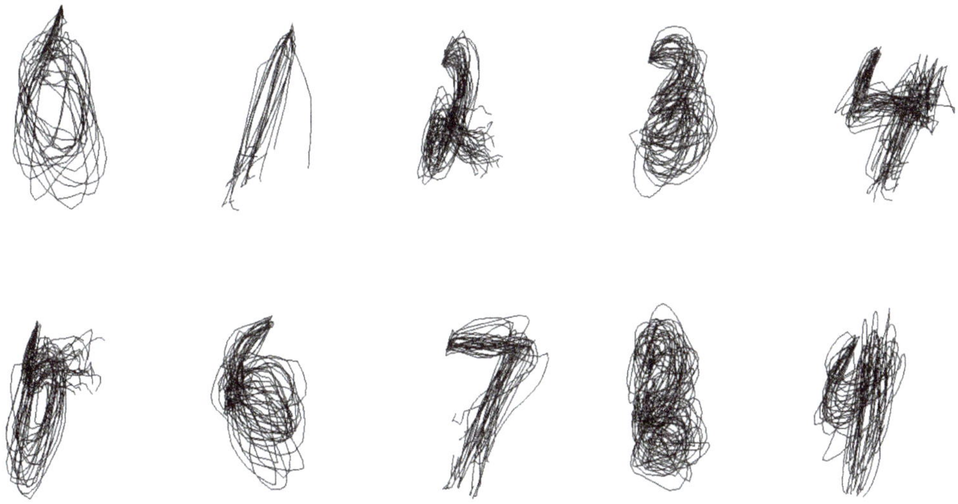

FIGURE 5 | Within-Group Reconstruction: several reconstructed trials of each symbol from cross-validation sample of one of the participants.

and, at times, inaccurate, the symbols are still identifiable and reproducible between trials.

Table 1 gives a detailed accuracy distribution for all symbols. Each of the entries in the table were found as follows: we computed accuracy of reconstruction for each test trial available for each symbol, then calculated the statistics within trial of the same symbol to determine the reported mean and standard deviation. Finally, we computed 95% confidence intervals for the average accuracy of every symbol reconstruction, based on the sample of 6 participants. We report reconstruction accuracy by coordinates independently, and as an average between the two coordinates.

Statistically speaking, we managed to achieve the average accuracy of 63 ± 17% and 73 ± 14% with 95% confidence, for the two reconstructed coordinates, as estimated for the six participants of the experiment. Note that the average accuracy in both coordinates is higher than that found by Linderman et al. (2009) (47 ± 2% and 63 ± 15% for the two coordinates, respectively), where non-causal Wiener Filter based reconstruction was employed. Additional improvement over that pioneering work lies in the use of the smaller number of measurement lags (L) (2 instead of 20, see Section 3.1) which reduces the response time of the system. These observations demonstrate the benefits brought in by the use of the dynamical properties of the process being identified.

3.3. Between-Group Design

In the Between-group design, we attempted to learn the parameters of the Kalman Filter for each symbol separately, and then reconstruct the traces of the same symbol. **Figure 6** shows the results of reconstruction of several trials of each symbol for one of the participants. As predicted, the separate Kalman Filters for each symbol perform a more specific and accurate reconstruction, which is visually evident from the figure.

The average reconstruction in the two coordinates between subjects was 78 ± 13% and 88 ± 7%, respectively. **Table 2** reports 95% confidence intervals for the average reconstruction accuracy of each symbol with separate Kalman Filters.

3.4. Comparison with the Wiener Filter

In the previous subsection we have shown that, as expected, the Kalman Filter improves the reconstruction performance, as compared to the previously proposed method (Linderman et al., 2009). The parameter search (Section 3.1) shows that adding non-zero autoregressive lag(s) to the model, and as a result, capturing the dynamical properties of the system, leads to the increase in accuracy of reconstruction for all subjects (**Figures 3, 4**).

To consider the increase in accuracy, specifically associated with the dynamical model, we reconstructed pen traces of several symbols by Within-group design (one set of parameters for all symbols), and then repeated the procedure on the same samples using the Wiener Filter, fixing all other external parameters, including those related to the training-testing split of the data and data preprocessing techniques.

On average, introduction of the KF framework leads to a significant increase in accuracy for both reconstructed coordinates across the six participants (**Figure 7**). The increase is more or less homogeneous between different symbols. **Figure 8** shows the distribution of the difference between the Kalman Filter accuracy and the Wiener Filter accuracy for separate symbols. For all symbols, the difference is significantly greater

TABLE 1 | Within-Group Reconstruction Performance: 95% confidence intervals for the average reconstruction accuracy of each symbol between the 6 participants.

	Average performance, R^2		
Symbol	**X-coordinate**	**Y-coordinate**	**Average: (X+Y)/2**
"0"	0.65 ± 0.15	0.57 ± 0.17	0.61 ± 0.15
"1"	0.49 ± 0.08	0.85 ± 0.08	0.67 ± 0.05
"2"	0.71 ± 0.14	0.75 ± 0.12	0.73 ± 0.13
"3"	0.59 ± 0.20	0.79 ± 0.09	0.69 ± 0.13
"4"	0.71 ± 0.15	0.63 ± 0.17	0.67 ± 0.13
"5"	0.67 ± 0.15	0.72 ± 0.05	0.70 ± 0.08
"6"	0.68 ± 0.18	0.71 ± 0.11	0.70 ± 0.12
"7"	0.59 ± 0.28	0.69 ± 0.22	0.63 ± 0.25
"8"	0.61 ± 0.15	0.74 ± 0.12	0.77 ± 0.11
"9"	0.62 ± 0.22	0.71 ± 0.15	0.67 ± 0.17
All	0.63 ± 0.17	0.73 ± 0.14	0.68 ± 0.13

TABLE 2 | Between-Group Reconstruction Performance: 95% confidence intervals for the average reconstruction accuracy of each symbol between the 6 participants.

	Average performance, R^2		
Symbol	**X-coordinate**	**Y-coordinate**	**Average: (X+Y)/2**
"0"	0.84 ± 0.06	0.86 ± 0.05	0.85 ± 0.05
"1"	0.63 ± 0.15	0.97 ± 0.01	0.80 ± 0.08
"2"	0.82 ± 0.11	0.92 ± 0.06	0.87 ± 0.09
"3"	0.75 ± 0.12	0.93 ± 0.06	0.84 ± 0.08
"4"	0.81 ± 0.11	0.81 ± 0.03	0.81 ± 0.05
"5"	0.80 ± 0.10	0.86 ± 0.06	0.83 ± 0.07
"6"	0.83 ± 0.05	0.88 ± 0.05	0.85 ± 0.05
"7"	0.76 ± 0.20	0.88 ± 0.08	0.82 ± 0.14
"8"	0.76 ± 0.12	0.86 ± 0.07	0.81 ± 0.09
"9"	0.81 ± 0.09	0.84 ± 0.08	0.83 ± 0.08
All	0.78 ± 0.13	0.88 ± 0.07	0.83 ± 0.08

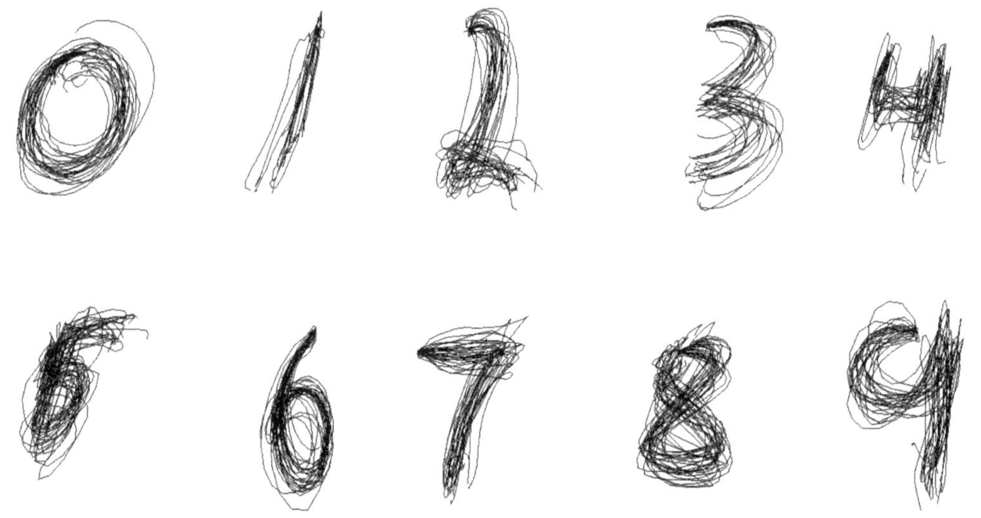

FIGURE 6 | Between-Group Reconstruction: several reconstructed trials of each symbol from cross-validation sample of one of the participants.

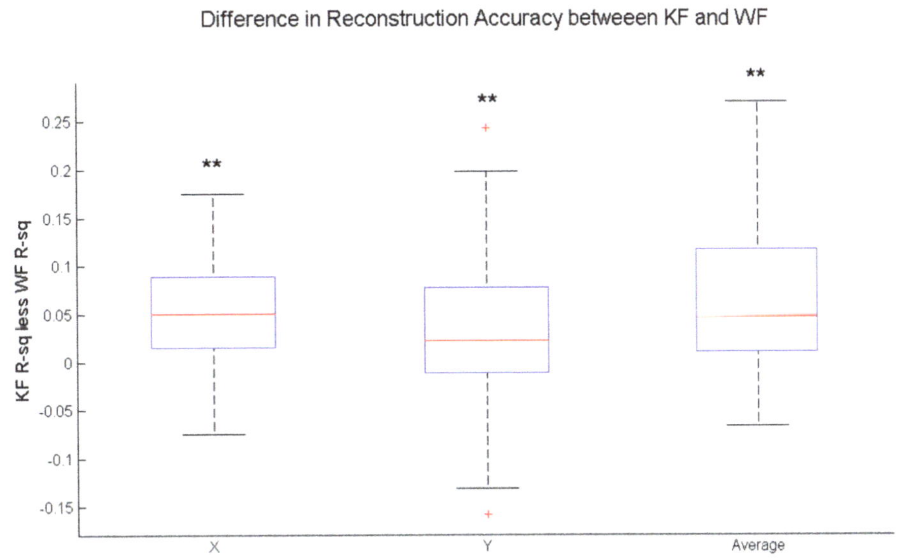

FIGURE 7 | Distribution of the difference in the average performance of the Kalman Filter (KF) and the average performance of the Wiener Filter (WF) for all written characters across subjects. Statistical Difference between the average KF and the average WF performance is measured by one-sided Wilcoxon matched-pair test for X-coordinate, Y-coordinate and the average of the two, i.e., (X+Y)/2: **significantly greater than zero at 1% significance level.

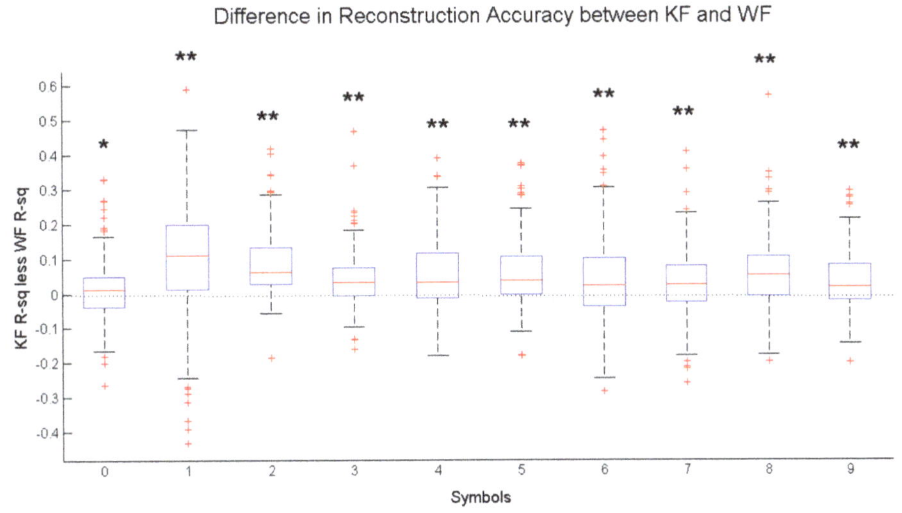

FIGURE 8 | Distribution of the difference between the Kalman Filter Accuracy (KF R^2) and the Wiener Filter Accuracy (WF R^2) between subjects, measured for each written character independently. Statistical Difference between the KF and the WF performance is measured by one-sided Wilcoxon matched-pair test for each character: *significantly greater than zero at 5% significance level, **significantly greater than zero at 1% significance level.

than zero with at least 95% confidence, guaranteed by the one-sided Wilcoxon test for matched pairs.

The ergonomics of the reconstructed handwriting traces plays an important role. The use of the dynamical model to enforce natural smoothness of handwriting yielded improved ergonomics of the recovered traces. **Figure 9** allow to visually compare the reconstruction of the pen traces for each symbol obtained with the two methods (left—the Kalman Filter reconstruction, right—the Wiener Filter reconstruction). As we can see from the figures, the use of the Kalman filter furnishes a smoother coordinate reconstruction than that based exclusively on the measurements. While both filters make it possible to visually discriminate between different symbols, the smoothness of the traces, obtained with the Kalman filter, makes them more natural and ergonomically plausible.

4. DISCUSSION

In this work we applied the Kalman Filter approach to reconstruction of handwritten pen traces on the basis of EMG

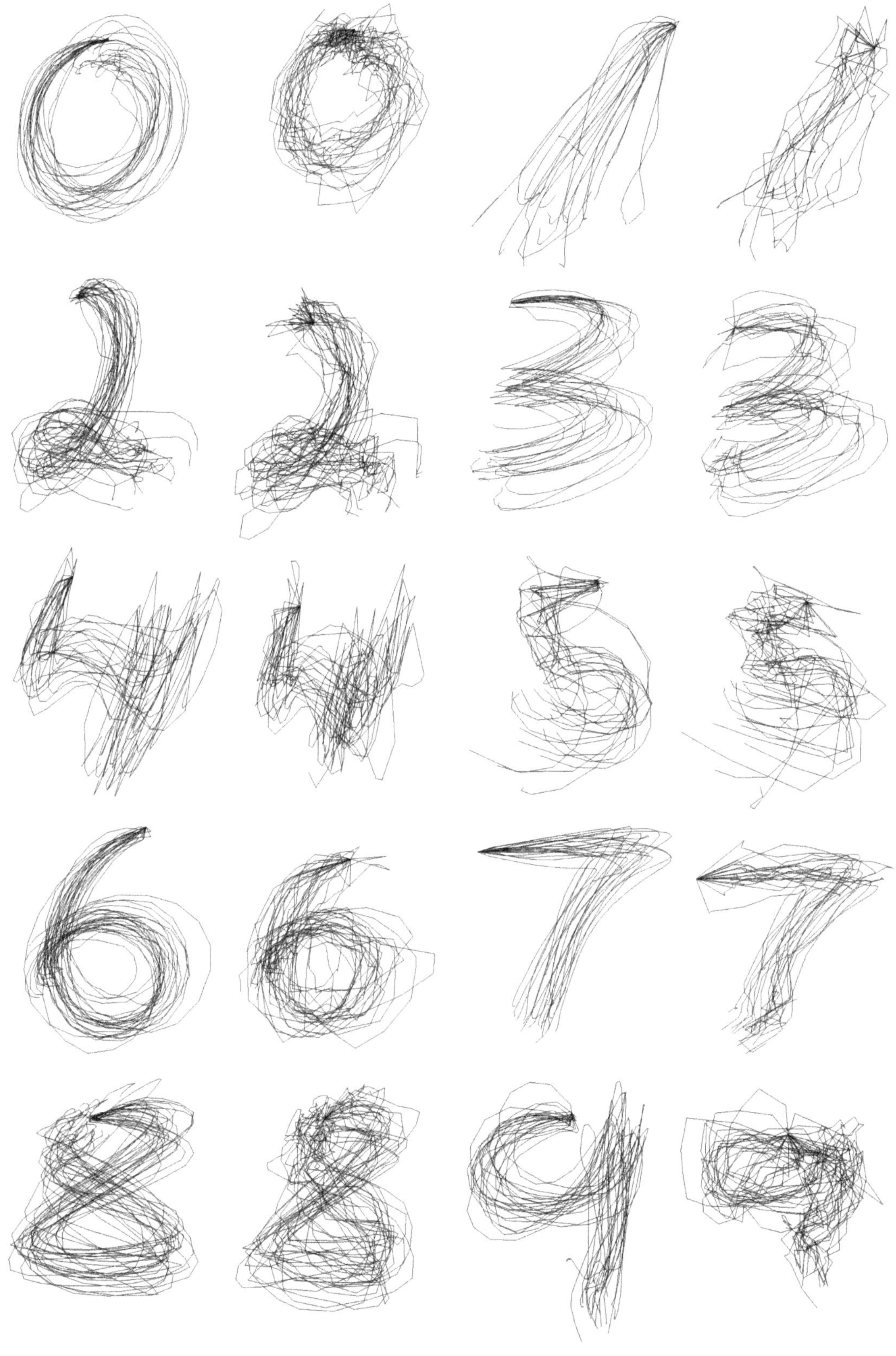

FIGURE 9 | Pen trace reconstruction of digits zero to nine with the Kalman Filter (left) and the Wiener Filter (right), Within-Group Method for several cross-validation trials of one of the participants.

measurements. We have demonstrated that it is possible to obtain accurate and ergonomic reconstruction of pen traces and still remain in the linear framework to utilize all the benefits associated with it. Our results show a significant improvement over the figures, previously reported by Linderman et al. (2009). In contrast to that pioneering work, we used only causal filtering and exploited fewer past samples of the EMG signals.

Although the accuracy of reconstruction does not generally go above 90%, in terms of the coefficient of determination, the method still offers a reliable and ergonomic reconstruction for all symbols. Approximately 25 trials of each symbol were enough to learn the parameters of the filter and yield comparable results in testing samples.

The method works well for both specific (Between-Group design) and general (Within-Group design) models, which reveals its potential for a wide range of applications. The Between-group design, although quite limited at first sight, is not entirely unrealistic, due to the fact that handwritten figures are very well discriminated between each other on the basis of EMG signals (Linderman et al., 2009; Huang et al., 2010). It means that separate Kalman filters can be applied as a second-stage algorithm in the off-line experiments, after another algorithm (such as the Hidden Markov Model of Linear Discriminant Analysis) is used to classify the symbols into groups.

The Within-group design, on the other hand, is more applicable to on-line handwriting reconstruction, when no prior information about the class of the symbol being written is available. In this framework the causality of our approach offers additional benefits and makes the EMG-controlled handwriting feel natural to the user. Also, the natural smoothness of the traces, recovered with the use of the KF, provides for an improved feedback, which is crucial in the real-life on-line scenario.

While our method has shown improvement over the previously proposed technique, it still requires thorough consideration before it can be reliably applied in neuroprosthetic devices and rehabilitation practices. One of the main difficulties in applying the Linear Kalman filter is the high variability of results across subjects. The confidence intervals in **Tables 1**, **2** clearly show very high margins of error, which indicate that handwriting is very person-specific.

Such heterogeneous performance across individuals apparently stems from a combination of behavioral and physiological factors, which we could not control in this study. Participants vary in the style and neatness of handwriting, including the way they hold and press the pen, and the strategies they apply to write the same symbol. Anatomical differences, such as the individual muscle length, muscle size and attachment to the bones and the differences in the amount of subcutaneous fat might be significant factors influencing the patterns of the recorded neuromuscular activity (EMGs). Additional source of variability may come from the variation in electrode placement sites.

The problem of EMG variability has received significant attention in the recent experimental literature (Linssen et al., 1993; Araújo et al., 2000; Nordander et al., 2003). Fundamentally, one and the same movement can be reproduced by different force patterns in multiple agonist and antagonist muscles. This phenomenon, called *motor redundancy* (Bernstein, 1967; Guigon et al., 2008) allows a certain kinematic pattern to be reproduced by virtually infinite number of distinct muscular activation patterns (Amis et al., 1979). The EMG recordings which we used captured relatively consistent EMG patterns in individual subjects, which were, however, different from subject to subject. The approach proposed in this paper appears to have sufficient generalization power to capture the within subject variability (both natural and the one that stems from instructed variations of symbol writings to be produced). However, initial training of the algorithm is required for each individual subject independently.

Additionally, the results can be further improved by individually tuning the latent parameters, such as the model orders, filter cut-off frequency and sensor locations. In this work, however, we intentionally used a single set of latent variable values in order to emulate the out-of-box performance of such a system. Methods for non-supervised on-line adaptation and individual tuning of the latent variables need to be developed to address these issues and make the fine-tuning seamless to the user.

The linear framework of the filter offers significant benefits, such as stability and good generalization ability. However, the non-linear nature of the relation between the recorded EMG signals and the actuator trajectory prompts to explore the use of non-linear models in this application. The benefits brought in by the non-linearity, however, have to be leveraged against the additional complexity and potential instability associated with the use of such models.

5. CONCLUSIONS

In this paper we investigated the relationship between handwriting and neuromuscular activity measured by electromyography. We built and optimized the Kalman filter in order to reconstruct the pen coordinates based on the dynamical characteristics of handwriting and the corresponding EMG measurements.

We showed that the Kalman filter significantly outperforms previously proposed method (Linderman et al., 2009) and yields a mean accuracy of 68% in Within-Group design and 83% in Between-Group design, measured by the coefficient of determination, averaged for the two reconstructed coordinates. Our method is suitable for real-time applications as it is causal and utilizes only the EMGs from the past. The dynamical nature of the Kalman filter provides for the time-varying optimal fusion of the information and allows to take into account not only the EMG activity, but also the physical properties of handwriting.

The main attraction of the proposed method is its ability to smooth the noise and, as a result, provide a comprehensible and realistic reconstruction. Further progress in this field would potentially create intelligent rehabilitation techniques for patients with hand injuries, as well as become useful in human-computer interfaces, associated with handwriting.

ACKNOWLEDGMENTS

The authors are grateful for the fruitful comments of Dr. Igor Furtat related to the algorithmic portion of the work. The experimental portion (Section 3) was funded by the government subsidy for improving competitiveness of National Research University Higher School of Economics among the leading world centers for research and education. The data fusion algorithm for reconstruction of pen traces (Section 2) was adapted to the use with the EMG data solely under support of RNF (grant 14-29-00142) in IPME RAS.

REFERENCES

Ahsan, M. R., Ibrahimy, M. I., and Khalifa, O. O. (2009). Emg signal classification for human computer interaction: a review. *Eur. J. Sci. Res.* 33, 480–501.

Amis, A., Dowson, D., and Wright, V. (1979). Muscle strengths and musculoskeletal geometry of the upper limb. *Eng. Med.* 8, 41–48. doi: 10.1243/EMED/JOUR/1979/008/010/02

Araújo, R. C., Duarte, M., and Amadio, A. C. (2000). On the inter-and intra-subject variability of the electromyographic signal in isometric contractions. *Electromyogr. Clin. Neurophysiol.* 40, 225–230.

Arulampalam, M. S., Maskell, S., Gordon, N., and Clapp, T. (2002). A tutorial on particle filters for online nonlinear/non-gaussian bayesian tracking. *Signal Process. IEEE Trans.* 50, 174–188. doi: 10.1109/78.978374

Bernstein, N. (1967). *The Coordination and Regulation of Movements.* Oxford: Pergamon Press.

Bu, N., Okamoto, M., and Tsuji, T. (2009). A hybrid motion classification approach for EMG-based human-robot interfaces using bayesian and neural networks. *Robot. IEEE Trans.* 25, 502–511. doi: 10.1109/TRO.2009.2019782

Carter, J. L., and Russell, H. L. (1985). Use of EMG biofeedback procedures with learning disabled children in a clinical and an educational setting. *J. Learn. Disabil.* 18, 213–216. doi: 10.1177/002221948501800406

Castellini, C., and van der Smagt, P. (2009). Surface EMG in advanced hand prosthetics. *Biol. Cybern.* 100, 35–47. doi: 10.1007/s00422-008-0278-1

Chan, F. H., Yang, Y.-S., Lam, F. K., Zhang, Y.-T., and Parker, P. A. (2000). Fuzzy emg classification for prosthesis control. *Rehabil. Eng. IEEE Trans.* 8, 305–311. doi: 10.1109/86.867872

Faragher, R. (2012). Understanding the basis of the kalman filter via a simple and intuitive derivation. *IEEE Signal Process. Mag.* 29, 128–132. doi: 10.1109/MSP.2012.2203621

Guigon, E., Baraduc, P., and Desmurget, M. (2006). Computational motor control: redundancy and invariance. *J. Neurophysiol.* 97, 331–347. doi: 10.1152/jn.00290.2006

Guigon, E., Baraduc, P., and Desmurget, M. (2008). Optimality, stochasticity, and variability in motor behavior. *J. Comput. Neurosci.* 24, 57–68. doi: 10.1007/s10827-007-0041-y

Henderson, H. V., and Searle, S. R. (1981). On deriving the inverse of a sum of matrices. *Siam Rev.* 23, 53–60. doi: 10.1137/1023004

Huang, G., Zhang, D., Zheng, X., and Zhu, X. (2010). "An EMG-based handwriting recognition through dynamic time warping," in *Engineering in Medicine and Biology Society (EMBC), 2010 Annual International Conference of the IEEE* (Shanghai: IEEE), 4902–4905.

Jazwinski, A. H. (2007). *Stochastic Processes and Filtering Theory.* Mineola, NY: Courier Corporation.

Julier, S. J., and Uhlmann, J. K. (1997). "New extension of the kalman filter to nonlinear systems," in *AeroSense'97*, ed I. Kadar (Orlando, FL: International Society for Optics and Photonics), 182–193.

Kalman, R. E. (1960). A new approach to linear filtering and prediction problems. *J. Fluids Eng.* 82, 35–45. doi: 10.1115/1.3662552

Li, C., Ma, Z., Yao, L., and Zhang, D. (2013). "Improvements on emg-based handwriting recognition with dtw algorithm," in *Engineering in Medicine and Biology Society (EMBC), 2013 35th Annual International Conference of the IEEE* (IEEE), 2144–2147.

Linderman, M., Lebedev, M. A., and Erlichman, J. S. (2009). Recognition of handwriting from electromyography. *PLoS ONE* 4:e6791. doi: 10.1371/journal.pone.0006791

Linssen, W. H., Stegeman, D. F., Joosten, E. M., Binkhorst, R. A., van't Hof, M. A., and Notermans, S. L. (1993). Variability and interrelationships of surface emg parameters during local muscle fatigue. *Muscle Nerve* 16, 849–856. doi: 10.1002/mus.880160808

McKeague, I. W. (2005). A statistical model for signature verification. *J. Am. Stat. Assoc.* 100, 231–241. doi: 10.1198/016214504000000827

Nordander, C., Willner, J., Hansson, G.-Å., Larsson, B., Unge, J., Granquist, L., et al. (2003). Influence of the subcutaneous fat layer, as measured by ultrasound, skinfold calipers and bmi, on the emg amplitude. *Eur. J. Appl. Physiol.* 89, 514–519. doi: 10.1007/s00421-003-0819-1

Ohnishi, K., Weir, R. F., and Kuiken, T. A. (2007). Neural machine interfaces for controlling multifunctional powered upper-limb prostheses. *Expert Rev. Med. Devices* 4, 43–53. doi: 10.1586/17434440.4.1.43

Plamondon, R., and Maarse, F. J. (1989). An evaluation of motor models of handwriting. *Syst. Man Cybern. IEEE Trans.* 19, 1060–1072. doi: 10.1109/21.44021

Reaz, M., Hussain, M., and Mohd-Yasin, F. (2006). Techniques of EMG signal analysis: detection, processing, classification and applications. *Biol. Proced. Online* 8, 11–35. doi: 10.1251/bpo115

Rencher, A. C. (2003). *Methods of Multivariate Analysis*, Vol. 492. John Wiley & Sons. Available online at: https://books.google.ru/books?hl=ru&lr=&id=SpvBd7IUCxkC&oi=fnd&pg=PR5&dq=methods+of+multivariate+analysis&ots=ItWFsHM9w3&sig=K7-D_CG8CgdDkrVrYX0wFYmBY-8&redir_esc=y#v=onepage&q=methods%20of%20multivariate%20analysis&f=false

Shenoy, P., Miller, K. J., Crawford, B., and Rao, R. P. N. (2008). Online electromyographic control of a robotic prosthesis. *Biomed. Eng. IEEE Trans.* 55, 1128–1135. doi: 10.1109/TBME.2007.909536

Shimkin, N. (2009). Derivations of the discrete-time kalman filter. *Estim. Ident. Dyn. Syst.*

Silveri, M. C., Corda, F., and Di Nardo, M. (2007). Central and peripheral aspects of writing disorders in alzheimer's disease. *J. Clin. Exp. Neuropsychol.* 29, 179–186. doi: 10.1080/13803390600611351

Stanford, V. (2004). Biosignals offer potential for direct interfaces and health monitoring. *Pervas. Comput. IEEE* 3, 99–103. doi: 10.1109/MPRV.2004.1269140

Van Gemmert, A., Teulings, H.-L., Contreras-Vidal, J., and Stelmach, G. (1999). Parkinsons disease and the control of size and speed in handwriting. *Neuropsychologia* 37, 685–694. doi: 10.1016/S0028-3932(98)00122-5

Wan, E., and Van Der Merwe, R. (2000). "The unscented kalman filter for nonlinear estimation," in *Adaptive Systems for Signal Processing, Communications, and Control Symposium 2000. AS-SPCC. The IEEE 2000* (Beaverton, OR: IEEE), 153–158.

Xiao, Z. G., and Menon, C. (2014). Towards the development of a wearable feedback system for monitoring the activities of the upper-extremities. *J. Neuroeng. Rehabil.* 11, 1–13. doi: 10.1186/1743-0003-11-2

APPENDIX

Parameters of the State Transition Model

Equation (A3) shows the distribution of the estimate of the State Transition Model given by Equation (1).

The mean of the distribution is

$$\boldsymbol{\mu}_{1t} = E[\boldsymbol{s}_t] = \boldsymbol{A}\hat{\boldsymbol{s}}_{t-1} = \boldsymbol{A}\boldsymbol{\mu}_{1(t-1)}. \tag{A1}$$

The covariance matrix is derived the following way:

$$\begin{aligned}
\boldsymbol{\Sigma}_{1t} &= E[(\boldsymbol{s}_t - \boldsymbol{\mu}_{1t})(\boldsymbol{s}_t - \boldsymbol{\mu}_{1t})^T] = \\
&= E[(\boldsymbol{A}\boldsymbol{s}_{t-1} + \boldsymbol{v}_t - \boldsymbol{A}\hat{\boldsymbol{s}}_{t-1})(\boldsymbol{A}\boldsymbol{s}_{t-1} + \boldsymbol{v}_t - \boldsymbol{A}\hat{\boldsymbol{s}}_{t-1})^T] = \\
&= E[(\boldsymbol{A}(\boldsymbol{s}_{t-1} - \hat{\boldsymbol{s}}_{t-1}) + \boldsymbol{v}_t)(\boldsymbol{A}(\boldsymbol{s}_{t-1} - \hat{\boldsymbol{s}}_{t-1}) + \boldsymbol{v}_t)^T] = \\
&= E[(\boldsymbol{A}(\boldsymbol{s}_{t-1} - \hat{\boldsymbol{s}}_{t-1}) + \boldsymbol{v}_t)((\boldsymbol{s}_{t-1} - \hat{\boldsymbol{s}}_{t-1})^T\boldsymbol{A}^T + \boldsymbol{v}_t^T)] = \\
&= \boldsymbol{A}E[(\boldsymbol{s}_{t-1} - \hat{\boldsymbol{s}}_{t-1})(\boldsymbol{s}_{t-1} - \hat{\boldsymbol{s}}_{t-1})^T]\boldsymbol{A}^T + \boldsymbol{A}E[(\boldsymbol{s}_{t-1} - \hat{\boldsymbol{s}}_{t-1})\boldsymbol{v}_t^T] \\
&\quad + E[\boldsymbol{v}_t(\boldsymbol{s}_{t-1} - \hat{\boldsymbol{s}}_{t-1})^T]\boldsymbol{A}^T + E[\boldsymbol{v}_t\boldsymbol{v}_t^T].
\end{aligned}$$

Since the state estimate noise $\boldsymbol{v}_t$ is uncorrelated with the estimate,

$$E[\boldsymbol{v}_t(\boldsymbol{s}_{t-1} - \hat{\boldsymbol{s}}_{t-1})^T] = E[(\boldsymbol{s}_{t-1} - \hat{\boldsymbol{s}}_{t-1})\boldsymbol{v}_t^T] = 0$$

and the covariance matrix reduces to:

$$\begin{aligned}
\boldsymbol{\Sigma}_{1t} &= \boldsymbol{A}E[(\boldsymbol{s}_{t-1} - \hat{\boldsymbol{s}}_{t-1})(\boldsymbol{s}_{t-1} - \hat{\boldsymbol{s}}_{t-1})^T]\boldsymbol{A}^T + E[\boldsymbol{v}_t\boldsymbol{v}_t^T] = \\
&= A\boldsymbol{\Sigma}_{1(t-1)}\boldsymbol{A}^T + \boldsymbol{Q}.
\end{aligned} \tag{A2}$$

The Fusion

Under the normality assumption the probability density function (pdf) of the state space vector $\boldsymbol{s}_t$ can be written as

$$f_1(\boldsymbol{s}_t|\boldsymbol{s}_{t-1}) = (2\pi)^{-3K}|\boldsymbol{\Sigma}_{1t}|^{-1/2}\exp\left(-\frac{1}{2}(\boldsymbol{s}_t - \boldsymbol{\mu}_{1t})^T \boldsymbol{\Sigma}_{1t}^{-1}(\boldsymbol{s}_t - \boldsymbol{\mu}_{1t})\right) \tag{A3}$$

Since the additive noise term $\boldsymbol{w}_t$ in Equation (2) is assumed to be Gaussian, while each of the observed EMG signals are not modeled as stochastic processes, the state vector follows the Gaussian distribution

$$f_2(\boldsymbol{s}_t|\boldsymbol{z}_t) = (2\pi)^{-4L}|\boldsymbol{\Sigma}_{2t}|^{-1/2}\exp\left(-\frac{1}{2}(\boldsymbol{s}_t - \boldsymbol{\mu}_{2t})^T\boldsymbol{\Sigma}_{2t}^{-1}(\boldsymbol{s}_t - \boldsymbol{\mu}_{2t})\right). \tag{A4}$$

By multiplying pdf in Equation (A3) by pdf in Equation (A4) we get a scaled fused Distribution of the state estimate:

$$\begin{aligned}
&f_{fused}(\boldsymbol{s}_t|\boldsymbol{s}_{t-1}, \boldsymbol{z}_t) = f_1(\boldsymbol{s}_t|\boldsymbol{s}_{t-1})f_2(\boldsymbol{s}_t|\boldsymbol{z}_t) = \\
&\mathcal{N}(\boldsymbol{\mu}_{1t}, \boldsymbol{\Sigma}_{1t}) \cdot \mathcal{N}(\boldsymbol{\mu}_{2t}, \boldsymbol{\Sigma}_{2t}) = c\mathcal{N}(\boldsymbol{\mu}_{fused}, \boldsymbol{\Sigma}_{fused}),
\end{aligned} \tag{A5}$$

with parameters

$$\boldsymbol{\Sigma}_{Fused} = (\boldsymbol{\Sigma}_{1t}^{-1} + \boldsymbol{\Sigma}_{2t}^{-1})^{-1} \tag{A6}$$

$$\boldsymbol{\mu}_{Fused} = \boldsymbol{\Sigma}_{Fused}(\boldsymbol{\Sigma}_{1t}^{-1}\boldsymbol{\mu}_{1t} + \boldsymbol{\Sigma}_{2t}^{-1}\boldsymbol{\mu}_{2t}) \tag{A7}$$

and a normalization constant

$$\begin{aligned}
c = \frac{1}{(2\pi)^{k/2}}\frac{|\boldsymbol{\Sigma}_{Fused}|^{1/2}}{|\boldsymbol{\Sigma}_{1t}|^{1/2}|\boldsymbol{\Sigma}_{2t}|^{1/2}}\exp\Bigg(-\frac{1}{2}\Big(&\boldsymbol{\mu}_{1t}^T\boldsymbol{\Sigma}_{1t}^{-1}\boldsymbol{\mu}_{1t} \\
&+ \boldsymbol{\mu}_{2t}^T\boldsymbol{\Sigma}_{2t}^{-1}\boldsymbol{\mu}_{2t} + \boldsymbol{\mu}_{Fused}^T\boldsymbol{\Sigma}_{Fused}^{-1}\boldsymbol{\mu}_{Fused}\Big)\Bigg)
\end{aligned} \tag{A8}$$

Let us reformulate the expressions for the mean and Covariance matrix of the new distribution in such a way that they separate the influence of the two fused distributions.

Using the Matrix Inversion lemma (the Woodbury matrix identity) for two matrices of the same dimension ($\boldsymbol{\Sigma}_{1t}$ and $\boldsymbol{\Sigma}_{2t}$) and setting $\boldsymbol{K}_t = \boldsymbol{\Sigma}_{1t}(\boldsymbol{\Sigma}_{1t} + \boldsymbol{\Sigma}_{2t})^{-1}$ the parameters of the fused Gaussian can be neatly rewritten in the form of Equations (8) and (9), i.e.,

$$\boldsymbol{\Sigma}_{Fused} = \boldsymbol{\Sigma}_{1t} - \boldsymbol{\Sigma}_{1t}(\boldsymbol{\Sigma}_{1t} + \boldsymbol{\Sigma}_{2t})^{-1}\boldsymbol{\Sigma}_{1t} = \boldsymbol{\Sigma}_{1t} - \boldsymbol{K}_t\boldsymbol{\Sigma}_{1t}. \tag{A9}$$

$$\begin{aligned}
\boldsymbol{\mu}_{Fused} &= (\boldsymbol{\Sigma}_{1t} - \boldsymbol{K}_t\boldsymbol{\Sigma}_{1t})(\boldsymbol{\Sigma}_{1t}^{-1}\boldsymbol{\mu}_{1t} + \boldsymbol{\Sigma}_{2t}^{-1}\boldsymbol{\mu}_{2t}) = \\
&= \boldsymbol{\mu}_{1t} + \boldsymbol{\Sigma}_{1t}\boldsymbol{\Sigma}_{2t}^{-1}\boldsymbol{\mu}_{2t} - \boldsymbol{K}_t\boldsymbol{\mu}_1 - \boldsymbol{K}_t\boldsymbol{\Sigma}_{1t}\boldsymbol{\Sigma}_{2t}\boldsymbol{\mu}_{2t} = \\
&= \boldsymbol{\mu}_{1t} + \boldsymbol{K}_t(\boldsymbol{K}_t^{-1}\boldsymbol{\Sigma}_{1t}\boldsymbol{\Sigma}_{2t}^{-1}\boldsymbol{\mu}_{2t} - \boldsymbol{\mu}_{1t} - \boldsymbol{\Sigma}_{1t}\boldsymbol{\Sigma}_{2t}^{-1}\boldsymbol{\mu}_{2t}) = \\
&= \boldsymbol{\mu}_{1t} + \boldsymbol{K}_t((\boldsymbol{\Sigma}_{1t} + \boldsymbol{\Sigma}_{2t})\boldsymbol{\Sigma}_{1t}^{-1}\boldsymbol{\Sigma}_{1t}\boldsymbol{\Sigma}_{2t}^{-1}\boldsymbol{\mu}_{2t} - \boldsymbol{\mu}_{1t} - \boldsymbol{\Sigma}_{1t}\boldsymbol{\Sigma}_{2t}^{-1}\boldsymbol{\mu}_{2t}) = \\
&= \boldsymbol{\mu}_{1t} + \boldsymbol{K}_t(\boldsymbol{\Sigma}_{1t}\boldsymbol{\Sigma}_{2t}^{-1}\boldsymbol{\mu}_{2t} + \boldsymbol{\mu}_{2t} - \boldsymbol{\mu}_{1t} - \boldsymbol{\Sigma}_{1t}\boldsymbol{\Sigma}_{2t}^{-1}\boldsymbol{\mu}_{2t}) = \\
&= \boldsymbol{\mu}_{1t} + \boldsymbol{K}_t(\boldsymbol{\mu}_{2t} - \boldsymbol{\mu}_{1t}) = (\boldsymbol{I} - \boldsymbol{K}_t)\boldsymbol{\mu}_{1t} + \boldsymbol{K}_t\boldsymbol{\mu}_{2t}.
\end{aligned} \tag{A10}$$

Testing the Assumptions of the Model

We ran the Royston test for multivariate normality on the residuals of each training sample and concluded that for most samples the assumption of normality is not violated (at 1% significance level). **Table A1** summarized the percentages of

TABLE A1 | Percentages of trials across participants, in which the assumption of multivariate normality of the error term is not violated at 1% significance level.

	Participants						
	1 (%)	2 (%)	3 (%)	4 (%)	5 (%)	6 (%)	Average (%)
State transition model	92	79	92	96	83	73	86
Measurement model	93	85	92	94	80	77	87
Joint model	89	72	89	93	76	67	81

TABLE A2 | Percentages of trials across participants, in which the test for uncorrelatedness of residuals of the two fused models was not rejected at 5% significance level.

	Participants						
	1 (%)	2 (%)	3 (%)	4 (%)	5 (%)	6 (%)	Average (%)
Independent trials	83	72	76	80	67	68	74

samples, in which the assumption of normality of the error term holds in the two reconstructed models and in the joint model.

The fusion of the two information sources described in this paper is heavily based on the assumption that the two merged sources are independent.

Then, we checked to what extent the two information sources can be considered independent. Taking into account the results of the test for multivariate normality, we checked for the absence of correlation between the error terms of the two merged models (Equations 1 and 2). We used the residuals of the two models to calculate the sample cross-correlation matrix and assessed the significance of its elements for each trial.

Given the sample size and the multiplicity of the tested hypothesis (36), we could not reject the null-hypothesis of no-correlation at 5% group level significance for the majority of trials (74%). Detailed distribution of the test performance across the participants is given in **Table A2.**

23

The elephant in the mirror: bridging the brain's explanatory gap of consciousness

Jasmine A. Berry[1]* *and Alice C. Parker*[2]

[1] *Biomimetic Real-time Cortex Project, Computer Science Department, University of Southern California, Los Angeles, CA, USA,* [2] *Biomimetic Real-time Cortex Project, Ming Hsieh Department of Electrical Engineering, University of Southern California, Los Angeles, CA, USA*

Keywords: self-recognition, self-awareness, consciousness, machine intelligence, hard problem

Edited by:
Mikhail Lebedev, Duke University, USA

Reviewed by:
Mazyar Fallah, York University, Canada
Paul Manger, University of the Witwatersrand, South Africa
Alexander Fingelkurts, BM-SCIENCE Brain & Mind Technologies Research Centre, Finland

****Correspondence:***
Jasmine A. Berry
jasminab@usc.edu

INTRODUCTION

The successes of the artificial retina and cochlea have lent encouragement to researchers in the general field of brain augmentation (Gantz et al., 2005; Dagnelie, 2012). However, in order for brain augmentation to progress beyond conventional sensory substitution to comprehensive augmentation of the human brain, we believe a better understanding of self-awareness and consciousness must be obtained, even if the "hard" problem of consciousness (Chalmers, 2007) remains elusive. Here we propose that forthcoming brain augmentation studies should insistently include investigations of its potential effects on self-awareness and consciousness. As a first step, it's imperative for comprehensive augmentation to include interfacing with the biological brain in a manner that either distinguishes self (biological brain) from other (augmentation circuitry), or incorporates both biological and electronic aspects into an integrated understanding of the meaning of self. This distinction poses not only psychological and physiological issues regarding the discrepancy of self and other, but raises ethical and philosophical issues when the brain augmentation is capable of introducing thoughts, emotions, memories and beliefs in such an integrated fashion that the wearer of such technology cannot distinguish his biological thoughts from thoughts introduced by the brain augmentation.

A consideration of self begins with the conventional mirror self-recognition test (MSR) (Gallop, 1970) that has been successfully executed with Eurasian magpies (Prior et al., 2008), bottlenose dolphins (Reiss and Marino, 2001), orca whales (Delfour and Marten, 2001), human infants typically between 18 and 24 months (Amsterdam, 1972; Rochat, 2003), and notably the Asian elephant (Plotnik et al., 2006). The only primate species reported to pass the Gallup Mirror Test, albeit controversially, were orangutans and chimpanzees (Suárez and Gallup, 1981). For years, MSR has been the designated litmus test for determining whether a species possesses self-awareness (SA), ultimately raising the question of whether the animal is then a conscious entity as a result of passing this test (De Veer and van den Bos, 1999). "Mirror self-recognition is an indicator of self-awareness," proclaims Gallup et al. (2002). If indeed so, then the subsequent query to raise is whether self-awareness, the ability to differentiate oneself among others, is a precursor to or derivative of consciousness, and whether the mirror test is necessary and sufficient (Morin, 2011).

In light of brain research like the Blue Brain Project (Markram, 2006), BRAIN Initiative (Kandel et al., 2013), and development of neural prosthetics, the interest in consciousness is steadily growing. Here, we not only encourage the study of and suggest methods for addressing science's "*elephant in the room*," which asserts consciousness is neither physical nor functional, but also place the *Elephas maximus* in our proverbial mirror to obtain a perspective toward forming a cohesive alliance between philosophical studies of consciousness and neural engineering's augmentative innovations. As MSR is purposed to grant the animal subject personal physical inspection from an objective viewpoint, resulting in self-cognizance, so shall we take the approach to examine our modern scientific methods in conceptual mirrors, to appraise our consciousness dilemma and propose an assertion for progression in augmentative technologies. Following here is a succinct primer of consciousness and SA. We also issue a proposition as to how brain augmentation can influence the arrival of machine consciousness. Overall, we state our opinion for (1) why SA must be systematically examined in conjunction with brain augmentation approaches and (2) how such a merger could become a tool for investigating consciousness.

Ineffable Consciousness

The first pitfall encountered with consciousness is the inability to derive a functional explanation for what it means to *experience*. Chalmers (2007) lists the "easy" problems of consciousness as "the ability to discriminate, categorize, and react to environmental stimuli; the integration of information by a cognitive system; the reportability of mental states; the ability of a system to access its own internal states; the focus of attention; the deliberate control of behavior; the difference between wakefulness and sleep." These phenomena are relatively feasible to exploit and can be described in computational model terms and neural operation derivations. Chalmers then counteracts them with the "hard" problem of lacking competency to explain why and how we have phenomenal experiences when being entertained by a movie, exhibiting a sensation toward classical music, or having feelings when watching a sunset. Explaining how the brain processes visual and auditory signals is trivial in comparison to how those same signals translate to *qualia*, subjective phenomenal experiences.

Explanatory Gap Dilemma

The term *explanatory gap*, coined by philosopher Joseph Levine (1983), notes our inability to connect physiological functions with psychological experience, thus creating the *gap*. Although Levine synonymizes consciousness with subjective feelings, the explanatory gap additionally alludes to reasoning, desires, memory, perception, beliefs, emotion, intentions, and human behavior/action. Correlating physical brain substrates to thoughts and feelings is the base of dispute between two parties: materialist reductionists and non-reductionists (Sawyer, 2002). Materialists' chief view, representative of most neuroengineers, on the matter involves the belief that "when the brain shuts off, the mind shuts off" and the brain is the sole causative driver for consciousness. However, non-reductionists (typically philosophers) embrace a holism approach of mandating that the brain's cortical components are insufficient in capturing consciousness, undertaking the possibility of supernatural properties. It's an inquiry of necessity and sufficiency. The brain may be necessary for mental functions, but is it sufficient? Earlier analytical inspections on conscious experience have implied that an exclusive reductive justification is not satisfactory in delineating its emergence (Churchland, 1988; Kim, 2005; Clayton, 2006; Feinberg, 2012). A novel approach is needed to explain such experience. Our explanatory gap needs an explanatory bridge.

UNRAVELING SELF-AWARENESS TOWARD AUGMENTATION

Although many facets of consciousness are difficult to investigate, the development of objective tests for SA could be utilized for brain augmented technologies. With SA comes the sense of *agency*. Agency imparts a sense of who is the owner of an action/trait, the self, and who represents any entities excluding self, the other(s). Self-other dichotomy processing in the brain is essential to consciousness due to the necessary implications the embodiment of "self" must have to form body ownership. Once an agent gains the ability to discern when its own body is the source of sensory perceptions, it will form body awareness that entails proprioceptive information. We can look to working experiments that attempt to showcase how the brain augments the "self" when necessary to complete a task (**Figure 1**). Perceptual parametric information builds a premeditated awareness of (1) body part locations and (2) the manipulation of those same parts in space. Body awareness was demonstrated by a machine via Gold and Scassellati (2007) who built a robot named Nico that successfully distinguished its own "self" from "other." Nico observably achieved self-recognition by completing mirror-aided tasks expending inverse kinematics. Nevertheless, it's believed Nico lacked consciousness.

Before the sense of agency becomes fully refined through experiences over time, there must be a repertoire built for perceptions and actions. Whether, action and perception are interdependent or each fundamentally isolated has been the focus of another ongoing debate. It's not yet concretely understood how the representation of self is formed during the initial stages of life. Either an agent first uses perception to motivate their

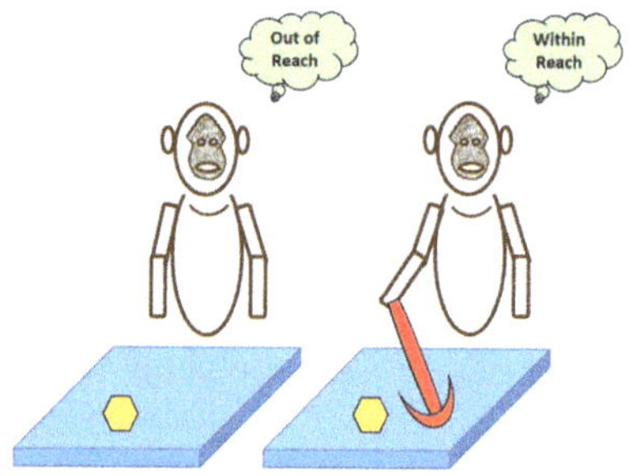

FIGURE 1 | Extension of self-representation. Here are two depictions of macaque monkeys that exhibit a case of the body making use of tools as an extension of the "self." If given a task to retrieve an object (yellow hexagonal shape) that is outside the peripersonal space and the immediate reach of an extended limb (left macaque), the body relies on its physical limitations to define the "self" and its aptitude for success of the task. However, when an apparatus is introduced (right macaque) that can help achieve the task's goal, the brain's neural correlates are able to augment themselves to psychophysically merge tools that were formerly considered to be of "other" classification into the "self" body schematic and permit optimal behavioral actions to take place (Hihara et al., 2006; Carlson et al., 2010). The paradigm for "self" is malleable to accept the dynamic interplay necessary to achieve an aim for biological function that was once previously unattainable. As tool-use changes the brain's representations of the body and alters proprioception, we subsequently believe it parallels how enriched brain augmentation can alter an individual's self-awareness and consciousness.

actions in the world or it first directs their actions to help drive perception of the sensory world or both occur simultaneously. In either method bodily awareness is eventually acquired which contributes to defining subjective cognitive attributes. Two opposing views attempt to solve this problem: the action-oriented theory of visual perception, which suggests that perception results from sensorimotor dynamics in an *acting* observer (Gibson, 1966; Noë, 2004; Mandik, 2005), and the dual-visual systems hypothesis, which advocates independent streams of perception and action (Schneider, 1969; Goodale and Milner, 1992; Jacob and Jeannerod, 2003; Milner and Goodale, 2006). Self-awareness uses expectation of impending perceptions and actions to gauge the assimilation of inner experience and external reality. Building a self-aware framework in augmentative technologies requires integration of an *expectancy intuition*, which is the capability to critique on the basis of differences between reality and internal experience. This is our tactic for creating systems with faculties for using perception and action to make predictions of self-sensory states, become self-adaptable to new environmental stimuli, and set objectives for self-improvement.

Crucial for understanding agency is determining how the embodied senses fuse to form self-referential experience (Fingelkurts et al., 2016a,b). It's our opinion that future advances of brain augmentation hinges on the application of such knowledge. Once we bridge this gap of the unknown we'll be challenged to use computational intelligence to create consciousness artificially and to integrate synthetic qualia with that produced in the brain. Presently, artificial devices can create various aspects of consciousness. Artificial perception is made available via cochlear, retinal, and tactile implants. But they simply work alone as replacements for sensory organs with consciousness and SA arriving later in the brain's neural processing. Applications for augmenting consciousness would contribute to studies relating to emotions, attention, supplementing memory capacity, personality alteration, experience enrichment, sensory perception enhancement, and hypernormal brain plasticity for self-repair.

PROPOSED TRANSITION TO MACHINE CONSCIOUSNESS

The marvel of human intelligence is its ability to eclipse physical limitations and overcome our biological constraints to form an ever-evolving existence (Jerison, 1973). One primary goal for reverse-engineering the human brain is to recreate the same functional mechanisms that underlie human consciousness in our software infrastructures, neurorobotic agents, and computational systems. However, prosthetic memory, sensory implants, neurofeedback (EEG Biofeedback) and brain computer interfaces (BCIs) are all working examples of fusing such "intelligent" systems with the brain, leading to conceivable prospects for consciousness-altering devices. Although BCIs commonly target disability treatments and brain function recovery from lesion, the amalgamation of computational devices with the cortical brain itself (Fingelkurts et al., 2012) may even prompt increasing developments of an operational "exobrain" (Bonaci et al., 2014) for the purposes of better understanding how our brain works. For example, in a scenario where a split-brain condition is present within a subject, we now have the option to look toward interfacing artificial exobrains with the cerebrum; such an interface can either serve as a replacement for neurological issues or supplement features the brain does not naturally comprise. If these exobrains have a modicum of manipulability, then we can explore the plausibility of mind transfer from device to organ and vice versa; thus, providing speculation for a conscious machine that can affect how we can perceive, act, express emotion, feel, and adapt. This poses ethical concerns as it opens the door for alterations of an individual's SA when augmentation is capable of modifying reasoning skills and subjective judgment. Successful augmentation of the sort might render the individual powerless in discriminating actual characteristics and thoughts from those that are mock and introduced artificially outside the cortex. Combining the precision and information processing speed of a computer with the intrinsic non-computational attributes of a human may provoke discoveries of the mind (e.g., consciousness) that we as humans are currently incapable of resolving. We suggest efforts made toward an augmentative interface between brain and machine that prompts the human mind to think beyond its unknown limits for the construction of our explanatory bridge.

CHALLENGES MOVING FORWARD

Many people view an in-depth exploration into consciousness and its emergence as a gamble, considering decades already spent on the matter with a void of consensus (Dennett, 1991; Jibu and Yasue, 1995; Hameroff and Penrose, 1996; Stapp, 2001; Crick and Koch, 2003; Tononi, 2008; De Sousa, 2013; Seager, 2016). Before we attempt to create another hypothesis, our approach needs to change; it's our suggestion to further refine the constructs and emergence of SA and to use brain augmentation as an instrument for inspection. We need to define an objective test for determining whether an entity is a sentient being. This test in addition to advances in neural engineering provide optimism that disputes within the consciousness field can be resolved. Augmentation has a promising future as an enhancement to our brains and will hopefully influence our centuries-old methods of thinking about consciousness toward an answer for science's greatest mystery.

AUTHOR CONTRIBUTIONS

JB: This author was responsible for providing the overall opinion of the topic and crafting the outline of the article. JB contributed most of the text and references supplied in the document. JB also primarily conducted the necessary research to develop this article. JB supplied the latter sections of the text with original ideas to add to the discussion of the Brain Augmentation research topic. AP: This author assisted in crafting the thesis of the article and provided additional topic of discussion to implement within the text. AP provided introductory material for the article and also made revisions to each section to ensure a coherent message about our opinion was made. AP also restructured the format of the article to enhance comprehension to an audience with varying backgrounds.

REFERENCES

Amsterdam, B. (1972). Mirror self-image reactions before age two. *Dev. Psychobiol.* 5, 297–305. doi: 10.1002/dev.420050403

Bonaci, T., Herron, J., Matlack, C., and Chizeck, H. J. (2014). "Securing the exocortex: a twenty-first century cybernetics challenge," in *Norbert Wiener in the 21st Century (21CW)* (Boston, MA), 1–8.

Carlson, T. A., Alvarez, G., Wu, D. A., and Verstraten, F. A. (2010). Rapid assimilation of external objects into the body schema. *Psychol. Sci.* 21, 1000–1005. doi: 10.1177/0956797610371962

Chalmers, D. (2007). "The Hard Problem of Consciousness," in *The Blackwell Companion to Consciousness,* ed M. Velmans and S. Schneider (Malden, MA: Blackwell Publishing), 225–235.

Churchland, P. S. (1988). "Reduction and the neurobiological basis of consciousness," in *Consciousness in Contemporary Science,* ed A. J. Marcel and E. Bisiach (New York, NY: Oxford University Press), 273–304.

Clayton, P. (2006). *Mind and Emergence: From Quantum to Consciousness.* New York, NY: Oxford University Press.

Crick, F., and Koch, C. (2003). A framework for consciousness. *Nat. Neurosci.* 6, 119–126. doi: 10.1038/nn0203-119

Dagnelie, G. (2012). Retinal implants: emergence of a multidisciplinary field. *Curr. Opin. Neurol.* 25, 67–75. doi: 10.1097/WCO.0b013e32834f02c3

Delfour, F., and Marten, K. (2001). Mirror image processing in three marine mammal species: killer whales (*Orcinus orca*), false killer whales (*Pseudorca crassidens*) and California sea lions (*Zalophus californianus*). *Behav. Processes* 53, 181–190. doi: 10.1016/S0376-6357(01)00134-6

Dennett, D. C. (1991). *Consciousness Explained.* Boston, MA: Little, Brown and Company.

De Sousa, A. (2013). Towards an integrative theory of consciousness: part 1 (neurobiological and cognitive models). *Mens Sana Monogr.* 11, 100–150. doi: 10.4103/0973-1229.109335

De Veer, M. W., and van den Bos, R. (1999). A critical review of methodology and interpretation of mirror self-recognition research in nonhuman primates. *Anim. Behav.* 58, 459–468. doi: 10.1006/anbe.1999.1166

Feinberg, T. E. (2012). Neuroontology, neurobiological naturalism, and consciousness: a challenge to scientific reduction and a solution. *Phys. Life Rev.* 9, 13–34. doi: 10.1016/j.plrev.2011.10.019

Fingelkurts, A. A., Fingelkurts, A. A., and Kallio-Tamminen, T. (2016a). Long-term meditation training induced changes in the operational synchrony of default mode network modules during a resting state. *Cogn. Processes* 17, 27–37. doi: 10.1007/s10339-015-0743-4

Fingelkurts, A. A., Fingelkurts, A. A., and Kallio-Tamminen, T. (2016b). Trait lasting alteration of the brain default mode network in experienced meditators and the experiential selfhood. *Self Identity* 15, 381–393. doi: 10.1080/15298868.2015.1136351

Fingelkurts, A. A., Fingelkurts, A. A., and Neves, C. F. (2012). "Machine" consciousness and "artificial" thought: an operational architectonics model guided approach. *Brain Res.* 1428, 80–92. doi: 10.1016/j.brainres.2010.11.079

Gallop, G. G. Jr. (1970). Chimpanzees: self recognition. *Science* 167, 86–87. doi: 10.1126/science.167.3914.86

Gallup, G. G. Jr., Anderson, J. L., and Shillito, D. P. (2002). "The mirror test," in *The Cognitive Animal: Empirical and Theoretical Perspectives on Animal Cognition,* eds M. Bekoff, C. Allen, and G. M. Burghardt (Cambridge, MA: MIT Press), 325–334.

Gantz, B. J., Turner, C., Gfeller, K. E., and Lowder, M. W. (2005). Preservation of hearing in cochlear implant surgery: advantages of combined electrical and acoustical speech processing. *Laryngoscope* 115, 796–802. doi: 10.1097/01.MLG.0000157695.07536.D2

Gibson, J. J. (1966). *The Senses Considered as Perceptual Systems.* Boston, MA: Houghton Mifflin.

Gold, K., and Scassellati, B. (2007). "A Bayesian robot that distinguishes "self" from "other"," in *Proceedings of the 29th Annual Meeting of the Cognitive Science Society* (Nashville, TN), 1037–1042.

Goodale, M. A., and Milner, A. D. (1992). Separate visual pathways for perception and action. *Trends Neurosci.* 15, 20–25. doi: 10.1016/0166-2236(92)90344-8

Hameroff, S., and Penrose, R. (1996). Orchestrated reduction of quantum coherence in brain microtubules: a model for consciousness. *Math. Comput. Simul.* 40, 453–480. doi: 10.1016/0378-4754(96)80476-9

Hihara, S., Notoya, T., Tanaka, M., Ichinose, S., Ojima, H., Obayashi, S., et al. (2006). Extension of corticocortical afferents into the anterior bank of the intraparietal sulcus by tool-use training in adult monkeys. *Neuropsychologia* 44, 2636–2646. doi: 10.1016/j.neuropsychologia.2005.11.020

Jacob, P., and Jeannerod, M. (2003). *Ways of Seeing: The Scope and Limits of Visual Cognition.* Oxford: Oxford University Press.

Jerison, H. J. (1973). *Evolution of the Brain and Intelligence.* New York, NY: Academic Press.

Jibu, M., and Yasue, K. (1995). *Quantum Brain Dynamics and Consciousness.* Amsterdam; Philadelphia, PA: John Benjamins Publishing.

Kandel, E. R., Markram, H., Matthews, P. M., Yuste, R., and Koch, C. (2013). Neuroscience thinks big (and collaboratively). *Nat. Rev. Neurosci.* 14, 659–664. doi: 10.1038/nrn3578

Kim, J. (2005). *Physicalism, or Something Near Enough.* Princeton, NJ: Princeton University Press.

Levine, J. (1983). Materialism and qualia: the explanatory gap. *Pac. Philos. Q.* 64, 354–361.

Mandik, P. (2005). "Action-Oriented Representation," in *Cognition and the Brain: The Philosophy and Neuroscience Movement,* eds K. Akins and A. Brook (Cambridge: Cambridge University Press), 284–305.

Markram, H. (2006). The blue brain project. *Nat. Rev. Neurosci.* 7, 153–160. doi: 10.1038/nrn1848

Milner, A. D., and Goodale, M. A. (2006). *The Visual Brain in Action.* Oxford: Oxford University Press.

Morin, A. (2011). Self-recognition, theory-of-mind, and self-awareness: what side are you on? *Laterality* 16, 367–383. doi: 10.1080/13576501003702648

Noë, A. (2004). *Action in Perception.* Cambridge, MA: MIT press.

Plotnik, J. M., de Waal, F. B. M., and Reiss, D. (2006). Self-recognition in an Asian elephant. *Proc. Natl. Acad. Sci. U.S.A.* 103, 17053–17057. doi: 10.1073/pnas.0608062103

Prior, H., Schwarz, A., and Gunturkun, O. (2008). Mirror-induced behavior in the magpie (pica pica): evidence of self-recognition. *PLoS Biol.* 6:e202. doi: 10.1371/journal.pbio.0060202

Reiss, D., and Marino, L. (2001). Mirror self-recognition in the bottlenose dolphin: a case of cognitive convergence. *Proc. Natl. Acad. Sci. U.S.A.* 98, 5937–5942. doi: 10.1073/pnas.101086398

Rochat, P. (2003). Five levels of self-recognition as they unfold early in life. *Conscious. Cogn.* 12, 717–773. doi: 10.1016/S1053-8100(03)00081-3

Sawyer, R. K. (2002). Emergence in psychology: lessons from the history of non-reductionist science. *Hum. Dev.* 45, 2–28. doi: 10.1159/000048148

Schneider, G. E. (1969). Two visual systems: brain mechanisms for localization and discrimination are dissociated by tectal and cortical lesions. *Science* 163, 895–902. doi: 10.1126/science.163.3870.895

Seager, W. (2016). *Theories of Consciousness: An Introduction and Assessment.* New York, NY: Routledge.

Stapp, H. P. (2001). Quantum theory and the role of mind in nature. *Found. Phys.* 31, 1465–1499. doi: 10.1023/A:1012682413597

Suárez, S. D., and Gallup, G. G. (1981). Self-recognition in chimpanzees and orangutans, but not gorillas. *J. Hum. Evol.* 10, 175–188. doi: 10.1016/S0047-2484(81)80016-4

Tononi, G. (2008). Consciousness as integrated information: a provisional manifesto. *Biol. Bull.* 215, 216–242. doi: 10.2307/25470707

24

Task-dependent calibration of auditory spatial perception through environmental visual observation

*Alessia Tonelli, Luca Brayda and Monica Gori**

Robotics, Brain and Cognitive Sciences Department, Fondazione Istituto Italiano di Tecnologia, Genoa, Italy

Edited by:
Mikhail Lebedev, Duke University, USA

Reviewed by:
Nicholas Altieri, Idaho State University, USA
Caterina Bertini, University of Bologna, Italy
Patrick Bruns, University of Hamburg, Germany

***Correspondence:**
Monica Gori, Robotics, Brain and Cognitive Sciences Department, Fondazione Istituto Italiano di Tecnologia, via Morego 30, 16163 Genoa, Italy
monica.gori@iit.it

Visual information is paramount to space perception. Vision influences auditory space estimation. Many studies show that simultaneous visual and auditory cues improve precision of the final multisensory estimate. However, the amount or the temporal extent of visual information, that is sufficient to influence auditory perception, is still unknown. It is therefore interesting to know if vision can improve auditory precision through a short-term environmental observation preceding the audio task and whether this influence is task-specific or environment-specific or both. To test these issues we investigate possible improvements of acoustic precision with sighted blindfolded participants in two audio tasks [minimum audible angle (MAA) and space bisection] and two acoustically different environments (normal room and anechoic room). With respect to a baseline of auditory precision, we found an improvement of precision in the space bisection task but not in the MAA after the observation of a normal room. No improvement was found when performing the same task in an anechoic chamber. In addition, no difference was found between a condition of short environment observation and a condition of full vision during the whole experimental session. Our results suggest that even short-term environmental observation can calibrate auditory spatial performance. They also suggest that echoes can be the cue that underpins visual calibration. Echoes may mediate the transfer of information from the visual to the auditory system.

Keywords: audio, vision, bisection, multisensory, calibration, space perception, echoes

Introduction

The visual system is the most accurate sense to estimate spatial properties. Many studies involving adult individuals support this idea, showing that when the spatial locations of audio and visual stimuli are in conflict, vision usually dominates, generating the so-called "ventriloquist effect" (Warren et al., 1981; Mateeff et al., 1985). This effect is possibly due to an optimal combination of cues performed by the human brain, where modalities are weighted by their statistical reliability. Vision dominates over audition in localization tasks (Alais and Burr, 2004). When visual and auditory systems are simultaneously presented to get spatial information, the final multisensory estimate tends to be more precise than either unisensory estimate (Clarke and Yuille, 1990; Ghahramani et al., 1997; Ernst and Banks, 2002; Alais and Burr, 2004; Landy et al., 2011). Interestingly, vision can interact with audition even when a visual stimulus is not provided during an auditory task: specifically. For example, although the angle of incidence of a sound source can be estimated with the use of only auditory cues, performance improves when vision is also present (Jackson, 1953; Shelton and Searle, 1980). A recent study by Tabry et al. (2013) has shown that the mere possibility of observing the setup by keeping eyes open during auditory horizontal and vertical localization tasks can improve audio accuracy, even if no visual cues of the stimuli are provided.

Another example of the connection between audio-spatial and visuo-spatial information is given by a technique used by some blind people, called echolocation. Some studies have shown that this technique can operate as a crude substitute for vision, because some purely visual phenomenona, such as size constancy (Milne et al., 2015) or size-weight illusion (Buckingham et al., 2015), are present in expert echolocators, who use echoes to navigate in unknown environments.

However, it is still unknown which are the visual cues that allow an improvement in audio-spatial tasks, nor it is understood how long visual cues should last to determine such improvement. As well, it is unknown whether this phenomenon can be task-specific, i.e., if audio-spatial abilities are improved in general or if the influence of vision depends on the complexity of the audio task. Can it be argued that increased audio-spatial abilities are due to a transfer of information from the visual to the auditory system? Which is the information that is transferred? Is vision more informative for some aspects than for others?

In this paper we tested two audio tasks under various environmental conditions and visual feedbacks to answer these questions. In particular we investigated: (i) whether the environmental visual cues (i.e., prior short observation of the environment and full vision during the tasks) can improve auditory precision; (ii) whether this improvement is task-specific; and (iii) which are the environmental cues that mediate the auditory improvement due to the interaction between vision and audition.

To investigate the first point about whether environmental visual cues can improve auditory precision we tested a sample of blindfolded sighted participants twice: the first time with no visual input of the environment where the auditory task was performed; the second time after they observed for 1 min the environment. We compared the performance with no visual input of the environment with that with 1 min observation. We also tested a different group of sighted participants, who performed the two tasks with a full vision of the room but without being blindfolded. We compared the performance of this last sample with the other. Our hypothesis was that if the visual cues coming from the environmental observation can help to improve the auditory precision, then the improvement should occur at least with full vision and possibly with short-term observation.

The second question was about whether auditory precision improvement was task-specific. We tested all participants in two audio tasks: the minimum audible angle (MAA) task and the spatial bisection. In the MAA task the participant had to judge which of the two sounds generated by an array of loudspeakers was more from the right. Instead, in the spatial bisection task the participant heard three sounds coming from three distinct locations and had to judge whether the second sound was closer to the first or third sound coming from the array. The difference between these two tasks is that the spatial bisection task requires subjects to encode the position of three sounds, remember them over a period of 1 s and compare their remembered positions. Contrarily, in the MAA task, the subject has to compare the position of the two sounds relatively to the subject's position. Moreover while MMA requires estimating a relation of order between two acoustic directions; bisection requires estimating a relation of order between two estimated acoustic distances. To summarize, while the space bisection requires a Euclidian representation of space and involves higher abstraction capabilities, for the MMA task a topological representation of space is sufficient.

Moreover, we chose these two tasks because we recently reported that the visual information is fundamental for the bisection task and not essential for the MAA task (Gori et al., 2014). A visual dominance over audition during development was observed for the space bisection task (Gori et al., 2012), while the absence of visual input in congenitally blind individuals negatively impacts their performance on audio space bisection tasks (Gori et al., 2014). However the absence of vision does not affect the ability of performing the MAA task in visually impaired individuals (Gori et al., 2014; in agreement with Lessard et al., 1998).

The apparent influence of the visuo-spatial knowledge on space bisection tasks leads to our second hypothesis: if the environmental visual information can improve acoustic spatial precision, then the improvement should be bigger for the space bisection task than for the MAA task.

With regard to the third point, which consists in investigating the environmental cues that possibly mediate the auditory improvement after observation, we replicated all audio tests in an anechoic room. In such a room, the walls absorb part of the sound energy; therefore the auditory system almost exclusively acquires the direct path of the sound, i.e., not reflected by walls. Conversely, in the normal room, a wall reflects sounds and generates echoes. Our hypothesis is that if the interpretation of echoes is triggered by visual observation, an improvement of acoustic precision should occur only in the normal room, while not in the anechoic chamber.

Materials and Methods

Participants

We measured auditory spatial discrimination in 33 sighted individuals with normal or corrected to normal vision (an average age of 28, 5 years, with 18 females and 15 males), all with normal hearing (assessed by Ear Test 1.0 software) and no cognitive impairment. All participants gave informed consent before starting the tests. The study was approved by the ethics committee of the local health service (*Comitato Etico, ASL3, Genova*).

Apparatus and Stimuli

The participants sat 180 cm away from the center of a bank of 23 speakers, 161 cm long (see **Figure 1**), and spanning ±25° of visual angle.

During the auditory space bisection task, three stimuli, each having a duration of 75 ms, were presented at interval of

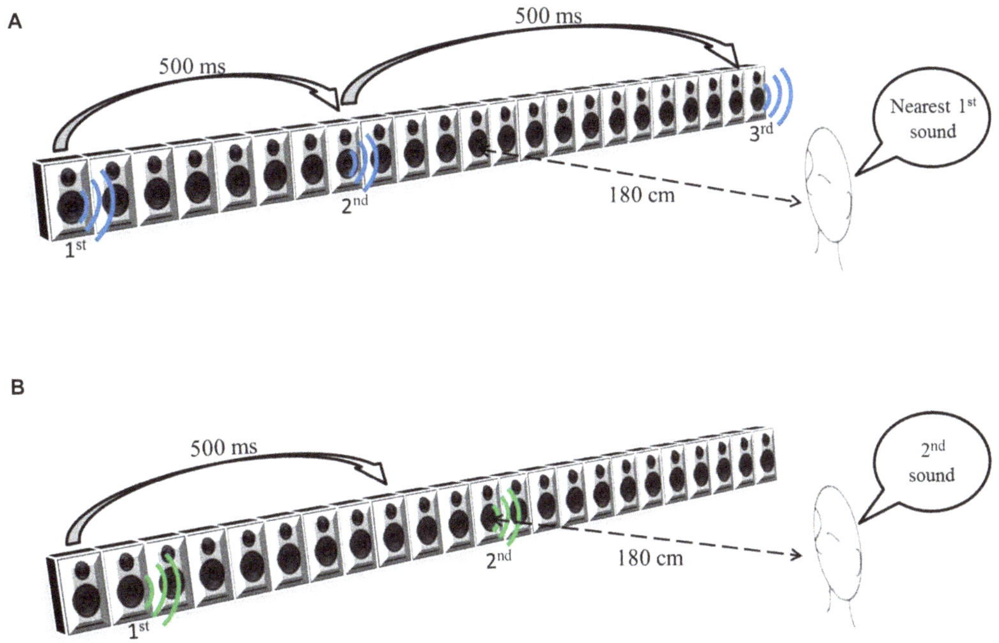

FIGURE 1 | (A) Space Bisection Task. **(B)** Minimum audible angle (MAA) task.

500 ms (see **Figure 1A**). The first stimulus was always at −25°, the third always at +25° and the second at an intermediate speaker position which was determined by QUEST (Watson and Pelli, 1983), an adaptive algorithm which estimates the best stimulus value to be presented after each trial, given the current participant's estimate. To ensure that a wide range of positions was sampled, that estimate was jittered by a random amount, drawn from a Gaussian distribution of space covering the full width of the loudspeaker's array, and the nearest speaker to that estimate chosen. In the MAA task, two 75 ms pink noise (Will and Berg, 2007) stimuli were presented with a 500 ms interval. One sound came from the central loudspeaker (12th speaker) and the other one at a random distance from center on its left or on its right (**Figure 1B**). Also in this case, the QUEST algorithm determined the position of the second stimulus. For both tasks, the proportion of rightward responses was calculated for each speaker distance. Gaussian functions by means of the Maximum Likelihood method were used to estimate both the mean, or PSE (Point of Subjective Equality), and the standard deviation, or JND (Just Noticeable Difference). The standard deviation of the fit was taken as an estimate of the threshold, indicating the precision of the task.

To better generalize our results, in 15 participants we used three different sound sources (randomized across trials), all with a 75 ms duration and a 60 dB SPL intensity (measured at the participant's position): a 500 Hz sound (for which interaural time differences are more important for sound localization); a 3000 Hz sound (for which interaural level differences are more important); and pink noise (ranging from 0 to 5 KHz) for which both are important. As the precision in sound localization varied very little among the three sounds, only pink noise burst data were considered.

Procedure

Two audio spatial tasks were considered: an auditory space bisection task and a MAA task. The entire group of participants were divided into three groups. The first group (composed of 11 participants) performed four audio tasks (two times the bisection task and two times the MMA task) in an anechoic chamber (3 m × 5 m), the second groups (composed of 11 participants) performed four audio tasks (two times the bisection task and two times the MAA task) in a normal room (7, 20 m × 3, 5 m). The participants of these two groups were blindfolded before entering the room; during the first two audio tasks (one audio bisection and one MAA task), they had no notion of the room or the acoustic stimulation setup. After having performed both the audio tasks, the participants were allowed to remove the blindfold and observe for 1 min the room: in one case an anechoic chamber (first group) and in the other case a normal room (second group). Afterwards they were blindfolded again to repeat both audio tasks again. The last group (composed of 11 participants) was not blindfolded, so they had a full vision of the room and the setup during the tasks. They performed two audio tasks (one time the bisection task and one time the MAA task) just on the normal room. For all the groups the bisection and MAA tasks were presented in a random order.

In the auditory space bisection, participants reported verbally whether the second sound was spatially closer to the first sound (produced by the first speaker on the left, number 1) than the last sound (produced by the last speaker on the right, number 23). Each subject performed 60 trials.

In the MAA task, the participants had to verbally report which sound was more from the right, choosing between the first or the second sound. Each subject performed 60 trials for each task.

Results

Figure 2 show psychometric functions of the proportion of trials judged "closer to the right sound source", plotted against speaker position (in cm). On the top of the figure are shown the results obtained by one of the participant took as an example of the global trend in the anechoic chamber for the space bisection (**Figure 2A**) and the MAA (**Figure 2C**). In the same way, on the bottom, the **Figure 2** show the results of one of the participant for the normal room in the space bisection (**Figure 2B**) and the MAA (**Figure 2D**).

Figure 3 shows the thresholds obtained before and after having observed the environment, it also shows the performance with eyes open for both the tasks: the MAA (**Figure 3A**) and the space bisection (**Figure 3B**). In both figures, the solid colors refer to the performance before room observation, while the colors with reticulus refer to the performance after the room observation.

We conducted a mixed model 2-way (2 × 2) ANOVA for both MAA and Space Bisection tasks with a between factor, *room kind* (normal room vs. anechoic chamber), and within factor, *room observation* (before environmental observation vs. after environmental observation). For the space bisection task the ANOVA revealed significant main effect for both factors, *room observation* ($F_{(2,22)} = 6.55$, $p < 0.02$) and *room kind* ($F_{(2,22)} = 7.35$, $p < 0.01$). It has been observed a significant *room observation* × *room kind* interaction ($F_{(4,11)} = 6.86$, $p < 0.01$). Then we ran Student's *t*-test that indicate a significant difference between the groups who performed the space bisection task in the normal room and anechoic chamber before observing the room (two tailed two-sample *t*-test, $t_{(20)} = 3.44$, $p < 0.01$) and in the normal room between before environmental observation and after environmental observation (two tailed pair-sample *t*-test, $t_{(10)} = 5.46$, $p < 0.001$). On the other hand, for the MAA, no significant effect was found (*room observation*, $F_{(2,22)} = 0.48$, $p = 0.49$; *room kind*, $F_{(2,22)} = 1.49$, $p = 0.28$; *room observation* × *room kind* $F_{(4,11)} = 0.506$, $p = 0.481$).

No significant difference was obtained in the precision after environmental observation and full vision (violet bars) for the space bisection task (two tailed two-sample *t*-test, $t_{(20)} = 1.279$,

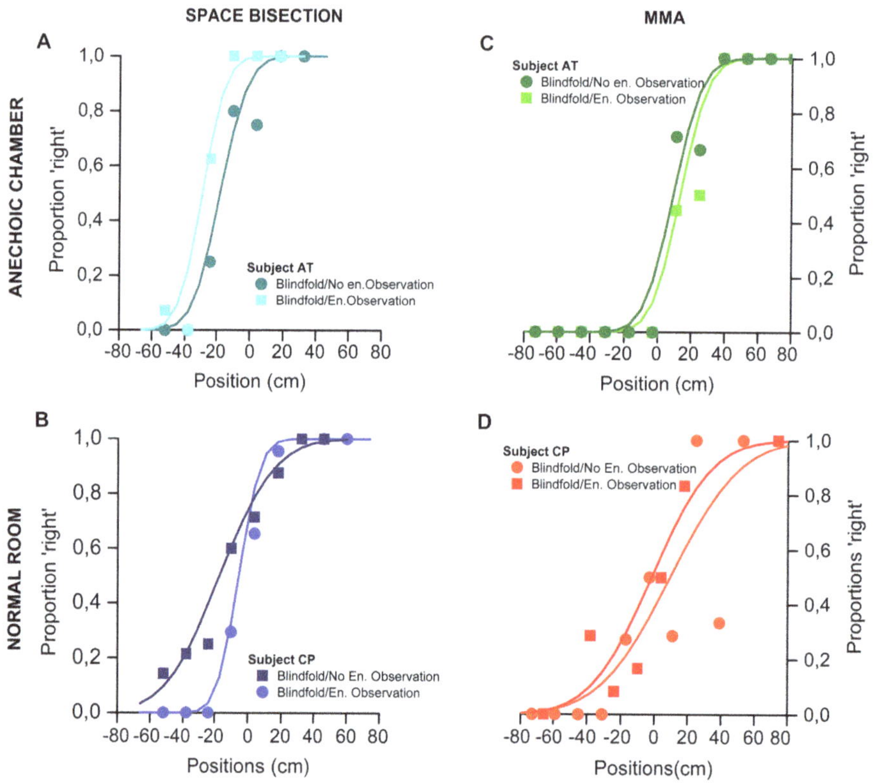

FIGURE 2 | Results of the Space Bisection Task and MAA of two participants, one for each group (normal room and anechoic chamber) as example. (A,B) Space bisection: proportion of trials judged "closer to the right sound source", plotted against speaker position (in cm). The area of the dots is the proportion of trials at that position, normalized by the total number of trials performed by each participants. At the top-left the results obtained in the anechoic chamber by participant AT **(A)**; at the bottom-left the results obtained in the normal room by participant CP **(B)**. Both sets of data are it with the Gaussian error function. **(C,D)** MAA: proportion of trials where the second of a two-sound sequence was reported to the right of the first, plotted against difference in speaker position. At the top-right the results obtained in the anechoic chamber by participant AT **(C)**; at the bottom-right the results obtained in the normal room by participant CP **(D)** Again the fits are the Gaussian error function.

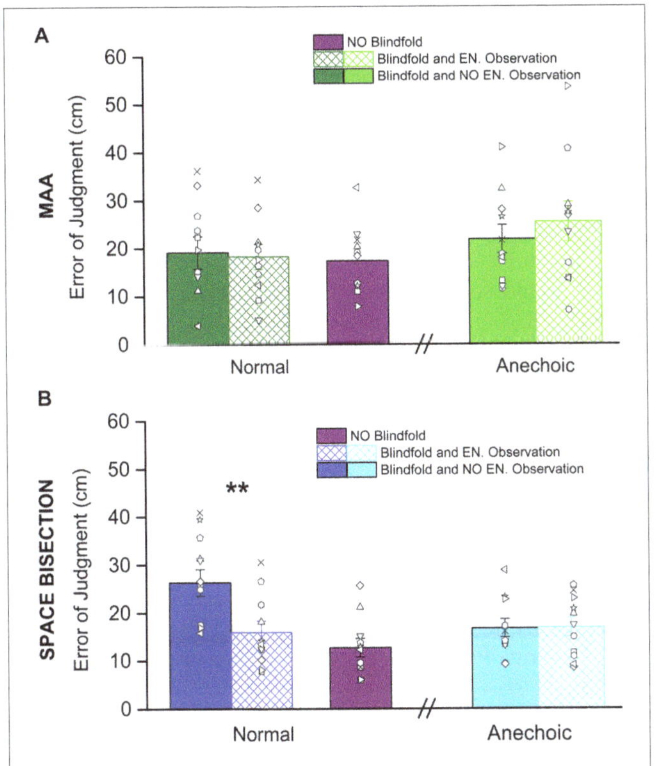

FIGURE 3 | Shown here are the average precision thresholds obtain in the MAA (A) and Space Bisection (B) tasks. **(A)** The dark green bars, on the left, represent the average precision thresholds obtained in the normal room before (fill in dark green bar) and after (reticulus dark green bar) environmental observation. On the right the light green bars are the average precision thresholds obtained in the anechoic chamber before (fill in light green bar) and after (reticulus light green bar) environmental observation. The violet bar is the average precision obtained by the subject in full vision in the normal room. The dots represent individual data. **(B)** For the space bisection, dark blue bars, on the left, represent the average precision thresholds obtained in the normal room before (fill in dark blue bar) and after (reticulus dark blue bar) environmental observation. On the right the light blue bars are the average precision thresholds obtained in the anechoic chamber before (fill in light blue bar) and after (reticulus light blue bar) environmental observation. Also in this case the violet bar represent the average precision obtained by the subject in full vision in the normal room. The dots represent individual data. (**) Indicates a significant difference of precision between before and after environmental observation in the normal room ($p < 0.01$).

$p = 0.27$) and for the MAA (two tailed two-sample t-test, $t_{(20)} = 0.257, p = 0.799$).

No change was observed in the localization bias (PSE) for both groups and tasks (bisection task: 2-ways (2 × 2) ANOVA with factors *room observation*—$F_{(2,22)} = 0.79, p = 0.38$—and *room kind*—$F_{(2,22)} = 1.48$, $p = 0.23$—and *room observation* × *room kind* interaction, $F_{(4,11)} = 0.088$, $p = 0.77$; MAA task: 2-ways (2 × 2) ANOVA with factors *room observation*—$F_{(2,22)} = 0.373$, $p = 0.545$—and *room kind*—$F_{(2,22)} = 1.91, p = 0.175$—, and *room observation* × *room kind* interaction, $F_{(4,11)} = 0.001, p = 0.97$).

Discussion

Recent works suggest that vision can interact with the auditory modality even when visual information is not useful for the auditory task, by improving the accuracy of auditory localization judgments (Jackson, 1953; Shelton and Searle, 1980; Tabry et al., 2013). For example acoustic performance has been found to be better when participants were allowed to observe the setup by keeping eyes open even if no visual cues were provided (Tabry et al., 2013). Thus even the simple observation of the setup and the environment during the task can improve auditory performance.

Why does this process occur? Which are the visual cues used by the visual system that allow for such an auditory improvement?

In this paper we investigated these issues by studying: (i) the environmental visual cues that are involved in auditory precision improvement; and (ii) whether this improvement is task related.

We tested the first point by asking the participants to perform two audio tasks twice. The first time the tasks were performed without observing the room; the second time, after having observed the room for 1 min. The results suggest that the observation of the environment for a brief period improves the auditory space precision and that the improvement is environment dependent. The improvement was only found after the observation of a natural environment, while, when the test was replicated in an anechoic chamber, no improvement was obtained. Besides, the improvement was task dependent. Two tasks were tested: a MAA task and an audio spatial bisection task; the improvement was observed only for the space bisection task but not for the MAA.

The first question that arises from these results is why the improvement is task-specific, giving that it occurs only for the audio space bisection task. We think that this specificity can be related to the role of visual information on the calibration of the auditory system.

Most recent works on multi-sensory interactions concentrated on sensory *fusion*, investigating the efficiency of the integration of information from different senses. Equally important, but somewhat neglected aspect, is sensory *calibration*.

Our idea is that, while *precision* has the highest weight for sensory integration, the most important property for sensory calibration is *accuracy*. Precision is a relative measure defined as the degree of reproducibility or repeatability between measurements, usually defined as the standard deviation of the distribution. Accuracy, conversely, is defined in absolute terms as the vicinity of a measurement to its true physical value.

We have recently observed that during an audio-visual bisection task, sighted children show a strong visual dominance before multisensory integration occurs (Gori et al., 2012). It is reasonable that for the audio bisection task, the sense of vision is the most accurate for estimating the space. Therefore, it may be used to calibrate the audio system for this spatial task. An important question inferring from our cross-modal calibration theory is: what happens when the calibrating sense is impaired or absent, as is the case of visually impaired adults? We recently tackled this question by testing blind adults in an spatial audio bisection task demonstrating that, in absence of visual input, they have deficits in understanding the spatial relationship between sounds (Gori et al., 2014). The audio deficit was not observed, in agreement with previous studies (Lessard et al., 1998), for the MAA task.

Several physiological works confirm that vision is fundamental for some kind of auditory spatial localization: a series of experiments on animals have documented that displacing vision (Knudsen and Knudsen, 1985) or producing total visual deprivation (King and Carlile, 1993) often lead to systematic and persistent biases in auditory tasks. In the same way, transitory visual distortions in humans produce dramatic changes in auditory spatial maps (Recanzone, 1998; Zwiers et al., 2003).

On the basis of this evidence we can infer that the visual environmental information is not directly involved in the calibration of acoustic system in tasks such as the MAA. This idea would explain why we found a specific audio improvement after environment observation only for the audio bisection task and not for the MAA task.

A second interesting result is that: (i) before the environment observation, audio space bisection performance was worse in the normal room than in the anechoic room; and (ii) after the environment observation, an audio improvement was observed in the normal room and not in the anechoic room. Why performance for the space bisection task did not improve in the anechoic chamber and why it was worse before environment observation in the normal room than in the anechoic chamber? The observed null effect of the short environmental observation in the anechoic room might have been caused by a ceiling effect, i.e., performance was best already before room observation. However, this was not the case in the normal room, suggesting an alternative interpretation: in an anechoic chamber part of the energy of sounds produced by the loudspeakers is absorbed by the walls, therefore the hearing system acquires almost exclusively the direct sound. This is not true in the normal room, where the sound produced by the speakers is reflected by the walls, therefore producing echoes. This results in stimuli with scattering patterns or spectral coloration, or both, which are as much different as source locations are far apart. These echoes add perceptual information to the direct path of the sound, which may not be immediately interpretable without visual input, therefore causing a mismatch and worse performance in the normal room than in anechoic condition. However, the visual system could help the auditory system to compensate for such mismatch and obtain performance again comparable to those obtained in anechoic condition.

For similar reasons, observing an anechoic room does not improve acoustic precision because visual knowledge of the room structure is by no means related to any acoustic cue. Obtaining improvements in both rooms (or in the anechoic room only) would have supported the hypothesis that vision helps in estimating mainly the direction of arrival of acoustic direct paths, i.e., the only cue present in an anechoic room. However, this did not happen, supporting instead the hypothesis that visual cues related, even if implicitly, more to a global footprint given by room acoustics than to the local and specific acoustical feedback of our stimulation setup.

As discussed above, the fact that only the space bisection task results improved after room observation suggests that the transfer of information from the visual system toward the auditory one occurs only for those aspects for which the visual system can be used to calibrate the auditory one. In this vein, gaining knowledge about room acoustics through vision seems to be involved much more when estimating complex relationship between sound sources: while estimating audible angles requires comparison between the estimated direction of two sound sources, space bisection requires establishing a specific ordering relation between the direction of three sound sources, of which two are far apart in space. This operation may require Euclidian representation of space (Gori et al., 2014) and involve more spatial processing, possibly related to cues linked to the room structure that visual input helps to interpret.

A final interesting result is that no difference was observed between the performance obtained for the space bisection task after 1 min of environment observation and in the condition in which the eyes were maintained open for the entire experimental session. This suggests that the visual system needs only a brief period of environment observation to allow an improvement in this audio task.

In our past works we suggested that a process of cross-modal calibration might occur during development (Gori et al., 2008). During this process the visual system seems to be involved in the calibration of auditory space bisection (Gori et al., 2012, 2014). A possible interpretation of the results presented in this paper is that vision can calibrate audition also in a short-term form in adult individuals. It can indeed improve auditory space precision through a transfer of information about environmental cues from the visual system. In particular our results suggest that visual information might help the hearing system to compensate for the mismatch produced by echoes, and that visual knowledge of the room structure is linked to understanding of room acoustics.

If this interpretation is correct, then our results can be discussed in relation to the echolocation technique. Some blind individuals use the echoes produced by the environment to their advantage, thanks to echolocation. Human echolocation is an ability of humans to detect objects in their surroundings by sensing echoes from those objects. By actively creating sounds, such as clicks produced by rapidly moving the tongue in the palatal area behind the teeth (Rojas et al., 2009) or sounds produced by external mechanical means such as tapping a cane against the floor (Burton, 2000), people trained to orientate with echolocation can interpret the sound waves reflected by nearby objects. Many studies conducted under controlled experimental conditions have shown that echolocation improves blind people's spatial sensing ability.

For example a recent study (Vercillo et al., 2015) has compared the performance of expert echolocators, blind and sighted people with no previous experience of echolocation, in a space bisection task. It was found that blind expert echolocators performed the spatial bisection task with similar or even better precision than the sighted group. Moreover, in several studies were demonstrated that echolocation improves the ability to determine other characteristics as distance (Kolarik et al., 2013), motion (Thaler et al., 2011, 2014), size (Teng and Whitney, 2011; Teng et al., 2012), shape (Thaler et al., 2011; Milne et al., 2014).

Therefore we can assume that echolocation could serve to recalibrate the ability of blind individuals to represent sounds in some spatial configurations and compensate the lack of vision. Our results support the idea that the visual system might in some form compensate for the mismatch produced by echoes in unknown environments by helping to interpret them. Visual information and spatio-acoustic representation appear therefore intertwined. If this is correct then the use of the echolocation technique can be a way of substituting the role of the visual system on this process. This would partially explain the improved spatial skills of blind expert echolocators. To conclude, the current findings suggest that vision is not only important for the auditory system during the development of space auditory representation, but also during adulthood. Although the mechanisms that subtend this process still have to be completely understood, our results suggest that the visual system can improve some forms of auditory spatial perception also in adults and after short-term environmental observation.

Acknowledgments

This research is partly funded by the FP7 EU STREP project BLINDPAD (www.blindpad.eu), under grant 611621, by the FP7 EU STREP project ABBI (www.abbiproject.eu), under grant 611452, and by the Fondazione Istituto Italiano di Tecnologia (www.iit.it). The authors would like to thank all the participants to this study.

References

Alais, D., and Burr, D. (2004). The ventriloquist effect results from near-optimal bimodal integration. *Curr. Biol.* 14, 257–262. doi: 10.1016/s0960-9822(04)00043-0

Buckingham, G., Milne, J. L., Byrne, C. M., and Goodale, M. A. (2015). The size-weight illusion induced through human echolocation. *Psychol. Sci.* 26, 237–242. doi: 10.1177/0956797614561267

Burton, G. (2000). The role of the sound of tapping for nonvisual judgment of gap crossability. *J. Exp. Psychol. Hum. Percept. Perform.* 26, 900–916. doi: 10.1037/0096-1523.26.3.900

Clarke, J. J., and Yuille, A. L. (1990). *Data Fusion for Sensory Information Processing.* Boston: Kluwer Academic.

Ernst, M. O., and Banks, M. S. (2002). Humans integrate visual and haptic information in a statistically optimal fashion. *Nature* 415, 429–433. doi: 10.1038/415429a

Ghahramani, Z., Wolpert, D. M., and Jordan, M. I. (1997). "Computational models of sensorimotor integration," in *Self-Organization, Computational Maps and Motor Control*, ed. P. G. M. A. V. Sanguineti (Amsterdam: Elsevier Science Publ), 117–147.

Gori, M., Del Viva, M., Sandini, G., and Burr, D. C. (2008). Young children do not integrate visual and haptic form information. *Curr. Biol.* 18, 694–698. doi: 10.1016/j.cub.2008.04.036

Gori, M., Giuliana, L., Sandini, G., and Burr, D. (2012). Visual size perception and haptic calibration during development. *Dev. Sci.* 15, 854–862. doi: 10.1111/j.1467-7687.2012.2012.01183.x

Gori, M., Sandini, G., Martinoli, C., and Burr, D. C. (2014). Impairment of auditory spatial localization in congenitally blind human subjects. *Brain* 137, 288–293. doi: 10.1093/brain/awt311

Jackson, C. (1953). Visual factors in auditory localization. *Q. J. Exp. Psychol.* 5, 52–65. doi: 10.1080/17470215308416626

King, A. J., and Carlile, S. (1993). Changes induced in the representation of auditory space in the superior colliculus by rearing ferrets with binocular cyclid suture. *Exp. Brain Res.* 94, 444–455. doi: 10.1007/bf00230202

Knudsen, E. I., and Knudsen, P. F. (1985). Vision guides the adjustment of auditory localization in young barn owls. *Science* 230, 545–548. doi: 10.1126/science.4048948

Kolarik, A. J., Cirstea, S., and Pardhan, S. (2013). Evidence for enhanced discrimination of virtual auditory distance among blind listeners using level and direct-to-reverberant cues. *Exp. Brain Res.* 224, 623–633. doi: 10.1007/s00221-012-3340-0

Landy, M. S., Banks, M. S., and Knill, D. C. (2011). "Ideal-observer models of cue integration," in *Book of Sensory Cue Integration*, ed. K. K. A. M. S. L. Julia Trommershauser (Sensory cue integration: Oxford University Press), 5–29.

Lessard, N., Paré, M., Lepore, F., and Lassonde, M. (1998). Early-blind human subjects localize sound sources better than sighted subjects. *Nature* 395, 278–280. doi: 10.1038/26228

Mateeff, S., Hohnsbein, J., and Noack, T. (1985). Dynamic visual capture: apparent auditory motion induced by a moving visual target. *Perception* 14, 721–727. doi: 10.1068/p140721

Milne, J. L., Anello, M., Goodale, M. A., and Thaler, L. (2015). A blind human expert echolocator shows size constancy for objects perceived by echoes. *Neurocase* 21, 465–470. doi: 10.1080/13554794.2014.922994

Milne, J. L., Goodale, M. A., and Thaler, L. (2014). The role of head movements in the discrimination of 2-D shape by blind echolocation experts. *Atten. Percept. Psychophys.* 76, 1828–1837. doi: 10.3758/s13414-014-0695-2

Recanzone, G. H. (1998). Rapidly induced auditory plasticity: the ventriloquism aftereffect. *Proc. Natl. Acad. Sci. U S A* 95, 869–875. doi: 10.1073/pnas.95.3.869

Rojas, J. A. M., Hermosilla, J. A., Montero, R. S., and Espí, P. L. L. (2009). Physical analysis of several organic signals for human echolocation: oral vacuum pulses. *Acta Acust. United Acust.* 95, 325–330. doi: 10.3813/aaa.918155

Shelton, B. R., and Searle, C. L. (1980). The influence of vision on the absolute identification of sound-source position. *Percept. Psychophys.* 28, 589–596. doi: 10.3758/bf03198830

Tabry, V., Zatorre, R. J., and Voss, P. (2013). The influence of vision on sound localization abilities in both the horizontal and vertical planes. *Front. Psychol.* 4:932. doi: 10.3389/fpsyg.2013.00932

Teng, S., Puri, A., and Whitney, D. (2012). Ultrafine spatial acuity of blind expert human echolocators. *Exp. Brain Res.* 216, 483–488. doi: 10.1007/s00221-011-2951-1

Teng, S., and Whitney, D. (2011). The acuity of echolocation: spatial resolution in the sighted compared to expert performance. *J. Vis. Impair. Blind.* 105, 20–32.

Thaler, L., Arnott, S. R., and Goodale, M. A. (2011). Neural correlates of natural human echolocation in early and late blind echolocation experts. *PLoS One* 6:e20162. doi: 10.1371/journal.pone.0020162

Thaler, L., Milne, J. L., Arnott, S. R., Kish, D., and Goodale, M. A. (2014). Neural correlates of motion processing through echolocation, source hearing and vision in blind echolocation experts and sighted echolocation novices. *J. Neurophysiol.* 111, 112–127. doi: 10.1152/jn.00501.2013

Vercillo, T., Milne, J. L., Gori, M., and Goodale, M. A. (2015). Enhanced auditory spatial localization in blind echolocators. *Neuropsychologia* 67C, 35–40. doi: 10.1016/j.neuropsychologia.2014.12.001

Warren, D. H., Welch, R. B., and McCarthy, T. J. (1981). The role of visual-auditory "compellingness" in the ventriloquism effect: implications for transitivity among the spatial senses. *Percept. Psychophys.* 30, 557–564. doi: 10.3758/bf03202010

Watson, A. B., and Pelli, D. G. (1983). QUEST: a Bayesian adaptive psychometric method. *Percept. Psychophys.* 33, 113–120. doi: 10.3758/bf03202828

Will, U., and Berg, E. (2007). Brain wave synchronization and entrainment to periodic acoustic stimuli. *Neurosci. Lett.* 424, 55–60. doi: 10.1016/j.neulet.2007.07.036

Zwiers, M. P., Van Opstal, A. J., and Paige, G. D. (2003). Plasticity in human sound localization induced by compressed spatial vision. *Nat. Neurosci.* 6, 175–181. doi: 10.1038/nn999

Permissions

All chapters in this book were first published in ABFFFCNP, by Frontiers; hereby published with permission under the Creative Commons Attribution License or equivalent. Every chapter published in this book has been scrutinized by our experts. Their significance has been extensively debated. The topics covered herein carry significant findings which will fuel the growth of the discipline. They may even be implemented as practical applications or may be referred to as a beginning point for another development.

The contributors of this book come from diverse backgrounds, making this book a truly international effort. This book will bring forth new frontiers with its revolutionizing research information and detailed analysis of the nascent developments around the world.

We would like to thank all the contributing authors for lending their expertise to make the book truly unique. They have played a crucial role in the development of this book. Without their invaluable contributions this book wouldn't have been possible. They have made vital efforts to compile up to date information on the varied aspects of this subject to make this book a valuable addition to the collection of many professionals and students.

This book was conceptualized with the vision of imparting up-to-date information and advanced data in this field. To ensure the same, a matchless editorial board was set up. Every individual on the board went through rigorous rounds of assessment to prove their worth. After which they invested a large part of their time researching and compiling the most relevant data for our readers.

The editorial board has been involved in producing this book since its inception. They have spent rigorous hours researching and exploring the diverse topics which have resulted in the successful publishing of this book. They have passed on their knowledge of decades through this book. To expedite this challenging task, the publisher supported the team at every step. A small team of assistant editors was also appointed to further simplify the editing procedure and attain best results for the readers.

Apart from the editorial board, the designing team has also invested a significant amount of their time in understanding the subject and creating the most relevant covers. They scrutinized every image to scout for the most suitable representation of the subject and create an appropriate cover for the book.

The publishing team has been an ardent support to the editorial, designing and production team. Their endless efforts to recruit the best for this project, has resulted in the accomplishment of this book. They are a veteran in the field of academics and their pool of knowledge is as vast as their experience in printing. Their expertise and guidance has proved useful at every step. Their uncompromising quality standards have made this book an exceptional effort. Their encouragement from time to time has been an inspiration for everyone.

The publisher and the editorial board hope that this book will prove to be a valuable piece of knowledge for researchers, students, practitioners and scholars across the globe.

List of Contributors

Satoko Koganemaru
Brain Integrative Science, Kyoto University School of Medicine, Sakyo-ku, Kyoto, Japan
Human Brain Research Center, Kyoto University School of Medicine, Sakyo-ku, Kyoto, Japan

Hidenao Fukuyama and Tatsuya Mima
Human Brain Research Center, Kyoto University School of Medicine, Sakyo-ku, Kyoto, Japan

Gelu Onose
Department of Physical and Rehabilitation Medicine, University of Medicine and Pharmacy "Carol Davila", Bucharest, Romania
Teaching Emergency Hospital "Bagdasar-Arseni", Bucharest, Romania

Vladimir Cârdei, Ştefan T. Crăciunoiu and Valeriu Avramescu
Research and Technological Design Institute for Machines Construction, Bucharest, Romania

Ioan Opriş
Miller School of Medicine, University of Miami, Miami, FL, USA

Mikhail A. Lebedev
Department of Neurobiology, Duke University, Durham, NC, USA

Marian Vladimir Constantinescu
Holistic Dental Medicine Institute - ROPOSTURO, Bucharest, Romania

Ryan McKendrick and Raja Parasuraman
Center of Excellence in Neuroergonomics, Technology, and Cognition (CENTEC), George Mason University, Fairfax, VA, USA

Hasan Ayaz
School of Biomedical Engineering, Science and Health Systems, Drexel University, Philadelphia, PA, USA

Giovanni Pezzulo
Institute of Cognitive Sciences and Technologies, National Research Council, Rome, Italy

Alessandro D'Ausilio
IIT - Istituto Italiano di Tecnologia, CTNSC@UniFe - Center of Translational Neurophysiology for Speech and Communication, Ferrara, Italy

Andrea Gaggioli
Department of Psychology, Università Cattolica del Sacro Cuore, Milan, Italy
Applied Technology for Neuro-Psychology Lab, I.R.C.C.S. Istituto Auxologico Italiano, Milan, Italy

Victor M. Pulgar
Biomedical Research and Infrastructure Center, Faculty of Natural and Physical Sciences, Winston-Salem State University, Winston-Salem, NC, USA
Hypertension and Vascular Research Center, Wake Forest School of Medicine, Winston-Salem, NC, USA
Department of Obstetrics and Gynecology, Wake Forest School of Medicine, Winston-Salem, NC, USA

Ki Yong Kwon and Wen Li
Department of Electrical and Computer Engineering, Michigan State University, East Lansing, MI, USA

Hyung-Min Lee and Maysam Ghovanloo
School of Electrical and Computer Engineering, Georgia Institute of Technology, Atlanta, GA, USA

Arthur Weber
Department of Physiology, Michigan State University, East Lansing, MI, USA

Robert Bauer and Alireza Gharabaghi
Division of Functional and Restorative Neurosurgery, Centre for Integrative Neuroscience, Eberhard Karls University Tuebingen, Tuebingen, Germany

Sungshin Kim and Thierri Callier
Department of Organismal Biology and Anatomy, University of Chicago, Chicago, IL, USA

Gregg A. Tabot
Committee on Computational Neuroscience, University of Chicago, Chicago, IL, USA

Francesco V. Tenore
Research and Exploratory Development Department, Johns Hopkins University Applied Physics Laboratory, Laurel, MD, USA

Sliman J. Bensmaia
Department of Organismal Biology and Anatomy, University of Chicago, Chicago, IL, USA
Committee on Computational Neuroscience, University of Chicago, Chicago, IL, USA

Adam G. Rouse and Marc H. Schieber
Department of Neurology, University of Rochester, Rochester, NY, USA
Department of Neurobiology and Anatomy, University of Rochester, Rochester, NY, USA
Department of Biomedical Engineering, University of Rochester, Rochester, NY, USA

Weiguo Song
Department of Neurobiology and Anatomy, Drexel University College of Medicine, Drexel University, Philadelphia, PA, USA

Iahn Cajigas
Brain and Cognitive Sciences, Massachusetts Institute of Technology, Cambridge, MA, USA

Emery N. Brown
Brain and Cognitive Sciences, Massachusetts Institute of Technology, Cambridge, MA, USA
Institute for Medical Engineering and Science, Massachusetts Institute of Technology, Cambridge, MA, USA
Department of Anesthesia, Critical Care and Pain Medicine, Harvard Medical School, Massachusetts General Hospital, Boston, MA, USA

Simon F. Giszter
Department of Neurobiology and Anatomy, Drexel University College of Medicine, Drexel University, Philadelphia, PA, USA
School of Biomedical Engineering, Drexel University, Philadelphia, PA, USA

Magteld Zeitler
Research Center Jülich, Institute of Neuroscience and Medicine, Neuromodulation (INM-7), Jülich, Germany

Peter A. Tass
Research Center Jülich, Institute of Neuroscience and Medicine, Neuromodulation (INM-7), Jülich, Germany
Department of Neurosurgery, Stanford University, Stanford, CA, USA
Department of Neuromodulation, University of Cologne, Cologne, Germany

Miri Benyamini and Miriam Zacksenhouse
Brain-computer Interfaces for Rehabilitation Laboratory, Department of Mechanical Engineering, Technion - Israel Institute of Technology, Haifa, Israel

Sean J. Nagel, Andre G. Machado and Darlene A. Lobel
Cleveland Clinic, Neurologic Institute, Center for Neurological Restoration, Cleveland, Ohio, USA
Department of Neurosurgery, Cleveland Clinic, Neurologic Institute, Cleveland, Ohio, USA

John T. Gale
Cleveland Clinic, Neurologic Institute, Center for Neurological Restoration, Cleveland, Ohio, USA
Department of Neuroscience, Cleveland Clinic, Lerner Research Institute, Cleveland, Ohio, USA

Mayur Pandya
Cleveland Clinic, Neurologic Institute, Center for Neurological Restoration, Cleveland, Ohio, USA
Department of Psychiatry, Cleveland Clinic, Neurologic Institute, Cleveland, Ohio, USA

E. Paul Zehr
Rehabilitation Neuroscience Laboratory, University Victoria, Victoria, BC, Canada
Human Discovery Science, International Collaboration on Repair Discoveries, Vancouver, BC, Canada
Centre for Biomedical Research, University of Victoria, Victoria, BC, Canada
Division of Medical Sciences, University of Victoria, BC, Canada
School of Exercise Science, Physical, and Health Education, University of Victoria, Victoria, BC, Canada
Zanshin Consulting, Inc., Victoria, BC, Canada

Lucia Billeci
Institute of Clinical Physiology, National Research Council of Italy, Pisa, Italy
Department of Clinical and Experimental Medicine, University of Pisa, Pisa, Italy

Alessandro Tonacci
Institute of Clinical Physiology, National Research Council of Italy, Pisa, Italy

Gennaro Tartarisco and Giovanni Pioggia
Institute of Applied Sciences and Intelligent Systems "Eduardo Caianiello", National Research Council of Italy, Messina, Italy

Antonio Narzisi and Sara Calderoni
Department of Developmental Neuroscience, IRCSS Stella Maris Foundation, Pisa, Italy

Simone Di Palma
Department of Information Engineering, University of Pisa, Pisa, Italy

Daniele Corda and Giovanni Baldus
HelpyLife Technology, Oristano, Italy

Federico Cruciani
I+ srl, Florence, Italy

Salvatore M. Anzalone
Institute of Intelligent Systems and Robotics, University Pierre and Marie Curie, Paris, France

Filippo Muratori
Department of Clinical and Experimental Medicine, University of Pisa, Pisa, Italy
Department of Developmental Neuroscience, IRCSS Stella Maris Foundation, Pisa, Italy

Benjamin Blankertz and Matthias Schultze-Kraft
Neurotechnology Group, Technische Universität Berlin, Berlin, Germany
Bernstein Focus: Neurotechnology, Berlin, Germany

Laura Acqualagna, Irene Sturm, Marija Ušćumlic and Markus A. Wenzel
Neurotechnology Group, Technische Universität Berlin, Berlin, Germany

Sven Dähne
Machine Learning Group, Technische Universität Berlin, Berlin, Germany

Stefan Haufe
Bernstein Focus: Neurotechnology, Berlin, Germany
Machine Learning Group, Technische Universität Berlin, Berlin, Germany

Gabriel Curio
Bernstein Focus: Neurotechnology, Berlin, Germany
Neurophysics Group, Department of Neurology, Campus Benjamin Franklin, Charité - University Medicine Berlin, Berlin, Germany

Klaus-Robert Müller
Bernstein Focus: Neurotechnology, Berlin, Germany
Machine Learning Group, Technische Universität Berlin, Berlin, Germany
Department of Brain and Cognitive Engineering, Korea University, Seoul, South Korea

Lutz A. Krawinkel
BrainImaging and NeuroStimulation (BINS) Laboratory, Department of Neurology, University Medical Center Hamburg-Eppendorf, Hamburg, Germany

Andreas K. Engel
Department of Neurophysiology and Pathophysiology, University Medical Center Hamburg-Eppendorf, Hamburg, Germany

Friedhelm C. Hummel
BrainImaging and NeuroStimulation (BINS) Laboratory, Department of Neurology, University Medical Center Hamburg-Eppendorf, Hamburg, Germany
Department of Neurology, Favoloro University, Medical School, Buenos Aires, Argentina

Andrea Caria
Department of Psychology and Cognitive Science, University of Trento, Rovereto, Italy
Institute of Medical Psychology and Behavioral Neurobiology, Eberhard-Karls-University of Tübingen, Tübingen, Germany

Samar S. Ayache
EA 4391, Excitabilité Nerveuse et Thérapeutique, Université Paris-Est-Créteil, Créteil, France
Service de Physiologie – Explorations Fonctionnelles, Hôpital Henri Mondor, Assistance Publique – Hôpitaux de Paris, Créteil, France
Neurology Division, Lebanese American University Medical Center - Rizk Hospital, Beirut, Lebanon

Ulrich Palm
EA 4391, Excitabilité Nerveuse et Thérapeutique, Université Paris-Est-Créteil, Créteil, France
Department of Psychiatry and Psychotherapy, Ludwig-Maximilian-University, Munich, Germany

Moussa A. Chalah and Jean-Pascal Lefaucheur
EA 4391, Excitabilité Nerveuse et Thérapeutique, Université Paris-Est-Créteil, Créteil, France
Service de Physiologie – Explorations Fonctionnelles, Hôpital Henri Mondor, Assistance Publique – Hôpitaux de Paris, Créteil, France

Tarik Al-Ani and Marc Sorel
EA 4391, Excitabilité Nerveuse et Thérapeutique, Université Paris-Est-Créteil, Créteil, France

Arnaud Brignol
Département d'Informatique et de Recherche Opérationnelle, Université de Montréal, Montréal, QC, Canada

Mohamed Abdellaoui and Dalia Dimitri
Service de Neurologie, Hôpital Henri Mondor, Assistance Publique – Hôpitaux de Paris, Créteil, France

Alain Créange
EA 4391, Excitabilité Nerveuse et Thérapeutique, Université Paris-Est-Créteil, Créteil, France
Service de Neurologie, Hôpital Henri Mondor, Assistance Publique – Hôpitaux de Paris, Créteil, France

Sergei L. Shishkin, Yuri O. Nuzhdin, Evgeny P. Svirin and Anastasia A. Fedorova
Department of Neurocognitive Technologies, Kurchatov Complex of NBICS Technologies, National Research Centre "Kurchatov Institute," Moscow, Russia

Alexander G. Trofimov
Department of Cybernetics, National Research Nuclear University MEPhI, Moscow, Russia

Bogdan L. Kozyrskiy
Department of Neurocognitive Technologies, Kurchatov Complex of NBICS Technologies, National Research Centre "Kurchatov Institute," Moscow, Russia
Department of Computer Systems and Technologies, National Research Nuclear University MEPhI, Moscow, Russia

Boris M. Velichkovsky
Department of Neurocognitive Technologies, Kurchatov Complex of NBICS Technologies, National Research Centre "Kurchatov Institute," Moscow, Russia
Centre for Cognitive Programs and Technologies, Russian State University for Humanities, Moscow, Russia
Department of Psychology, Technische Universität Dresden, Dresden, Germany

Cheryl Ann Sexton
Department of Physiology and Pharmacology, Wake Forest University, School of Medicine, Winston-Salem, NC, USA

Mikhail Lebedev
Department of Neurobiology, Duke University, Durham, NC, USA

Elizaveta Okorokova
Centre for Cognition and Decision Making, National Research University Higher School of Economics, Moscow, Russia

Michael Linderman
Department of Biomedical Engineering, Norconnect Inc., Ogdensburg, NY, USA

Alex Ossadtchi
Centre for Cognition and Decision Making, National Research University Higher School of Economics, Moscow, Russia
Laboratory of Control of Complex Systems, Institute of Problems of Mechanical Engineering, Russian Academy of Sciences, St. Petersburg, Russia

Jasmine A. Berry
Biomimetic Real-time Cortex Project, Computer Science Department, University of Southern California, Los Angeles, CA, USA

Alice C. Parker
Biomimetic Real-time Cortex Project, Ming Hsieh Department of Electrical Engineering, University of Southern California, Los Angeles, CA, USA

Alessia Tonelli, Luca Brayda and Monica Gori
Robotics, Brain and Cognitive Sciences Department, Fondazione Istituto Italiano di Tecnologia, Genoa, Italy

Index

CPSIA information can be obtained
at www.ICGtesting.com
Printed in the USA
LVHW060854030122
707669LV00002B/147

9 781639 893607